DECISIONS IN
Nutrition

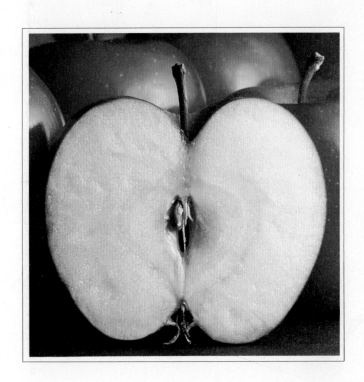

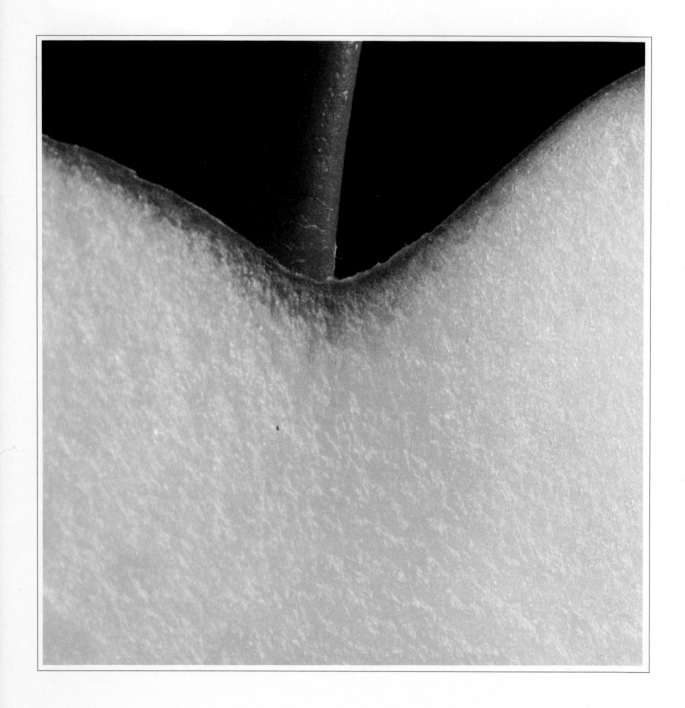

DECISIONS IN
Nutrition

Vincent Hegarty, Ph.D.

Professor

Department of Human Development
and Consumer Sciences
University of Houston
Houston, Texas

Illustrations by Donald O'Connor
St. Peters, Missouri

Times Mirror/Mosby College Publishing

ST. LOUIS • TORONTO • SANTA CLARA • 1988

Publisher   Nancy K. Roberson
Editor   Ann Trump
Developmental Editor   Kathy Sedovic
Project Manager   Teri Merchant
Production Editor   Robert A. Kelly
Design   John R. Rokusek
Editing   Editing, Design & Production, Inc.

Cover illustration   Penny & Stermer Group/Julia Noonan

Credits for all materials used by permission appear after the index.

Printed in the United States of America

Library of Congress Cataloging-in-Publication Data

Hegarty, P. Vincent.
    Decisions in nutrition.

    Bibliography: p.
    Includes index.
    1. Nutrition.   I.   Title.
TX354.T39   1988   613.2   87-18078
ISBN 0-8016-2195-X

GW/GW/VH 9 8 7 6 5 4 3 2 1   01/A/032

ABOUT THE AUTHOR

Vincent Hegarty was the Evans Medical Research Fellow at the University of London, England, where he obtained a Ph.D. in human nutrition. He also holds a B.Sc. and M.Sc. in biochemistry, and a B.A. in political economy, philosophy, and history from the National University of Ireland. He is author or co-author of over 100 papers in more than 30 different journals in basic, agricultural, and biomedical sciences. Winner of the Amoco-Morse Foundation Award for Outstanding Contributions to Undergraduate Education when he was a professor at the University of Minnesota, he is presently Professor and Department Chairman at the University of Houston. He is also affiliated with the University of Texas Health Sciences Center, Houston, where he is Adjunct Professor, School of Public Health, and member of the Graduate School of Biomedical Sciences. Dr. Hegarty has taught the introductory nutrition course for over 15 years.

Preface

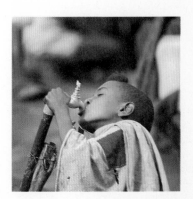

The health and well-being of individuals, families, and nations are determined by the quality of the diet. Likes and dislikes for food vary widely, as do dietary restrictions because of health, lifestyle, or religious or cultural reasons. *Decisions in Nutrition* emphasizes the importance of nutrition by capturing the student's personal involvement and illustrating the global consequences. It invites the reader to become actively involved in using basic nutrition information to make personal decisions and to examine national and global concerns in nutrition. Let me demonstrate how I will deliver on my promise of involving the student in the fascinating study of nutrition.

AUDIENCE

A typical introductory class in nutrition may have students with backgrounds as diverse as the components of nutrition itself. Students taking this course may be majoring in psychology, sociology, economics, nursing, science, premedicine, business, engineering, home economics, physical or health education, and many other areas. They will be male and female, young students and older ones returning to further their education. Some students will be athletes interested in the relationships between food and athletic performance. Others may be interested in keeping their weight under control. The course may be taught in a 2- or 4-year college or university, or as part of a continuing education workshop/course. *Decisions in Nutrition* is appropriate for all of the above. It could also be used by professionals in the health, recreation, food, and agricultural industries, as well as by individuals who are simply interested in learning about nutrition. *Most important, a background in nutrition or science is not needed to understand the concepts presented in this text.*

CONTENT HIGHLIGHTS

Some important features *unique* to *Decisions in Nutrition* make it distinctive from other texts.

Chapter 8: Oxygen, Water, and Other Fluids looks at nutrients frequently taken for granted—is it because air and water are free? Yet these are vitally important for the utilization of other nutrients in maintaining life and essential to the student's understanding of topics discussed throughout the text (e.g., iron deficiency anemia). Although other texts include coverage of water, *Decisions in Nutrition* provides a unique discussion of the role of oxygen as well.

Chapter 15: Nutrition and Current Lifestyles discusses circumstances that have arisen recently or become more common because of the pressures of today's lifestyles. It includes *unique* examinations of nutrition and stress, legal and illegal drug use,

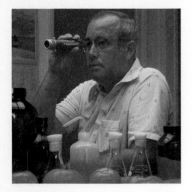

the effects of working patterns on food intake in families, the role of exercise, food faddism and food quackery, and the role of the federal government as a surrogate provider of food.

Chapter 16: Nutrition and the Future includes a *unique* and fascinating look at the role of biotechnology and bioengineering in providing new sources of food, the food-producing capabilities of the earth to provide enough food for an expanding population, and the nutritional requirements for prolonged space flights. This chapter offers an interesting and appropriate conclusion to the text, highlighting information and trends that may influence the future of food availability and consumption.

Consumer-Oriented and Practical

We are all consumers and users of food. This common factor is highlighted throughout the book through practical applications of nutrition concepts.

This text contains relevant, accurate, practical nutrition information. The production and consumption of food is an economic exercise. Therefore, the consumer must make correct food choices to maximize both the sensory satisfaction and nutritive value of the food dollar. This is done from birth until death—a fascinating lifelong challenge.

The reader will be given the tools needed to distinguish between real and false anxieties about the quality of our diet. The unbiased presentation found in *Decisions in Nutrition* will enable the student to make informed decisions in nutrition.

Personalized Information

It is not selfish to ask, "Is it good for *me?*" The "me" part of the answer requires consideration of the gender, age, socioeconomic status, health, and possibly race, religion, and occupation. The "is it good" part requires a knowledge of food production and preparation. This text presents the information necessary to address a wide range of needs, allowing students to make decisions or evaluate their own dietary practices.

Up-to-date Information

Nutrition is a rapidly changing and growing subject. A lot of effort was put into using the most up-to-date information from the widest range of journals, books, and reports. *Seventy-five percent of the references in each chapter are from 1985 or later.* Journal listings in each chapter are extensive, ranging from the behavioral and social sciences to the natural, agricultural, and medical sciences. These are provided in the hope that the reader will explore further, and also to demonstrate that the information in the text comes from far-ranging current sources.

ORGANIZATION

Decisions in Nutrition is organized into four sections. There is enough flexibility to allow instructors to change the sequence of chapters within each section.

The reader is introduced to nutrition in Part I—Food, Nutrients, and You. Chapter 1 sets the stage by examining the close relationship between the nutrients, the vehicle in which they are carried—food, and the consumer of the nutrients. In Chapter 2, methods of determining the nutritional quality of the diet, the nutritional status of individuals, present food consumption trends, and U.S. and Canadian guidelines for good eating practices are discussed. The student is also shown how to calculate nutrient values from food composition tables and how to apply RDAs.

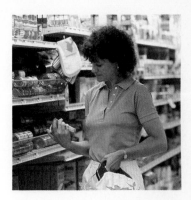

The nutrients are discussed in Part II—Nutrients: Their Sources and Functions. The energy nutrients are examined first. Carbohydrates, fats, and proteins are presented in Chapters 3, 4, and 5. These are followed by discussions of vitamins and minerals in Chapters 6 and 7.

Air (oxygen), water, and other liquids are discussed separately in Chapter 8. Both the importance of a number of nutrients in getting oxygen to the cells for energy release and the importance of water in metabolism are stressed. The negative effects of alcoholic drinks and the positive effects of milk and natural fruit drinks are discussed.

Energy requirements/energy balance and their application to obesity, eating disorders (anorexia nervosa and bulimia), and starvation from famine are evaluated in Chapters 9 and 10. This is more logical than the formats in other texts, which place energy and body weight problems immediately after the energy nutrient. Diets low in some vitamins and minerals cause health problems for some dieters. Athletes take vitamin and mineral supplements in a mistaken hope that their utilization of energy will be improved. Therefore, a knowledge of vitamins and minerals is necessary before one can understand their effect on energy balance and overeating or malnutrition. But it is, of course, possible to follow the more traditional format in this book also is you so desire. Chapter 11 examines the long process of bringing food from the farm to every cell in our body, including intermediate stops in the supermarket and the kitchen.

The varying need for nutrients throughout our life is discussed in Part III—Nutrition Throughout Life. The physiological need for nutrients is viewed in the context of developmental and behavioral changes, the effect of employment, recreation, family status, and other influences on our lives. Topics include the recommended diet for pregnancy and breastfeeding (Chapter 12), childhood obesity (Chapter 13), the diet of college athletes and nonathletes and diseases that may be related to diet—coronary heart disease, hypertension, cancer, and others (Chapter 14).

In Part IV—Applications and Implications we examine the role of nutrition in our modern lifestyles. Some topics that are becoming increasingly important as we cope with everyday pressures include the role of nutrition on stress, in the use of both legal and illegal drugs, and in excessive use of alcohol and tobacco. The significance of exercise and "eating on the run" on nutritional status is discussed. These topics and the impact of the changing structure of the family on dietary intake are examined in Chapter 15. In Chapter 16, future trends in nutrition research including food for space travel and new sources of food are addressed, a *unique* and upbeat way of ending an exciting subject.

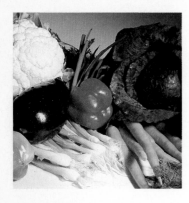

PEDAGOGICAL FEATURES

Decisions in Nutrition has a variety of learning aids to assist instructors and to enhance student learning.

Illustrations

Unique and visually appealing illustrations are presented in two and four color throughout the text, supporting important concepts and aiding student comprehension of the material. All of the line art has been specifically created for *Decisions in Nutrition.*

Connections

We eat mouthfuls of nutrients when we eat mouthfuls of food. However, nutrition information must be presented and "digested" one nutrient at a time. Every text presents the nutrients this way. In this text, a *unique* section, entitled Connections, is provided at the beginning of each chapter. This section incorporates information from preceding chapters into an overview of what is covered from one chapter to the next, and enables the student to form a clear understanding of the interrelationships of nutrition concepts.

Marginal definitions

Key terms are italicized in the narrative and repeated in the margin, along with the definition, to reinforce important nutrition concepts where they are presented in the text. The definitions are repeated in a comprehensive glossary at the end of the text.

Marginal notations

Keeping in touch with reality (a title we do not use because of its length) is the purpose of the marginal notes in each chapter. The information in the margin helps relate basic information with the real world. It is placed in the margin rather than "buried" in the text so that the reader can take time out to note and reflect on the implications.

Marginal discipline key

Relationships between nutrition and other disciplines are highlighted by referencing the appropriate discipline and a key symbol ⚷ in the margin to nutrition information being discussed (e.g., economics, sociology, medicine). This *unique* feature demonstrates for students the extensive interactions between nutrition and other disciplines and will increase their involvement in understanding the full implications of the information while making learning more interesting.

Debates

Nutrition information is constantly changing. New information is presented continuously, resulting in discussion and study about its basis in fact and potential implications for consumers. Topics may currently be debated by some nutrition experts, or new research may be presented that has not yet been proved or supported by additional study. In recognition of this fact, students are alerted to these topics by the use of colored arrows ⤸⤹ in the text discussions, highlighting such topics while maintaining the narrative flow. This should prove to be a helpful feature that can be used to stimulate student discussion and encourage critical evaluation of new nutrition information as it becomes available from the scientific literature and media.

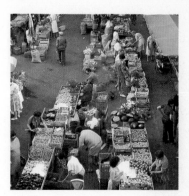

Section summaries

Each chapter contains brief summaries following major sections to reinforce student comprehension of the material before proceeding to the next secton. This should allow time for reflection and be useful for quick reviews.

Pictorial summaries

We live in a visual age. At the end of each chapter the *unique* visual summary provides an interesting and effective review of each chapter, as well as giving a visual break from a chapter of words. The supplementary package of transparency acetates includes the pictorial summaries from all 16 chapters.

Decisions

A *unique* feature of this text, each chapter contains several nutrition-related questions that directly involve the reader in using the information in the chapter in making decisions on many popular topics (e.g., What type of fiber, and how much, is good for me? Should supplements be taken during pregnancy?). In some instances, the student is then guided through the necessary steps involved in making a particular nutrition-related decision. In other cases, the student is simply given the factual information about a topic and asked to draw his or her own conclusions, incorporating or extending information contained in that chapter.

Documentation

It is important for both instructor and student that the information in a text is scientifically accurate, fully documented, and as current as possible. The reference list at the end of each chapter is a guarantee that this is so in this text. Seventy-five percent of the references in each chapter are from 1985 or later.

Metabolism notes

The reader who desires a deeper understanding of how nutrients work in the human body will find this information in the metabolism notes. This *unique* section is independent from the chapter and intended as an *optional* tool available to instructors who require that their students obtain additional information about how nutrients are used in our bodies. It is separated from the main body of the chapter and located at the end of the relevant chapters (1-10). Instructors who may be teaching this course to a class of combined majors and nonmajors may find this feature particularly useful.

Appendices

In addition to the standard reference tables, such as food composition and nutrient content of fast foods, some particularly helpful appendices have been provided for the student.

For students who would like to briefly review the basic anatomy and physiology of the digestive system, Appendix A, Nutrition and The Human Body, has been included.

Appendix B, Calculating Your Nutrient Intake, includes a description and

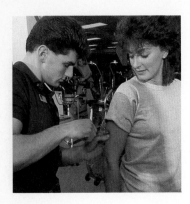

examples of the steps involved in measuring the student's nutritional status. The reader can refer to this appendix during or following the study of a particular topic, such as carbohydrates, to determine his or her own intake, and make comparisons with recommended intakes.

Appendix E provides a comprehensive listing of reliable Sources of Nutrition Information to which the student can refer for additional information.

The end papers include conversion factors, height and weight tables, and the RDAs.

SUPPLEMENTS

A complete package of supplements is available for use with *Decisions in Nutrition*. As with the text itself, producing supplements of extraordinary quality and utility was a primary objective of the author and publisher. All supplements accompanying this text that are to be used with students, from the test items to the study guide, have been reviewed by many of the same instructors who critiqued the text.

Instructor's Manual and Test Bank

Prepared by Evelyn Day of Weber State College, the Instructor's Manual and Test Bank provides text adopters with substantial support in preparing for and teaching introductory nutrition with this text. The manual is perforated and three-hole punched for convenience.

Conversion notes. Each chapter of this manual begins with a section entitled "What's Different and Why." This *unique* feature indicates how the coverage of each chapter in *Decisions in Nutrition* differs from other introductory nutrition texts. These conversion notes enable the instructor to make a convenient transition to *Decisions in Nutrition* from other texts.

Chapter overview. A brief summary of the major concepts presented in each chapter.

Dietary assessments. Self-evaluation exercises are provided in each chapter and can be easily photocopied to be used as handouts to the student.

Related issues. Each chapter includes current issues for class discussion related to the chapter topic.

Transparency masters. Key illustrations and charts appearing in the text are reproduced as full-page transparency masters at the back of the manual. Masters are also provided for supplemental material not appearing in the textbook.

Test bank. An extensive test bank, including over 2000 multiple-choice, completion, true-false, and essay questions, is contained in the manual. Test questions have been carefully evaluated by reviewers of the text for clarity, accuracy, and level of difficulty.

Transparency Acetates

A set of 50 overhead transparency acetates in 2-color is available to adopters of the text for use as teaching aids. These include the most important illustrations from the text (including all the pictorial summaries), as well as additional illustrations that have been developed to supplement the text and help teach important concepts.

Computerized Test Bank

A computerized version of the test bank (Microtest II) is available to instructors on disks for IBM-PC, Apple II+, Apple IIe, Apple IIc, and IBM-compatible computers. Microtest II also provides instructors with the opportunity to add questions of their own, as well as to modify or rearrange existing questions.

Nutrient-Analysis Software

This interactive software allows students to assess their dietary intake for multiple days. The data disk contains over 1500 food items, including fast foods and fad diet preparations. Unlike any other software available with introductory nutrition texts, *this program allows the student to enter food items by their names.*

Study Guide

Prepared by Joanne Spaide of the University of Northen Iowa, the study guide is uniquely designed to help students become involved in the learning process. It encourages students to apply what they have learned in the text. Features in the study guide include key terms and definitions, guidepoints targeting the key points of each chapter, a chapter outline, student activities, self-quizzes, enrichment activities, and a comprehensive resource directory.

ACKNOWLEDGMENTS

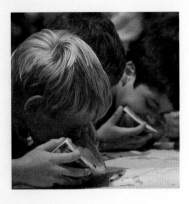

My thanks go to the following people who can take part in the credit for what I think is an exciting and refreshing introduction to nutrition text:

▪ Students in universities in different parts of the world where I was fortunate to experience the excitement of teaching nutrition. Their challenging questions were the inspiration for this book.

▪ Teachers and colleagues for their wisdom and guidance. Special thanks go to the reviewers listed below. Their suggestions were invaluable. Their efforts indicated to me that there is a place for this text in introductory courses in nutrition. Thanks are also extended to the many other professors contacted by Times Mirror/ Mosby College Publishing in preliminary surveys of the characteristics of a good introductory text in nutrition.

Nancy Betts
University of Nebraska

Carol Bishop
Solano College

Virginia Campbell
Acadia University

Evelyn Day
Weber State College

Ethel Fowler
Palm Beach Junior College

Betty Friedman
Southwest Texas State University

Margarette Harden
Texas Tech University

Margaret Hedley
University of Guelph

Paula Howat
Louisiana State University

Jan Johnson
Illinois State University

Sooja Kim
Bowling Green State University

Melinda Manore
Arizona State University

Jacquelyn McClelland
North Carolina State University

Susan Mellinger
SUNY, Cortland

Mary Nelson
Southeastern Louisiana State University

Joanne Ossell
University of Minnesota, Duluth

Helen Reid
Southwest Missouri State University

Jean Skinner
University of Tennessee

Helen Smith
Ball State University

Joanne Spaide
University of Northern Iowa

Susan Strahs
California State University, Long Beach

Kathryn Sucher
San Jose State University

Sheron Sumner
University of North Carolina, Greensboro

Anna Svacha
Auburn University

Billie Wood
Daytona Beach Community College

Franklin Young
West Chester University

Joan Yuhas
Ohio University

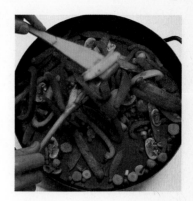

The staff at Times Mirror/Mosby College Publishing have left their mark of excellence on this book. Special thanks go to Kathy Sedovic—she is any author's dream of a developmental editor. Her professional wisdom, patience, and good humor were most helpful. Nancy Roberson, Ann Trump, and Jean Babrick helped in innumerable ways.

The text was carefully crafted by Brian Williams who brought his unique writing skills to refine the final draft. Ralph Zickgraf tidied up my editorial loose-ends, and Donald O'Connor translated my amateur attempts at art into the fine line art throughout the text.

Some special people in my life deserve thanks—my sons Adrian and Neal did the word processing, my wife Maura provided support, nutrients, and encouragement, and my parents gave me the great gift of an education.

AN INVITATION

If you have any comments or suggestions for revisions after using this text, I invite you to share them with me for consideration in the second edition. Send your comments to the publisher—I will be glad to respond to all letters.

Vincent Hegarty

To the Student

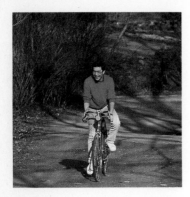

Nutrition has fascinated me for over 25 years. I want to transfer that fascination to you through the pages of this book.

Our partnership starts with many advantages. We know the foods we like and dislike, and we can list some reasons why—taste, appearance, cultural/ethnic preferences, happy personal experiences associated with food, and many others. We will draw on these shared experiences to understand all aspects of nutrition. We will learn about its history: if you were reading this book in 1900 there would be no information on the vitamins, little on the minerals, and a poor understanding of the workings of the human body. We will get to know each individual nutrient and understand how nutrients interact with our bodies. We will be startled by the effects of too much and too little food. We will taste the great joy food brings to our lives and feel the suffering of those less fortunate without food. We will appreciate why nutrition is important to our modern lifestyles, in health promotion, and in disease prevention. We will look to the future and see the possibilities of eating in space and of getting foods from new sources.

We will distinguish between information accepted by nutrition scientists and information still debated. More important, you will be given reasons for the debate. You will be involved in the decision-making process on some nutrition issues at the end of each chapter.

We must remember that we are social animals, made up of a bunch of chemicals called nutrients, dependent on the fruits of the soil for our survival, and on medical science for our health and well-being. Come with an inquiring mind ready to explore all of these fascinating interactions between so many disciplines. The personal satisfaction and the intellectual excitement obtained from the study of nutrition will ensure your own personal health and well-being and ideally heighten your sensitivity to the nutritional circumstances of others.

Contents In Brief

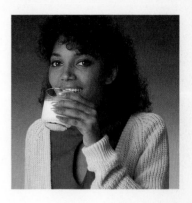

Contents

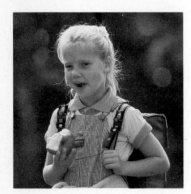

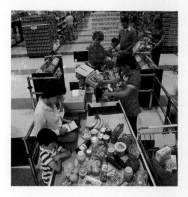

PART II   NUTRIENTS: THEIR SOURCES AND FUNCTIONS

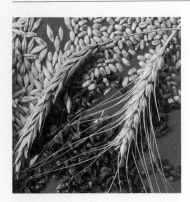

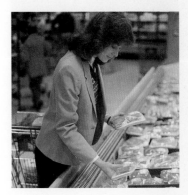

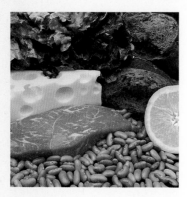

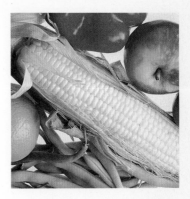

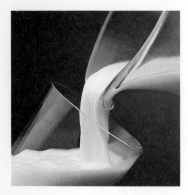

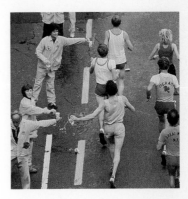

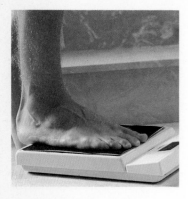

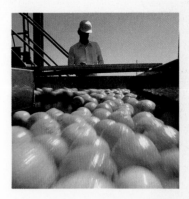

PART III NUTRITION THROUGHOUT LIFE

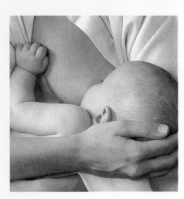

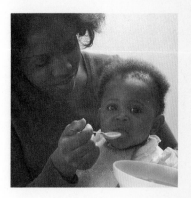

PART IV   APPLICATIONS AND IMPLICATIONS

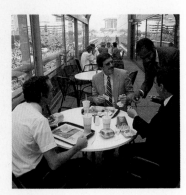

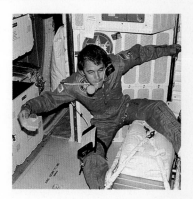

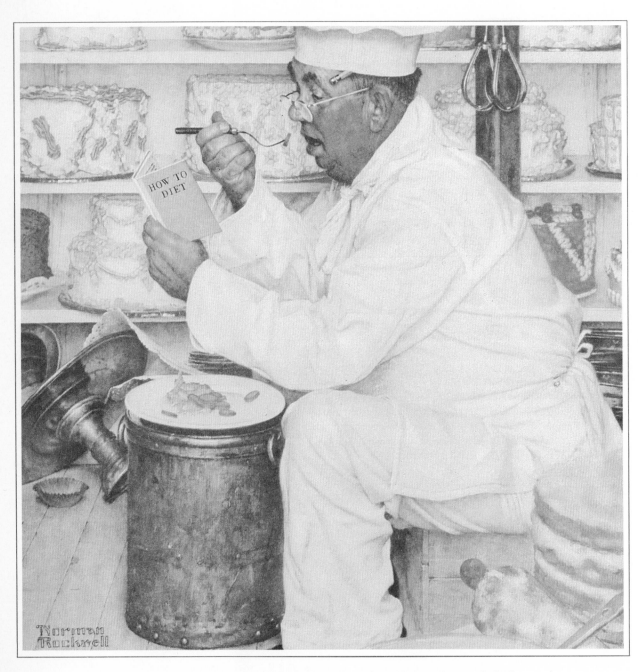

PART I

Food, Nutrients, and You

On some level, people everywhere worry about food—probably always have and probably always will.

There you are, along with perhaps 60 other human beings, camped in the middle of an area 20 miles long and 20 miles wide, occupied by different kinds of animals and plants. "Every so often," says writer Desmond Morris in *The Human Zoo*, "the men in your group set off in pursuit of prey. The women gather fruits and berries." If these roles seem highly traditional, it is because they are; that's the way our prehistoric ancestors acted in response to their worries about whether there would be enough wild animals and plants to eat.

Or maybe there you are strapped into your seat, the rim of the earth outside your window, ballpoint pens and notepads drifting crazily in the weightless atmosphere inside the cabin of the space capsule. Will eating be a bizarre and difficult experience? As Joseph Allen describes it in *Entering Space*, "Bread, it was guessed, might break into thousands of pieces; vegetables would disintegrate; soups might explode out of their bowls." Experience proved, however, that eating in orbit was much like eating on earth.

Such concerns show that people have always worried and still worry about food— about getting enough of it, about its being palatable, and about its being nutritious. Many people in the world can only worry about getting food at all. We expect that you are more fortunate—that food is something you can not only obtain but even *celebrate*.

In the first two chapters of this text, we will first explore *why* we eat as we do and then begin to lay the background for dietary guidelines.

1

How Food Becomes You

CONNECTIONS

Good-tasting, affordable, healthful—or simply the only thing available? What *is* the reason you chose the last food you ate?

The choice of food may seem to be strictly a personal decision, but that decision is actually affected by age, gender, genetic makeup, lifestyle, and sociocultural background. We tend to make choices about food for reasons that have to do with how we grew up, what's most pleasurable or what's usually affordable, and what is available. Availability in turn depends on agricultural practices, the environment, climate, food processing, political and economic decisions, and cultural preferences. Sometimes what we eat is influenced by health reasons, as may be true of athletes on the one hand and diabetics on the other.

But there is more to eating than this. Without diminishing the pleasure that so many people associate with food, this book will show you how you can eat in ways that will bring the greatest benefits possible: lack of disease, presence of good health, and long life.

Consciously or—perhaps more likely—unconsciously, several times a day you need to make three decisions. When should you eat? What should you eat? Is the food you eat good or bad—or, more specifically, is it *nutritious*, based on the information you currently have?

Do you, for instance, dutifully eat three square meals a day, starting with cereal and orange juice at 7:00 a.m.? Or do you plunge through the day without eating and then have a gargantuan dinner of hamburgers and fries? Are you concerned about how you look, so that you find yourself dipping into popular books and magazines for diet tips? Some people are nearly indifferent to food, giving eating no more thought than they give to putting gas in a car, while others are obsessed by it, agonizing over calories and fat content. Still, the fact remains that each of us every day still makes the same three decisions about what to put in our mouths. These decisions are important—and the last part of each chapter, the "Decisions" section, will help you evaluate yours.

WHY IS NUTRITION SUCH A PUZZLE?

Clearly, the human race has had a lot of experience with eating. And nutrition, which is concerned with examining the production and acceptance of sufficient food to provide *nutrients*—chemicals in food needed to maintain life—for good health, is an established scientific discipline. Yet it seems that hardly a month passes without some new discovery or scare relating to food—a disturbing matter, when you think of the possible consequences to people's well-being.

Although the point of this book is to give you the best nutrition advice possible, it is not going to be able to solve all the food controversies. In this respect, nutritionists are no different from members of other scientific disciplines—from physicists who argue the pros and cons of nuclear power to physicians who disagree on appropriate treatments for certain diseases. In a way, however, the lack of reliable nutrition information may bother people more: perhaps they can't do much individually about nuclear power or treatment of diseases, but every day they are obliged to make personal decisions about food—and about what those decisions mean for their moods, their performance, their looks, and other matters of high individual importance.

To return to the question raised above—why is nutrition such a puzzle?

1. We all tend to be our own experts on "what is good for us," since we have been living with the same body and know our likes and dislikes in foods.
2. We forget that the human body is far more complex than a rocket engine or computer—that more chemical reactions are taking place within you right now than in the largest chemical laboratory in the world, yet the role of some nutrients in these chemical reactions is not understood.
3. Even if we want to understand some of these chemical reactions, we cannot always do so. Ethics sometimes prevents us from examining human beings (for, say, the causes of malnutrition) in a way that is never a problem with examining rocket engines.
4. How food actually works to fuel and repair our body is not always understood. A single mouthful of food, after all, may contain hundreds of different chemicals and nutritional values, and these chemicals are distributed through the body in different ways.

⟾ Thus, for all these reasons, this book will not always be able to give firm recommendations on the best nutritional decisions. However, we will lay our cards on the table and tell you whenever a particular statement or idea is considered controversial. Whenever you see arrows in the text, such as these, you will know that the matter is under debate among nutritionists. ⟾

Throughout this book, we will stop every so often—between major sections—and summarize what has just been said. We hope you will find these summaries useful for reviewing. The first summary follows.

Nutrients
Chemicals in food needed to maintain life.

Medicine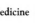

Nutrition is a puzzle because we are all our own experts on food. We overlook the facts that the human body consists of many complex chemical reactions, that the role of nutrients in these reactions is not well understood, that ethics prevents us from examining human beings in certain ways that might yield more knowledge about nutrition, and that how food works to fuel and repair our bodies is not well understood.

WHERE DOES NUTRITION INFORMATION COME FROM?

Does the study of food and nutrition sound dull? Perhaps, you suspect, delving into nutritional information as an academic subject isn't going to be as much fun as reading about it in a popular magazine or book. But suppose you were the star reporter for matters of food and health on a major newspaper. Here are the kinds of areas you would be looking into for sources of nutrition information.[1]

- *Natural disasters and travelers' tales:* The 1985 earthquake in Mexico City showed that newborns can live up to nine days without food and fluids—much longer than was expected. Explorers in past centuries, prisoners of war, and astronauts have described the reactions of the body to food in unusual circumstances.
- *Comparative and evolutionary studies:* Knowledge from archeological records and from studies on hunter-gatherer people living today in remote parts of the world can provide information that can be compared with our present diet.
- *Epidemiological studies:* Correlations between diets of different people and the incidence of disease such as heart disease or cancer are studied in epidemiology. Care must be exercised because these correlations may not prove cause and effect. The present emphasis on the positive effects of high-fiber diets comes from the observation that Africans have high-fiber intakes and low incidences of colon cancer. In North America fiber intakes are lower, and a higher proportion of people suffer from colon cancer.
- *Clinical records:* People with diseases (such as coronary or kidney diseases), either in hospitals or in the community, provide information on nutritional changes during the onset and recovery from disease. Healthy volunteers (such as athletes) provide information on the amount of each nutrient required by the body.
- *Human experiments and trials:* These may be as short as a few hours, as in experiments on the absorption of nutrients from the diet into the blood, or they may last several years, as in studies about the relationship of diet to heart disease and cancer. Ethical considerations limit the scope of many trials.
- *Animal experiments:* The big advantage in nutrition experiments on animals is that variables can be controlled more effectively than in human beings. Much of the knowledge on vitamins and minerals, for instance, was obtained originally from experimental animals. We have learned much about how our genetic background influences our nutritional status by studying the interaction between genetics and nutrition in animals. For example, genetics influences the amount of body fat in farm animals. This knowledge has been used to produce meat with more lean and less fat than at the turn of the century. Consumer demand for leaner meat encouraged these changes.
- *Food analysis:* Our food supply continually changes—over 1,400 food products were introduced in 1985—so food analysis is an ongoing task for nutritionists. Methods of chemically analyzing nutrients are always improving.

Thus, you can see that the search for nutritional information can take you into many different areas. Nutritional research is detective work at its best.

Medicine

Food Chemistry

Nutritional information comes from natural disasters and travelers' tales, comparative and evolutionary studies, epidemiological studies, clinical records, human experiments and trials, animal experiments, and food analysis.

WHY DOESN'T EVERYBODY EAT THE SAME FOODS?

Indeed, why *doesn't* everybody in the world eat the same foods? This may seem like a stupid question (like "Why is grass green?"), but stupid questions are often a starting point for creativity and insights. If you know why you don't eat like, say, a Japanese factory worker or a farmer in Africa, you may be in a better position to evaluate whether your diet is any better or worse than anyone else's.

As a way of getting into this subject, consider the following reasons offered by Daphne Roe of Cornell University as to why people will eat and won't eat certain foods[2]:

Preferences are for foods used for rewards, prestige, or foods having special properties; foods believed to be tasty, good sensory appeal, filling, cheap, sweet; foods that you can't get at home, foods that are easily prepared or available; foods promoted by the media, familiar foods, ethnic or regional foods; foods that are easy to chew.

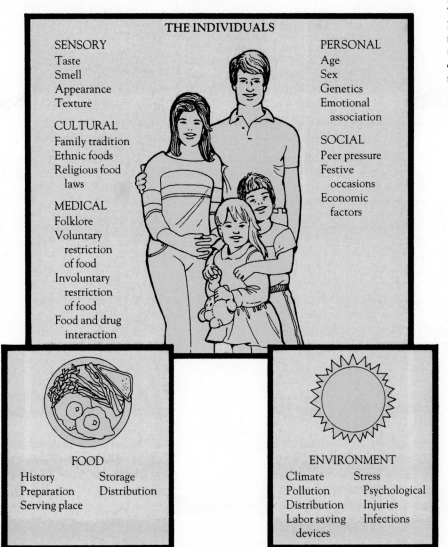

THE INDIVIDUALS

SENSORY
Taste
Smell
Appearance
Texture

CULTURAL
Family tradition
Ethnic foods
Religious food
  laws

MEDICAL
Folklore
Voluntary
  restriction
  of food
Involuntary
  restriction
  of food
Food and drug
  interaction

PERSONAL
Age
Sex
Genetics
Emotional
  association

SOCIAL
Peer pressure
Festive
  occasions
Economic
  factors

FOOD
History   Storage
Preparation   Distribution
Serving place

ENVIRONMENT
Climate   Stress
Pollution   Psychological
Distribution   Injuries
Labor saving   Infections
  devices

FIGURE 1-1
What influences the choice of food? Differences in environment, differences in food, and differences in people affect individual nutrient intake. Compare each of these with those affecting your family and friends.

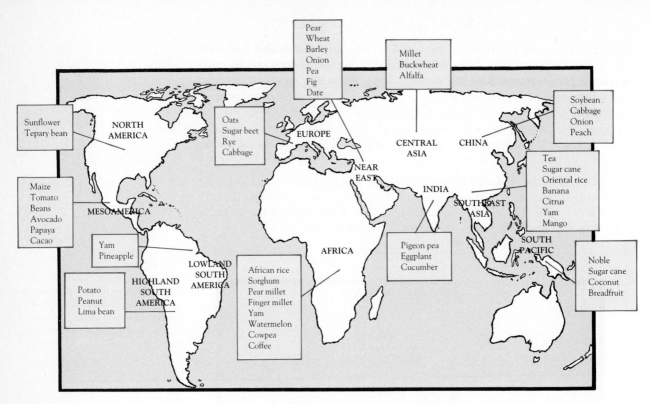

FIGURE 1-2
Areas where plants were domesticated. The rest of the world has made a huge contribution to the composition of the North American diet.

Dislikes include foods enforced by parents, foods that are unfamiliar, badly prepared, causing allergic reactions, difficult to cook or prepare; for substances not considered edible, for foods that are bland, or not filling or satisfying; for foods having peculiar smell, taste, or consistency; for foods difficult to chew; for foods that are considered to be "good for you."

Actually, the first food eaten by almost everyone in the world *is* the same: human milk, cow's milk, or infant formula. From childhood onward, however, the 5 billion people of the world go completely separate ways, although many of their diets may be nutritionally balanced. Let us, then, examine why people differ in their choice of food, which in turn may determine their intake of nutrients. There are three principal reasons (Figure 1-1):

- Environmental factors
- Differences in food
- Differences between people

Environmental Factors

Without question, food differences are heavily affected by environmental factors like history and climate and pollution.

History

The potential variety of our diet is taken for granted sometimes. There are about 20,000 edible plants in the world, of which about 100 have been developed as significant food crops. The top seven—none originally domesticated in North

America, by the way—are wheat, rice, corn (maize), potato, barley, sweet potato, and cassava.

The areas where many plants were domesticated are shown in Figure 1-2, and clearly their importance varies with their availability to certain regions. Some of these crops are fed to farm animals in order to increase the supply of meat, milk, and eggs.

One crop important in history is the potato. Originally from South America, it was brought to Europe several centuries ago. However, because potatoes were believed to be poisonous and to cause syphilis and leprosy, it was 200 years before they were accepted into the European diet. Although not the most nutritious of foods, it became a staple of poor people because a small patch of ground could provide high yields. As a result, Ireland became particularly dependent on potatoes, so much so that when the crop failed in that country as a result of potato blight, over 1 million people perished from famine, and thus began the great waves of Irish emigration to North America. Nowadays, of course, you certainly know that you cannot get leprosy from potatoes, although their fat-dipped variations (like French fries and hashbrowns) may not be the healthiest of foods.

History

Climate and pollution

Low rainfall or floods affect food production. So do temperature, elevation, wind, and other climatic factors. Industrial and household waste can make food dangerous to eat. Untreated sewage may also contribute to the problem of unsafe food. Eating raw shellfish, for instance, can be risky when the shellfish are harvested from water exposed to sewage that has not been properly treated.[3]

Differences in Food

Foods themselves are different, of course. Foods differ according to how they are stored, prepared, and distributed, as well as according to the place in which they are served.

Storage

Improved methods for preserving and storing food give us year-round availability of nutrients that our forebears could only dream about. Freezing, salting, canning, smoking, drying, fermentation, radiation, and certain additives can be used to preserve food. Clearly, modern appliances such as refrigerators affect people's ability to store food.

The nutritional advantages of modern storage techniques are obvious. Nevertheless, some of these processes are cause for concern. Some nutrients are quite sensitive to heat and are lost during canning. Too much salt consumption may lead to *hypertension.* Smoking of meats may produce cancer-causing agents. Improper canning, particularly home canning, may lead to food poisoning.

Hypertension
High blood pressure.

People living in countries without as many food preservation techniques not only have less food available but also lose existing food to spoilage, rodents, insects, and molds.

Preparation

The nutritive value of a food may be changed by peeling, dividing, washing, refining, fortification, and sprouting. It may also be changed by the amount and

FIGURE 1-3
Ethnic foods. Figure at base of graph represents percentage of the population that has repeatedly tried a particular ethnic food. For example, 90% of the population has tried Italian food more than once. Growth in sales will change the composition of the national diet.

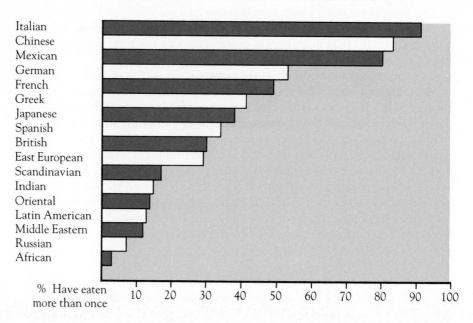

POPULARITY OF ETHNIC FOOD IN RESTAURANTS

Italian
Chinese
Mexican
German
French
Greek
Japanese
Spanish
British
East European
Scandinavian
Indian
Oriental
Latin American
Middle Eastern
Russian
African

% Have eaten more than once   10   20   30   40   50   60   70   80   90   100

type of heat applied to the food, whether by boiling, steaming, roasting, frying, grilling, pressure cooking, or microwave cooking. How long a food is kept at a particular temperature is also important; some nutrients, including vitamin C and thiamin, are destroyed by heat, which means that keeping food on a steam holding table, while allowing a restaurant to operate efficiently, may well cause nutrient loss.

Distribution

Geographical isolation or lack of suitable roads or other means of transportation may affect the distribution of food. This is one problem with famine relief in Africa; in remote areas food has had to be air-dropped. Inadequate transportation hinders food distribution in poor countries, while the air, rail, and trucking systems in the United States permit a well-stocked supermarket to carry as many as 13,000 different food items.

Food distribution can also be subject to political problems, as has happened in programs to alleviate famines in impoverished nations when food supplies have been held up by local officials who are diverting it for blackmarket purposes or for other reasons. Food distribution may also be affected by government regulation of prices or the supply of foods important in the diet.

Serving place

Whether the food comes from a vegetable garden in your back yard or is imported from abroad and sold through a supermarket or health food store, what happens to it next affects its nutritive values. Besides the home, the serving place may be an institutional setting like a hospital or hotel kitchen, work or school cafeteria,

Political Science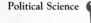

Thailand

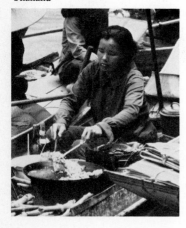

or any of a number of restaurants: steakhouse, seafood, vegetarian, health food, and so on.

Two types of restaurants that have become particularly significant in recent years are ethnic food and fast food. As Figure 1-3 shows, sales of ethnic foods in the United States are expected to increase sharply in the future. This will influence the kinds of nutrients that people take in. As for fast food, more meals than ever before are eaten away from home. Indeed, 40 million Americans eat fast food every day—and that's counting only those who eat *out* in hamburger, fried chicken, and pizza restaurants, and the like. Clearly, many more people also bring home easy-to-prepare convenience foods—the kinds once upon a time referred to as "TV dinners," now much more elaborate. The problem with so many fast foods, however, is that they are often prepared with fat, which is why one magazine headlined a story *Warning: Fast foods are hazardous to your health*[4]—a reference to the dangers of fat as a contributor to heart disease and possibly to certain types of cancer.

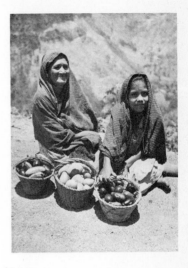

Mexico

Differences Between People

"One man's meat is another man's poison," the expression goes. Why is this? The differences in food preferences between people are based on at least five different reasons: sensory, personal, cultural, social, and medical. Let us examine these.

Sensory differences

Sensory differences have to do with all those reasons that advertisers like to tell us about in those 30-second program interruptions on our television screen: taste, smell, appearance, and texture.

Taste. We are all aware that foods taste different when we have a cold. But people also have individual differences in their tolerance for sweet and salty tastes. From a nutrition standpoint, this means that if you like a lot of sugar, you may be more susceptible to tooth decay. If you dislike salt, you may be less likely to suffer hypertension. Deficiencies of zinc and vitamin A cause a loss of the sense of taste. Pregnancy causes a change in how certain foods taste and smell to many women, and may cause a higher preference for salt.[5]

Smell. Does camembert cheese smell "stinky" to you? To other people, it smells wonderful. Tibetans may love the smell of yak oil or butter, but many Westerners cannot stand it. Spices came into being partly because they obscured the odor of aging meats, but they are now, of course, used to increase the attractiveness of food by creating attractive odors.

Appearance. Chefs and food packagers pay special attention to the appearance or "architecture" of food. Television advertising tries to make food appear even more attractive by the use of words such as "crisp," "wholesome," "fresh," "juicy," "rich," and "finger-lickin' good." Nature is also expert in increasing our attention to foods by the use of bright colors, like the yellow of bananas. Once again, however, there are individual differences: a picture of a hot dog with melted cheese may look terrific to some people and awful to others.

Texture. There is no point in explaining to some people that raw oysters or sheep eyes are a gourmet delicacy; the "feel" of these items on the tongue will repel them. Similarly, although tough meat has the same amount of nutrients as tender meat, most people will not avail themselves of nutrients in this form.

Food preparation methods differ throughout the world, but for these people in Thailand (opposite page), Mexico, and Israel, the nutrient requirements are the same.

Israel

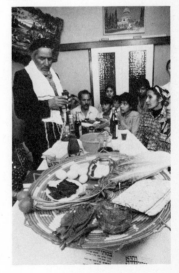

Personal differences

What kind of person are you? Young or old, male or female, blessed or cursed in genetic inheritance, happy or sad or stressed—all these qualities have a lot to do with the food choices you make.

Osteoporosis
Loss of bone in adults, especially women.

Anemia
Low blood hemoglobin, or low concentration of red blood cells.

Age and gender. One's ability to taste and to smell food changes with age. Older people detect bitter and sour better than, and sweet and salty not as well as, when they were younger. Some nutrition problems are more common at certain ages. For example, *osteoporosis* occurs in elderly women, whereas iron deficiency *anemia* ("iron-poor blood") is more common in women during their child-bearing years. Coronary heart disease is highest in men between 35 and 55 years of age. Dietary and nondietary factors throughout life may influence whether a person will get coronary heart disease. As these examples show, some nutrition problems are more common in one sex than in the other. Women, of course, have additional nutrition demands during periods of pregnancy and lactation.

Genetics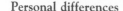

Genetic inheritance. Recently it was confirmed that genetics plays an important role in human obesity.[6] When the obesity of adopted children was compared with the obesity of both their adoptive parents and their biological parents, a relationship was found between the children's body mass and that of their biological parents but not of their adoptive parents.

Diet and genetics may also affect people with phenylketonuria (PKU), a problem affecting about 1 out of every 8,000 babies (although in the United States most babies are tested for this problem at birth). In this disorder, mental retardation results because a person cannot process an essential amino acid in foods known as phenylalanine. Phenylalanine is also part of the molecule of aspartame (Nutra-sweet), a sweetener in many diet drinks and foods.

Emotions. Emotions are, of course, a big factor in individual food choice (as we explain in detail later in the book). Your choice or rejection of foods is quite often related to state of mind. Grief, fear, and anxiety usually decrease food intake. Disappointments and rejections cause some people to seek emotional rewards by eating more, which may lead to obesity. Some young women and teenage girls respond to stress with such eating disorders as anorexia nervosa (self-induced denial of food) or bulimia (binge eating followed by vomiting). Sometimes emotions affect food choices in ways that seem more "principled," as when people avoid eating meat because of an emotional aversion toward killing animals.

Cultural, social, and economic factors

Your family, ethnic, and religious background have everything to do with why you choose certain foods. So do social and economic factors.

Family and religious background. Eating patterns of first- and second-generation immigrants vary depending on country of origin. For instance, persons of Chinese descent tend to retain their food patterns longer than do other immigrants. Dinner is the meal with the least amount of change from the pattern of eating in the old country.

Anthropology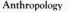

Many religions have specific food laws. Hindus, for example, avoid beef, and many Jews and Muslims avoid pork. Seventh Day Adventists avoid meat, fish, poultry, alcohol, tea, and coffee. Certain times of the year are reserved for fasting (Lent for Roman Catholics, Ramadan for Muslims). An anthropologist suggests that many religious food laws grew out of practical considerations of climate and agricultural restrictions rather than from any fundamental principles of these religions.[7]

For instance, it was difficult for early societies to preserve meat with absolute safety. There was a lot of food poisoning, which increased, of course, with the age of the meat. It was easier to get people to abstain from eating meat and other such risky foods by using the force of religious law, however, than by explaining cause and effect relationships that were not clearly understood by anyone at the time.

Social factors. Social factors include peer pressure and economic matters. Peer group pressure works in many different ways. Of course, peer pressure lies behind the kind of foods brought out on festive occasions, such as white cake at wedding receptions, turkey at Thanksgiving, and fruitcake at Christmas. The mass media keeps up a constant drumbeat of peer pressure that "thin is in" and often dispenses dietary advice (such as the "Drinking Man's Diet" or the all-protein diet) that is just plain wrong. Peer pressure may also lie behind the sudden popularity of certain kinds of foods, such as white wine and Brie cheese among certain fashion-conscious people. Peer pressure may also account for the attractiveness of certain foods labeled "natural," "organic," or "health"—although in point of fact there is no official definition of any of these terms.

Economic factors influence where people shop, what they buy, and how they store and cook food. People who shop in small "Mom and Pop" stores tend to buy in small quantities, thus missing the kind of savings that come with shopping in bulk at supermarkets. Low incomes clearly determine how well, both in quantity and in quality, people eat. A change in a family's status from two incomes to one will usually have a bearing on the family's eating habits.

Medical factors. Medical factors most certainly affect why different people eat different foods. Sometimes medical cures are prescribed by folklore,[8] like the prescription of homemade chicken soup as a remedy for colds and the flu. Sometimes medical concerns dictate voluntary restriction on certain kinds of foods; recent public awareness of the importance of fat, cholesterol, and salt in contributing to heart disease has caused many people to try to cut foods heavy in these substances from their diets. Sometimes medical matters force people *involuntarily* to restrict their diet, as is the case for people afflicted by certain allergies, diabetes, or kidney disease; in advanced cancer, some patients become deficient in some nutrients because of a loss of taste for food. Certain drug and food interactions may also affect diet; for example, orange juice can destroy the effectiveness of penicillin; zinc supplements may increase blood cholesterol and increase the risk of heart attacks; regular use of aspirin causes anemia in menstruating women and elderly people.[9]

Injuries and infections clearly affect diet. People suffering from broken bones, burns, and surgery need more nutrients for satisfactory recovery. *Antibodies*, which fight infection within the body, are made of protein, which must be provided by the diet. Infections causing fever require a higher energy intake in the diet because of the increased amount of body heat produced. Infections causing diarrhea can lead to the body's excreting water and certain nutrients such as minerals.

Emotionally loaded words will not automatically make a food nutritious

Natural Food
Unprocessed food.

Organic Food
Food produced without artificial fertilizers, pesticides, or additives.

Health Food
These foods have no special health-giving properties.

If you must take medication, be aware of possible interactions with nutrients.

Antibodies
Blood proteins protecting the body from foreign proteins.

Everybody in the world does not eat the same kinds of food. There are regional differences in the production, storage, preparation, and place of serving food. People from different cultures have different responses to the taste, smell, and appearance of food. Finally, each individual's choice of food is affected by such factors as age, gender, genetics, emotions, or medical condition.

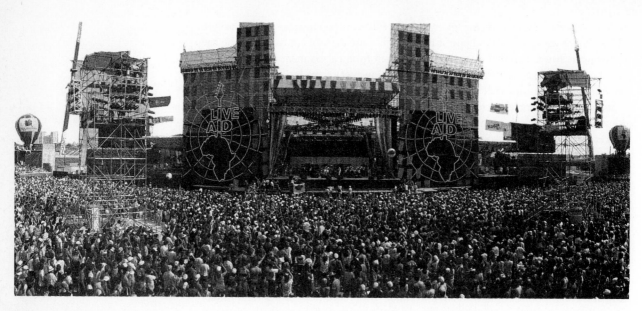

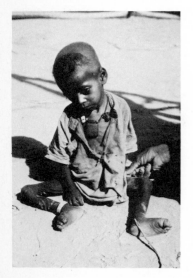

Music and famine. Rock music concerts have been used to call attention to the problems of hunger and malnutrition.

WHAT IS NUTRITION?

We have tried to show why people have different eating habits, whether they're sitting at different ends of the table or different ends of the earth. Now let us get down to basics, and ask the fundamental question: *What is nutrition?*

The Council of Food and Nutrition of the American Medical Association has offered the following definition of nutrition. This is important, and you may wish to mark this page or write the statement out on a separate sheet of paper, since we will then go through it step by step. Nutrition is defined as

the science of food, the nutrients and other substances therein, their action, interaction, and balance in relation to health and disease, and the processes by which the organism ingests, digests, absorbs, transports, utilizes and excretes food substances.

Let us examine this definition, which forms the basis for all further discussion about the subject in this book.

The Science of Food, the Nutrients and Other Substances Therein

Nutrition, says the AMA definition, begins as "the science of food, nutrients and other substances therein. . . ." Let us examine this first part word by word.

The science of food

The statement that nutrition is *the science of food* means that it is the study of the chemistry, physics, biology, and economics of food and food production. As everyone knows (some, unfortunately, all too well), hunger, nutrition deficiencies, and eventually death result if insufficient food is produced. Food production involves all branches of agricultural and veterinary science. As we indicated in the preceding section, the amount and type of food on your plate may depend on geographical location and climate, species of animals and plants, soil quality, use of fertilizer, presence or absence of diseases, presence or absence of pests like insects and rodents, handling of food after harvesting, transportation, economic and political factors, and preservation and preparation methods.

Recently, there have been attempts to publicize many of these factors in food production. In 1985, the "Live Aid" rock music concert helped focus the world's attention on areas suffering from famine—where desert had claimed much of the farmland and what remained was threatened by drought. Such conditions are made worse because poor countries cannot afford adequate fertilizers to increase crop yields, or to control diseases in plants and animals. Even some of the food aid from other countries never gets to the starving people because of poor transportation and political problems. Much of the food rots in the ports or is eaten by insects and rodents. Lack of money or political indifference frequently means that starving people never get the available food.

All these factors are important in industrialized countries but are usually less critical. Because food production is not generally a problem, more attention is given to food preservation and preparation. In the United States, we seldom see newspaper and magazine articles about lack of food commodities; most are concerned with such issues as food additives or fat content.

Nutrients

Nutrition is "the science of food, *the nutrients and other substances therein . . .*" *Nutrients* means the chemicals in food needed to maintain life. *Substances* means other chemicals, which may include nonessential nutrients; chemicals involved in color, flavor, odor, and texture; naturally occurring *toxicants*, additives, and environmental contaminants; bacteria, fungi, and molds.

Toxicants
Chemicals that harm the human body.

Let us consider these elements.

Essential nutrients. How many nutrients do you think you need to live? Ten? One hundred? Actually, as the result of increased research about nutrition, most experts now accept the number of essential nutrients to be about 46. These 46 nutrients are listed in Table 1-1. (The exact number is still in some dispute: microminerals have been found essential for certain experimental animals, which does not mean they are proven essential for humans; however, most scientists accept that they are.) These 46 nutrients must be provided by the food you eat, that is, they cannot be generated by your body.

For convenience, we will describe the nutrients individually, in the order that they are listed in Table 1-1. However, of course, if you eat a meal consisting of a wide variety of foods, a single mouthful may well contain most of these nutrients.

Other substances

This category includes nutrients, such as some other forms of carbohydrates, lipids, and amino acids, that are not essential. It also includes chemicals involved in the color, flavor, odor, and texture of food. Finally, it includes naturally occurring toxicants, additives, and environmental contaminants.

Nonessential nutrients. Most meals you eat will contain a large number of other

TABLE 1-1 The Essential 46 Nutrients*

Major Category	Essential Nutrient	
Carbohydrate	Glucose	
Lipid or fat	Linoleic acid	
Protein	Amino acids:	lysine, methionine, phenylalanine, threonine, tryptophan, leucine, valine, isoleucine, histidine
	Nonessential nitrogen	
Vitamins	Fat-soluble:	A† (retinol) D (cholecalciferol, ergocalciferol) E (tocopherol) K (menadione)
	Water-soluble:	C (ascorbic acid) B (thiamin§ [vitamin B_1], riboflavin [vitamin B_2], niacin§ [nicotinamide, nicotinic acid], vitamin B_6 [pyridoxine, pyridoxal, pyridoxamine], pantothenic acid, biotin, folacin† [folic acid, folate], cobalamin [cyanocobalamin])
Minerals	Macrominerals:	calcium, phosphorus, sodium‡, potassium, magnesium, chlorine, sulfur
	Microminerals:	iron†, zinc†, iodine§, selenium, copper, manganese, cobalt, chromium, molybdenum, vanadium, tin, nickel, silicon

*Experts disagree on the exact number of essential nutrients. This is because our knowledge on the role of some nutrients in the human body is less than perfect. This list is agreed on by most experts to be the *known* essential nutrients.
†Intake may be too low among some people in the United States.
‡Intake may be too high among some people in the United States.
§Intake was low in the recent past in the United States. The problem has been corrected.

chemicals occurring naturally in—that is, inherent in—food. Did you have cantaloupe for breakfast? If you exclude the essential nutrients in Table 1-1 and any additives, the minimum number of naturally occurring chemicals in a breakfast of cantaloupe is 10. For toast and coffee cake, there are 22 naturally occurring chemicals. For scrambled eggs, 15.

Some of the chemicals of this sort that you might find in foods eaten at breakfast are nonessential forms of carbohydrates (fiber, starch, sucrose, or table sugar), lipids, and amino acids.

Chemicals for color, flavor, odor, and texture. Naturally occurring also are chemicals that give foods their particular color, flavor, odor, and texture.

Naturally occurring toxicants. Bananas and broccoli each have five potentially harmful chemicals—naturally occurring toxicants. Coffee has three; apples and potatoes each have two. The list of foods with naturally occurring toxicants is long.[10] However, there is no real cause for concern. These toxicants are present in such small amounts in the plant that they cause no known harm to the body.

Additives. The subject of food additives is an emotionally charged issue, and we examine this in detail later. For now, we will speak of them as part of the

Toxicology

category of "other substances"—chemicals used for various functions in food.

Some food additives, preservatives, extend shelf life; *antioxidants* prevent spoilage from the air. Other additives are nonnutritive sweeteners. Some prevent the loss of moisture, prevent caking, keep food firm, or act as whipping agents.

Antioxidants
Protect other chemicals from damaging effects of oxygen.

Public concern about food additives has grown in recent years. Yet all of the evidence shows that the majority are safe.[11] The Food and Drug Administration publishes a list of additives considered safe in human foods. Unsafe additives are not permitted. However, constant testing for harmful effects is necessary.

Environmental contaminants. Environmental and industrial contaminants affect nutrient intake by making some foods dangerous to eat. The Chernobyl nuclear reactor disaster in the Soviet Union in April 1986, which showered radioactive material over much of Europe, resulted in warnings about radioactivity in milk and other foods in that part of the world. Other warnings in recent years have been issued about high levels of toxic minerals such as lead, arsenic, and mercury (especially in fish). Industrial wastes have also caused problems in foods, as have antibiotics given to farm animals produced for meat consumption.

Bacteria, fungi, and molds. Microorganisms in food may be helpful or harmful. The making of sour cream, yogurt, cheese, and wine and the baking of bread all require the action of what we might call "good" microorganisms. Microorganisms are also needed to produce riboflavin, vitamin K, and several antibiotics (including penicillin). However, bacteria that cause food spoilage or food-borne diseases are certainly not welcome. Food-borne diseases may take the form of bacteria-induced food infections. These produce vomiting, diarrhea, and fever. They may take the form of food poisoning, such as staphylococcal infection, which also causes vomiting and usually diarrhea. Another food-borne disease is botulism, a pernicious and, in the past, often fatal disorder resulting from eating home-canned nonacid vegetables (such as corn or beans) or inadequately cooked home-canned meat. Today, deaths from botulism are not common, owing to better understanding about canning methods and treatment.

Some molds and fungi can be deadly. Most dangerous are the cancer-causing aflatoxins, which occur in peanuts, grains, and some vegetables—foods now screened by government regulatory agencies for contamination by such molds.

Be aware of the nutrients and other chemicals at least in foods eaten often.

Action, Interaction, and Balance in Relation to Health and Disease

Nutrition, to resume our definition, is "the science of food, the nutrients and other substances therein, *their action. . . .*"

Action

One example of the action of nutrients is as sources of energy. Another action is the growth and maintenance of tissues. Still another example is the regulation of body processes. Let me give some examples.

Sources of energy. As we are all personally aware, an important action of nutrients is as sources of energy—the amount of energy available for physical work, athletic performance, growth rate in children, and recovery from illness. It is, of course, possible to have too much or too little of energy-supplying nutrients: too much can cause overweight, too little can cause starvation.

The nutrients that provide energy are carbohydrates, lipids, and protein (terms that will be defined shortly) (Figure 1-4). But what about vitamins and minerals? What about all those ads that tell us vitamins and minerals (particularly iron) "give us energy"? The answer is that they do not have energy to *give*. Rather, they help "liberate" the energy locked up in carbohydrates, lipids, and proteins.

Growth and maintenance of tissues. Protein, vitamins, minerals, and water are all nutrients that help in the growth and maintenance of tissues. Children who do not get enough food or who eat food low in nutrients may experience slower growth because some tissues require more specific nutrients for growth. Bone formation, for example, requires calcium, phosphorus, and vitamin D.

Regulation of body processes. The same nutrients required for growth—proteins, vitamins, minerals, and water—also help regulate body processes. There are hundreds of such processes, but one familiar example is blood clotting—the factor that keeps most people from bleeding to death when accidentally cut; blood clotting requires sufficient vitamin K in the diet. Another body process is eye function, which requires adequate vitamin A.

Interaction

Nutrition is "the science of food, the nutrients and other substances therein, their action, *interaction* . . ."

Nutrient interactions follow laws of chemistry and physiology. Bone formation requires calcium, phosphorus, and vitamin D. Lack of enough of any *one* of these means bone will not form properly, because the three nutrients interact. The interaction may also change periodically; marathon runners, for example, use different amounts of carbohydrate and fat for energy as the race progresses.

FIGURE 1-4
Dietary energy sources.

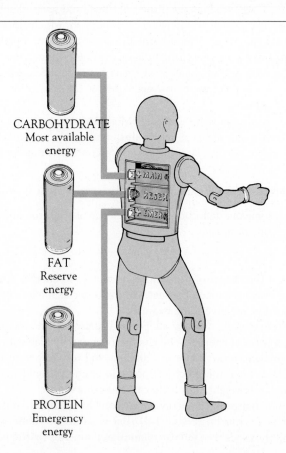

CARBOHYDRATE
Most available
energy

FAT
Reserve
energy

PROTEIN
Emergency
energy

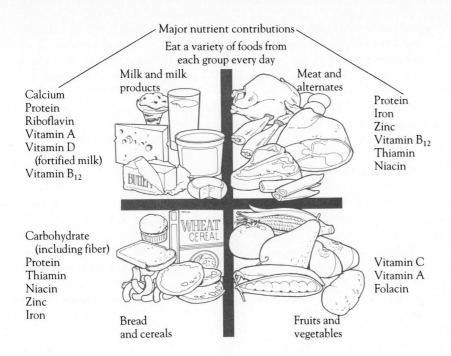

Major nutrient contributions
Eat a variety of foods from
each group every day

Milk and milk products

Meat and alternates

Calcium
Protein
Riboflavin
Vitamin A
Vitamin D
  (fortified milk)
Vitamin B$_{12}$

Protein
Iron
Zinc
Vitamin B$_{12}$
Thiamin
Niacin

Carbohydrate
  (including fiber)
Protein
Thiamin
Niacin
Zinc
Iron

Vitamin C
Vitamin A
Folacin

Bread
and cereals

Fruits and
vegetables

FIGURE 1-5
Major nutrient contributions. You
should eat a variety of foods from each
of the four food groups every day.

Balance

Nutrition is "the science of food, the nutrients and other substances therein, their action, interaction, *and balance . . .*"

"Eat a balanced diet." Does this sound like the advice of several generations of mothers talking to their children? It is, however, excellent advice.

In general, your diet is probably balanced if it consists of a *wide variety* of foods, of the sort indicated in Figure 1-5. Unbalanced means too few or too many of specific nutrients. Whether your diet is unbalanced depends on what foods you eat, on whether you take nutrition supplements, and on your general health status. Too little of a nutrient can produce unpleasant deficiency symptoms; lack of iron, for instance, can produce weakness. Too much of a nutrient can often be even worse; too much iron will cause death. Some other examples are as follows. Fluoride: too little—increased tooth decay; too much—mottled teeth (brown spots). Protein: too little—death; too much—gout (a type of arthritis). Magnesium: too little *or* too much—abnormal nerve function.

These unpleasant consequences suggest that, if you take nutrient supplements, there are some important "survival rules":

- Use nutrient supplements correctly. Because they are available over the counter (that is, without a doctor's prescription), vitamin A capsules or iron tablets may seem "safe." However, swallowing half a bottle of these supplements may well be fatal.
- Read the labels on nutrient supplements. You should know exactly how much extra you are adding to your normal dietary intake.
- Ask yourself: Do I really need this nutrient supplement? Of course you might want to look better or have less stress in your life, as the ads state; you might wonder if you are really nutrient-deficient. But try to analyze the information critically and beware of false promises.

Fortunately, if you live in an industrialized country, your diet is probably reasonably well balanced. If your diet *is* deficient in any of the 46 essential nutrients, the deficient nutrient is likely to be vitamin A, thiamin, vitamin B_6, folacin, calcium, iron, or zinc—or so studies have shown for the typical American diet. On the other hand, the availability of over-the-counter nutrient supplements has caused problems. One problem is taking in nutrients in too large amounts; we will cover that in detail in this book.

In relation to health and disease

Nutrition is the science of food, and so on, "*. . . in relation to health and disease. . . .*"

In the early 1900s, people were concerned about nutrition deficiencies, but in industrialized countries today many medical disorders are probably due to high intakes of certain types of food. Often called "diseases of affluence"—heart disease, obesity, hypertension, and stroke—these disorders may be traceable to diets high in salt and in meat and other foods of animal origin that are high in cholesterol and certain types of fat. (We say they *may* be traceable to these food items because experts are not in total agreement on the importance of diet in some of these diseases.)

Processes by Which the Organism Ingests, Digests, Absorbs, Transports, Utilizes, and Excretes Food Substances

Nutrition, to continue the definition, is not only the science of food, the nutrients, and so on, but also the study of several *processes*—that is, the activities "by which the organism"—meaning you—"ingests, digests, absorbs, transports, utilizes, and excretes food substances." Let us now proceed to describe what is meant by these processes.

Ingestion and digestion

When you swallow food, the nutrients it contains are not "within you" in a biological sense—at least not yet. Swallowing is only the *beginning* of the chain of several activities in which nutrients are taken from the food and delivered to the cells in your body.

Ingestion—eating and swallowing—is only the first step. *Digestion* is the next step, and the first phase of extracting the nutrients from food. As food moves down the hollow tube of the digestive tract (Figure 1-6), the digestive juices break large complex molecules of carbohydrate, lipid, and protein into small, basic building blocks. The small molecules of water and individual vitamins and minerals are then ready for absorption into the blood.

Absorption

Most nutrients are absorbed in the duodenum (the upper part of the small intestine) (Figure 1-6). You might picture this area as consisting of hundreds of different chemicals lining up to squeeze through tiny openings between the cells. If the movement of food along the digestive tract is too fast (as happens with excessive use of laxatives), the amount of nutrients absorbed is reduced. Any unabsorbed nutrients and other chemicals move on to the large intestine, and most are finally eliminated in the feces.

Transportation

After the nutrients are absorbed from the duodenum, they are *transported*—that is, taken in the blood—to the liver. This wonderful multipurpose organ puts some nutrients (such as carbohydrates, lipids, fat-soluble vitamins, and iron) through some chemical changes so that they can be stored more efficiently—which explains why liver from farm animals is such a good source of many nutrients. The liver is also the detoxification center for alcohol and drugs.

From the liver, the blood transports nutrients to every cell in the body. The critical last step is the transporting of nutrients through the membrane surrounding each cell; if this does not happen, the cell may die from lack of nutrients.

Utilization of food substances

After all is said and done, a nutrient can only be said to be "good for you" when it performs its function in your body—when it is actually *utilized*. For example, plenty of vitamin A may be stored in a person's liver, but during starvation he or she may go blind from vitamin A deficiency—simply because the vitamin A is

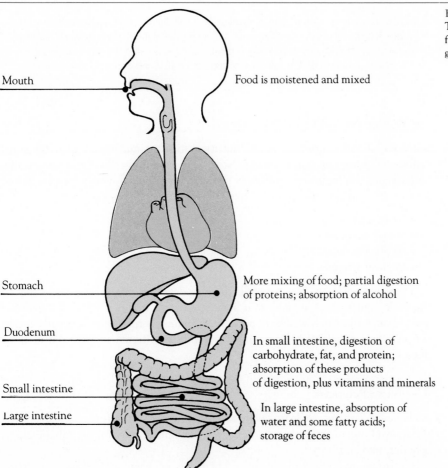

FIGURE 1-6
The human digestive tract. The major functions of each of the principal organs are described.

Mouth — Food is moistened and mixed

Stomach — More mixing of food; partial digestion of proteins; absorption of alcohol

Duodenum

Small intestine — In small intestine, digestion of carbohydrate, fat, and protein; absorption of these products of digestion, plus vitamins and minerals

Large intestine — In large intestine, absorption of water and some fatty acids; storage of feces

not utilized: there are transportation problems that prevent vitamin A from getting from the liver to the eye.

Excretion

As mentioned, nutrients and other chemicals in food that are not absorbed from the digestive tract, plus some of the digestive secretions, are eliminated in the feces. However, once substances have been absorbed into the body, the methods of waste disposal are more limited.

Urination is the method of excreting water-soluble waste products and excess water-soluble vitamins that are filtered out of the blood by the kidney. Perspiration is excretion through the skin, which allows the loss of water and salt. Exhalation is the method by which the lungs expel carbon dioxide and water vapor. Even milk through the breast is considered a kind of excretion according to some authorities, since antibiotics and other toxic substances, if taken in the diet, are later excreted in human breast milk.

Some materials are simply not excreted. Fat and fat-soluble substances, including fat-soluble vitamins and some toxic substances, remain in the body, stored in fat.

> In this section, we have looked at the details of the definition of nutrition. Nutrition is the science of food, the nutrients and other substances therein, their action, interaction, and balance in relation to health and disease, and the processes by which the organism ingests, digests, absorbs, transports, utilizes and excretes food substances.

HOW DO WE STUDY NUTRITION?

We have all, of course, "studied" nutrition in what might be called the usual "hands-on" sense: by simply eating. Now let us look at food more systematically.

As Figure 1-7 indicates, the study of nutrition is linked with a lot of different subjects or academic disciplines. They fall in four general categories:

- Basic sciences
- Social sciences
- Applied sciences
- Medical sciences

There is no way we can cover all these in detail, of course, but let us suggest the basic constituents of these four areas. Although it is not a task for amateurs and although there may well be opportunities for misinterpretation between experts, you may find it helpful to know how to gather nutritional information in these disciplines.

The Basic Sciences

As Figure 1-7 shows, at least seven basic sciences provide distinct approaches to the study of nutrition: chemistry, biology, biochemistry, physiology, microbiology, genetics, and statistics.

Nutrition involves the transfer of chemicals between two biological systems: food and you. Therefore, *chemistry* and *biology* clearly are important. One effect of

Chemistry

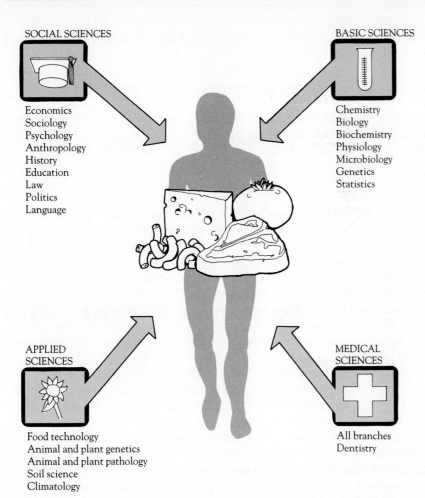

SOCIAL SCIENCES

Economics
Sociology
Psychology
Anthropology
History
Education
Law
Politics
Language

BASIC SCIENCES

Chemistry
Biology
Biochemistry
Physiology
Microbiology
Genetics
Statistics

FIGURE 1-7

The study of nutrition. Four basic areas make up the interdisciplinary study of food in relation to you.

APPLIED SCIENCES

Food technology
Animal and plant genetics
Animal and plant pathology
Soil science
Climatology

MEDICAL SCIENCES

All branches
Dentistry

these sciences is seen whenever a TV commercial trumpets that a certain margarine is "high in polyunsaturates." What's going on here? From chemistry and biology we have learned that a certain group of chemicals called polyunsaturated fats may be helpful in controlling coronary heart disease (although experts still debate how important this connection is).

Biochemistry describes the chemical reactions taking place within the body. From this academic discipline, nutritionists can learn how nutrients are involved in the buildup and breakdown of human tissue. In turn, this can help you understand the effects of taking in low amounts of certain nutrients.

Physiology describes the normal workings of the human body. This field can teach us how much the body departs from normal functioning when nutrient intake is low. *Microbiology* includes the study of food spoilage, nutrient production by bacteria, and certain illnesses with nutritional implications, such as diarrhea.

Genetics is quite important: through genetic selection, more efficient food-producing plants and animals can be bred. Moreover, genetics may show us how certain diseases with possible genetic bases may be avoided or treated by a change in diet—for example, high blood pressure can sometimes be controlled by a low-salt diet.

Biology

Biochemistry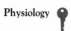

Physiology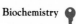

Genetics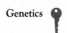

Statistics

Statistics helps quantify information about food and determine normal nutritional values. For example, if your weight and height, blood pressure, serum cholesterol level, and blood sugar significantly differ from the ordinary, you need to revise your eating habits. Statistics also, of course, help researchers establish national trends. In fact, the U.S. Department of Agriculture found that it could predict the nutritional intake and status of the entire country of over 250 million people with access to hundreds of different foods merely by surveying only 34,000 people and only 200 different foods.[12]

The Social Sciences

As Figure 1-6 shows, nine social sciences have an important bearing on the study of nutrition: economics, sociology, psychology, anthropology, history, education, law, politics, and language.

Economics

The majority of people in industrialized countries do not, needless to say, hunt or even grow their own food. Therefore, food is an article of commerce, which is to say it is a subject of scarcity and supply and demand (though it is argued that everyone should have food as a basic human right).[13] Thus, *economics* studies how people allocate their money among food and other commodities and how government policies of food assistance and food subsidy programs affect the distribution of food to people.

Sociology

Social attitudes toward food are influenced by marketing, advertising, food fads, and even mystical concerns, all subjects of study for *sociology.* This is a fascinating area. Consider, for instance, how attitudes toward food have changed with time. Would you ever think that the aristocracy would prefer beans and the peasants would prefer salmon instead of the other way around? Yet indeed this was the case in nineteenth-century London. Or consider the importance of meat. Since the beginning of time, meat has been associated with strength and virility. Even today, the availability of meat is thought to be a measure of the success of a political system: beef, lamb, and pork are easily found in an American supermarket, but in Russia and Eastern Europe people stand in line for hours to buy meat.

Psychology

Psychology, too, has a great deal of insight to offer about nutrition. Overweight and obesity or underweight and anorexia are conditions that have psychological causes.[14] Diet may also have some relationship to such psychological matters as mood changes, hyperactivity in children, and even criminal behavior.

Anthropology

Anthropology—specifically that branch called "nutrition anthropology"—uses information from archeology and accounts of explorers and missionaries to evaluate food-related behavior, diet, and nutritional consequences on societies.[15] *History* also offers insights about nutrition—the explorations in search of new sources of food, and the nutritional deficiencies suffered during those long sea voyages, the acceptance of hunger as the inevitable human condition for many centuries.[16]

Education

Education, especially nutrition education, has become a highly visible field. Nutrition education in schools and universities may be the least of it. Dietary advice appears to be everywhere: in weight-reducing programs, in government pamphlets on dietary goals, in hospital regimens, and certainly everywhere in the mass media.[17] An important area of research is the effects of severe undernutrition on the ability of children to learn.[18]

Law

The role of the *law* in food standards has changed since Upton Sinclair's book *The Jungle* highlighted unsanitary conditions in meat-packing plants at the beginning of this century. Now the law emphasizes truth in labeling and control of misleading or false medical and nutritional claims.[19]

Politics is concerned with a great many food and nutrition issues, ranging from grain embargoes against the Soviet Union to whether tomato ketchup should be considered a "vegetable" for nutrition purposes in school lunch programs.

Political Science

The social sciences concerned with *language,* such as linguistics, examine the emotional power of words and such issues as whether nutrition terms are truly descriptive and correct. As mentioned, the terms "health food," "natural," and "organic" have no legal definition but are used by food manufacturers to suggest a "healthy" quality to their products. Newspapers and magazines sometimes misrepresent factual matters about nutrition—even medical journals, one of which ran the headline "Hidden Dangers of Sliced Bread" on an article not about additives or toxic chemicals, as one might suspect, but on the gastrointestinal problems of two people who accidentally swallowed the bread wrapper clip.[20]

Language

The Applied Sciences

As Figure 1-6 indicates, the applied sciences cover food technology, animal and plant genetics, animal and plant pathology, soil science, and climatology.

Food Technology

Inasmuch as over half of the typical American diet consists of processed food, it is clear that *food technology* has played an important role in changing our food preferences. However, although this technology has made food more readily available, some critics question whether processed food is really wholesome. *Animal and plant genetics* has increased the efficiency of food production, and *animal and plant pathology* has helped control diseases. Specialists in *soil science* have helped farmers and livestock growers evaluate soils in order to avoid raising food products in earth with harmful constituents.

Animal and Plant Genetics

Animal and Plant Pathology

Soil Science

The Medical Sciences

All branches of the medical sciences have some interaction with nutrition, but I can suggest only a few of the specialties here. *Obstetrics* gives attention to the nutritional status of pregnant women and their unborn children. *Pediatrics* deals with child growth and development, including nutrition-related disorders. *Psychiatry* is involved with treating food-related neuroses—for example, anorexia nervosa and bulimia in teenage girls. Nutritional deficiencies may be quantified by specialists in *pathology*. *Geriatrics* is concerned with the problems of the elderly, including special nutritional needs and problems. *Dentistry* is related to nutrition because one's choice of foods is limited unless one has the teeth or dentures to eat with. And of course we are interested in knowing which substances cause tooth decay.

Medicine

Dentistry

Dietetics involves monitoring diets for possible nutrient deficiencies. People in this specialty also modify diets to help treat or ease certain disorders, such as diabetes or heart disease, or to help the body with increased nutrient demands while recovering from stresses such as surgery or burns.

Dietetics

There are many interactions between nutrition and other disciplines in the basic sciences, social sciences, applied sciences, and medical sciences, and nutritionists should be aware of how to obtain nutrition information from these sources. However, gathering such information is not a task for amateurs and one must be alert for possible misinterpretations between experts in different disciplines.

WHAT ARE THE BEST WAYS TO MAKE DECISIONS ABOUT FOOD?

With this overview of nutrition behind you, you are now in a position to begin to make some personal decisions about what you eat on some basis other than "it tastes good" or "it's available." Thus, at the end of every chapter you will find a section headed "Decisions" that shows you step by step how to evaluate your own eating behavior and food choices. The first such section follows immediately below.

DECISIONS

1. What Foods Are "Good" for Me?

It is better to think of *combinations* of food, like those in the "four food groups" illustration back in Figure 1-5, rather than individual foods.

Correct combination of two foods can improve nutritive value significantly.

To appreciate this, consider a simple experiment in which three different groups of laboratory rats were fed three different kinds of "sole food": hamburger meat, breakfast cereal, and spinach. The results are shown in Figure 1-8. The group that ate only hamburger meat (without bun or other food) experienced a better rate of growth than did the groups that ate only breakfast cereal (without milk) or spinach. However, after 13 weeks, the animals fed hamburger died of nerve and musculo-skeletal problems (paralysis, fragile bones), owing to the absence of calcium in the diet—which would not have happened if they had been fed cheeseburgers. Five of the six rats fed only breakfast cereal survived to 13 weeks, but they experienced loss of hair and showed an unkempt appearance—which would not have happened if milk had been added to the cereal. The rats fed spinach died after only a week. (So much for Popeye the sailor man's favorite food.)

Lessons

Two lessons may be drawn from this experiment. First, nutrition information may differ depending on how long the experiment lasts (compare what happened at 4 and 13 weeks in Figure 1-8). Second, although all three foods make useful nutrient contributions to the total diet, if only one food is the sole source of nourishment it can lead to problems.

2. When Should I Eat?

The answer is straightforward: When you are hungry. There is no rule that says you need to eat three (or two or one) meals per day. After all, your ancestors certainly did not have food available continuously as we do today. Whatever admonitions you may have heard against snacking, you should be aware that snacks are not a problem provided (1) they are nutritious and (2) the total amount of food from meals plus snacks for the day is not so high as to cause obesity. Once I participated in an experiment in malnutrition (while visiting the University of the West Indies in Jamaica) in which nutrients in liquid form were piped continuously into my stomach for 36 hours. After that day and a half, I had received all the nutrients I required, but I had a headache and felt nauseated—simply because my body was not used to being continuously fed. Also, as you might expect, although I was not hungry, because my nutrient needs certainly had been met, I had a powerful yearning for tasty food. You see, I had not tasted the food because it was piped directly into my stomach.

What and when to eat is often a subject of misinformation. The best-selling (2 million copies) diet book *Fit For Life* by Harvey and Marilyn Diamond has been roundly condemned by the American Medical Association and the American Dietetic Association because, among other reasons, it erroneously tells you that you should eat at a certain time of day so that food will not rot in your digestive tract!

Lessons

Whether you will become over- or undernourished depends on your *total* food intake every day, not when or how far apart the meals are. Moreover, as my experiment showed, we may need nutrients but we also *want* food: the taste, smell, and sight of "real food" are important. Finally, beware of those who come bearing the gifts of nutritional advice packaged in best-selling books until you've had a chance to verify the advice with someone who has some knowledge of physiology and biochemistry.

3. How Do I Know if Nutrition Information Is Correct?

Despite our caution in the last sentence above, you should be aware that differences in interpretation of experimental data and even disputes sometimes appear in the scientific literature on nutrition. You should not be surprised or disappointed by this. A science as young and as complex as nutrition gets reliable information only after repeated testing of a result.

Perhaps of more personal interest to you, however, is how to evaluate nutrition

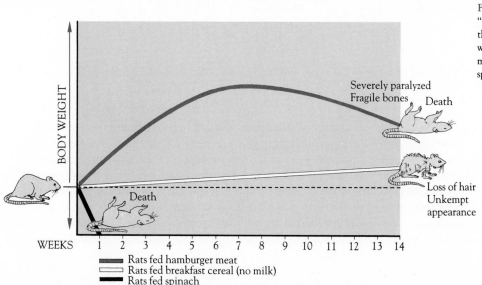

FIGURE 1-8
"Sole food." This shows the results of three groups of laboratory rats that were each fed a diet of hamburger meat, breakfast cereal, and spinach, respectively.

TABLE 1-2 ACSH Ratings of Nutrition Coverage in 19 Major Magazines*

Magazine	Circulation	Articles Reviewed: Accurate	Articles Reviewed: Inaccurate	Percent Accurate
Generally Reliable				
50 Plus	180,000	14	0	100
Parents	1,500,000	30	1	97
Redbook	4,200,000	28	1	97
Reader's Digest	18,000,000	20	1	95
Good Housekeeping	5,400,000	37	3	93
Inconsistent				
Glamour	1,800,000	41	10	80
Vogue	1,100,000	19	5	79
Woman's Day	7,500,000	35	12	74
Ms.	490,000	8	3	73
Seventeen	1,500,000	15	6	71
Family Circle	7,400,000	24	17	59
McCall's	6,300,000	17	13	57
Ladies' Home Journal	5,400,000	14	14	50
Unreliable				
Mademoiselle	920,000	17	20	46
Essence	600,000	10	17	37
Cosmopolitan	2,800,000	14	24	37
Harper's Bazaar	630,000	12	29	29
Organic Gardening	1,300,000	2	6	25
Prevention	2,000,000+	3	28	10

*Values may change from year to year for some magazines. This is usually the result of a change in writers or editorial policy.

and diet information in popular magazines. I would hope, of course, that you will find this text to be of true value in that it will help you sort fact from fiction in the food-related information you read in other places. For the moment, however, you may find Table 1-2 helpful. This table reflects the American Council on Science and Health (ACSH) ratings of nutrition coverage in 19 major American magazines. Note that some general-interest magazines such as *Reader's Digest* and *Good Housekeeping* are considered "generally reliable," whereas some special-interest magazines such as *Organic Gardening* and *Prevention* are considered "unreliable" by the ACSH.

Lesson

You should learn the basic facts about nutrition so that *you* can be a sound judge of nutrition information and won't have to rely on someone else.

Summary

QUALITY AND QUANTITY OF FOOD AND DRINK DEPENDS ON:

Location
Climate
Soil
Species
Fertilizer
Disease
Pests
Storage
Transportation
Economics
Politics
Preservation
Preparation

Storage
Distribution
Serving place

FOOD IS ACCEPTED BECAUSE:

Taste
Appearance
Color
Texture

FOOD CONTAINS: Nutrients, naturally occurring toxicants, food additives, environmental contaminants

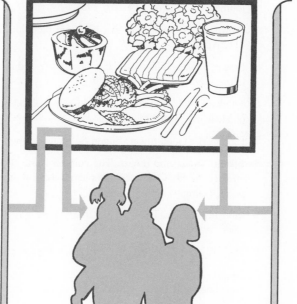

PEOPLE ARE INFLUENCED IN FOOD CHOICES BY:

Age
Gender
Genetics
Emotions

Family traditions
Ethnic foods
Religious food laws

Peer group pressure
Festive occasions
Economic factors

Folklore
Voluntary and
   involuntary
   food restrictions

Climate
Pollution
Food distribution
Labor-saving
   devices
Stress

Information on the action and interaction of each of the above comes from one or more of the following:

   Food analysis
   Comparative and evolutionary records
   Natural disasters and travellers' tales
   Epidemiological studies
   Animal experiments
   Clinical records

REFERENCES

1. Truswell, A.S.: ABC of nutrition: Some principles, British Medical Journal **291**:1486, 1985.

2. Roe, D.A., Clinical nutrition for the health scientist, CRC Press, Inc., Boca Raton, Fla., 1979.

3. DuPont, H.L.: Consumption of raw shellfish: Is the risk now unacceptable? New England Journal of Medicine **314**:707, 1986.

4. Brown, M.H.: Warning: Fast foods are hazardous to your health, Science Digest, p. 311, April 1986.

5. Brown, J.E., and Toma, R.B.: Taste changes during pregnancy, American Journal of Clinical Nutrition **43**:414, 1986.

6. Stunkard, A.J., and others: An adoption study of human obesity. New England Journal of Medicine, **314**:193, 1986.

7. Harris, M.: Good to eat, Simon & Schuster, Inc., New York, 1986.

8. Bryant, C.A., and others: The cultural feast, West Publishing Co., St. Paul, 1985; and Lee, W.H.: Customers and pharmacists pay attention to herbs, American Druggist, p. 99, February 1986.

9. Morgan, B.L.G.: The food and drug interaction guide, Simon & Schuster, Inc., New York, 1986.

10. Hall, R.L.: Safe at the plate, Nutrition Today, p. 6, November/December 1977.

11. Levine, A.S., Labuza, T.P., and Morley, J.E.: Food technology: a primer for physicians, New England Journal of Medicine **312**:628, 1985.

12. Swan, P.B.: Food consumption by individuals in the United States: Two major surveys. Annual Review of Nutrition **3**:413, 1983.

13. Eide, A., and others: Food as a human right, The United Nations University, Tokyo, 1984.

14. Stunkard, A.J., and Stellar, E., editors: Eating and its disorders, Raven Press, New York, 1984.

15. Grivetti, L.E.: Cultural nutrition: Anthropological and geographic themes, Annual Review of Nutrition **1**:47, 1981.

16. Rotberg, R.I., and Rabb, T.K., editors: Hunger and history, Cambridge University Press, New York, 1985.

17. Symposium: Teaching nutrition to the public and the professions. Proceedings of the Nutrition Society, **43**:205, 1984.

18. Grantham-McGregor, S.: Chronic undernutrition and cognitive abilities, Human Nutrition: Clinical Nutrition **38**(C):83, 1983.

19. Hutt, P.B.: Government regulation of the integrity of the food supply, Annual Review of Nutrition **4**:1, 1984.

20. Bundred, N.J., and others: Hidden dangers in sliced bread, British Medical Journal **288**:1723, 1984.

METABOLISM NOTES: *An Introduction*

It is not the food you eat that gets to your cells. Rather, it is the *nutrients* in the food you eat. In the cells, specific nutrients are involved in storing and using energy; in building, maintaining, and repairing tissue; and in communications, transportation, and defense. Metabolism is the name given to all of the chemical reactions involved in these processes. Most reactions take place within cells. The transfer of nutrients from cells in plants and animals to human cells is shown in Figure 1-9. Within the billions of cells in your body are a number of organelles

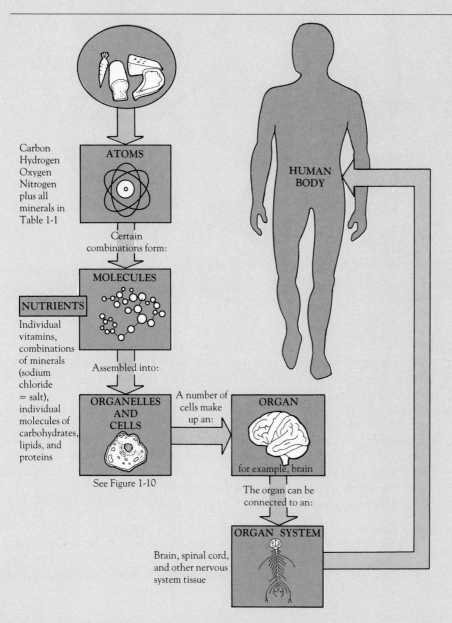

FIGURE 1-9
Cell to cell. The transfer of nutrients from cells in plants and animals—the food we eat—to human cells is shown here. Note that within the cells are a number of organelles—see Figure 1-10

FIGURE 1-10
The cell. The cell is a complex structure that relies heavily on nutrients for normal functioning.

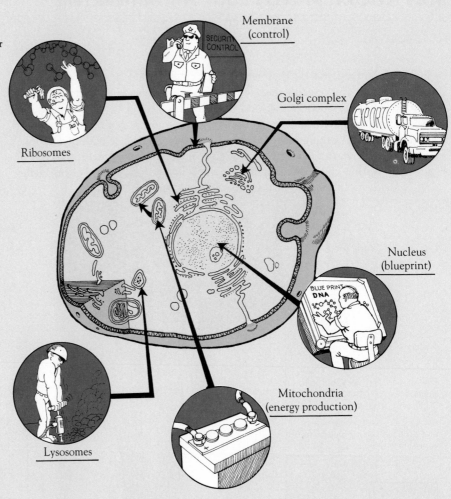

(Figure 1-10), each with a specific function. Notice how each function relies on energy. In starvation, severe weight-reducing diets, and certain eating disorders, there is little or no energy entering the body from the diet. Therefore, some of these functions are performed at below maximum capacity.

Within the cell the nucleus draws up the master plans. It has deoxyribonucleic acid (DNA), the genetic material controlling heredity. Proteins are made by ribosomes and packaged and exported from the cell by the Golgi complex. Lysosomes can break down cell components and some foreign matter that may enter the cell. The plasma membrane controls what enters and leaves the cell. Mitochondria supply energy for all of this activity within the cell.

Factors that *increase* energy metabolism in a person include the following:

- Gender—men have a slightly higher metabolic rate than women do
- Body surface area—smaller people have proportionately higher energy expenditure
- Hormones—for example, the iodine-containing hormone, thyroxin, regulates energy metabolism

- Environmental temperatures—the colder the temperature, the more energy that must be burned to maintain body temperature
- Type of food eaten—metabolic rate is higher after a meal of protein than one with carbohydrate or fat
- Increased body temperature—as in fevers
- Emotional state—such as anger or fear
- Pregnancy and lactation
- Exercise

Factors that *decrease* energy metabolism in a person include:

- Age—metabolism rate declines from young adulthood into old age
- Undernutrition—during certain eating disorders, severe weight-reducing diets, and starvation.

For additional information on metabolism, *see* W.J. Bettger and W.L. Mc-Keehan: Mechanisms of cellular nutrition, *Physiological Reviews* **66:**1, 1986.

2

Eating Right
A Matter of Balance

Obesity
More than 20% over ideal body weight.

CONNECTIONS

Recall from the last chapter all the factors that make you and all other individuals unique in making food choices. Now let us apply these factors to matters that contribute to an adequate diet.

What nutrients are low in the diet of North Americans and people in developing countries? Why are both quantity and quality of food important in determining adequate nutrition? How can foods be grouped to provide a guide to a balanced diet—so that, for example, it is perfectly healthy to exclude meat, as vegetarians do? The answers to these questions, described in this chapter, will give you practical reasons for altering your own diet, if you wish.

This chapter will also show how to calculate nutrient values from tables of food composition, how to apply RDAs (recommended dietary allowances) when you are reading food labels, and how to measure the quantity of food eaten. In addition, the harmful consequences of eating too much are discussed, and guidelines for healthiest eating patterns are described. All these topics will provide solid links to the discussion in the chapters that follow.

Let me make a guess: you probably had something to eat within the last four hours. No? Then you'll probably have something to eat within the *next* four. Indeed, you probably take eating pretty much for granted if you live in North America, because the people who live there are among the best fed in the world.

That said, it may come as a surprise to learn that some doctors believe hunger in the United States is "a national epidemic." After traveling around the country, the Physician Task Force on Hunger in America stated in 1985, "We believe that today hunger and malnutrition are serious problems in every region of the nation. We have, in fact, returned from no city and no state where we did not find extensive hunger." On the other hand, undernutrition is not our only problem. Overnutrition is also a problem. "Obesity is the most prevalent and serious nutritional disease in the United States," writes one researcher. "From 5% to 25% of children and adolescents may be affected."[2]

The extremes of both conditions are not very pretty. Later we will describe how these conditions come about and how they may be prevented, but here let us ask, "How are undernutrition and overnutrition measured?" Once we understand these measurements, we may be in a position to do something about nutritional suffering. Let us begin with a subject of personal interest to you: you and food.

FOOD BECOMES YOU: THE VITAL RELATIONSHIP

You may think of food as having a one-way relationship to you, since we mainly think of it as substances we take in. However, it is actually a two-way relationship. On the one hand, it involves a transfer of nutrients from food to you. On the other hand, we are attracted to certain foods because of sensory, sociocultural, economic, or health reasons. The food sources, and the functions each nutrient performs in your body, are given in Table 2-1. I hope you'll take the time to look through this table, for three reasons:

- So that you can get an overview of the functions of each specific nutrient in the body.
- So that you can see that severe dietary deficiency usually involves alterations in these functions.
- So that you can see the important nutrient contribution of various food groups.

TABLE 2-1 The Major Nutrients, Their Functions and Dietary Sources

Nutrient	Body Functions	Major Food Sources
Carbohydrate	Supplies energy; spares protein	Cereals, fruits, some vegetables, milk
Lipid (Fat)	Provides *essential fatty acid*; supplies energy; absorbs and transports fat-soluble vitamins (A, D, E, and K); insulates; protects vital body tissues	Fats and oils, meats, fish, nuts, some seeds, dairy products
Protein	Growth and repair of tissues; supplies energy; fluid and acid-base balance; all *enzymes*, antibodies, and some *hormones* (insulin) are proteins	Meats, fish, legumes, nuts, dairy products, eggs, cereals
Vitamin A	Vision; health of skin; growth of teeth, nails, hair, bones, and glands	Dairy products, liver, carotene in deep green and orange vegetables
Vitamin D	Bones and teeth	Dairy products, egg yolk
Vitamin E	Antioxidant—prevents cell damage	Oils, nuts, seeds
Vitamin K	Blood clotting	Green leafy vegetables, meats
Vitamin C	Antioxidant; *collagen* formation; health of teeth and gums	Citrus fruits, green pepper, broccoli, cantaloupe
Thiamin (Vitamin B₁)	Nerve function; aids in energy metabolism	Whole grains and cereals, meats (especially pork)
Riboflavin (Vitamin B₂)	Aids in energy metabolism; protects against skin and eye disorders	Whole or enriched grains, milk, eggs, cheese, meats, green vegetables

Essential Fatty Acid
Linoleic acid. Cannot be made by the body in an amount sufficient for normal needs of the body.

Enzymes
Proteins that speed up biochemical reactions.

Hormones
Chemical messengers secreted by certain glands; may affect metabolism at other sites in the body.

Collagen
A protein; acts as the "scaffolding" around cells; a major part of tendons.

Continued.

TABLE 2-1 The Major Nutrients, Their Functions and Dietary Sources—cont'd

Nutrient	Body Functions	Major Food Sources
Niacin	Aids in energy metabolism	Lean meats, fish, whole grains, cheese, peanuts, vegetables, eggs
Vitamin B_6	Aids in *amino acid*–protein metabolism; nerve function	Liver, fish, nuts, meats, potatoes, some vegetables
Pantothenic acid	Aids in energy metabolism; nerve function	Most foods of plant and animal origin
Biotin	Aids in energy metabolism	Most foods of plant and animal origin
Folacin	Synthesis of *DNA*, *RNA* (genetic material); prevents a type of anemia; red blood cell formation	Liver, green leafy vegetables, peanuts
Vitamin B_{12}	Red blood cell formation; synthesis of DNA and RNA; component of sheath around nerves	Foods of animal origin, microorganisms (fermented foods)
Calcium	Bones and teeth; blood clotting; nerve function	Dairy products, legumes
Phosphorus	Bones and teeth; part of *coenzymes*	Dairy products, meats, cereals
Sodium	Nerve-muscle function; body fluid balance	Salt (sodium chloride), salted foods (meats, pickles, some crackers), cheese, butter
Potassium	Nerve-muscle function; body fluid balance	Fruits and vegetables (especially bananas), meats, dairy products, whole grains
Magnesium	Nerve-muscle function; part of coenzymes	Green vegetables, whole grains
Chlorine	Hydrochloric acid in the stomach; acid-base balance	Salt
Sulfur	Part of proteins in tendons and hair; acid-base balance	Dietary proteins high in sulfur amino acids
Iron	Oxygen transport (mainly in *hemoglobin* in blood)	Meats, legumes, cereals
Zinc	Protein synthesis; coenzymes; wound healing; taste	Meats, fish, whole grains
Iodine	*Thyroid hormones*	Seafood, iodized salt, dairy products
Selenium	Coenzymes; acts with vitamin E	Seafood, whole grains, meats
Fluoride	Prevents tooth and bone loss	Drinking water, seafood, tea
Manganese	Coenzymes	Whole grains, fruits and vegetables, nuts

Amino Acids
The "building blocks" of proteins. There are 20 different amino acids.

DNA
Deoxyribonucleic acid. It is found in the nucleus of cells; determines the hereditary make-up of an individual.

RNA
Ribonucleic acid. It is found mainly outside the nucleus of the cell; controls manufacture of body proteins, including enzymes.

Coenzymes
Substances needed by some enzymes before enzyme activity occurs. Several are B-complex vitamins.

Hemoglobin
Iron-containing protein in red blood cells; carries oxygen to the cells and carbon dioxide back to the lungs.

Thyroid Hormones
Produced by thyroid gland in neck; require iodine for activity; control energy metabolism.

It is fairly easy to learn the nutrient composition of various foods—see, for example, the table in Appendix P. Wouldn't it be nice if you could look up the amount of each nutrient in your *body* the same way? Unfortunately, there are no such simple methods. All methods of determining the amount of nutrients in the human body come from indirect measures, and some are difficult, costly, and even unpleasant to perform (as in measuring the chemical composition of cadavers). Be that as it may, we can get some idea of the percentage of water, protein, fat, and minerals in the human body by looking at Table 2-2. This table also shows the percentages of these substances for certain foods—hamburger, bread, whole milk, and minced ham. Note that the percentages for the minced ham are almost the same as those for the human body. Does this mean that if you ate nothing but minced ham day after day you would have a healthy diet? Of course not. As shown in Chapter 1, what is important is the *total* nutrient contribution of *all* food you eat.

> Nutrient intake from the entire diet is more important than the nutrient intake from individual foods.

HOW DO YOU MEASURE HOW MUCH AND WHAT KIND OF FOOD WE EAT?

Establishing nutritional standards means, first of all, finding out what people eat—and how much. Imagine a researcher asking you questions about this. The accuracy of the results will, of course, depend on that researcher's attention to detail and on his or her knowledge of food.[3] It will also depend a lot on you.

Diet Histories Are Used To Establish Nutrition Standards

"What do you eat on a typical day?" you are asked. To help you answer, you may find utensils and plates useful to identify portion sizes. Models or replicas of certain foods may also be helpful. Indeed, young adults frequently cannot quantify food portion sizes if they are not shown food models.[4]

TABLE 2-2 You Are What You Eat, Or Are You?

	Percent of Total Body Weight			
	Water	Protein	Fat	Minerals
Human body*	62	16	15	5.7
Hamburger	54	24	20	1.3
Bread	36	9	3	1.9
Milk (whole)	87	4	3.5	0.7
Ham (minced)	62	14	17	3.3

NOTE: Contributions of the various minerals to total body weight are:
  2.3%-3.4%   calcium and phosphorus
  0.95%   sodium, potassium, magnesium, chlorine, sulfur
  0.004%   iron
  0.002%   zinc
  smaller amounts of all of the other minerals listed in Table 1-1
*The average, healthy person.

"What did you have yesterday?" the researcher presses. Trying to remember what you ate in the last 24 hours may be difficult. Moreover, the day may be unusual in that you consumed more or less than normal. "Yesterday" may have been a special day of eating out or partying or of skipping meals. Because this question depends on people's memories, it is valid only when asked of large numbers of people—which makes this form of research expensive.

"What did you eat last week and how much?" Keeping a food record or diary for a three-, four-, or seven-day period is one method. It works best, however, when food is weighed and the volume of liquids measured—exactly the kind of activity that may influence people to eat *less* once they see the amount of food they are taking in. Moreover, because they are aware of being "investigated," people may bias their choice of foods toward items that they think are more nutritious.

Most People Cannot Tell Accurately What Food They Eat

"How often do you eat, and what foods do you eat?" Again the problem of honesty and memory. There may be the temptation to hide a poor diet from the investigator.

In sum, most people do not eat exactly the same foods and the same amount of nutrients each day, which is not a problem if the diet is balanced over the long term. Still, it is a disquieting thought that most of us cannot tell accurately how much food we eat. For researchers trying to establish consumption patterns, however, all methods are time-consuming and many are not very accurate.

> The kinds and amount of food eaten can be measured by a diet history, a 24-hour diet recall, a written record, or by measuring food frequency—all time-consuming and generally not accurate methods.

THE ETHICS OF EVALUATING NUTRITIONAL STATUS

The preceding suggests the difficulties of establishing the nutritional status for people. As mentioned earlier, only indirect methods are available for determining nutritional status, and they must be used only by nutritionists and physicians, never amateurs.

As Figure 2-1 indicates, the trick is to measure dietary deficiency of a nutrient over the long term by measuring the dietary histories of people. How can one do this? Obviously, it would be unethical not to treat people in the early stages of nutrition deficiency, but how then can we know how the disorder will turn out? And if a nutrition problem is far advanced, not only should it be treated but observers may also have missed the early stages and thereby missed necessary information about the causes of the disorder.

Let me also describe some of the other difficulties of tracking nutrition deficiencies.

Is "Feeling Poorly" Caused by Nutritional or Nonnutritional Factors?

People may complain that they are not feeling well or that they lack energy: such feelings could well have a nutritional reason, such as low intakes of *kcalories*. The condition may also be a result of low intake of iron, thiamin, riboflavin, and niacin, which are involved in liberating energy, or low intake of folacin. Clearly, these represent a case for nutritional intervention.

However, feeling unwell may also be due to nonnutritional factors, such as certain illnesses, lack of sleep, overwork, even watching too much television. Obviously, some detective work by dietitians and physicians is necessary to determine the exact cause.

Kcalorie

A unit of heat, used to measure energy in food and in the body.

Poor Physical Appearance May Signal Poor Diet

Poor appearance of hair, eyes, skin, gums, and fingernails and abnormalities in bone shape could signal a poor diet in general and deficiencies of some nutrients in particular. These may be borne out if the researcher or physician has established that the person had a poor diet in the past.

Here, too, however, other factors can cause a person to look unwell. If you see any of these things about yourself, don't jump to conclusions on the basis of diet alone.

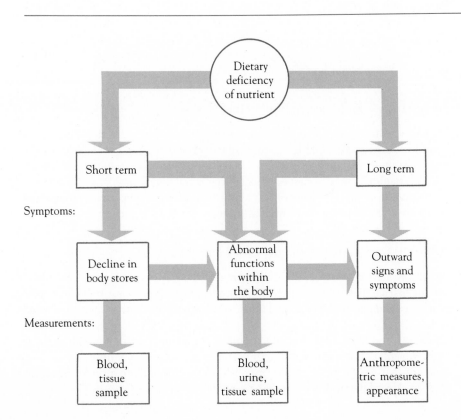

FIGURE 2-1
The course of dietary deficiency. The effect of the dietary deficiency of a nutrient ranges from short-term symptoms to long-term changes in appearance.

Tests on Blood Samples Can Reveal Nutrient Levels

Blood samples taken shortly after a meal, when nutrients are being absorbed from the digestive tract, will reveal high levels of many nutrients. Samples taken many hours after a meal give a more realistic indication of the body's store of some nutrients.

Diabetes
Inadequate insulin to control blood sugar levels.
    Type I—genetic, usually first seen in childhood
    Type II—adequate insulin is unable to help glucose into cells; usually in obesity

An example of a blood test is the blood sugar (glucose) test given for diabetes. Here the blood sample is usually drawn early in the morning before a meal. If the blood sugar level is high, the person is usually suffering from diabetes. Diabetes is of two types. In *type I diabetes*—also known as insulin-dependent or juvenile diabetes because it is a genetically inherited form usually first seen in childhood—the pancreas fails to produce enough of the hormone called insulin to control blood sugar levels. This means that the body is not producing enough insulin to take the glucose from the blood to the cells. Insulin is needed to get glucose into the cells for metabolism and energy release. (When no insulin is secreted, the body gets rid of the excess glucose in the blood by excreting it in the urine; this glucose is then lost from the body.) In *type II diabetes*—also called non-insulin-dependent or maturity-onset diabetes, which is seen especially in people with obesity—the pancreas does produce sufficient insulin, but there is interference in the delivery of glucose to the cells with the help of insulin.

Another test is a measure of hemoglobin levels in the blood as a test for how much iron is in the body. Low hemoglobin means you have, in that advertiser's phrase, "iron-poor blood." Measurement of the blood may also indicate the activity of metabolism in the kidneys, since blood takes wastes from the cells to the kidneys for excretion in urine.

In general, however, blood is not a good indicator of the body level of most nutrients. For example, even if your body is not effective in storing calcium, this will not show up in blood tests because a particular interaction between two hormones keeps blood levels of calcium stable.

Urine Tests Can Measure Nutritional Status

Unused chemicals in the body are filtered from the blood by the kidneys and dumped into the urine. This means that the urine contains two substances: (1) materials absorbed but not used by the body, such as excess amounts of water-soluble vitamins, and (2) waste products from metabolism, such as waste nitrogen compounds from protein metabolism. Urine tests, then, are effective measures with which to evaluate people's nutritional status.

Anthropometric Measurements Can Measure Fat

Anthropometric measurements include body weight, height, arm and head circumference, fatfold thickness.

"Anthropometric" refers to the study of human body measurements, especially on a comparative basis. *Anthropometric measurements*, then, may include weight, height, circumference of head and arms, and (using *calipers*) the thickness of folds of fat.

Weight and height are obviously useful for measuring growth in children. However, weight is not a good indicator of the nutritional status of an adult, since much of that weight can be either muscle or fat—hence the reason for measuring folds of skin to determine a person's fat content.

Nutritional status is determined by professionals, who use diet history, blood and urine tests, and anthropometric measurements. Reports of feelings are not reliable indicators of nutritional status.

WHAT FOODS AND NUTRIENTS ARE NORTH AMERICANS EATING?

To the extent that the difficulties of measurement have been overcome by nutrition professionals, what can we say about the contents of the North American diet?

The first thing to note is that the consumption of different foods is constantly changing, as a glance at Figure 2-2 shows. Note that egg consumption in the United States dropped from 300 eggs per person per year in 1965 to 250 in 1984. Soft drinks and vegetables, however, have gained in popularity, and yogurt has made significant gains compared with where it was. Clearly, a change in the kinds of foods consumed also changes the kind of nutrients taken in.

Note also that more food is being eaten now than was the case in 1965. Does this mean that the conclusions by the Physician Task Force on Hunger in America are misguided? Not at all. The fact that the *average* food intake has risen simply obscures the extremes in food intake. What is happening is that increasing numbers

FIGURE 2-2
Food trends in the United States: 1965 versus 1984. Note the changes in the amount of different foods eaten during this 19-year period.

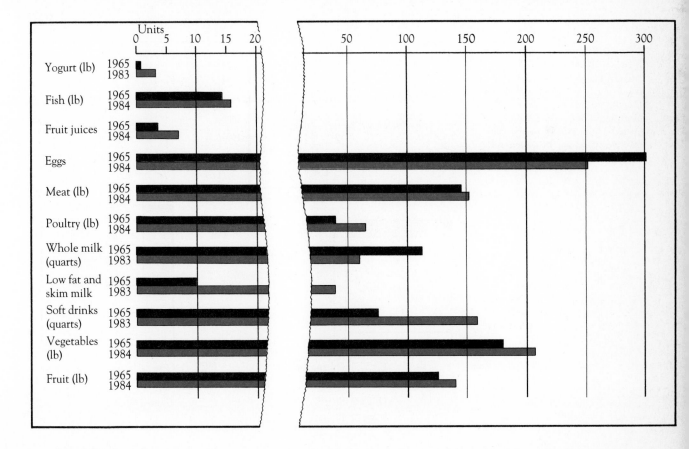

COST OF A WEEK'S FOOD
FOR A FAMILY OF FOUR

DIETS THAT MET THE RDA FOR ELEVEN NUTRIENTS

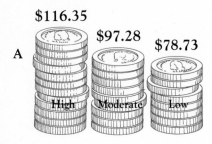

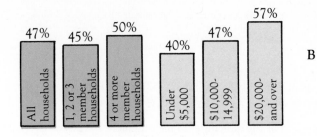

FIGURE 2-3
Incomes and intake. **A,** Cost of a week's food for a family of four. **B,** The higher the income, the greater the likelihood a household will meet the recommended dietary allowances for nutrients. The nine nutrients are protein, calcium, iron, magnesium, phosphorus, vitamin A, thiamin, riboflavin, and vitamin B_6.

of hungry people are simply not getting this extra food. The causes may be unemployment, cutbacks in federal food programs, or ignorance about such programs that still remain. In general, however, as Figure 2-3 shows, people's nutrient intake is related to their incomes; households making under $5000 a year are less apt to meet recommended dietary allowances (RDAs) than are those making $20,000 or more. Sadly, a great deal of the food that is available in the United States is simply wasted; as Figure 2-4 shows, the proportion of unused food in the United States is quite large compared with that in rural China. Food is wasted not only from being left uneaten on people's plates or spoiling in the refrigerator but also in the normal course of being processed, transported, and stored.

FIGURE 2-4
Food available and food wasted. The diet varies considerably between the two countries. Compared with the rural Chinese, Americans eat more animal foods (meat, fish, poultry, dairy products), oils and fats, sugars, and fewer vegetables and fruits, cereals, legumes, and tubers.

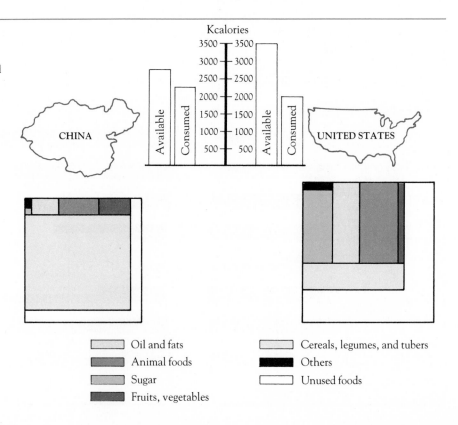

The most important information on the nutrition and health status of Americans is obtained from two surveys conducted by the federal government—the Nationwide Food Consumption Survey, conducted by the U.S. Department of Agriculture, and the Health and Nutrition Examination Survey (HANES).[5] Similar information was obtained on Canadians between 1970 and 1972.[6] These studies cover an enormous number of people, but their cost and time are also enormous, and the information is not complete.

What Nutrients Are Low in the North American Diet?

Vitamin A, vitamin B_6, folacin, calcium, magnesium, iron, and (according to some surveys) zinc have all been found to be low in some people's diets in the United States. Fortunately, physical signs of *severe* deficiency associated with these nutrients are rare, both in the U.S. and in Canada.

Some groups are particularly apt to have problems obtaining sufficient nutrient intake: pregnant women, preschool children, the elderly, the poor, and members of large families. People living in isolation may also be in this category; Eskimos in Canada, for instance, have a traditional diet low in citrus fruits (a source of vitamin C) and vegetables (a source of folacin).

Geography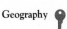

Despite such failings, there have been improvements. Seventy years ago, vitamin D deficiency was commonplace in northern industrial cities, niacin deficiency was common in the South, and vitamin C deficiency was found everywhere.

History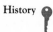

What Nutrients Are Low in Developing Countries?

Other countries in the world have different kinds of nutrient deficiencies. As Table 2-3 makes clear, four essential substances—protein and energy, vitamin A, iodine, and iron—tend to be in inadequate supply for many people in the developing nations of Asia, Africa, and Latin America. Although vitamin A intake is low in some North Americans, it is not so severe as to cause permanent blindness, as it does elsewhere in the world. Iron deficiency may also be a problem in some Americans and Canadians—indeed, it may be a problem in women of childbearing years in all countries, because it results from loss of blood in the monthly menstrual cycle. Iron deficiency produces anemia, a disorder characterized by low oxygen-carrying capacity in the blood.

TABLE 2-3 Estimates of the Total Number of Persons Affected by Currently Preventable Malnutrition in the World Today

Deficiency	Effects	Prevalence (Millions)	Age (Years)	Mortality Per Year
Protein and energy	Stunted growth	500	0-6	10 million
	Wasting of the body	1	1-4	
Vitamin A	Blindness	6	All ages	750,000
Iodine	Goiter	150	All ages	
	Cretinism	6	All ages	
Iron	Anemia	350	Women 18-45	

Goiter
Enlargement of the thyroid gland due to iodine deficiency.

Cretinism
Mental and physical retardation in children because of iodine deficiency during pregnancy.

Severe deficiencies of some nutrients cause death; others cause irreversible or reversible damage.

High intakes of some nutrients may cause death, as in overconsumption of certain vitamin supplements.

Anemia is reversible, but the irreversible problems associated with the deficiencies listed in the table are alarming: the shortage of protein and energy are responsible for the deaths of 10 million children *every year*, the equivalent of the entire population of a country like Belgium. Three quarters of a million people also die every year as a result of vitamin A deficiency. Deficiencies in iodine can produce *goiter*, an enlargement of the thyroid gland, and *cretinism*, mental and physical retardation in children. The tragedy is that such suffering is entirely preventable.

Most people in North America have adequate nutrient intakes, although some people show shortages in vitamin A, vitamin B₆, folacin, calcium, magnesium, iron, and zinc. Much of this deficiency is associated with low incomes. In other parts of the world, death, blindness, goiter, cretinism, and anemia are the result of deficiencies in protein and energy, vitamin A, iodine, and iron.

QUANTITY AND QUALITY: HOW TO AVOID NUTRIENT DEFICIENCIES

What does it mean to say the suffering caused by nutrient deficiencies is preventable? The answer can be expressed in two words: quantity and quality.

Quantity refers to the amount of nutrients in the diet, and quantity can also be expressed in two ways: deficient and toxic. *Deficient* means a nutrient is present in an amount less than that required by the body for normal functioning. *Toxic* (or harmful) means it is far in excess of the body's requirements, as when people consume too much of some vitamin supplements. At the extremes, too little or too much of a certain nutrient can cause death.

Quality has two meanings here. First, it means that nutrients are present in optimum balance for growth and health. Thus, you may eat food low in quantity but high in quality. Second, it means the food itself is "good"—palatable, attractive, socially acceptable, and containing no contaminants or harmful additives. Thus, a food may well be nutritionally balanced but will simply lack the popular features that would attract people to eat it.

How can we be assured of sufficient quantity and quality in our food? Actually, a system has been in existence since early in this century that attempts to do precisely this—to give us not only enough food and of nutritionally balanced quality but also to allow enough variety to keep our diets interesting. This system begins with the concept of *food groups*.

WHAT ARE FOOD GROUPS?

As suggested briefly in Chapter 1, balance in nutrient intake is obtained from four food groups: (1) meat and alternates, (2) milk and milk products, (3) bread and cereals, and (4) fruits and vegetables. In the United States, this is known as *The Four Food Group Plan* and in Canada it is called simply *The Food Guide;* both are shown in Figure 2-5.

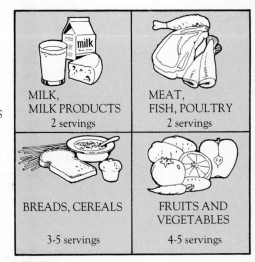

UNITED STATES

CANADA

A

B

FIGURE 2-5
Food groups for, **A,** the United States and, **B,** Canada. You should eat a variety of foods from each of the four food groups each day.

What both plans have in common is that the absence of one or more of these food groups from the regular diet may produce nutrient deficiencies. Still, the grouping was criticized by some nutritionists as providing low intakes of zinc, iron, magnesium, vitamin E, and vitamin B_6.

As a result, in the U.S. the Department of Agriculture in 1979 introduced a revised plan labeled *The Hassle-free Food Guide,* which emphasizes the use of nuts and *legumes,* plants of the bean and pea families, instead of enriched cereal products. Although this sytem provides sufficient nutrients, it is also high in kilocalories (kcalories), which causes problems for people trying to lose weight. This new food guide also introduced a fifth "food group"—one including alcohol, fats, and desserts. This was certainly not intended as an endorsement of these foods in the diet, only as a recognition that these substances are part of the diet of many people.

While we're on the subject of food groups, let's also introduce two other concepts: exchange systems and the Index of Nutrient Quality.

Legumes
Plants of the bean and pea families.

Exchange Systems Group Foods According to Kilocalories

Exchange lists are not the same as, and should not be confused with, the food group guides. Exchange lists are special lists created for the benefit of diabetics and others needing to regulate their dietary energy (kcalorie) intake. The lists consist of six food "exchanges" that group foods with the same number of kcalories from carbohydrate, fat, and protein. Table 2-4 summarizes the U.S. food exchange system. (Details of the U.S. and Canadian systems appear in Appendix M.)

TABLE 2-4 Food Exchange Groups

Exchange	Portion Size	Carbohydrate (g)	Protein (g)	Fat (g)	Energy (kcals)
Milk (nonfat)	1 cup	12	8	Trace	90
Vegetable	½ cup	5	2	0	25
Fruit	1 portion	15	0	0	60
Starch/bread	1 slice	15	3	Trace	80
Meat (lean)	1 ounce	0	7	3	55
Fat	1 teaspoon	0	0	5	45

Source: Adapted from Franz, M.J., and others, Exchange lists: Revised 1986. Journal of the American Dietetic Association 87, 28, 1987.

Notes: Canadian recommendations are in Good Health Eating Guide, Canadian Diabetes Association, Toronto, Ontario, 1981.

Consult the above source for details of modifications if the following are consumed:

Milk: low-fat and whole milk.

Vegetables: those low in kcalories, including cabbage, carrots, celery, cucumbers, spinach, green beans, tomatoes.

Starchy vegetables higher in kcalories are included in the bread group. They include dried beans, peas, lentils, potato, corn.

Bread: includes all cereal products, plus starchy vegetables.

Meat: Meat and cheeses fall into one of three categories, low-, medium-, or high-fat. Peanut butter is in the high-fat category.

Index of Nutrient Quality

A basic trick to eating is to take in enough food to provide for sufficient nutrients but not so much as to increase body weight. The ideal situation is a food high in nutrients and low in energy (kcalories).

To arrive at a measurement of such a food or portion of food, a calculation has been devised known as the Index of Nutrient Quality (INQ), which is computed as follows:

$$\frac{\text{Nutrient in food}}{\text{RDA of nutrient}} \div \frac{\text{Energy (kcalories) in food}}{\text{RDA of energy}} = \text{INQ}$$

Recommended Dietary Allowance (RDA) Recommended nutrient intake to maintain heath of people in the United States.

This number yields what is known as the nutrient density of food. The information for this formula is derived from the Recommended Dietary Allowance (RDA) table (inside front cover), Table of Food Composition (Appendix P), or the nutrition information on a food package label.

Here are two examples of how the INQ works.

Example 1: Suppose you want to compare the amount of protein between cheddar cheese and hamburger for a woman between 19 and 22 years old. You have 1 ounce of cheddar cheese. You have 2.9 ounces of ground beef patty (made up of 21% fat). Which is better?

Using the Table of Food Composition, we can use the formula as follows:

Cheese
$$\frac{7}{44} \div \frac{115}{2100} = 2.9$$

Ground beef
$$\frac{20}{44} \div \frac{235}{2100} = 4.1$$

The higher the INQ number—4.1 for ground beef versus 2.9 for cheese—the better the nutrient density, or nutritive value. Here the hamburger offers more protein yet fewer kcalories, even though the portion itself weighs considerably more than the portion for the cheese.

Example 2: Now suppose you want to compare the same portion of ground beef with a 2 ounce lean pork chop, this time to determine the thiamin INQ for a man of the same age:

$$\text{Pork} \qquad\qquad\qquad \text{Ground beef}$$

$$\frac{0.63}{1.5} \div \frac{150}{2900} = 8.1 \qquad\qquad \frac{0.07}{1.5} \div \frac{235}{2900} = 0.57$$

Pork is clearly the better choice. The high value for pork is a combination of a high concentration of thiamin and a low number of kcalories.

Choose foods of high nutrient density (larger INQ) for optimum nutrient intake.

WHAT ARE TABLES OF FOOD COMPOSITION?

Nutrients have always been in food, of course, but it is only in modern times that we have been able to measure them. Indeed, the first food composition tables were published in Germany in 1878 (the first U.S. tables appeared in 1896). As you might expect, such tables were limited in the number of nutrients analyzed—not surprising when you realize the first vitamin was discovered 30 years later.

History

By now there are sophisticated methods of chemical analysis for determining the amount of nutrients in food, and the equipment used is often quite complex.[7] Such tests are often expensive, and their cost is added to the price of food products—perhaps enough reason in itself why we should pay attention to the nutrition information on package labels.

Economics

It is worth becoming familiar with the Table of Food Composition provided in Appendix P because it is referred to frequently throughout this book. More detailed information on food composition tables is available.[7]

THE RECOMMENDED DIETARY ALLOWANCES (RDAs) ARE GUIDELINES FOR A BALANCED DIET

"How much food does man require?" This was the title of a 1973 paper by some well-known British nutritionists.[8] After over a century since the invention of tables of food composition and years after the establishment of the four food groups, this question seems wildly inappropriate. Yet, as these authors point out, "the measurement of normal daily food intake and energy expenditure poses many technical and logistic problems, requires large teams of skilled staff and is expensive; hence so far only small populations of individual men and women have been studied."

Although the interactions between food and ourselves may be complex, clearly we need *some* guidelines for how much we can eat and of what. Such guidelines are provided by the Recommended Dietary Allowances.

The RDAs

Most countries provide some version of the RDAs—the Recommended Dietary Allowances, which provide recommended intake of some of the essential nutrients.

In the United States, the RDAs are updated about every five years by the National Research Council, a part of the National Academy of Sciences.[9] Canada, most European countries, the United Nations World Health Organization and Food and Agricultural Organization provide their own set of dietary recommendations.[10]

History

The idea of RDAs has been developed over a long period of time. Indeed, attempts to set dietary standards were made in Biblical times and were refined by the Greeks and Romans.[11] By the nineteenth century, knowledge was advanced enough to allow recommendations to be made in terms of nutrients rather than foods. In the United States, the RDAs were first published in 1943 "to provide standards serving as a goal for good nutrition" and, because World War II was then in full swing, to act as a "guide for planning and procuring food supplies for national defense." The latest recommendations (still the subject of some controversy, as described at the end of this chapter) are presented on the inside cover at the front of this book. Included are recommended levels of intake of protein, ten vitamins, and six minerals considered adequate to meet the known nutritional needs of practically all healthy persons. Canadian values are inside the back cover.

Not all of the essential nutrients (see Table 1-1) appear in the RDA table. There is not sufficient knowledge of nutrients not listed to make specific recommendations at this time—another indication that nutrition is a young science. However, recent scientific advances enable us to make recommendations on estimated safe and adequate daily dietary intakes for three vitamins: vitamin K, biotin, and pantothenic acid. Recommendations can also be made on nine minerals: copper, manganese, fluoride, chromium, selenium, molybdenum, sodium, potassium, and chloride (Appendix F).

It must be pointed out that the RDAs should be achieved by eating a *variety* of foods. You should not achieve them either by adding nutrients to single foods or by taking supplements in pill or powdered form.

There Are Some Things the RDAs Don't Tell You

Since the RDAs were first published in World War II, their purpose has been expanded to accomplish the following:

- Interpret food consumption records of groups of people
- Evaluate whether food supplies are adequate in meeting nutritional needs— for example, in planning menus for the armed services, hospitals, mental hospitals, and penal institutions
- Plan and buy food supplies for groups of people
- Establish guides for public food assistance programs
- Develop new food products by industry
- Set guidelines for nutritional labeling of foods
- Develop nutrition education programs

The scope of these functions is ambitious. Nevertheless, there are a number of conditions that the RDAs do *not* cover—namely:

- Inherited metabolic disorders—such as genetically caused inability to use certain amino acids, vitamins, or carbohydrates in the diet

- Chronic diseases—for example, lung disease and some types of heart and kidney disease
- Special diets required by certain medications
- Infections
- Premature births
- Evaluation of *individual* diets—because the allowances deal only with *groups* of people

The final item—the lack of coverage of individual diets—is certainly worthy of further discussion.

Why Are RDAs for Groups, Not Individuals?

Individuals differ in their need for food. As the British nutritionists I cited above stated, "in any group of twenty or more subjects, with similar attributes and activities, food intake can vary as much as twofold."

A longer answer to the question is shown in an experiment in which food was withheld from 21 laboratory rats of the same age, sex, and body weight.[12] Because the animals were similar in all respects, you would expect them all to perish within a few days of each other. Yet their survival ranged from as few as 4 days to as many as 30 days, as shown in Table 2-5. Such individual variations in survival are also probably true of people, if the experiences of starvation during war and disasters are any indication, although the length of time would be different (in healthy adults, death usually occurs after 60 days without food).

TABLE 2-5 Survival Time of Rats from Whom Food Was Withheld

Survival time (days)	4	7	8	10	11	12	14	16	21	23	25	26	30
Number of rats dying	2	1	2	3	1	2	1	2	1	1	1	3	1

The essential point is that people vary widely in their need for nutrients, and this variation has been taken into account in the establishment of RDA values. Thus, the RDAs are supposed to cover the needs of 97.5% of the population—which is certainly quite likely to cover you as an individual, but not necessarily so.

As an example of the variations in RDA values, consider the case of vitamin C. There are a number of things to point out about this vitamin:

- Different countries have different RDAs, ranging from 30 to 100 mg per day. This is because of different interpretations by nutrition experts in those countries.
- However, only 10 mg per day is the amount of vitamin C needed to prevent scurvy (vitamin C deficiency). This is true for both adults and children.
- Even so, if *no* vitamin C is obtained, it will take different time periods for different individuals to deplete their vitamin C reserves, ranging from 60 to 120 days. These individual differences also apply for depletion of some other but not all nutrients, as shown in Table 2-6.

TABLE 2-6 Extent of Body Reserves of Nutrients and Nutrient/Health Consequences of Depletion

Nutrient	Time Required to Deplete Reserves	Nutrient/Health Implications
Amino acids	Few hours	No problems, you wake up every morning with these depleted and do not notice the difference!
Carbohydrate	13 hours	No problem because the body switches to protein or fat for energy. Long-term depletion is more serious—the brain and nervous system prefer carbohydrates for energy, but they now must use less preferential fat.
Sodium	2-3 days	Muscle cramps, death—usually only after prolonged sweating with no food intake. Sweating after a game or run is no problem because there is plenty of sodium in most foods.
Water	4 days	Contrast this with a survival time of 60 days without food for a healthy adult.
Fat	20-40 days	This is for a person with average amount of fat. Obese people have much longer, very thin people have shorter time.
Vitamin C	60-120 days	Water-soluble, so excess is excreted in urine rather than stored in tissues.
Vitamin A	90-360 days	Fat-soluble; excess cannot be excreted in urine; instead, it is stored in body fat.
Iron	125 days (women) 750 days (men)	Smaller reserves in women due to monthly loss of iron in blood during menstruation.
Calcium	2500 days	Most calcium in the body (99%) is in bone, so drawing on reserves affects bones—reason for present interest in osteoporosis in older women.

Body reserves can be drawn on if dietary intake of the nutrient is low. Deficiency symptoms occur when reserves are depleted.

Note that, as Figure 2-6 indicates, there are many sources of vitamin C. Although you can obtain vitamin C tablets containing 1000 mg—equivalent to eating more than 16 oranges—remember that vitamin C is *all* you get from that tablet. As I stated earlier, the best advice is to get your nutrients from *foods* rather than from supplements.

One point to note about the variability of RDA values: These values also allow for some nutrients not being absorbed from the digestive tract. For example, if you are a young woman, your actual requirement for iron is only 1.8 mg per day. However, the RDA is set at 18 mg per day to allow for the fact that only 10% of dietary iron is absorbed from the gastrointestinal tract.

The RDAs for Energy Are Halfway Between the Highest and Lowest Needs

If nutritionists allowed the same generous recommendations for energy intake as they do for nutrients, they would be building a nation of tremendously overweight people. Because excess kcalories convert to fat in the body, the RDAs for energy (see Table 9-5) are set halfway between the highest and lowest needs of people in each age and sex group. Moreover, these RDA values are not minimums but only *guidelines* because energy intake is related to amount of physical activity, which, of course, can vary greatly among people.

Note that we get our energy (kcalories) from carbohydrate, fat, protein, and alcohol. There are no RDA values for carbohydrate or fat, because these two nutrients are common in the typical diet. Alcohol is not a nutrient.

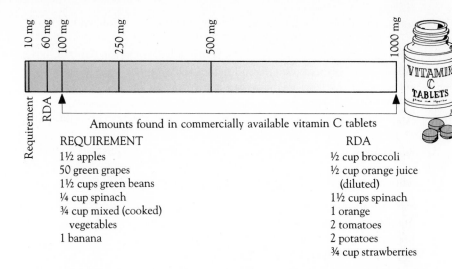

REQUIREMENT
1½ apples
50 green grapes
1½ cups green beans
¼ cup spinach
¾ cup mixed (cooked)
   vegetables
1 banana

RDA
½ cup broccoli
½ cup orange juice
   (diluted)
1½ cups spinach
1 orange
2 tomatoes
2 potatoes
¾ cup strawberries

FIGURE 2-6
Sources of vitamin C can be natural food sources or vitamin supplements, which can range in tablet form up to 1000 mg. This figure shows the amount of an individual food needed to meet requirements (10 mg) and the amount required to meet RDA, which is 60 mg per day in the United States.

If you should travel outside the country, you may find that international travel will change your need for energy intake. This is mainly caused by extreme changes in climate. In very warm climates, the requirement for energy decreases, and the need for vitamins involved in energy metabolism decreases also. In particular, the RDAs for thiamin, riboflavin, and niacin are tied to kcalorie intake.

Persons traveling abroad need to watch changes in energy intake, if they experience extreme changes in climate.

Why Do Individuals Vary in Their RDAs?

As I said above, the short answer is that individuals vary in their need for food because of individual differences in the body. However, the differences also have to do with the following:

- Body size—the larger the weight, the more nutrients are required.
- Growth and pregnancy—more nutrients are required during periods of rapid growth and during pregnancy and lactation than for normal maintenance.
- Gender differences—after age 10, because of differences in growth rate, body weight, or body composition, males and females have different nutrient requirements. Men, for instance, have increased lean body mass, whereas women have a higher proportion of body fat. Women also have a higher requirement for iron because this nutrient is lost through menstruation.

> RDAs are levels of intake of essential nutrients adequate to meet the known nutritional needs of almost all healthy people. RDAs are higher than the amount needed to meet requirements, energy (kcalories) being the one exception. Values differ according to age and gender.

The U.S. Recommended Daily Allowances (U.S. RDAs)

The U.S. RDA is *based on* the RDA values. Note that the "D" in RDA means Dietary, whereas in the U.S. RDA it means Daily. Both sets of values—RDA and U.S. RDA—are often misunderstood. (For further information on the history of dietary standards and their differences between nations, see Hollingsworth's essay.)[13]

Why the differences? Actually, the U.S. RDAs serve a practical purpose. If the labels on food packages were obliged to list the RDAs for each age group and for males and females, the label might be too large to fit on the package! Using the U.S. RDAs means food packagers can stick to one set of values—namely, a number that is expressed as a percentage of the U.S. RDA per *serving size*. This is illustrated in Figure 2-7.

Using serving size is an important idea because these sizes differ depending on the food.

In addition, each of the following groups have their own U.S. RDA:

- Infants up to one year.
- Children under four years.
- Children over four years of age and adults.
- Women who are pregnant or lactating.

The U.S. RDAs for the first two groups—infants and children under four—are used for infant formulas, baby foods, and vitamin-mineral supplements for children in these age groups. The highest RDA value within the age group is the U.S. RDA. Therefore, U.S. RDAs for many nutrients on food labels are derived from values for teenage boys since they have the highest RDA values (see RDA table). They can stand in front of an open refrigerator and make the contents disappear fastest!

Some practical ways of applying the information on RDAs and U.S. RDAs is described next.

> U.S. RDAs are used on food labels to indicate nutritional value.

HOW CAN FOOD LABEL INFORMATION BE USED?

What kind of information do you want to see on a food label? What kind of information do you think *other* people want to see?

Government

A glance at Table 2-7 shows the results of a survey of what people think is important. Most people, for instance, think a complete ingredient listing ought to appear on a food label, but only about half care about serving size (even though that is one of the first items listed), and very few care about recipes. In general, however, most people are concerned about the nutritional and economic value of food, and feel it is the government's responsibility to ensure health and economic protection of the food we eat. In any event, an understanding of how a nutrition label works is important, not only for nutrition and health, but also for economic reasons.[14,15]

Consumer Science

Government intervention in the regulation of the quality of food goes back to ancient times,[16] but in the United States it is the Food and Drug Administration that regulates the information on food labels. The real question is: does this

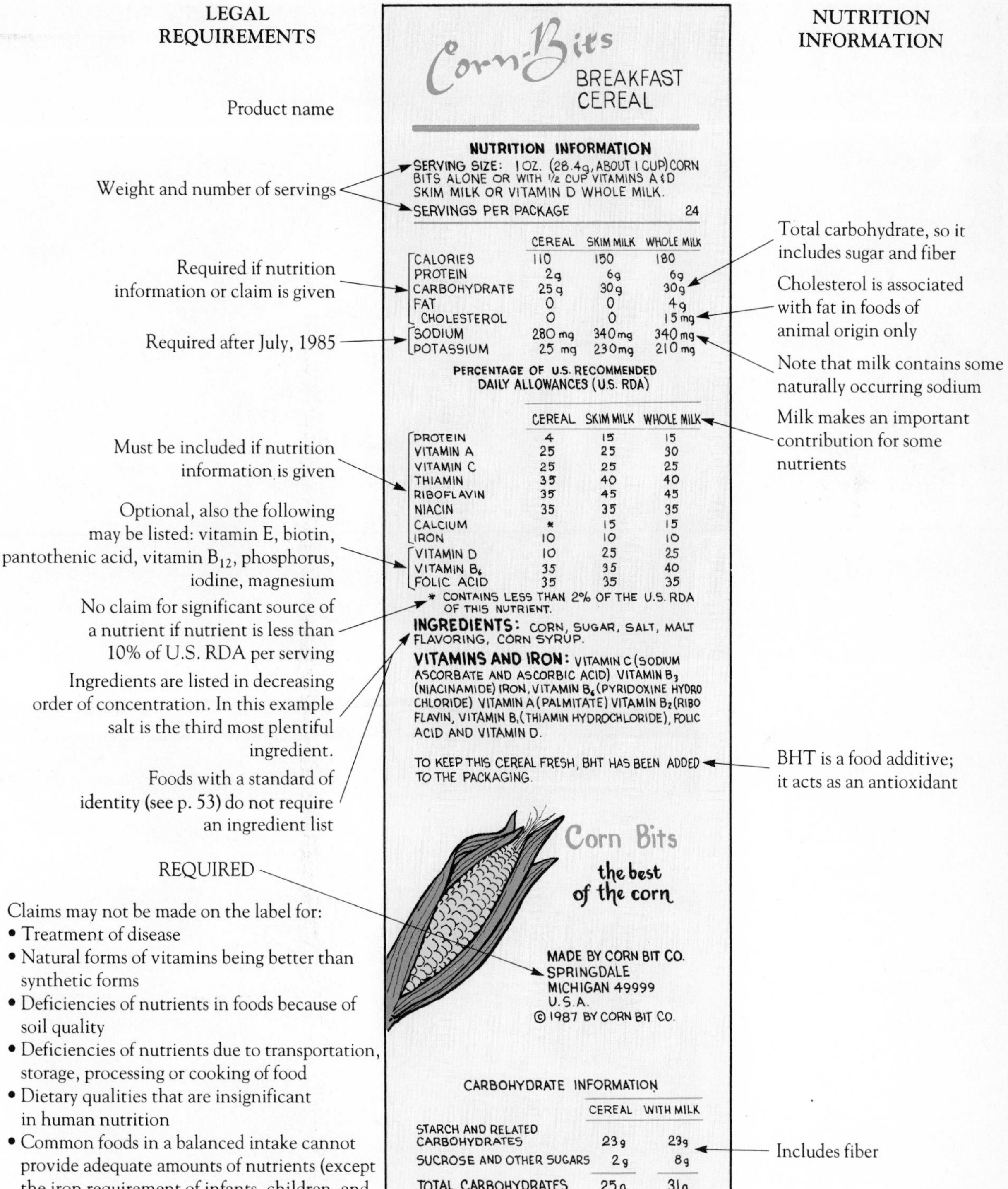

LEGAL REQUIREMENTS

NUTRITION INFORMATION

Product name

Weight and number of servings

Required if nutrition information or claim is given

Required after July, 1985

Must be included if nutrition information is given

Optional, also the following may be listed: vitamin E, biotin, pantothenic acid, vitamin B_{12}, phosphorus, iodine, magnesium

No claim for significant source of a nutrient if nutrient is less than 10% of U.S. RDA per serving

Ingredients are listed in decreasing order of concentration. In this example salt is the third most plentiful ingredient.

Foods with a standard of identity (see p. 53) do not require an ingredient list

REQUIRED

Claims may not be made on the label for:
• Treatment of disease
• Natural forms of vitamins being better than synthetic forms
• Deficiencies of nutrients in foods because of soil quality
• Deficiencies of nutrients due to transportation, storage, processing or cooking of food
• Dietary qualities that are insignificant in human nutrition
• Common foods in a balanced intake cannot provide adequate amounts of nutrients (except the iron requirement of infants, children, and pregnant and lactating women)

Total carbohydrate, so it includes sugar and fiber

Cholesterol is associated with fat in foods of animal origin only

Note that milk contains some naturally occurring sodium

Milk makes an important contribution for some nutrients

BHT is a food additive; it acts as an antioxidant

Includes fiber

Corn-Bits BREAKFAST CEREAL

NUTRITION INFORMATION

SERVING SIZE: 1 OZ. (28.4g, ABOUT 1 CUP) CORN BITS ALONE OR WITH ½ CUP VITAMINS A & D SKIM MILK OR VITAMIN D WHOLE MILK.

SERVINGS PER PACKAGE   24

	CEREAL	SKIM MILK	WHOLE MILK
CALORIES	110	150	180
PROTEIN	2g	6g	6g
CARBOHYDRATE	25g	30g	30g
FAT	0	0	4g
CHOLESTEROL	0	0	15mg
SODIUM	280mg	340mg	340mg
POTASSIUM	25mg	230mg	210mg

PERCENTAGE OF U.S. RECOMMENDED DAILY ALLOWANCES (U.S. RDA)

	CEREAL	SKIM MILK	WHOLE MILK
PROTEIN	4	15	15
VITAMIN A	25	25	30
VITAMIN C	25	25	25
THIAMIN	35	40	40
RIBOFLAVIN	35	45	45
NIACIN	35	35	35
CALCIUM	*	15	15
IRON	10	10	10
VITAMIN D	10	25	25
VITAMIN B_6	35	35	40
FOLIC ACID	35	35	35

* CONTAINS LESS THAN 2% OF THE U.S. RDA OF THIS NUTRIENT.

INGREDIENTS: CORN, SUGAR, SALT, MALT FLAVORING, CORN SYRUP.

VITAMINS AND IRON: VITAMIN C (SODIUM ASCORBATE AND ASCORBIC ACID) VITAMIN B_3 (NIACINAMIDE) IRON, VITAMIN B_6 (PYRIDOXINE HYDRO CHLORIDE) VITAMIN A (PALMITATE) VITAMIN B_2 (RIBO FLAVIN, VITAMIN B_1 (THIAMIN HYDROCHLORIDE), FOLIC ACID AND VITAMIN D.

TO KEEP THIS CEREAL FRESH, BHT HAS BEEN ADDED TO THE PACKAGING.

Corn Bits
the best of the corn

MADE BY CORN BIT CO.
SPRINGDALE
MICHIGAN 49999
U.S.A.
© 1987 BY CORN BIT CO.

CARBOHYDRATE INFORMATION

	CEREAL	WITH MILK
STARCH AND RELATED CARBOHYDRATES	23g	23g
SUCROSE AND OTHER SUGARS	2g	8g
TOTAL CARBOHYDRATES	25g	31g

FIGURE 2-7
Label contents.

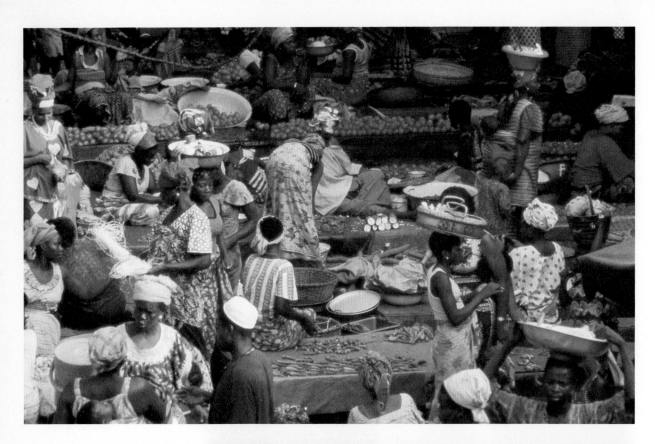

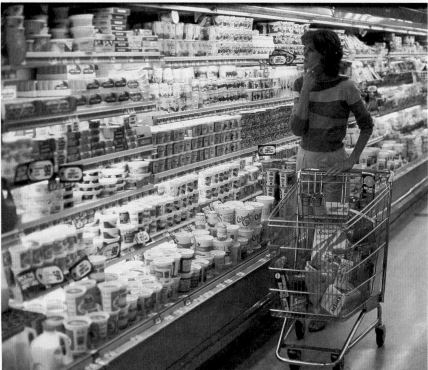

Food choices differ throughout the world. About three-quarters of the people in the world do not have the benefit of food labeling.

TABLE 2-7 Consumer Rating of Importance for 21 Items of Information on Food Labels

	Percentage Rating Item "Important" (In Decreasing Order Within Each Range)
90–80	Complete ingredient listing; sugar content; chemical additives; price
80–70	Principal ingredients; salt content; identity or name of the food; net weight of contents
70–60	Manufacturer's brand name; calorie count; vitamins and minerals
60–50	Cholesterol content; fat content; number of servings in container; protein information; fiber content
50–40	Carbohydrate information; serving size
40–30	Pictures of the food; manufacturer's name and address
20–10	Recipes on the package

information really help? Studies show that many consumers are confused by the present labels.[17] For some the information is too technical, or there is more information than they really want. Others want more information—what to avoid or not overconsume. As a result of these demands, nutrition labels have undergone extensive review to make them more easily understood.

But is nutrition labeling required on all products? Not at all. Labeling is voluntary—the packager may choose to do it or not do it—unless (1) nutrients are added to the food or (2) the label or advertising makes nutritional claims. Consequently, only about half of the food supply used daily by consumers in the United States *must* carry a nutritional label. Most breakfast cereals, for instance, must have a nutritional label because vitamins and minerals have been added (Figure 2-7). Note that a label has certain legal requirements such as listing the product name, weight, number of servings, and a list of ingredients in decreasing order of concentration. Some foods with a standard of identity (such as corn syrup) do not require an ingredient list. Certain claims are not permitted on the label, such as claims for treatment of disease or the statement that natural forms of vitamins are better than synthetic forms.

Advocates of tougher labeling requirements claim that the voluntary labeling we have now hides nutritional "evils" such as excessive amounts of sodium and cholesterol. For instance, legislation introduced in the U.S. Senate proposes that all processed foods must list the amount of sodium, potassium, cholesterol, and fat per serving; total kcalories per serving; and information on the type and source of fat. Food companies, however, claim such requirements would add up to $5000 in costs per product, would confuse consumers, and in any event are unnecessary because there are other means of educating the public.

Nutrition labels meet the demand for consumer protection and for providing information on nutrition and health.

TOO MUCH NUTRIENT: IS IT HARMFUL?

All those ads on TV and in print seem to suggest that the more nutritional supplements you take, the better. However, as suggested earlier, it is not just a lack of nutrients that cause problems. So can high intake, as Table 2-8 indicates. Too much of certain nutrients can lead to permanent injury and even death.

Consider the following issues:

- Heart disease, cancer, diabetes, stroke, and high blood pressure are the principal causes of death in developed countries like the United States. Could high intakes of certain nutrients (lipids, for example) be contributing factors? There are those who think so, although nondietary factors are also involved.
- Sodium often is added to food as table salt (sodium chloride) or as a flavor enhancer (such as monosodium glutamate). It also appears in food simply

TABLE 2-8 Harmful Effects from Prolonged High Intake of Nutrients*

Nutrient	Health Problems Caused by Excess
Total Energy (From High Intakes of Carbohydrate, Fat, Protein and/or Alcohol)	Obesity leading to increased mortality from coronary heart disease, stroke, cancer, diabetes, digestive disease
Carbohydrate	Dental caries if sucrose (table sugar) intake is high; malabsorption of minerals if fiber intake is high
Lipids	
Fat	(Cancer?)
Cholesterol	Coronary heart disease
Essential fatty acid	Increased requirement for vitamin E, increased growth of tumor cells, changes in the properties of cell membranes
Protein	*Gout*; loss of calcium in the urine
Vitamin A	Vomiting, headache, loss of appetite, dry and itchy skin, symptoms suggestive of brain tumor, blurred vision, menstrual disturbances, loss of hair
Vitamin D	Vomiting, wasting, kidney failure, irritability
Folacin	Nerve degeneration
Vitamin C	Kidney stones, rebound scurvy when intake of vitamin C is reduced to dietary levels
Iron	Altered liver function
Sodium	Hypertension (high blood pressure)
Fluorine	Brown discoloration of teeth
Cobalt	Heart failure

*For a more detailed account refer to: McLaren, D.S.: Excessive nutrient intakes.

Cholesterol
Substance found in the body; related to lipids; made in the body and consumed in some foods of animal origin. A human adult body has about 140 grams. Most kinds of cholesterol are found in all membranes. Cholesterol is the raw material in the synthesis of sex hormones, vitamin D₃, and bile salts.

Gout
A type of painful arthritis affecting especially the toes and fingers. May be genetic in origin, but associated usually with the "good life"—high intakes of protein and alcohol. Treated by diet change or with drugs.

because it was part of the original plant or animal or was added during food processing. The effects of sodium on people may vary—for about a quarter of the population, genetic differences mean it may cause high blood pressure— and so you now see a great deal of advertising stressing that products are "low salt" or "sodium-free."

- There *are*, of course, good reasons sometimes for taking nutritional supplements—people on weight-reducing diets, for example. But, as Table 2-8 makes clear, taking more and more of a nutrient—whether protein, vitamin, or mineral supplement—can be quite dangerous.[18]

Taking more of a nutrient does not necessarily mean better health.

DIETARY GUIDELINES SUGGEST WHAT FOODS WE SHOULD EAT

As the foregoing suggests, high blood pressure, heart disease, cancer, and diabetes may be diseases of "overnutrition," although experts are not unanimous in their conclusions about the exact role of diet in these diseases.[19] Scientists are very concerned about the *truth* of things. Therefore, they are cautious people; they don't like to impart information to the public until they are sure about its accuracy.

Public health professionals, on the other hand, are concerned about people's welfare. They argue that if certain dietary information will clearly do no harm, it should be given out.[20] However, if the information is incomplete, publicizing it upsets not only scientists but food producers whose products may be considered at risk. The experience of the United States and Great Britain in such matters shows, therefore, that any attempts to recommend changes in eating patterns will provoke numerous debates among scientists, food producers, and politicians.

Government

Cigarette packages in many countries carry government health warnings. Should food packages as well? Not long ago a British scientific journal carried an article headed "Why Eating Should Carry a Government Health Warning."[21] Whatever the pressures from scientists and food producers for caution, the governments of different countries have felt it best to produce dietary guidelines for their citizens. Two important examples are *Dietary Recommendations for Canadians* (1976) and *Dietary Goals for Americans* (1977). In Great Britain, the National Advisory Committee on Nutrition Education has also issued guidelines (1983). Although they differ in details, all concentrate on problems caused by excess intakes of sugar, fat, and sodium.

In the United States, the most recent set of recommendations is *Dietary Guidelines for Americans,* produced jointly by the U.S. Department of Agriculture and the Department of Health and Human Services.[22] Issued in 1980 and again in 1985, these guidelines try to acknowledge the concerns of both food producers and food consumers. Although not intended for people on special diets, these guidelines try to provide:

- Eating advice to all healthy Americans wanting to avoid nutritional deficiencies and to reduce the risks of obesity, hypertension, diabetes, cancer, and premature heart disease.
- Nutrition advice for people with a family history of risk factors of chronic diseases.
- Recommendations on how best to spend the food dollar (Figure 2-8).

FIGURE 2-8

The food dollar. How it is spent, how it might be better spent.

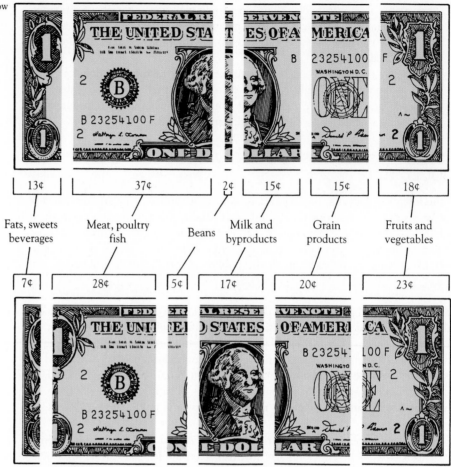

How it was spent...

| 13¢ | 37¢ | 2¢ | 15¢ | 15¢ | 18¢ |

Fats, sweets beverages · Meat, poultry fish · Beans · Milk and byproducts · Grain products · Fruits and vegetables

| 7¢ | 28¢ | 5¢ | 17¢ | 20¢ | 23¢ |

How it might be spent

If we try to distill the advice presented in these guidelines, we wind up with the following specific seven recommendations:

1. Eat a variety of foods.
2. Maintain reasonable weight.
3. Avoid too much fat, saturated fat, and cholesterol.
4. Eat food with adequate starch and fiber.
5. Avoid too much sugar.
6. Avoid too much sodium.
7. Drink alcoholic beverages in moderation if at all, and don't drive after drinking.

In future chapters, we will take up these points in detail.

All national dietary recommendations emphasize variety, balance, and moderation.

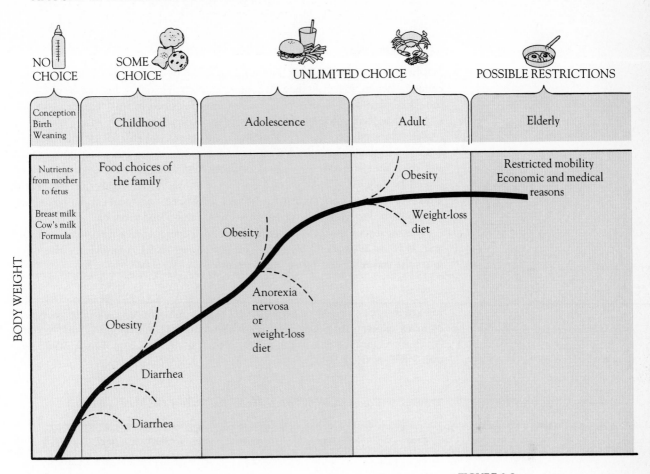

AMOUNT OF CHOICE ON FOOD INTAKE

NO CHOICE · SOME CHOICE · UNLIMITED CHOICE · POSSIBLE RESTRICTIONS

| Conception Birth Weaning | Childhood | Adolescence | Adult | Elderly |

Nutrients from mother to fetus

Breast milk Cow's milk Formula

Food choices of the family

BODY WEIGHT

Obesity

Obesity

Anorexia nervosa or weight-loss diet

Obesity

Diarrhea

Diarrhea

Obesity

Weight-loss diet

Restricted mobility Economic and medical reasons

LIFE-LONG EATING HABITS

Your eating patterns were far different when you were an infant and a child than they are now. Those were critical dietary periods in your life, and you were extremely dependent on others for nutrients (Figure 2-9). Your mother's decision as to what to eat during pregnancy and whether to breast- or bottle-feed you may have had important influences on your basic state of health.

You are probably now at an age at which you have potentially unlimited choices of foods. Your choices about quantity and quality can affect not only your basic health but also any propensity for being overweight or underweight. Aside from voluntary self-limitations such as fasting, factors that might decrease your weight (now or at any time during your life) are surgery, infections, malnutrition, and such diseases as diabetes, cancer, and diseases of the heart and kidney.

As you advance into old age, you may become dependent on others for food choices—not only because of economic reasons, but possibly because your mobility becomes more restricted or because of some medical reasons. The choices you make now, however, may well affect the choices you are able to make then: good nutritional habits have a lifelong payoff.

FIGURE 2-9

Life-long eating patterns. Food choices affect body weight and one's basic health. Whether a person has no choice or potentially unlimited choice varies throughout life.

The influences on, and composition of, your diet change throughout your life.

DECISIONS

1. How Do I Know If My Diet Is Nutritionally Adequate?

Self-help is a great concept, but it's important to know when self-help is not enough—when, in fact, it may cause more harm than good. A dietitian or physician should be consulted if some of the conditions described in this chapter make you suspect that your nutrient intake is less than satisfactory.

Before you go see these professionals, however, you should use the methods described in this chapter to determine how much food you eat, what kind of food and their nutrients (see the Table of Food Composition), and what your RDA should be (see the RDA tables). Table 2-9 shows how to compute the energy intake for a 19-year-old man and a 19-year-old woman of a meal consisting of roast beef, potato, broccoli, roll, margarine, low-fat milk, and an apple.

This meal provides 24% of the recommended energy intake for 19-year-old men and 33% for 19-year-old women. The percentage of RDA intake for the other nutrients varies depending on the nutrient.

Lessons

Intakes in excess of two thirds of the RDA of a nutrient are considered adequate by many experts; thus, this meal is sufficient in protein, vitamin C, and vitamin A. However, intake of calcium is low; providing another cup of milk would give over 100% of the RDA.

TABLE 2-9 Computation of Energy Intake for 19-Year-Old Male and Female

Food	Amount	Energy (Kcalories)	Protein (g)	Calcium (mg)	Vitamin C (mg)	Vitamin A (IU)
Roast beef (lean & fat)	3 oz	165	25	11	—	10
Baked potato	1 medium	145	4	14	31	Trace
Broccoli	½ cup	20	2.5	68	70	3,880
Roll	1	155	5	24	Trace	Trace
Margarine	1 pat	35	Trace	1	0	170
Milk, low-fat (1%)	1 cup	100	8	300	2	500
Apple	1 medium	80	Trace	10	6	120
Totals		700	44.5	417	109	4,680
RDA 19-Year-Old Woman		2,100	44	800	60	4,000
% RDA		33%	101%	52%	182%	117%
RDA 19-Year-Old Man		2,900	56	800	60	5,000
% RDA		24%	80%	52%	182%	94%

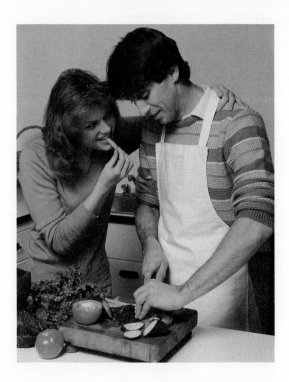

Be sure to use the correct measures (below) to determine your diet's nutritional adequacy.

Notice the important contribution of different foods to high intakes of specific nutrients—for example, beef and protein, milk and calcium, broccoli and vitamins C and A.

Note also that this example is for only *one* meal on a certain day, which means the low intakes here may be improved upon at other meals or even in meals eaten on other days. Because we have reserves of nutrients in our bodies (as shown in Table 2-6), it is not necessary to obtain one's complete RDA every single day. However, you should be concerned if the intake is less than two-thirds RDA for many days, for this suggests the diet is not in balance.

When determining the nutritional adequacy of your own diet, be sure to use the correct measures:

- Notice the different measures used in the Table of Food Composition: cup, teaspoon, tablespoon, ounces, slice, packet, etc.
- The nutrients are measured in different units of weight: 1 ounce = 28 grams; 1 gram (g) = 1000 milligrams (mg); 1 mg = 1000 micrograms (μg).
- Vitamin A is reported as retinol equivalents (RE) in the RDA table.
- International Units (IU) are the older method of measuring vitamin A used on labels on vitamin supplements.

Calculation of nutrient intake and comparisons with RDA values are now done easily and quickly by computers.

2. Is Hair Analysis an Appropriate and Accurate Measure of Nutritional Status in People?

The accuracy of commercial hair analysis has been brought into question.[23] Perhaps the opinion of most experts is summarized in the article title "Hair Analysis: Worthless for Vitamins, Limited for Minerals."[24] In other words, the article writer says, hair analysis has limited application for the status of some minerals, but is of no value for predicting overall nutritional status. In addition, values between different laboratories have been found to have large variations, suggesting that most of the values were worthless. This criticism, however, has been disputed by some of the providers and users of these services.[25]

Why wasn't hair analysis listed as one of the nutritional tests (along with blood and urine tests) earlier in this chapter? The principal reason is the lack of quality control when samples are taken. You pop a hair sample into an envelope requiring no protective packaging, no preservative, and little control against contamination and mail it off to the lab, so the results may be misleading. Because blood and urine, on the other hand, must be collected in a clinic setting and handled much more carefully, the results of their analyses are apt to be much more reliable.

3. Are New RDA Values That Have Been Proposed Useful to Me?

After costing $580,000 in government funds and taking five years of study, the National Academy of Sciences decided in 1985 not to issue new RDA values. Cancelling RDA values is the first time this has happened since RDA values were first issued in 1943. Among the changes considered were increased RDAs for protein and calcium, a reduction of fat reserve during pregnancy from 9 to 7 pounds, and (most controversial) reduction in RDA for vitamin A by about one third from the present values and of RDA for vitamin C by nearly one third for men and one half for women.

The reason for rejection—"scientific differences of opinion"—revolved around the question: should RDAs remain at their present high level to cover most healthy people in the population, or should they be set at a lower level sufficient to avoid deficiencies?

Lessons

Political Science

To understand the politics behind such a decision, consider the following information about vitamin C. The average American diet provides 100 mg of vitamin C per day, and the present RDA is 60 mg. It was proposed that the RDA be lowered to 40 mg. If you now consult the Table of Food Composition, you will see that the vitamin C content of one orange has about 66 mg; one cup of diluted frozen concentrate orange juice has 120 mg; one banana has 12 mg.

Those who opposed lowering the RDA for vitamin C complained that the real reason for the decrease was political: if the RDA values were lowered, they said, it could be shown that hungry, poor Americans were not as lacking in food as was previously claimed. In addition, critics said, a lowered RDA could be used to justify less federal money being spent on school lunches, food stamps, and such persons under institutional care as prisoners and hospital patients.

Why did the question of lowering the RDA for vitamin C (and also vitamin A) arise in the first place? One suggestion was that the present higher values lead Americans to think that their diets are inadequate, so that they mistakenly think they need to buy additional vitamin supplements—thus helping to artificially support the nutrient-supplement industry.

The debate is still going on.[26,27,28]

SUMMARY

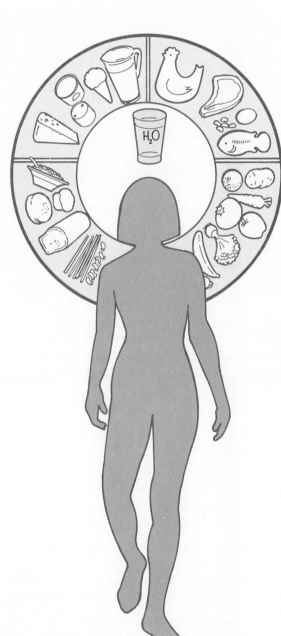

46 nutrients required

Source of these nutrients changes as food patterns change

Presently in the U.S. some people have low intakes of:
Vitamins A, B$_6$, and folacin
Calcium, magnesium, iron and zinc (in some surveys)

Quantity and quality of diet important
Food groups
Exchange systems
Nutrient density
Food composition tables
RDAs
U.S. RDAs
Required intakes

People most likely to have nutrition problems:
Elderly
Poor
Large-size families
Pregnant women
People in isolated communities

Ethical problems in measuring nutritional status. We must rely on:
Feeling poorly
Looking poorly
Blood levels of nutrients and metabolites
Urine sample
Anthropometric measurements
None of these give the complete picture

Measures of how much food we eat:
Diet history
24-hour diet recall
Food diary or record
Food frequency

Dietary guidelines aid in making wise food choices for optimum health

REFERENCES

1. Physician Task Force on Hunger in America: Hunger in America: The growing epidemic, Wesleyan University Press, Middletown, Conn., 1985.

2. W.H. Dietz: Childhood obesity: Susceptibility, cause, and management, Journal of Pediatrics **103:**676, 1983.

3. Truswell, A.S.: Measuring nutrition, British Medical Journal **291:**1258, 1985.

4. Guthrie, H.A.: Selection and quantification of typical food portions by young adults. Journal of the American Dietetic Association **84:**1440, 1984.

5. Swan, P.B.: Food consumption by individuals in the United States: two major surveys, Annual Review of Nutrition **3:**413, 1983.

6. Beaton, G.H.: Nutritional considerations in Canada. In Nutrition in the 1980s: Constraints on our knowledge, N. Selvey and P.L. White, editors, Alan R. Liss, Inc., New York, 1981.

7. Cooke, J.R.: Food composition tables: Analytical problems in the collection of data, Human Nutrition: Applied Nutrition **37(A):**441, 1983.

8. Durnin, J.V.G.A., and others: How much food does man require? Nature **242:**418, 1973.

9. Food and Nutrition Board, National Academy of Sciences–National Research Council: Recommended Dietary Allowances, revised 1980, Washington, D.C., 1980.

10. Wretlind, A.: Standards for nutritional adequacy of the diet: European and WHO/FAO viewpoints. American Journal of Clinical Nutrition **36:**366, 1982.

11. Davidson, S., and others: Dietary standards. In Human nutrition and dietetics, 7th edition. Churchill Livingstone, Edinburgh, 1979.

12. Kleiber, M.: The fire of life: An introduction to animal energetics. Robert E. Krieger Publishing Company, Huntington, N.Y., 1975, p. 11.

13. Hollingsworth, D.F.: Dietary standards. In Present knowledge in nutrition, 5th edition. The Nutrition Foundation, Washington, D.C., 1984, p. 711.

14. Marks, L.: What's in a label: Consumers, public policy and food labels, Food Policy **9:**252, 1984.

15. Taylor, D.L.: Regulating the nutrition label: Will lawmakers tighten the reins? Food Engineering, January, 1986, p. 19.

16. Hutt, P.B.: Government regulation of the integrity of the food supply, Annual Review of Nutrition **4:**1, 1984.

17. Lecos, C.: For food labels, better read = better fed, FDA Consumer, October, 1982, p. 8.

18. Dubick, M.A.: Dietary supplements and health aids: A critical evaluation, part 2: Macronutrients and fiber, Journal of Nutrition Education **15:**88, 1983.

19. Symposium: Report of the task force on the evidence relating six dietary factors to the nation's health, American Journal of Clinical Nutrition **32:**2621, 1979.

20. Miller, S.A., and Stephenson, M.G.: Scientific and public health rationale for the dietary guidelines for Americans, American Journal of Clinical Nutrition **42:**739, 1985.

21. Rivers, J., and Payne, P.: Why eating should carry a government health warning, Nature **279:**98, 1979.

22. Nutrition and your health: Dietary guidelines for Americans, 2nd edition, Home and Garden Bulletin No. 232, U.S. Department of Agriculture, and Department of Health and Human Services, Washington, D.C., 1985.

23. Barrett, S.: Commercial hair analysis: Science or scam? Journal of the American Medical Association **254:**1041, 1985.

24. Hambidge, K.M.: Hair analysis: Worthless for vitamins, limited for minerals. American Journal of Clinical Nutrition **36:**943, 1982.

25. Three letters taking a critical view of the data presented in reference 24, plus a reply by Dr. Barrett, Journal of the American Medical Association **255:**2603, 1986.

26. Marshall, E.: The Academy kills a nutrition report, Science **230:**420, 1985.

27. On withholding the RDA's. Letter from Frank Press, comment by Joan Gussow, comment by Helen Guthrie, Journal of Nutrition Education **17**(5):191, 1985.

28. A statement by the Food and Nutrition Board: Recommended dietary allowances: scientific issues and process for the future, Journal of Nutrition Education **18:**82, 1986.

29. Young, S.: A Christmas digest, New Scientist, p. 24, 19/26 December, 1985.

METABOLISM NOTES: *How Digestion Works*

The level of metabolic activity within the body is influenced by the amount and type of food eaten. This in turn depends on the efficiency of absorption. In the normal person, about 90% of the total diet is absorbed from the digestive tract into the blood. About 90% of carbohydrate, fat, and protein is absorbed. Some of the minerals are absorbed poorly. For example, in a healthy person only about 10% of iron and 20% to 40% of calcium gets into the blood. Dietary fiber is not absorbed. The percentage of the diet absorbed is lowered by diarrhea, abuse of

FIGURE 2-10
Areas of the digestive tract in which the nutrients extracted and digested from the food consumed pass through the tract wall and are absorbed into the bloodstream.

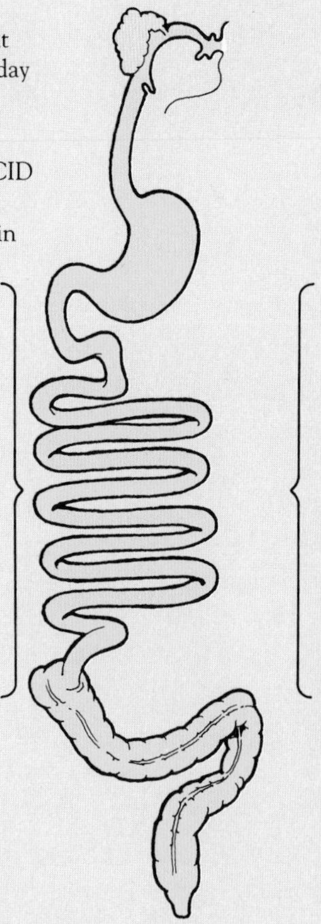

SECRETIONS

SALIVA
About 1½ liters = about
   2 pints produced per day

Amylase

HYDROCHLORIC ACID
Secretion stimulated
  by the hormone gastrin
Protease

BILE
From liver
AMYLASE
PANCREATIC AND
  MUCOSAL
  SECRETIONS
Amylase
Disaccharidases
Lipase
Protease
Enzymes that
  break down
  protein

Bacterial action

ABSORPTION

Water, alcohol

Calcium, magnesium,
  iron, glucose,
  galactose
Fat—soluble vitamins A and D
Fat: as short- and long-
  chain fatty acids,
  and partially split
  glycerides
Water-soluble vitamins:
  thiamin, riboflavin,
  pyridoxin, folacin,
  vitamin C
Bile salts
Vitamin B_{12}
Proteins and amino acids

Potassium, water, sodium
  chloride, short-chain
  fatty acids and gases from fiber
  digestion

Feces: 75% water; 25%
  bacteria, inorganic
  salt and fat

ENZYMES IN DIGESTION OF:
       Carbohydrate: Amylase
                       Disaccharidases
           Protein: Protease
        Lipid (fat): Lipase

laxatives, and excessive intakes of fiber (nature's natural laxative found in foods of plant origin). We have seen that these factors are responsible for the rapid movement of food through the digestive system. Therefore, there is not sufficient time for the nutrients to be absorbed.

The time from when food is swallowed until it is eliminated in the feces is called the transit time. This ranges from about 6½ hours to 98 hours.[29] Applying this term to the discussion above, we see that diarrhea, laxatives, and fiber will decrease the transit time. Fatty food stays in the stomach longer than foods rich in carbohydrate or protein. Warm drinks take longer than cold drinks to leave the stomach. Alcohol is absorbed at a slower rate from the stomach than from the intestine. Two useful terms in this discussion are: digestibility, referring to the amount of a diet that is absorbed, and bioavailability, which means the amount of a nutrient that is absorbed and used by the body.

Don't eat fatty foods shortly before intense exercise or athletic activity.

There are important nutrition messages in Figure 2-10. Various secretions are important in digestion. Saliva softens food; hydrochloric acid makes the stomach contents very acidic. Bile, which is made in the liver and stored in the gallbladder, is secreted into the small intestine for fat digestion. Enzymes play important roles in the breakdown of carbohydrate, fat, and protein. A malfunction of any one of these secretions decreases the bioavailability of the nutrients responsive to the secretion.

Your body is not 100% effective in absorbing many nutrients, but this is not a problem if the quantity and quality of the diet is satisfactory.

Other factors of importance include the action of muscles in moving the products of digestion downward toward the anus. In older people, the action of these muscles decreases, giving rise to problems with constipation. Hormones influence some secretions. One example is the hormone secretin, which stimulates the secretion of hydrochloric acid.

The site of absorption of each nutrient is important. Surgical removal of the stomach is not as important as loss of the duodenum or jejunum, which form the upper portion of the small intestine. Most of the nutrients are absorbed by the time the colon (large intestine) is reached. Water from the feces is reabsorbed into the blood. The longer the feces remain in the colon, the more water is taken from the feces, thus causing constipation. Colon cancer is a more common form of cancer in the United States than in other parts of the world. There is some evidence that this may be due to a low intake of fiber by many Americans.

Medicine

For an interesting account of the biochemical and physiological processes taking place in what is described as a "miraculous bit of bioengineering" (the digestive system), see Young, S.: A Christmas digest. *New Scientist,* page 24, 19/26 December, 1985.

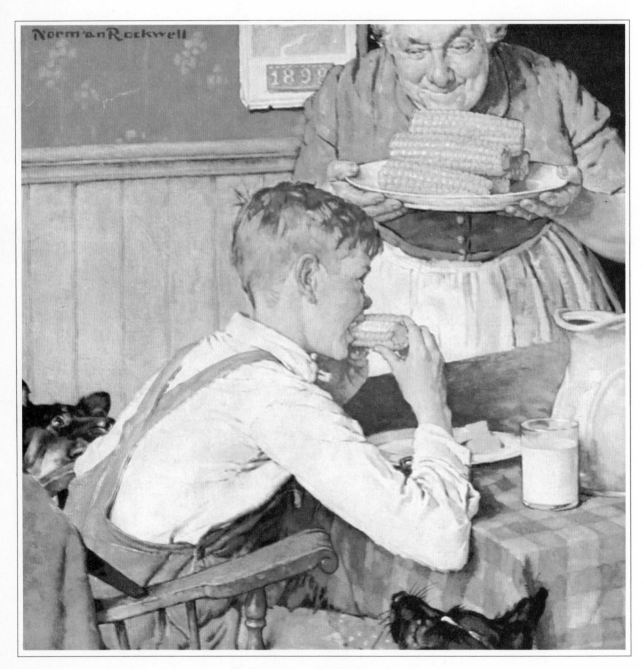

Printed by permission of Pillsbury, Minneapolis, MN

PART II

Nutrients
Their Sources and Functions

People are often curious to know whether certain foods are "good for you." You may have asked the question many times yourself, or been told by anxious parents to "eat up—it is good for you."

Some of the information needed to answer this question is provided in Part I, in which we explored the reasons why we eat the foods we do and discussed the background for dietary guidelines. There is other important information we must know about the nutrients in foods, and that is what we will explore in Part II.

Each nutrient is unique. Certain foods are good sources of individual nutrients. Each nutrient has unique chemical and physiological properties, so that if we consume too little or too much of the nutrient, specific deficiency or toxicity symptoms can occur in the body. Certain diseases of affluence, such as coronary heart disease, obesity, and hypertension, are also thought to be related to specific nutrient intakes.

In addition to examining the nutrients contained in foods, we must consider some other important factors. For example, is the energy content of your diet balanced with the energy expenditure in physical activity and the energy needed to maintain the body? If not, there may be serious problems with obesity, eating disorders, or starvation. Techniques used in the production and processing of foods may influence how safe and nutritious they are. These are some of the factors that we will now consider to help determine whether certain foods are "good for you."

3 Carbohydrates
Starches, Sugars, and Fiber

CONNECTIONS

Does sugar cause tooth decay and diabetes? Does fiber prevent constipation and cancer? Does "carbohydrate loading" really help athletes maintain endurance?

These are all popular ideas about carbohydrates: sugars, starches, and fiber. In this chapter, we will relate all the aspects of the definition of nutrition presented in Chapter 1, as well as the ideas of nutrient quantity and quality and nutrient density developed in Chapter 2, to carbohydrates.

Are carbohydrates fattening? Not if the kcalories from carbohydrates taken in are balanced by kcalories of energy going out. Well, then, is *sugar* more fattening than other carbohydrates, fat, or protein with the same number of kcalories? Actually, no. The problem is that refined sugar is of low nutrient density—it contributes kcalories but no vitamins or minerals to the diet—which is why you can see the importance of reading food labels, as described in Chapter 2. Also, as discussed in Chapter 2, carbohydrates do not have RDA values unlike protein, most vitamins, and minerals.

Let us see, then, what carbohydrates are all about.

When it comes to sugar, everyone wants to get in on the act.

"Probably no single food commodity on the world market has been subjected to so much politicking as sugar," writes one observer. "The study of this universally popular food is the province of the historian, economist, demographer, geographer, anthropologist and sociologist, as well as the clinician and scientist."[1]

Sugar, then, seems to get all the attention, which is why it's not surprising that so many people are confused or concerned about it. There are several other kinds of nutrients in the category of *carbohydrates* besides table sugar—including other sugars, starches, and fiber.

CARBOHYDRATES: MORE THAN SUGAR

Individual carbohydrates vary greatly in where they come from and what they do in the body. They also vary in the amount of misinformation people have about them. To clear up much of the confusion about carbohydrates, let us look at Table 3-1 on naturally occurring carbohydrates and then study the following six propositions.

FIGURE 3-1
Three carbohydrate molecules. The differences are explained in the text.

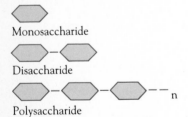

Monosaccharide

Disaccharide

Polysaccharide

(n = up to several thousand)

Carbohydrates Are Classified by the Size of Their Molecules

Three types of molecules constitute carbohydrates (Figure 3-1). The kinds of carbohydrates they make up are shown in Table 3-1.

- The *monosaccharides*, the building blocks of which other carbohydrate molecules are built, are molecules with five or six carbon atoms. The monosaccharides include the simple sugars glucose, fructose, and galactose.
- *Disaccharides*, which include the sugars sucrose, lactose, and maltose, consist of two monosaccharide molecules linked together.
- The *polysaccharides* are very large molecules formed from many hundreds or thousands of glucose molecules joined together. They include starch, dextrin, glycogen, and cellulose (which is one of the chemicals included in the term *fiber*).

Monosaccharide
Simple sugar with five or six carbon atoms—glucose, fructose, galactose (mono = one).

Disaccharide
Simple sugars with two monosaccharides linked together—sucrose, lactose, maltose (di = two).

Polysaccharides
Complex carbohydrates formed from many monosaccharides linked together—starch, dextrin, glycogen, cellulose (poly = many).

TABLE 3-1 Naturally Occurring Carbohydrates Important in Nutrition—What They Are and Where They Are Found

		Some Concepts About Carbohydrates	
Classification	**Common Food Sources**	**Correct**	**Untrue or Unproven**
Simple Sugars			
Monosaccharides:			
Glucose	Fruits; honey; maple sugar; traces in most plant foods	Main source of energy for brain and nerves	
Fructose	Honey; fruits; traces in most plant foods	Sweeter than sucrose	Better sugar substitute for diabetics and in weight-reducing diets
Galactose	Part of lactose, which is the sugar in milk		
Disaccharides:			
Sucrose	Table sugar (cane or beet); fruits; maple sugar	Sugar in certain foods causes tooth decay	Causes "sugar blues" and behavioral problems; fattening
Lactose	Milk and some dairy products	Nausea and diarrhea caused by lactose in people with lactase deficiency	Prevalence of lactase deficiency in the world debated
Maltose	Sprouted seeds; produced in digestion of starch		
Complex Carbohydrates or Polysaccharides			
Starch	Starchy plants, grains		Fattening
Glycogen	Liver (in very small amounts)	May help long-distance athletes; controversial	Benefits all athletes
*Cellulose	Wheat bran; part of cell walls	Relationship between high fiber intake and lower incidence of colon cancer	Some mystical properties now attributed to high fiber intakes
*Hemicellulose	Plant walls		
*Pectins	Fruits		

*These, together with lignin and gums, form what is commonly called "fiber."

FIGURE 3-2
Our bodies have many sources of the
essential carbohydrate, glucose.

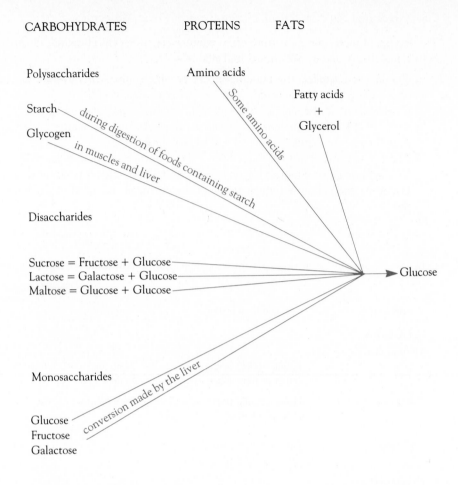

Of the Several Carbohydrates, Only Glucose Is Essential

Glucose is a simple sugar derived from fruits, honey, and maple sugar, and found in small amounts in most plant foods. It is an essential nutrient; that is, it must be provided in the diet, either directly or indirectly. Glucose is the main source of energy for your brain and nerves. Although your body makes most of its supply of glucose from other carbohydrates in your diet, some comes from amino acids and from the glycerol part of fat, as shown in Figure 3-2.

Plant Foods Provide Most of the Carbohydrates in Our Diet

As Table 3-1 shows, the common food sources of most carbohydrates are fruits, plants, seeds, and grains. However, there are some exceptions:

- Milk and some dairy products, which provide lactose and its constituent monosaccharides galactose and glucose
- Liver and some shellfish, which contain a small amount of glycogen

Carbohydrates Vary in Sweetness

Ever noticed how bananas and apples increase in sweetness as they ripen? This is because during the ripening process the starch in these fruits is converted into sugars. In peas and corn, however, the opposite happens: sugars are converted into starch as these plants mature.

Sugars are not the only sweeteners in food. Since sugary snacks are a major cause of *dental caries* (or cavities), in which the tooth enamel is destroyed by acid produced by the fermentation of dietary carbohydrates by oral bacteria, it may be advisable to use sugar substitutes instead of sucrose to sweeten some foods.[2] Food may be sweetened by any of a variety of carbohydrates, sugar alcohols, and artificial sweeteners. *Sugar alcohols* have chemical structures similar to simple sugars; the most widely used of these sugar substitutes are sorbitol and mannitol, which are used in chewing gums and candies labeled "sugarless."

The differences in sweetness among carbohydrates can be compared if sucrose is given a sweetness rating of 1, as shown in Table 3-2. Note that fructose is 1.7 times sweeter and aspartame (Nutrasweet) 180 times sweeter than sucrose. Thus, in diet drinks, for example, artificial or nonnutritive sweeteners can replace sugar and reduce kcalories without reducing sweetness. For instance, the same amount of sweetness that is in 5 grams (1 teaspoonful) of sugar (sucrose, which, at 4

Dental Caries
Cavities, one of the most common health problems in the world. Oral bacteria produce acid by fermenting dietary carbohydrates; the acid destroys tooth enamel.

Sugar Alcohols
Structures similar to simple sugars that are used as sweeteners.

Nonnutritive sweeteners give taste but few if any kcalories.

TABLE 3-2 How Sweet It Is: Sugars Compared with Artificial Sweeteners

Substance	Sweetness Rating
Carbohydrates	
Sucrose	1
Fructose	1.7
Invert sugar	1.3
Glucose	0.7
Maltose	0.4
Galactose	0.3
Lactose	0.2
Starch	0
Sugar alcohols	
Xylitol	0.9
Mannitol	0.7
Sorbitol	0.6
Noncarbohydrates	
Saccharin (artificial)	500
Aspartame [Nutrasweet] (2 amino acids)	180
Cyclamate (artificial)	100
Tryptophan (amino acid)	30

* Formed by the splitting of sucrose. It is a mixture of half glucose and half fructose. Honey has the same sweetness as invert sugar.

kcalories per gram, is 20 kcalories) is provided by only 0.027 grams of aspartame, because aspartame is 180 times sweeter than sugar (5 grams divided by 180 is 0.027 grams). Aspartame is two amino acids (aspartic acid and phenylalanine) joined together; amino acids are the building blocks of protein. Since 1 gram of protein contains 4 kcalories, then 0.027 grams of aspartame contains only 0.108 kcalories. Compare this approximately one tenth of a kcalorie of aspartame with 20 kcalories of sugar for the same degree of sweetness.

"Fiber" and "Roughage" Are Popular Words for Some Carbohydrates

Fiber

Part of plants indigestible to humans, but digestible by bacteria, cattle, and some other animals—example, cellulose.

Fiber—also called "roughage," "bulk," "nature's broom," or "nature's natural laxative"—has probably been a staple in the diet since time immemorial. Although first discussed in the last century in German scientific literature, it was "rediscovered" in the 1960s. You see the word *fiber* used a lot in advertising; it refers to the part of plants (including cellulose) that is indigestible to humans, though it may be digestible by bacteria and animals like cattle. Fiber is a generic term that includes some or all of the following: three different polysaccharides—cellulose, hemicellulose, and pectin, plus the noncarbohydrate lignin. Actually, the term *fiber* is a misnomer because these compounds are not all fibrous or stringy.

An association between low fiber intakes in the diet and colon cancer has been proposed. This association has resulted in great scientific and public interest in fiber. There was a 40-fold increase in the number of published scientific papers on fiber in the decade 1968-1978, and there is still much to be learned about it.

Popular Understanding of Carbohydrates Is Incomplete or Inaccurate

The media have made many people aware of the nutritional importance of fiber. But what about cellulose, hemicellulose, and pectin? Not many know that these are kinds of dietary fiber. Galactose and maltose are also not mentioned much in magazine articles, but both are important sources of the essential carbohydrate glucose.

Many people also have mistaken ideas about carbohydrates—that they are unnecessary and fattening, for instance, which is why some popular weight-reducing diets are low in carbohydrates. Actually, kcalories from carbohydrates are no more fattening than the same number of kcalories from fat or protein.

Another popular belief is that sucrose (table sugar) is the cause of behavioral or emotional problems. This notion comes from unscientific, anecdotal observations; little evidence supports it.[2] More long-term studies are needed before any such association between diet and the emotions is proven or disproven.

Most carbohydrates come from plant food. Milk and liver are the only animal sources. The essential carbohydrate is glucose. Carbohydrates are grouped by the size of the molecule. Sweetness varies among different carbohydrates. Fiber is a generic term that includes three different carbohydrates.

CHEMICAL STRUCTURES OF THE CARBOHYDRATES

If you understand the chemical structures of carbohydrates, you can also begin to understand the reasons for their nutritional characteristics.

Consider the following general facts about the structure of carbohydrates:

- All carbohydrates contain carbon, hydrogen, and oxygen.
- When energy is liberated from carbohydrates, the carbon and oxygen atoms form carbon dioxide (CO_2), which is excreted in the expired air. Hydrogen and oxygen are excreted as water (H_2O) in urine and perspiration.
- One gram of any digestible carbohydrate provides 4 kcalories of energy—no matter whether the gram comes from the sucrose in table sugar, the fructose in honey, the lactose in milk, or the starch in pasta.
- All carbohydrates except for dietary fiber are broken down fully into their constituent monosaccharides during digestion. Dietary fiber includes cellulose, hemicellulose, and pectin.
- Only monosaccharides are absorbed from the gastrointestinal tract into the blood. The molecules of disaccharides and polysaccharides are too large to be absorbed. Therefore, they must be broken down into their constituent monosaccharides during digestion in order to be absorbed into the blood.

Now let us look at the chemical structures of the monosaccharides, disaccharides, and polysaccharides.

The Monosaccharides

The structure of glucose, the essential carbohydrate, is shown in Figure 3-3. Fructose and galactose have the same number of carbon, hydrogen, and oxygen atoms, but their arrangement in galactose molecules is different from that in glucose molecules.

The Disaccharides

The chemical structure of this group of carbohydrates is as follows:

Sucrose = Glucose + Fructose

Lactose = Glucose + Galactose

Maltose = Glucose + Glucose

Digestion breaks disaccharides into their monosaccharide components. For example, one molecule of lactose in milk will be digested into one molecule each of glucose and galactose.

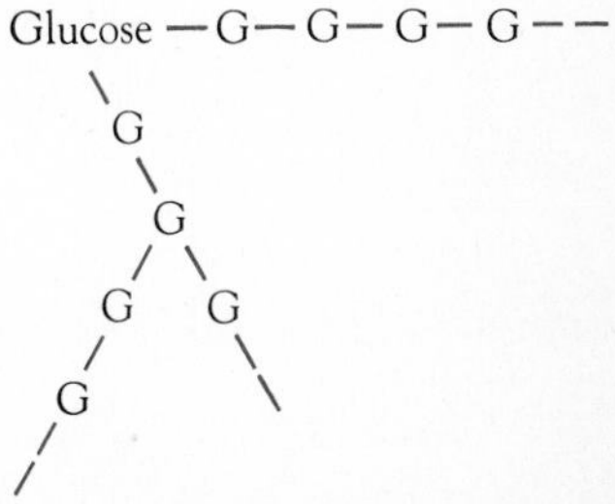

The Polysaccharides

The polysaccharides are called complex carbohydrates because they may consist of hundreds or thousands of monosaccharides, usually glucose units, linked together. The makeup of starches, fiber, and glycogen is as follows.

Starches

The chains of glucose units may be in a straight line or branched, as shown in Figure 3-4, but this structure makes no difference to nutritional value. Digestion breaks the starch into individual glucose units.

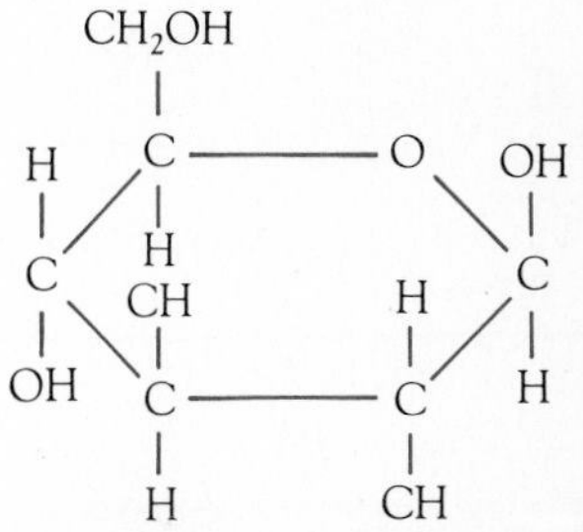

FIGURE 3-3
The structure of glucose. Note the arrangement of carbon, hydrogen, and oxygen groups, which become H_2O and CO_2 when energy is released from glucose.

FIGURE 3-4
Starch from the diet is digested into glucose units.

Fiber

Cellulose is hundreds of glucose units joined together. Hemicellulose and pectin are related structurally to cellulose. Because of the type of linkages, cellulose, hemicellulose, and pectin are not digested by the enzymes in the human digestive system. Recent evidence suggests that bacteria in the large intestine can release some components of fiber. These monosaccharides can be absorbed and used for energy.

How much is digested, and under what conditions, is debated by the experts. However, most of the different components of fiber are eliminated in the feces.

Glycogen

Also known as animal starch, glycogen is the reserve form of carbohydrate in human beings and other animals. It is not found in plants. It consists of up to thousands of glucose molecules joined together.

WHERE CARBOHYDRATES COME FROM

As Table 3-3 points out, plants and milk are the major sources of carbohydrates, which means carbohydrates are an inexpensive source of dietary energy. Let's discuss the food sources of monosaccharides, disaccharides, and polysaccharides.

TABLE 3-3 Principal Carbohydrate and Energy Contribution from Different Foods

	Principal Carbohydrate	% Energy from Carbohydrate
Plant Foods		
Cereals	Starch	65-90
Potatoes	Starch	80
Vegetables	Starch, sucrose	60-90
Fruits and berries	Fructose, glucose, sucrose	80-95
Animal Foods		
Milk		
Human	Lactose	50
Cow's	Lactose	30-50
		(depending on fat content)
Shellfish		
Oysters	Glycogen	20-25
Lobster/crab/shrimp	Glycogen	2-4
Liver	Glycogen	about 10
Meat and fish	—	Negligible

Food Sources of Monosaccharides

The three principal monosaccharides are glucose, fructose, and galactose.

Glucose

Also known as dextrose, glucose is found in honey and fruits, especially grapes. *Chlorophyll*, a green pigment, enables plants to use energy from sunlight to make glucose from water and carbon dioxide.

Chlorophyll
Green pigment in plants; uses sunlight to make carbohydrates from CO_2 and H_2O.

The typical diet contains less than 20 grams of free glucose per day. This is much less than the daily requirements of the body. This is not a problem because the body makes glucose from many other sources, as we saw in Figure 3-2.

Fructose

Sometimes called "fruit sugar," fructose occurs naturally in the highest concentrations in the following foods; the percentages express how much of the edible portion of each food is fructose.

- Honey—40%
- Apples, grapes, pears, bananas—6%
- Oranges, strawberries—2 to 2.5%
- Plums, tomatoes, asparagus—1.5%

Fructose is also produced by the breakdown of the sucrose molecule. Fructose may be converted into glucose in the body, regardless of dietary source (see Figure 3-2).

Increasing amounts of fructose in our diet come from high-fructose corn syrups (abbreviated HFCS). These are produced by the breakdown of cornstarch. Their fructose content is 55% to 90% of total sugars. HFCS have sweetened soft drinks, canned foods, jams, jellies, and salad dressings since the early 1970s.

Food Technology

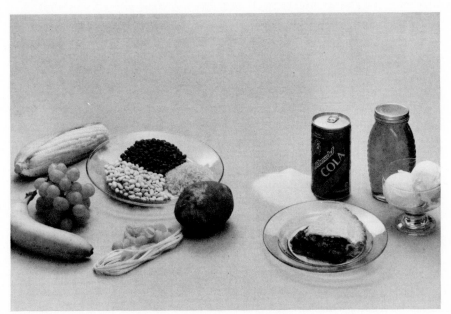

Carbohydrate-rich foods. Complex carbohydrate foods, high in starch and in fiber are on the left; high sugar foods are on the right. All are high in carbohydrate, but only foods high in complex carbohydrates are recommended.

Galactose

Galactose comes mainly from the digestion of lactose (glucose plus galactose). It is not found free in nature except in digested milk.

Food Sources of Disaccharides

The most important disaccharides are sucrose, lactose, and maltose.

Sucrose

Sucrose is considered by many people to be the dietary enemy among carbohydrates. Are they right? Before you decide, let's discuss the function of sucrose in foods.

First, note that the term *sugar* is not being used indiscriminately in this book. There are particular kinds of sugar, namely:

- Table sugar—sucrose
- Blood sugar, dextrose, grape sugar—glucose
- Milk sugar—lactose
- Fruit sugar—fructose

Nutritionists use the more technical terms—sucrose, glucose, lactose, fructose.

TABLE 3-4 Examples of Sugar Content of Foods

Food	% Total Sugar by Weight	Nutrition Comments
Grapes, fresh green	16	Removal of water in the conversion of grapes into raisins concentrates sugar
Raisins	66	
Apple, fresh	11	Buy unsweetened applesauce if you are controlling sugar intake
Applesauce, canned, unsweetened	10	
Applesauce, canned, sweetened	23	
Natural rolled oats	0	Some breakfast cereals have *no* sugar
Cream of Wheat	0	
Nabisco Shredded Wheat	1	
Cheerios	3	
Special K	7	
Total	9	
Quaker 100% Natural, raisin and date*	26	
Sugar Frosted Flakes	41	Some breakfast cereals are very high in sugar
Sugar Smacks	58	
Raisin bran*		Many people are turning to bran cereals to increase their fiber intake; note how the amount of sugar varies among different brands
Kellogg	33	
Post	32	
Ralston	12	
Ralston instant oatmeal		
plain	0	Use of the word "sugar" does not always mean the highest sugar content
with maple and brown sugar	17	
with cinnamon and spice	27	

* Includes sugars occurring naturally in dried fruits.

Most commercial sugar is obtained from sugar cane or sugar beets, with small amounts produced from maple and sorghum. White table sugar consists of about 99.9% sucrose. Brown sugar has a little less sucrose. Both, together with honey, have a low index of nutrient quality (INQ) for all vitamins and minerals. Because nutrient content is so low, these concentrated sources of sugar are sometimes referred to as "empty calories."

Sugar consumption is decreasing in the United States, with per-person consumption at 71 pounds in 1983, significantly lower than the 103 pounds per capita in 1972. Unfortunately, during the same period the use of corn sweeteners doubled, to about 39 pounds per person. The truth is, then, that only the source of the sugars has changed.

Growers and food producers increase the sugar content of foods in two ways:

Be careful in interpreting consumption data for individual foods.

- *Drying:* Fresh fruits may range from 6% to 25% in sugar content, depending on the dilution provided by a fruit's water content (the watermelon has only 5% sugar content, compared with 20% in bananas). The sugar content of certain fruits—grapes, dates, figs, prunes, and apricots—can be raised to as much as 50% to 90% by drying.

Microbiology

- *Adding sugar:* Food processors add sugar to increase sweetness, add bulk (in some baked goods), and to prevent spoilage (as an antimicrobial agent in jams, jellies, and fermented sausages). Many foods have sugar added to increase sweetness: catsups, peanut butter, potato chips, some drinks, even some medications—including children's vitamin supplements. Though used as an additive in these examples, sucrose is considered safe at present levels of consumption.[3,4]

The sugar contents of some foods are shown in Table 3-4.

Lactose

Found naturally only in milk and certain other dairy products (Table 3-5), lactose is removed in the processing of some cheeses, including cheddar. Lactose also appears in several nondairy products, to which lactose or dairy products have been added during processing. Because the chemical has a number of properties useful

TABLE 3-5 Lactose Content of Some Foods

Food	Serving Size	Lactose (grams)
Milk, human	1 cup	17
Milk, cow's, skim or whole	1 cup	12
Buttermilk	1 cup	12
Yogurt	1 cup	11
Cottage cheese	1 cup	6
Ice cream	1 cup	6
Swiss, brick cheese	1 ounce	1
Cream cheese	1 ounce	0.8
Butter	1 stick	0.04

in food processing, lactose may be included in bread, soups, salad dressings, cereals, breakfast drinks, cake mixes and confectionary, and some meat products.

Lactose is also useful in making tablets; it appears in about 21% of all prescription drugs (over 1,000) and in 6% of all over-the-counter drugs.[5]

Maltose

Maltose occurs less commonly in nature than either sucrose or lactose. It is found in germinating seeds or is prepared commercially by the partial hydrolysis (breaking apart with water) of starch.

Food Sources of Polysaccharides

Polysaccharides include starch, glycogen, dextrin, and fiber.

Starch

The storage form of energy in plants, starch is the main source of dietary energy for adults in many developing countries because of their dependence on starch-rich foods such as cereals. Starch has also been used as a food additive (for instance, in soups) because it thickens foods.

In recent years, a controversy developed over the use of modified food starch in baby foods.[6] It was removed by one manufacturer from a line of baby foods, who then turned the event into a commercial advantage by an extensive marketing campaign highlighting the fact that the starch is modified chemically—the word "chemically" was emphasized in television commercials. However, there is no medical evidence at present that modified food starch has any harmful effects. Indeed, it has been used for around 50 years to make food more palatable and to improve the thickening properties of foods. You will find modified food starches in many canned, frozen, baked, or dry foods. The amount in baby foods is small, amounting to only about 8% of total kcalories.

Glycogen

As Table 3-3 indicates, glycogen is found only in liver and some shellfish and in negligible amounts in meat. Natural chemical changes lead to the loss of glycogen after meat animals are slaughtered.

Dextrin

Dextrin is formed when heat (toasting) or enzymes (during digestion) act on starch. The molecule is a little smaller than starch. Dextrimaltose is a mixture of dextrin and maltose. It is easily digested by infants.

Fiber

Fiber content may vary widely within a food category—for example, bread.

Fiber content is highest in beans, vegetables, nuts, and unrefined cereals, as indicated in Figure 3-5; no fiber is obtained from foods of animal origin. In the figure, notice that the amount of fiber in foods can vary considerably—even the amount of fiber in bread. Indeed, research has shown that specialty breads and breads labeled "wheat" can vary greatly in fiber content.[7] Refining of grain removes the part of the seed richest in fiber. If edible skins of fruits are removed, fiber values are reduced.

DIETARY FIBER

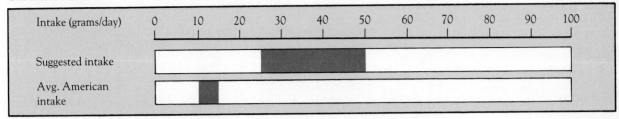

SOURCE

GRAMS OF FIBER
(Approximate)

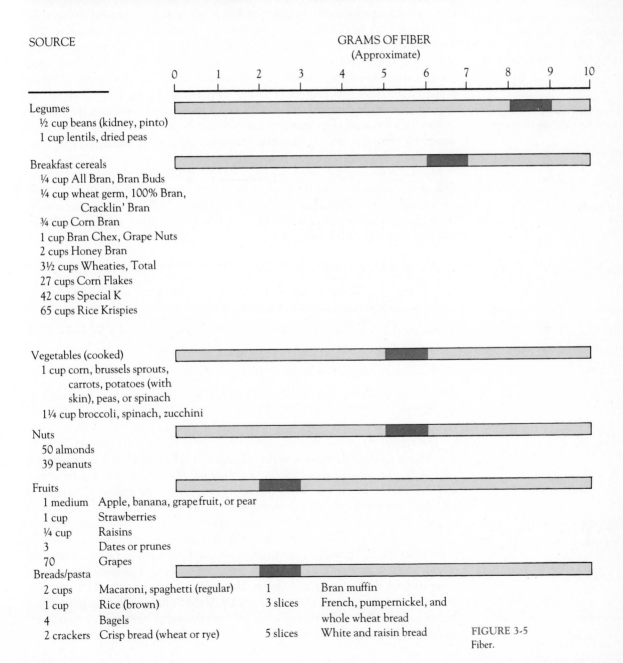

Legumes
  ½ cup beans (kidney, pinto)
  1 cup lentils, dried peas

Breakfast cereals
  ¼ cup All Bran, Bran Buds
  ¼ cup wheat germ, 100% Bran,
        Cracklin' Bran
  ¾ cup Corn Bran
  1 cup Bran Chex, Grape Nuts
  2 cups Honey Bran
  3½ cups Wheaties, Total
  27 cups Corn Flakes
  42 cups Special K
  65 cups Rice Krispies

Vegetables (cooked)
  1 cup corn, brussels sprouts,
        carrots, potatoes (with
        skin), peas, or spinach
  1¼ cup broccoli, spinach, zucchini

Nuts
  50 almonds
  39 peanuts

Fruits
  1 medium   Apple, banana, grapefruit, or pear
  1 cup   Strawberries
  ¼ cup   Raisins
  3   Dates or prunes
  70   Grapes

Breads/pasta
  2 cups   Macaroni, spaghetti (regular)   1   Bran muffin
  1 cup   Rice (brown)   3 slices   French, pumpernickel, and
  4   Bagels   whole wheat bread
  2 crackers Crisp bread (wheat or rye)   5 slices   White and raisin bread

FIGURE 3-5
Fiber.

Most plant foods have varying proportions of the following two categories of fiber, classified by their solubility in water:

- *Water-insoluble fibers:* Cellulose, hemicellulose, and lignin—in plant walls, skins, peels, and in the outer, or bran layer, of whole grains.
- *Water-soluble fibers:* Pectin—from soft fruits and in vegetables; gums—from the stems and seeds of some tropical plants. Gums are used as a food additive.

In general, vegetables are higher in cellulose, and fruits are higher in pectin. Cooking, canning, and freezing do not seem to decrease the fiber content of foods. However, scientists are still struggling to find accurate ways to measure the amount and type of fiber in the diet. Older methods of measurement underestimated the amount of fiber in foods because strong acids were used in the testing—not a realistic representation of people's normal chemical processes in digestion—and some of the water-soluble fiber was lost in these methods. The resulting values expressed the *crude fiber* content of a food. This outdated term may still appear on some food labels, leading to confusion because it usually underestimates the amount of fiber in a food. Modern methods measure *dietary fiber*, which duplicates more accurately the processes of digestion. However, even these methods have their problems.[8]

Medical claims for the beneficial effects of fiber in foods are monitored carefully. The only claims that have been accorded recognition to date are that (1) fiber reduces available kcalories and (2) it produces a laxative effect.[9] Boasts that certain cereals prevent colon cancer should give you fair warning about advertising claims, a matter that will be discussed at the end of this chapter.

Chemistry

Crude Fiber
A number expressing the fiber content of a food; obtained from older methods. This value should not be used now, although it is still found on labels.

Dietary Fiber
More realistic measure of what happens to fiber in the digestive tract.

In calculating your fiber intake, use the *dietary fiber* value.

Carbohydrates are inexpensive sources of dietary energy. Food sources of sucrose, starch, and fiber are of most interest to the public.

THE NORMAL DIET: TOO MANY OR TOO FEW CARBOHYDRATES?

There is no RDA for carbohydrates. However, it is recommended that over half of your total kcaloric intake should come from carbohydrates, especially from complex carbohydrates.

The typical American diet provides about 300 grams of total carbohydrate per day. This is 1,200 kcalories of energy (300 grams × 4 kcalories). If you are between 19 and 22, the recommended intake of energy is 2,900 kcalories if you are a man and 2,100 kcalories if you are a woman. Thus, if you are eating 300 grams of carbohydrates every day, you are getting 41 percent (men) and 57 percent (women) of total dietary energy intake from carbohydrates.

Some popular weight-reducing diets require carbohydrate intakes considerably lower than the 100 grams of carbohydrate per day considered to be safe. There are serious medical dangers associated with these low-carbohydrate diets. Some best-seller diets in this category include Dr. Robert Atkin's *Superenergy Diet,* and *The Doctor's Quick Weight-Loss Diet* by the late Dr. Irwin Stillman. The dangers include loss of body fluid, high intakes of kcalories from fat and protein, and, for pregnant women, possible danger to the fetus.

Medicine

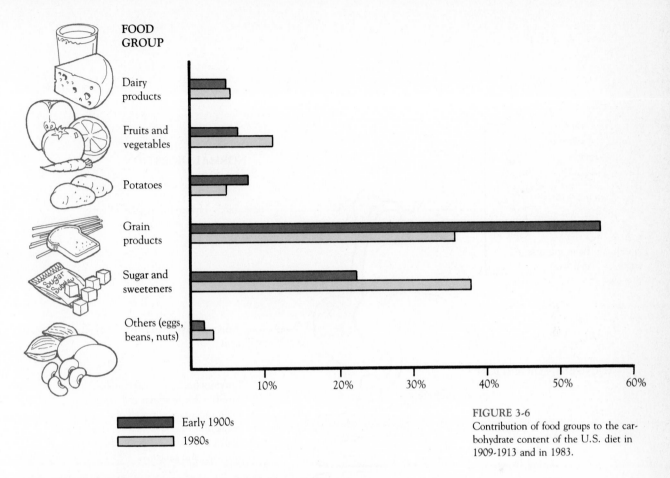

FIGURE 3-6
Contribution of food groups to the carbohydrate content of the U.S. diet in 1909-1913 and in 1983.

People Throughout the World Eat Different Amounts of Carbohydrates

Dietary intake of carbohydrates varies throughout the world—from about 40% of energy intake in the United States, up to 80% to 90% in Southeast Asia, down to about 10% to 15% among the Eskimos. Within a given country, poorer people usually have higher intakes of dietary carbohydrates because carbohydrates are an inexpensive source of dietary energy.

Economics

Carbohydrate sources in the American diet have changed since the beginning of this century, as Figure 3-6 shows. Americans eat fewer complex carbohydrates mainly because of a decreased intake of grain products. Many of the present-day grain products are highly refined. This leads to a lower intake of fiber. The average daily intake of starch in the U.S. is about 180 grams (which amounts to 720 kcalories). More sugar and other sweeteners are eaten in greater quantities now.

How Carbohydrates Are Digested, Absorbed, and Used

Suppose, for the sake of example, you have a breakfast of cereal, milk, sugar, and bean sprouts—an odd combination, but it includes all the important carbohydrates. Figure 3-7 shows how these carbohydrates are digested, absorbed, and transported to the cells.

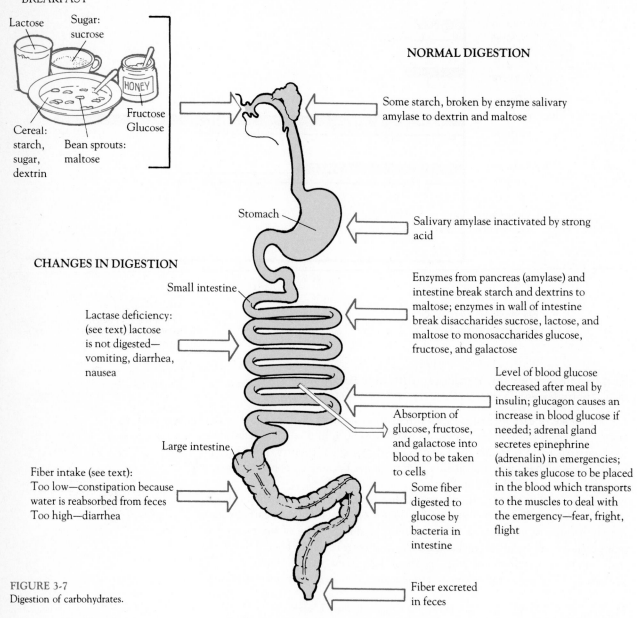

BREAKFAST

Lactose

Sugar: sucrose

Cereal: starch, sugar, dextrin

Bean sprouts: maltose

Fructose Glucose

NORMAL DIGESTION

Some starch, broken by enzyme salivary amylase to dextrin and maltose

Stomach

Salivary amylase inactivated by strong acid

CHANGES IN DIGESTION

Small intestine

Lactase deficiency: (see text) lactose is not digested— vomiting, diarrhea, nausea

Enzymes from pancreas (amylase) and intestine break starch and dextrins to maltose; enzymes in wall of intestine break disaccharides sucrose, lactose, and maltose to monosaccharides glucose, fructose, and galactose

Level of blood glucose decreased after meal by insulin; glucagon causes an increase in blood glucose if needed; adrenal gland secretes epinephrine (adrenalin) in emergencies; this takes glucose to be placed in the blood which transports to the muscles to deal with the emergency—fear, fright, flight

Absorption of glucose, fructose, and galactose into blood to be taken to cells

Large intestine

Fiber intake (see text): Too low—constipation because water is reabsorbed from feces Too high—diarrhea

Some fiber digested to glucose by bacteria in intestine

Fiber excreted in feces

FIGURE 3-7
Digestion of carbohydrates.

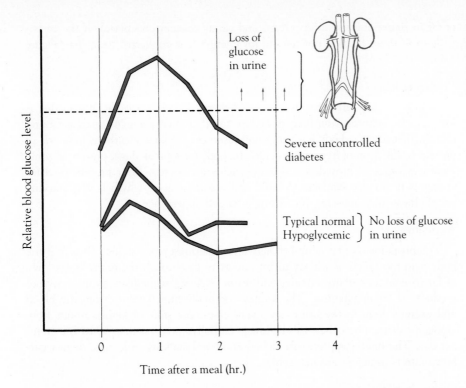

Relative blood glucose level

Loss of glucose in urine

Severe uncontrolled diabetes

Typical normal ⎱ No loss of glucose
Hypoglycemic ⎰ in urine

Time after a meal (hr.)

FIGURE 3-8
Typical response of blood glucose after a meal taken by a diabetic and nondiabetic person. Dangerously low levels of blood glucose may occur in hypoglycemia.

The metabolism of glucose is an example of the influence of hormones on a nutrient. In this case, *insulin*—a hormone produced by the pancreas—removes glucose from the blood, helps it enter the cells, and stores the excess as glycogen or fat. People who secrete insufficient insulin cannot use or store the glucose in the blood. This results in high blood glucose levels. The kidneys reduce the high levels of glucose by excreting excess glucose in the urine (Figure 3-8). *Glucagon*—another hormone secreted by the pancreas—has the opposite effect to that of insulin: by stimulating the liver to break down glycogen, it prevents the level of blood glucose from reaching dangerously low levels. The adrenal gland produces the hormone *epinephrine*. This has the same effect as glucagon. Epinephrine is important in emergency situations of fear or fright. It makes glucose available quickly for immediate energy use.

Carbohydrates Are Important in the Diet and the Body

Although carbohydrates make up only about 1% of body weight, they are important in both the diet and the body. As mentioned above, some carbohydrates (sucrose, for example) provide sweetness in foods and drinks, but carbohydrates also have more important functions.

Energy

Available carbohydrates have 4 kcalories per gram. The body has enough glycogen to meet normal energy requirements for about half a day. Any excess dietary carbohydrate is converted into fat. If you go to the Table of Food Composition (Appendix P) and check on the amount of fat in high-carbohydrate foods commonly called "fattening," notice that there is no fat in sugar, and only a small amount

Biochemistry

Insulin
Hormone produced by the pancreas. It removes excess glucose from blood, helps glucose enter cells, and helps in storing excess as glycogen or fat.

Glucagon
Hormone secreted by the pancreas. It has the opposite function of insulin—helping the breakdown of glycogen and fat.

Epinephrine
A hormone secreted by the adrenal gland in emergencies to speed the release of glucose. Better known as adrenaline.

Foods are fattening only if total kcalorie intake exceeds total kcalorie expenditure—regardless of whether the kcalories come from carbohydrates, fats, or protein.

of fat in rice, potatoes, most breads, and candy (except chocolate). If the carbohydrate in these foods is not needed for energy, it is converted to fat (see Figure 3-1).

Protein sparing

Some weight-reducing diets rely on the protein-sparing concept, providing enough carbohydrate to prevent wasting of muscles.

Your body uses carbohydrate first as its energy source. However, if your diet is low in carbohydrates, your body must turn to other energy sources, such as fat and protein. Because the body has very small reserves of available carbohydrate and of protein in the form of free amino acids, the body must break down protein in some tissues in order to provide extra amino acids for energy. Body protein used for energy is no longer available to build and repair tissues—which is why starving people have small muscles, presenting a wasted appearance.

Antiketogenic action

Low-carbohydrate weight-reducing diets require the dieter to reach a state of ketosis, which is when ketones can be measured in the urine, indicating that fat is being broken down.

The breakdown of fat described above is sometimes not complete. It is as if the body is in too much of a hurry to get energy to go through the entire breakdown of fat to energy, carbon dioxide, and water. *Ketones* accumulate as intermediate products of fat metabolism. The kidneys normally filter ketones from the blood and excrete them in the urine. In severe cases, the state of ketosis results from ketogenic diets. These diets can be low in carbohydrate, less than 50 to 100 grams per day. The main symptoms are dehydration and acidosis. Adequate dietary carbohydrate is therefore antiketogenic.

Ketones
When carbohydrates are not available, fat is broken down incompletely to ketones. The presence of high levels in urine and blood is known as ketosis.

Other contributions

Carbohydrates provide the following:

- Fat metabolism—from a small amount of carbohydrate
- Bulk—by fiber in the diet
- Specialized functions—such as structural "scaffolding" of cells, part of the DNA and RNA molecules, and part of the skeleton for some amino acids.

> Regular diets provide sufficient carbohydrates. In general, poorer people have higher carbohydrate intakes. Digestion involves breaking dietary carbohydrates into their constituent monosaccharides. Some carbohydrates provide flavor and bulk in the diet. In the body, carbohydrate functions include: provision of energy, protein sparing, antiketogenic activity, help in fat metabolism, and involvement in certain specialized functions.

CARBOHYDRATES, HEALTH, AND DISEASE

High carbohydrate intake has been recommended in a number of recent health fads, including "carbohydrate loading" for athletes and high-fiber diets. High carbohydrate intake has also been related (though causation has not always been proved) to a number of diseases and disorders: obesity, diabetes, hypoglycemia, coronary heart disease, behavioral and learning problems, lactase deficiency, and dental caries. Let's evaluate the links to disease first, then evaluate the benefits of the high-fiber diet and carbohydrate loading.

Obesity Has No Specific Link to Sugar

At a May 1986 conference on the link between sugar and obesity, Dr. John Durnin of the University of Glasgow stated that although much of the research was inconclusive, in his opinion sugar intake did not play an important part in the development of obesity. However, this should not be taken as a guarantee that you can treat yourself to sugar and sugar-rich foods and stay slim, since many sweet foods are high in kcalories. All digestible carbohydrates, including sugar, have 4 kcalories per gram, regardless of food source, but refined sugar comes with no other nutrients. Foods that contribute vitamins, minerals, and fiber along with kcalories are a better deal from a nutrition standpoint than foods high in refined sugar.

Diabetes Is Related in Several Ways to Carbohydrate Intake

Diabetes involves hyperglycemia, usually accompanied by altered fat and protein metabolism. There are four forms of diabetes:

- Insulin-dependent, or type I, or juvenile diabetes mellitus
- Non-insulin-dependent, or type II, or adult-onset diabetes mellitus
- Gestational diabetes
- Tropical or malnutrition-related diabetes

Insulin-dependent diabetes mellitus (IDDM)

About 10% of all cases of diabetes must be treated with injections of insulin. Insulin-dependent diabetes mellitus (also known as type I or juvenile diabetes) can occur at any age. IDDM results from an interplay of genetic and environmental factors including certain viruses. The patient's pancreas does not produce sufficient insulin to control blood glucose levels (Figure 3-8). Treatment requires the injection of insulin, but food intake must be coordinated with these injections so as to keep levels of blood glucose within safe ranges. A recent study showed that many teenage diabetics do not monitor their blood glucose properly.[10] This kind of inattention can have serious ill effects.

Glycemic Index (GI)
Measures changes in blood glucose caused by different foods eaten by diabetics. High GI values means higher blood glucose levels.

The good news, however, is that there are no longer rigid restrictions on carbohydrate intake by diabetics. Many diabetes associations now recommend an increase in carbohydrate intake to about 50% of total kcalories. This can be done because much progress has been made in recent years in understanding the blood glucose response caused by different carbohydrate-containing foods. Consider Table 3-6. The lower the index number in this list of foods, the lower the blood glucose response. You will notice that starchy foods and foods high in fiber have a low *glycemic index (GI)*, the measure of changes in blood glucose caused by different foods eaten by diabetics. Increasing the proportion or absolute amount of high-starch, low-fat, low–glycemic-index foods in the diet of diabetics is encouraged.

As Table 3-6 shows, fructose has a low glycemic index and is independent of insulin. This can be misleading because a major portion of ingested fructose will be converted to glucose within the body (see Figure 3-1). This adds to the body's problems in controlling glucose levels.

Small amounts of sugar (sucrose) eaten with high-fiber foods such as whole meal bread or whole grain breakfast cereals cause no problems for the diabetic person. In fact, this combination may have a lower glycemic effect than any low-fiber, sugar-free equivalents.

TABLE 3-6 Carbohydrates for Insulin-dependent Diabetics

Food	Glycemic Index*
Bread	
White (wheat)	100
Whole meal (wheat)	99
Whole grain (rye)	58
Cereal Products	
Millet	103
Sweet corn	87
Rice (white)	83
Spaghetti (white)	66
Breakfast Cereals	
Cornflakes	119
All-Bran	73
Root Vegetables	
Potato (instant)	116
Potato (new, boiled)	81
Potato (sweet)	70
Dried Legumes	
Beans (baked, kidney, haricot)	45-60
Soy beans (tinned)	20
Fruit	
Raisins	93
Bananas	79
Oranges and orange juice	66
Apples	53
Cherries, grapefruit, plums, peaches	30-40
Dairy Products	
Yogurt, ice cream	52
Skim milk	46
Sugars	
Maltose	152
Glucose	138
Honey	126
Sucrose	86
Fructose	30

*The lower the index number, the lower the blood glucose response. Proportionally adjusted so that white bread = 100.

Exercise is important therapy for IDDM because physical activity increases the utilization of glucose along with producing an insulin-like effect.

Non-insulin-dependent diabetes mellitus (NIDDM)

In individuals with non-insulin-dependent diabetes mellitus (NIDDM), insulin is produced by the pancreas. The problem is that glucose does not get into cells. This extra glucose remains in the blood and is finally excreted in the urine. However, there is no evidence that total carbohydrate intake should be restricted greatly.

Because most people with NIDDM are obese, weight loss and exercise are the best remedies for the problem. It has been suggested that short-term treatment (36 days) with very low kcalorie diets of about 300 kcalories will provide safe, effective weight loss for people with NIDDM.[11] However, before we can subscribe to this recommendation, we should await further experiments over longer periods of time; after all, 300 kcalories a day is very low indeed.

The incidence of NIDDM increases with age. At ages 30 to 50, the disease is present in only 3% to 5% of the population, but by age 80, it has risen to 16% to 20%.[12] There is also an association between NIDDM and vascular disease, as is discussed elsewhere in this book.

Gestational diabetes

Caused by a resistance to insulin, gestational diabetes develops in women during about 2% to 3% of pregnancies, especially during the third trimester. The disease occurs mainly in women who are obese before the pregnancy, or in those with a family history of diabetes. Treatment involves a restricted intake of simple sugars, although some women may require insulin. Weight loss should not be recommended during pregnancy. Gestational diabetes usually disappears after delivery of the infant.

Tropical or malnutrition-related diabetes

This kind of diabetes strikes people who are malnourished and who live in tropical countries.[13] It is thought that toxic or infective agents may damage the pancreas in people with low protein intakes.

Hypoglycemia Is Rare

"Even in a large institution, really significant hypoglycemia is rare," says a past president of the American Diabetes Association.[14] Why, then, does hypoglycemia seem so fascinating to the general public?

Many people "self-diagnose" this disorder, because hypoglycemia has been popularized in magazine articles and on television talk shows and related to symptoms that most of us experience now and then anyway. However, there is no good evidence that hypoglycemia causes the catalog of problems attributed to it: depression, chronic fatigue, allergies, nervous breakdowns, alcoholism, juvenile delinquency, childhood behavior problems, drug addiction, or inadequate sexual performance.[15] We should be wary about interpreting the many reports associating reactive hypoglycemia with criminality and delinquency, since the accuracy of the analytical methods used has been questioned.[16] Some psychiatrists are concerned

Changing your diet after self-diagnosis from nonspecific symptoms may be dangerous.

that some people are being incorrectly treated for hypoglycemia who instead should be treated for panic attacks, a treatable neurological disorder.[17]

Hypoglycemia means a low level of blood glucose. The symptoms are sweating, shakiness, trembling, anxiety, fast heart action, headache, hunger sensations, brief feelings of weakness, and sometimes seizures and coma. These symptoms, which may be caused by many factors, including low blood glucose, are useful because they may signal the need for food. Glucose, as mentioned earlier, is the primary fuel for the brain and nervous system. If drops in blood glucose did not trigger appetite, the brain could be damaged because of lack of glucose.

What triggers low blood glucose is what is important in a study of nutrition. In 1973, the American Medical Association distinguished between reactive or fed hypoglycemia and spontaneous or fasting hypoglycemia, and the distinction is still valid today.[15]

> Hypoglycemia can occur in diabetics if they do not eat a meal after insulin injections. Alcohol can also decrease blood glucose level.

In *reactive* or *fed hypoglycemia,* which is the most common form of hypoglycemia, symptoms occur several hours after a meal because of a rapid fall in blood glucose levels, the result of a temporary overproduction of insulin by the pancreas. This form of hypoglycemia is found most frequently in nervous, thin women, people with mild diabetes, and patients who have had stomach operations. It is rare in normal infants and children. Treatment is usually a diet low in carbohydrates and high in protein, sometimes with multiple feedings. *Spontaneous* or *fasting hypoglycemia* occurs at night or before breakfast in adults and children. This type is serious and requires medical treatment.

Sugar Does Not Cause Coronary Heart Disease

To date there is no consistent evidence that high sugar (sucrose) intake is directly responsible for coronary heart disease. However, indirectly, sugar could be a cause by contributing excess kcalories and contributing to obesity.[18] Higher incidence of coronary heart disease occurs in obese people.

Evidence That Sugar Causes Behavioral Problems Is Weak

> Learn to distinguish between good and poor evidence in nutrition research.

Although the evidence suggests sucrose does not contribute to hyperactivity or to behavior and learning problems,[19] there have been reports in the media that it does. One experiment found that adults eating high-carbohydrate food items had reduced powers of concentration compared with adults who ate a high-protein meal; however, this study was poorly designed. This is an area requiring much more detailed studies before any definite relationships between behavior and diet, including carbohydrates, are established.[19]

Why Milk Is Not for Everybody: Lactase Deficiency

> Hydrolyze
> **To use water in the chemical breakdown of a substance. For example, digestion is the hydrolysis of carbohydrate, fat, and protein.**

The enzyme called lactase *hydrolyzes*—that is, uses water in a chemical breakdown of a substance—lactose into glucose and galactose in the small intestine, as shown in Figure 3-7. This is important in early life because of the high intake of lactose from human or cow's milk. Since a large part of the world's population becomes lactase deficient in the first or second decade of life,[20] we should take note of the following.

The incidence of lactase deficiency varies

Only people from northern and western Europe and their overseas descendants have a low incidence of lactase deficiency. Lactase deficiency is more common among blacks, Native Americans, Jews, Arabs, most Africans, Japanese, Chinese, and other Asians.

Symptoms

The symptoms of lactase deficiency include abdominal discomfort, bloating, and diarrhea. These occur for two reasons: first, undigested lactose draws a lot of water into the large intestine; second, bacteria in the large intestine act on the undigested lactose. The symptoms occur 30 to 90 minutes after taking lactose, and all are gone within 2 to 6 hours. The severity depends on the amount of lactase in the system, on the amount of lactose taken, the rate of emptying of the stomach, and intestinal transit time. There is a great degree of variation in the response of people within the groups who may be lactase deficient; some, for instance, may be able to tolerate one, but not two, glasses of milk.[20] Most people either learn quickly how much milk they can tolerate or they eliminate milk from their diet.

Eating lactose-rich food

There are ways that the lactase-deficient person may now eat some lactose-rich food without discomfort. For instance, yogurt is a rich source of lactose (Table 3-5), but this amount is well tolerated because lactase from bacteria in yogurt is activated when the yogurt is heated to body temperature.[21] This yogurt only requires minor changes from the normal production procedures. Much of the lactose is hydrolyzed into glucose and galactose by the time the yogurt is swallowed. In addition, some markets carry lactose-reduced milk, which tastes slightly sweeter than untreated milk. You can buy lactase through the mail or in pharmacies and add it to milk yourself.

Food Science

Is lactase deficiency abnormal?

It has long been argued whether lactase deficiency is a genetic defect. Might people with the ability to digest milk after infancy be the abnormal group? These questions cause some experts to question whether recurring abdominal pain in children may be caused by lactase deficiency. There are differing opinions,[20] but the latest evidence suggests that children can recover from mild acute gastroenteritis regardless of the dietary carbohydrate source.[22] If confirmed by further studies this finding would mean that families would no longer face the confusion and inconvenience resulting from a child's being automatically placed on non-lactose-containing formulas. For low-income families this may result in an important financial saving.

Genetics

Economics

Nutrition implications

Dairy products contribute about 75% of the calcium, 40% of the riboflavin, and 23% of the protein available for dietary consumption in the United States. Milk powder is the most effective way to transport high-quality protein to areas of severe undernutrition. Elimination of milk and dairy products from the diet would have serious nutrition implications (see Figure 3-7).

Note: *Lactase deficiency* is now the preferred term instead of *lactose intolerance.*[20]

Is Sugar the Great Rotter of Teeth?

Dental caries occurs when acids are formed from the bacterial metabolism of carbohydrates in the mouth. Successful prevention of dental caries involves considerations of the person, the oral bacteria, and the diet.

The individual

Saliva
The fluid in the mouth.

What is the person's genetic background, tooth structure, and rate of production of *saliva* (the fluid in the mouth—the more the better)? What is the person's "food clearance"? This term means that if high-sugar, sticky foods are kept in the mouth for long periods, more acid is produced by the oral bacteria.

Oral bacteria

Streptococcus mutans causes most of the acid production in the mouth. It will only cause tooth decay if all factors are present, especially fermentable carbohydrates.

The diet

Dental caries has long been associated with high sugar intakes. All carbohydrates contribute to dental caries, but sucrose and glucose are the most responsible. The texture of the food and the length of time it is in the mouth determine how harmful a food may be to the teeth.[23]

Arguments continue as to the role of sugar in dental caries.[24] There is evidence that not all countries with a high sugar intake also have high incidences of dental caries, and that many factors, including sugar, contribute to the incidence of dental caries in a community.

Some components in the diet actually may protect teeth from dental caries. These include calcium, phosphorus, fluoride, protein, and fats and oils. Certain cheeses such as aged cheddar, Swiss, and Monterey jack may reduce the incidence of dental caries.[23]

There is good news in that the incidence of dental caries has decreased in Western countries within the past 10 to 15 years.[25] Among the reasons are the following:

- Change in the diagnostic criteria of dental caries
- Oral microorganisms responsible for dental caries have become less active, or have been affected by the widespread use of antibiotics
- Decreased sugar consumption by children, though there is no meaningful evidence to support this speculation
- Widespread fluoridation of water—fluoride strengthens teeth against decay
- Increased dental health education, including the advertising of toothpaste with fluoride

Fiber Has Become One of the Great Nutrition Revolutions

Epidemiology

We could say that fiber represents the nutrition revolution that is "Out of Africa." For much of history, fiber was known only for its laxative properties. In the 19th century, Sylvester Graham, a clergyman who gave his name to a cracker, and William K. Kellogg, who started a breakfast cereal empire, advocated increased use of bran and whole grain cereals. However, their advice did not receive much attention until the 1960s, when British doctors discovered that the incidences of certain diseases were much lower in Africa than in Western countries and credited the high fiber content of the African diet.

As a result of recent research, fiber has been found to have laxative and anti-diarrheal effects, because of the increased water-holding capacity of many types of dietary fiber. This in turn has been said to lead to decreases in the incidence of colon cancer, appendicitis, varicose veins, hemorrhoids, and diverticulosis (inflammation in pouches called diverticula in the intestine). The reason for these effects is that the faster movement of the intestinal contents allows less time for carcinogens to interact with the colon, for bacterial infection of the appendix, and for the increased pressure that brings about varicose veins, hemorrhoids, and diverticulosis.

Evidence suggests that fiber may also provide the following health benefits.

Detoxification. Fiber binds with some toxic substances present in food or produced by the action of bacteria on food. These are then eliminated with the fiber in the feces.

Diabetes therapy. High-fiber foods have a lower glycemic index, as mentioned earlier.

Lowering of cholesterol. *Bile*—a liquid made in the liver and stored in the gallbladder—is secreted into the small intestine and aids in fat digestion. After digestion, the bile is reabsorbed from the intestines and transferred to the liver to be recycled. It contains cholesterol, some of which is bound by certain types of fiber in the gastrointestinal tract. The bound cholesterol is eliminated with the feces, thus reducing the amount that is reabsorbed into the blood.

Bile
A liquid made in the liver, stored in the gallbladder and secreted into small intestine. Bile aids in fat digestion.

⟵ ***Prevention of gallstones.*** Certain types of fiber are thought to prevent gallstones, although the evidence is far from complete. ⟶

Weight control. The bulking effect of fiber in the stomach is thought to make people less hungry. Furthermore, high-fiber foods are low in fat. A study with human volunteers showed that a diet high in refined carbohydrate foods resulted in increased intake of kcalories, decreased intake of dietary fiber, and decreased intake of many minerals and vitamins.[26]

Is fiber too good to be true?

The health benefits described above make up an impressive list, but caution is needed in evaluating these claims. The medical problems cited above are caused by many factors, of which the amount of fiber in the diet is just one. For instance, perhaps there are genetic differences between African and Western countries in the incidence of some of these diseases. However, a recent study showed that diverticular disease and hiatus hernia are as common in black as in white Americans; this suggests an environmental rather than a genetic cause.[27]

Increasing fiber intake is just one of many ways serum cholesterol can be lowered.

⟵ Should you permit yourself high intakes of fiber? That may not be advisable. Apart from causing the personal discomfort of loose stools, very high fiber intakes may interfere with the absorption of some nutrients. Some evidence suggests that the absorption of iron, zinc, and calcium may be impaired by a high-fiber diet, although further research is necessary before we can be sure. In the meantime, many medical experts doubt the long-term benefits from diets that are very high in fiber.[28] ⟶

Carbohydrate loading is a controversial method by some long-distance runners to avoid "hitting the wall."

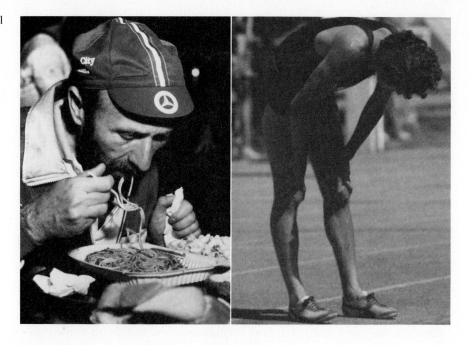

Carbohydrate Loading Helps Long-distance Runners Run Farther, Not Faster

The activity known as carbohydrate loading has become popular among athletes who participate in endurance events lasting more than 60 minutes, such as marathon running and cross-country skiing. It is of no benefit to sprinters or football or basketball players.

Carbohydrate loading means that for three days before the event the athlete eats a diet in which 70% to 80% of the kcalories come from carbohydrate. This diet provides extra glycogen to be loaded into muscles—the extra glycogen may make the difference between finishing a marathon race or "hitting the wall" after 18 miles.

Carbohydrate loading can have harmful effects. Incomplete absorption of the carbohydrate in macaroni and wheat flour may cause diarrhea. The depletion-loading cycle may cause chest pain, depression, lethargy, and abnormal heart patterns. People with heart or kidney disease or adult-onset diabetes could develop severe medical problems from carbohydrate loading. It should not be undertaken by adolescent and preadolescent athletes. In a later chapter the risks and benefits of carbohydrate loading will be explained in more detail.

Sugar is associated with dental caries. A cause and effect relationship between carbohydrate intake and obesity, diabetes, hypoglycemia, and learning or behavior problems has not been proved. Some people cannot digest lactose. Fiber is a laxative and may be involved in lowering the incidence of colon and rectal cancer, appendicitis, and hemorrhoids. Carbohydrate loading may help in endurance athletic events, but it may be harmful in some people.

DIETARY GUIDELINES

The dietary guidelines for carbohydrates are simple:
- Eat foods with adequate starch and fiber
- Avoid too much sugar

DECISIONS

Many personal decisions relating to carbohydrate nutrition involve the following: How can I reduce sugar intake? How safe are artificial sweeteners? What type of fiber, and how much, is good for me?

Let us deal with these practical decisions in that order.

1. How Can I Reduce Sugar Intake?

First you should learn the "smokescreen" words for sugar on food labels. This is becoming increasingly important because of the rapid changes in the consumption of various types of sweeteners, as shown in Figure 3-9. All of the following are sugar, and have about the same nutritive value and contain 4 kcalories per gram: sucrose, brown sugar, confectioner's sugar, granulated sugar, invert sugar (a mixture of glucose and fructose), raw sugar (residue when sugar cane juice is evaporated), high fructose corn sweetener, corn sweeteners, corn syrup, glucose (a.k.a. dextrose), fructose (a.k.a. levulose), lactose, honey, molasses, maple sugar, sorbitol, mannitol, xylitol, and natural sweetners. Quite a mouthful—literally!

An example of three forms of sugar in the same food is the following ingredients label:

INGREDIENTS: Bleached flour, *sugar*, partially hydrogenated vegetable shortening, *dextrose*, water, *corn syrup*, carob, whey blend, cornstarch, salt, sodium bicarbonate, lecithin, artificial flavorings, and artificial colors.

Note that sugar, meaning sucrose, is the primary source of sugar in this food, followed by dextrose and corn syrup.

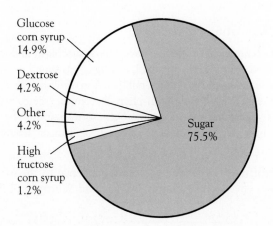

FIGURE 3-9
Per capita consumption of high fructose/corn syrup gains at sugar's expense. Corn syrups are replacing sugar in many foods.

TABLE 3-7 How Much Sugar in Certain Foods?

Food	Sugar (teaspoons)	kcalories*	% RDA kcalories for a 19- to 22-year-old Woman (2100 kcalories)
12-ounce cola	9	180	9%
12-ounce fruit drink, ade, or punch	12	240	11%
1-ounce chocolate bar	5	100	5%
½ cup fruit canned in heavy syrup	4	80	4%

* Approximate

The second way to reduce your sugar intake is to eat unsweetened foods:

- Eat fewer sweetened breakfast cereals, canned fruits
- Eat less candy, cookies, and high-sugar desserts
- Eat more fresh fruit, because the sugar content is lower than when the same fruit is dried or canned
- Eat less jelly
- Drink pure fruit juices, not imitation
- Avoid high-sugar drinks
- Use spices such as cinnamon, coriander, nutmeg, ginger, instead of sugar to flavor foods
- Do not put sugar in tea or coffee

Note that a teaspoonful of sugar has about 20 kcalories. If you did not add one teaspoonful of sugar per day for one year to your coffee, it means 7,300 less kcalories from that one teaspoonful during one year (20 kcalories × 365 days). We will see soon that it requires a loss of 3,500 kcalories to lose one pound of body fat. Therefore, you would lose just over 2 pounds of body fat per year (7,300/3,500) if you did not replace these kcalories from other food sources.

Sugar also makes surprisingly high contributions of kcalories to some foods, as shown in Table 3-7. Be careful here because this is the amount of kcalories coming only from *sugar*. Some of these foods will have other contributors to kcaloric content. For example, the chocolate bar also has fat, so the total amount of kcalories would be higher.

2. How Safe Are Artificial Sweeteners?

The two most common nonnutritive sweeteners, saccharin and aspartame (Nutrasweet) are safe according to the available evidence, as stated in an extensive report on each of these artificial sweeteners published in 1985 by the American Medical Association (AMA).[29,30] People with phenylketonuria (see p. 10) should monitor the amount of aspartame they consume because it contains the amino acid phenylalanine. There was no evidence found of cancer formations caused by aspartame.

This report has not slowed the correspondence to the medical journals on possible harmful effects of aspartame. Dr. Richard Wurtman of the Massachusetts

Institute of Technology is convinced that aspartame intake is associated with seizures.[31] A scientist working for the manufacturer claims that this is not the case.[32] The latest complaint is that aspartame increases motivation to eat, and decreases ratings of fullness.[33] It is predicted that this may lead to disordered patterns of eating even in some people of normal weight.

Aspartame has been approved by the FDA, World Health Organization (WHO), and the regulatory agencies in nearly 50 countries, but some people feel so strongly against its use that they formed a group called Aspartame Victims and Their Friends. If you have a concern about aspartame, you should continue to follow the debate in the medical/scientific literature.

Saccharin in high doses has produced bladder cancer in rats. However, the AMA concludes that there is no evidence of its causing any cancer in humans. The AMA points out some advantages of saccharin use. Saccharin helps in maintaining desirable body weight, in reducing body weight, in preventing dental caries, and in controlling diabetes.[30] You now have the latest evidence, and the decision of whether to consume either of these sweeteners is yours.

3. What Type of Fiber, and How Much, Is Good for Me?

Evidence was presented earlier in this chapter that fiber may play a role in prevention or control of many diseases. The fiber content of different foods is given in Table 3-7. How much of which type of fiber is good for you is still a matter for debate.

Fiber is often classified by its solubility in water:

- Soluble fiber is found in fruit, oat bran, and beans—lowers serum cholesterol and helps control diabetes.
- Insoluble fiber occurs in fruit, vegetables, wheat bran, whole wheat, and beans—may prevent colon and rectal cancer, helps control diverticulosis, and has laxative effect.

The National Cancer Institute in 1984 stated that bran and cellulose fiber may have a protective effect against colon and rectal cancer. This prompted a major manufacturer of breakfast cereals to try to cash in on these benefits of bran. Trade journals point out that sales of this well-known breakfast cereal increased dramatically after this line of advertising was started. This has raised a major issue about claims for disease prevention properties in certain foods.[34] The FDA is investigating such practices.

Marketing

Beware of words on labels about the amount of fiber in the food. These words are misleading frequently. "More fiber," and "high fiber" mean different amounts, depending on the manufacturer. Regulatory agencies have not issued rules that put a level above which high, good, or similar words can be applied to a fiber source.

Finally, decide if the source of fiber is important to you. For example, in the mid-1970s a bread was marketed as being high in fiber and low in kcalories. Sound terrific? Many consumers thought so. Then the media announced that the source of fiber was wood pulp. Within four weeks sales fell to about 15% of their original level. A U.S. Senator was outraged that wood pulp was in our bread. You decide whether the source of the fiber is important to you. From a nutritional point of view, the cellulose is cellulose regardless of whether the source is vegetables or trees.

Summary

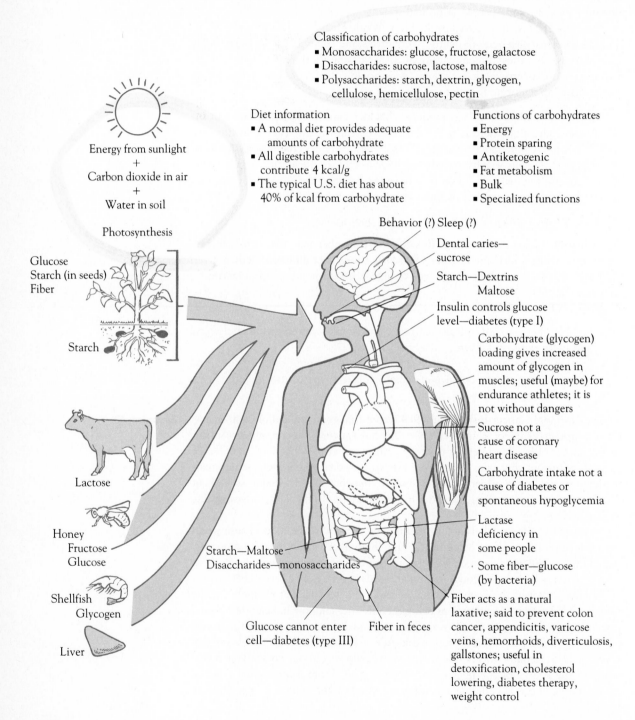

Classification of carbohydrates
- Monosaccharides: glucose, fructose, galactose
- Disaccharides: sucrose, lactose, maltose
- Polysaccharides: starch, dextrin, glycogen, cellulose, hemicellulose, pectin

Diet information
- A normal diet provides adequate amounts of carbohydrate
- All digestible carbohydrates contribute 4 kcal/g
- The typical U.S. diet has about 40% of kcal from carbohydrate

Functions of carbohydrates
- Energy
- Protein sparing
- Antiketogenic
- Fat metabolism
- Bulk
- Specialized functions

Energy from sunlight
+
Carbon dioxide in air
+
Water in soil

Photosynthesis

Glucose
Starch (in seeds)
Fiber

Starch

Lactose

Honey
Fructose
Glucose

Shellfish
Glycogen

Liver

Behavior (?) Sleep (?)

Dental caries—sucrose

Starch—Dextrins
Maltose

Insulin controls glucose level—diabetes (type I)

Carbohydrate (glycogen) loading gives increased amount of glycogen in muscles; useful (maybe) for endurance athletes; it is not without dangers

Sucrose not a cause of coronary heart disease

Carbohydrate intake not a cause of diabetes or spontaneous hypoglycemia

Lactase deficiency in some people

Some fiber—glucose (by bacteria)

Starch—Maltose
Disaccharides—monosaccharides

Glucose cannot enter cell—diabetes (type III)

Fiber in feces

Fiber acts as a natural laxative; said to prevent colon cancer, appendicitis, varicose veins, hemorrhoids, diverticulosis, gallstones; useful in detoxification, cholesterol lowering, diabetes therapy, weight control

REFERENCES

1. Yudkin, J.: Sweet—and sour (book review), Nature **316:**770, 1985.

2. Conners, C.K.: In Nutrition and behavior, J.R. Galler, editor, Plenum Publishing Corporation, New York, 1984.

3. Dahlqvist, A.: Carbohydrates. In Present knowledge in nutrition, 5th edition, Washington, D.C., The Nutrition Foundation, Inc., p. 116, 1984.

4. Federation of American Societies for Experimental Biology, S.C.O.G.S.-69: Evaluation of the health aspects of sucrose as a food ingredient, The Food and Drug Administration, Washington, D.C., 1976.

5. Brown, J.L.: The health hazard of unlabeled ingredients in pharmaceuticals, Pediatrics **73:**402, 1984.

6. Barry, H.M.: Addressing confusion over the role of modified starches, Food Engineering, January, 1986, p. 56.

7. Patrow, C.J., and Marlett, J.A.: Variability in the dietary fiber content of wheat and mixed–grain commercial breads, Journal of the American Dietetic Association **86:**794, 1986.

8. Lanza, E., and Butrum, R.R.: A critical review of food fiber analysis and data, Journal of the American Dietetic Association **86:**732, 1986.

9. Vanderveen, J.E.: Federal regulations. In Dietary fiber: Basic and clinical aspects, G.V. Vahouny and D. Kritchevsky, editors, Plenum Press, New York, 1986.

10. Wilson, D.P., and Endres, R.K.: Compliance with blood glucose monitoring in children with type 1 diabetes mellitus, Journal of Pediatrics **108:**1022, 1986.

11. Henry, R.R., and others: Metabolic consequences of very-low-calorie diet therapy in obese non-insulin-dependent diabetic and nondiabetic subjects, Diabetes **35:**155, 1986.

12. Lipson, L.G.: Diabetes in the elderly: a multifaceted problem, American Journal of Medicine **80**(Suppl 5A):1, 1986.

13. Abu-Bakare, A., and others: Tropical or malnutrition-related diabetes: A real syndrome? Lancet **1:**1135, 1986.

14. Allan, F.N., quoted by Rynearson, E.H.: Americans love hogwash, Nutrition Reviews **32**(Suppl 1):1, 1974.

15. Editorial: Statement on hypoglycemia, Journal of the American Medical Association **223:**682, 1973.

16. Gray, G.E.: Diet, crime and delinquency: A critique, Nutrition Reviews **44**(Suppl): 89, 1986.

17. Schweizer, E., and others: Insulin-induced hypoglycemia and panic attacks, American Journal of Psychiatry **143:**654, 1986.

18. Danowski, T.S., and Sunder, J.H.: Sugar and disease. In Controversies in nutrition, L. Ellenbogen, editor, Churchill Livingstone, New York, 1981, p. 85.

19. Diet and Behavior Symposium proceedings: Summary. Nutrition Reviews **44**(Suppl): 252, 1986.

20. Newcomer, A.D., and McGill, D.B.: Clinical importance of lactase deficiency, New England Journal of Medicine **310**:42, 1984.

21. Kolars, J.C., and others: Yogurt—an autodigesting source of lactose, New England Journal of Medicine **310**:1, 1984.

22. Groothuis, J.R., and others: Effect of carbohydrate ingested on outcome in infants with mild gastroenteritis, Journal of Pediatrics **108**:903, 1986.

23. Anonymous: Diet, nutrition, and oral health, Journal of the American Dental Association **109**:19, 1984.

24. Walker, A.R.P.: Diet and dental caries: A skeptical view, American Journal of Clinical Nutrition **43**:969, 1986.

25. Jenkins, G.N.: Recent changes in dental caries, British Medical Journal **291**:1297, 1985.

26. Heaton, K.W., and others: Not just fibre: The nutritional consequences of refined carbohydrate foods, Human Nutrition: Clinical Nutrition **37C**:31, 1983.

27. Burkitt, D.P., and others: Prevalence of diverticular disease, hiatus hernia, and pelvic phleboliths in black and white Americans, Lancet **ii**:880, 1985.

28. Anonymous: The bran wagon. Lancet **i**:782, 1987.

29. American Medical Association, Council on Scientific Affairs: Aspartame: Review of safety issues, Journal of the American Medical Association **254**:400, 1985.

30. American Medical Association, Council on Scientific Affairs: Saccharin: Review of safety issues, Journal of the American Medical Association **254**:2622, 1985.

31. Wurtman, R.J.: Aspartame: possible effect on seizure susceptibility (letter to the editor), Lancet **2**:1060, 1985.

32. Gaull, G.E.: Aspartame and seizures (letter to the editor), Lancet **2**:1431, 1985.

33. Blundell, J.E., and Hill, A.J.: Paradoxical effects of an intense sweetener (aspartame) on appetite (letter to the editor), Lancet **1**:1092, 1986.

34. Anonymous: Cereal maker's health claims raise broad issues, Tufts University Diet and Nutrition Letter, **4**(4):1, June 1986.

METABOLISM NOTES: *Metabolism of Carbohydrates*

METABOLISM OF CARBOHYDRATES AFTER DIGESTION

Why are carbohydrate-rich foods fattening if we eat a lot of food, and do not exercise? This very practical question is answered in the diagram in Figure 3-10.

Consider what may happen to glucose after it is absorbed from the gastrointestinal system. It may be: (1) used for energy by the cells, (2) converted to glycogen in the liver, (3) stored as fat in the liver, (4) taken to adipose tissue, where it is stored as fat (triglycerides), (5) taken up by muscle cells for either immediate use for energy or for storage as glycogen for future use in energy expenditure.

Some details from Figure 3-10:
1. The body is clever in obtaining the essential carbohydrate, glucose, from several sources after carbohydrates are digested—glucose itself, fructose, galactose, glycogen. Glucose can be obtained also from some amino acids, but that is not shown here.
2. Carbohydrates are fattening irrespective of food source if kcalorie intake is in excess of kcalorie expenditure. For example, Figure 3-10 shows how sugar is fattening. Remember that the sugar has been digested into glucose plus fructose when it enters the diagram here. The fat formed from carbohydrate may be stored in the liver or exported to the adipose tissue. This is done by means of very low density lipoprotein (VLDL). In VLDL the fat is combined with a

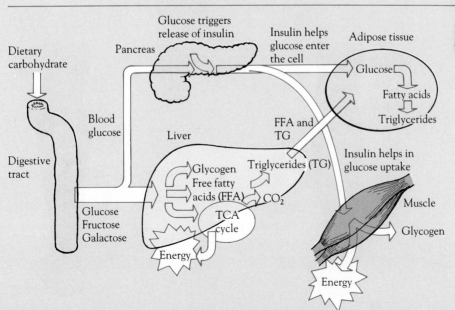

FIGURE 3-10
How dietary carbohydrate is used or stored by the body.

FIGURE 3-11

People with type II, or noninsulin-dependent, diabetes produce adequate insulin in their bodies. Problems arise in obesity because the insulin cannot attach to receptors on the cell membranes, which allows glucose to enter the cell.

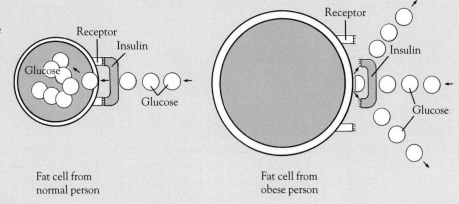

Fat cell from normal person

Fat cell from obese person

FIGURE 3-12

How muscles use glucose and glycogen during fasting, exercise, and carbohydrate loading.

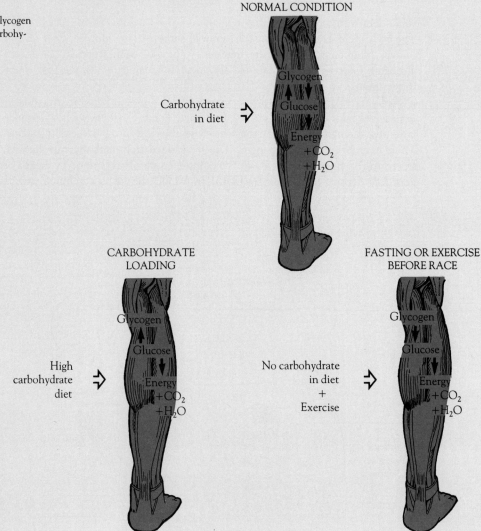

NORMAL CONDITION

Carbohydrate in diet

Glycogen
Glucose
Energy
$+CO_2$
$+H_2O$

CARBOHYDRATE LOADING

High carbohydrate diet

Glycogen
Glucose
Energy
$+CO_2$
$+H_2O$

FASTING OR EXERCISE BEFORE RACE

No carbohydrate in diet + Exercise

Glycogen
Glucose
Energy
$+CO_2$
$+H_2O$

protein, which makes it more easily transportable. We will have much more to discuss about VLDL and some other lipoproteins in Chapter 4.

3. The role of insulin is important in removing glucose from the blood and in helping it enter cells, including the muscle and adipose tissue cells.

Why Must Diabetic People Take Insulin?

Only people with type I or insulin-dependent diabetes mellitus (IDDM) must take injected insulin. The word *mellitus* comes from the Latin meaning "sweet" because of the high amount of glucose in the urine of untreated diabetics.

People with type II or non-insulin-dependent diabetes mellitus (NIDDM) need not take insulin, as seen in Figure 3-11. There is an increase in glucose in the blood, and an increase in circulating insulin at the receptor site in the fat cell. When the fat cell size decreases after weight loss through diet or exercise, insulin can again bind with receptors to get glucose into the cells. About 15% to 20% of the people with type II diabetes are not overweight.

How Does Carbohydrate Loading Help the Endurance Athlete?

The larger arrows in Figure 3-12 indicate the direction of greatest activity. But why does the body go to so much trouble to make glycogen when glucose is the most readily available source of energy? There are three good reasons. First, sufficient glucose is not always available from the blood supply during strenuous exercise. Blood flow through exercising muscles is not continuous. Therefore, reserve of energy in muscles is an advantage. Second, getting glucose ready biochemically for breakdown to energy is slower when the glucose comes from the blood than when the glucose comes from the glycogen in the muscles. Third, the energy yield is 50% greater from glycogen than from glucose. This may seem odd since glycogen is a collection of glucose molecules joined together, but the glucose molecules in glycogen are primed for energy release through different metabolic pathways. It takes more energy input to release the energy in glucose than that in glycogen. The body therefore has a system of allocating energy effectively. It spends the extra energy during times of high energy intake in the diet to make reserves of glycogen for use in times of high energy expenditure.

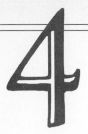

4

The Lipids
Fats and Oils

CONNECTIONS

Do you need all your body fat? Perhaps not, but many people have survived famines on their fat—a form of stored energy, unlike carbohydrates, which are a source of immediate energy. We saw in Chapter 3 how excess carbohydrate is converted into body fat.

Fats, oils, and related substances such as cholesterol have no RDA, but there are still many dietary recommendations about them. High intakes of saturated fat and cholesterol are associated with heart disease. High intakes of total lipids are related to certain cancers, especially cancer of the breast.

Earlier you saw that carbohydrates are sometimes "hidden" in foods; fat presents a similar problem. Whereas you can see the fat in oils and on meats and avoid it, invisible fat, which amounts to half of Americans' fat intake, is more difficult to avoid.

BODY FAT: OLD LIFESAVER, MODERN NUISANCE

How much electrical power does this country really need? An odd question in a nutrition book, but consider this report from the *Wall Street Journal*:

> Two scientists at the University of Illinois at Urbana recently did some calculations and reported that if the 110 million adult Americans who are overweight would slim down and stay slim, the energy that would be saved in planting, cultivating, harvesting, processing, transporting, selling, storing, and cooking the food that now keeps them plump would more than supply the annual residential electrical requirements of Chicago, Boston, San Francisco, and Washington.

This may be a novel way of looking at the problem of overweight and obesity. To the energy costs one could also add costs of diet aids and the costs of medical treatments for obesity-related disorders.

Yet fat does perform vital functions in the body. When your ancestors were forced to endure without food for long periods between harvests, their reserve supply of energy, body fat, made the difference between life and death. Today, of course, with modern agriculture and food processing, this survival mechanism is no longer as important in industrialized countries. Instead, Americans are often concerned with consuming too much fat.

Economics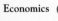

Total intake of a nutrient should not be based on the intake of a few foods rich in the nutrient.

102

Has the public awareness of fat paid off in healthier eating habits? You would think so, if you believe "futurist" John Naisbitt's 1982 statement that "We've reduced our fat intake mightily: butter consumption is down 28%—milk and cream, down 21%—since 1965." Unfortunately, Naisbitt assumes that, since the intake of three fat-containing foods has decreased, total fat intake has decreased. On the contrary, average intake of fat for every man, woman, and child in the United States rose from 55.8 pounds per year during the period from 1970 to 1974 to 61.6 pounds per year in 1984 (Figure 4-1).

More kcalories in the American diet are coming from fat now than at any time since the beginning of this century. The contribution of the various food groups to this intake is interesting. Fats and oils contribute 43%, meats, fish, and poultry 36%, and dairy products only 12% of the total kcalories coming from dietary fat. The proportion of fat from animal and vegetable foods (Figure 4-2) shows that estimating national fat intake based on how much butter, milk, and cream we eat is inaccurate. Our first task, then, must be to consider what the term *fat* means to nutritionists.

> Dietary fat now contributes 43% of total kcalories in the American diet, compared with 32% at the beginning of this century. More fat from plants and less from animal sources is the recent pattern of fat intake.

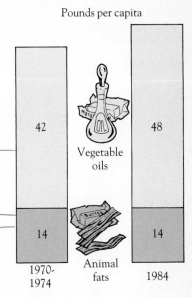

Pounds per capita

FIGURE 4-1
We continue to eat more fat.

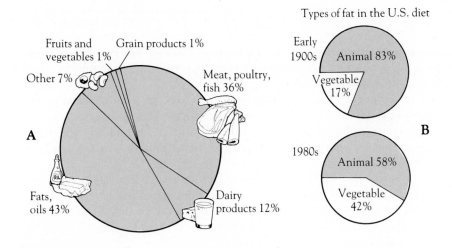

Types of fat in the U.S. diet

A

Fruits and vegetables 1%   Grain products 1%

Other 7%

Meat, poultry, fish 36%

Fats, oils 43%

Dairy products 12%

Early 1900s — Animal 83% / Vegetable 17%

B

1980s — Animal 58% / Vegetable 42%

FIGURE 4-2
A, Contribution of different food groups to the fat content in the U.S. diet. **B,** Types of fat in the diet 1909–1980.

THE CHEMISTRY OF LIPIDS: THEIR ROLE IN HEALTH AND DISEASE

Many familiar terms used to describe the health benefits and hazards of fat will be more understandable after some definitions and a little chemistry. These will enable you to understand information about fat on food labels, to evaluate advice in reducing the quantity and type of fat in your diet, and to understand whether suggested relationships between fat intake and heart disease, cancer, and other health problems apply to you.

Foods high in fat. Food containing hidden fat (left), and some obvious fatty foods (right).

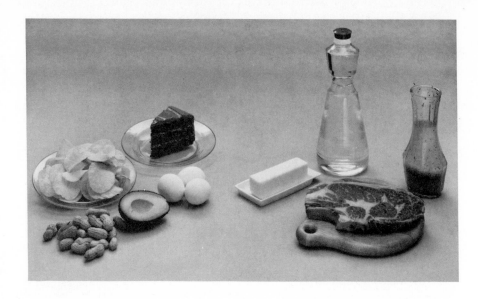

Lipids
Fats, oils, and related substances, including cholesterol and phospholipids

Glycerol
All fats and oils have glycerol as part of their structure; has three-carbon-atom chain that can attach to three fatty acids.

Sterols
Fat-related substances, including cholesterol, sex hormones, and vitamin D; soluble in fat solvents.

Phospholipids
A fat-related substance, in which one of the three fatty acids in a triglyceride is replaced by a phosphorus-containing unit.

Lecithin
A phospholipid, made in the liver; an important part of cell membranes, and an emulsifier in the body and in foods; found in high amounts in soy and egg yolks.

Emulsifier
Allows water and fatty substances to mix; breaks large fat globules into many smaller ones.

Cell Membrane
The cell wall around the outside of cells.

Some Definitions Will Help You Understand What Fat Is

Some of the most important terms related to fats are defined below.

Lipid

Lipid is a generic term that includes fats, oils, and fat-related substances. All are usually insoluble in water but soluble in fat solvents. Note that there is a difference between the popular and the scientific use of the word *fat*. Popular use refers to all of the components described here under the term *lipid*. Scientifically, the following distinction is made:

Fat. To scientists, fat is a solid and oil a liquid at room temperature. Both consist of *glycerol* bonded to one, two, or three fatty acids.

Fat-related substances. Other lipids differ from fats and oils in their chemical makeup, but are classified as lipids because they are also insoluble in water, and soluble only in fat solvents.

The best known fat-related substances are *sterols* and *phospholipids*.

Sterols. These substances occur in foods from plants and animals. The most famous (or infamous) is cholesterol, which is in foods of animal origin only, but other sterols include sex hormones and vitamin D. Sterols are discussed in detail in this chapter.

Phospholipids. A phosphorus-containing unit replaces a fatty acid chain in a fat molecule to form a phospholipid. The best known phospholipid is *lecithin*. It is an important *emulsifier*—a substance that allows water and fatty substances to mix—in our bodies and in foods. Lecithin helps transport fat from one part of the body to another. As part of the *cell membrane*—the wall around the outside of cells—lecithin helps regulate what gets into cells. The highest concentration of lecithin in the body is in nerve cells; the highest concentrations in foods are in eggs and soybeans. You will find lecithin listed as an ingredient in cake mixes and salad dressing, in which it acts as an emulsifier.

A Little Chemistry Also Helps You Understand Fat

Fat and oil molecules consist of carbon, hydrogen, and oxygen atoms. Both fats and oils are made up of one molecule of glycerol combined with one, two, or three fatty acids. These combinations are called mono-, di- or triglycerides.

Over 40 different fatty acids are found in nature. Therefore, a great number of different fatty acids can be joined in different combinations to the glycerol molecule. *Triglycerides*—three fatty acids bonded to one molecule of glycerol—are the most important in nutrition. Over 90% of the lipids in food and in the body are triglycerides. Therefore, when we talk of fat in the body or in food we are really referring to triglycerides. Serum triglyceride measurements indicate the amount of fat in blood. Some research indicates that high triglyceride values may be warning signs for coronary heart disease. The other lipids are monoglycerides and diglycerides, individual or "free" fatty acids, and lipid-related substances.

Different fatty acids are involved in the formation of triglycerides. Two chemical properties of fatty acids are of interest to nutritionists. These are the length of the carbon-atom chain, and the way the carbon atoms are linked together. The latter is called the *degree of saturation* of the fatty acid.

Each fatty acid consists of a chain of carbon atoms. The length of the chain allows fatty acids to be grouped as short-, medium-, and long-chain. Short-chain fatty acids are not important in nutrition. Of interest to trivia fans is the fact that butyric acid (4 carbon atoms) occurs in butter, hence its name. Medium-chain fatty acids of 8 to 12 carbon atoms comprise 10% of the lipid in our food. The long-chain fatty acids of 14, 16, 18, or 20 carbons are the most important in nutrition.

There Are Three Degrees of Saturation

We will use examples of three different fatty acids, each with a chain length of 18 carbon atoms, to demonstrate the three degrees of saturation—saturated, monounsaturated, and polyunsaturated. The fat in the typical American diet is about 37% saturated, 41% monounsaturated, and 12% polyunsaturated. Note that the numbers do not add up to 100%. The difference is made up of other minor fat components in the diet. For health reasons, it is suggested that the percentage of saturated fat should be reduced. Notice that it takes only one or two double bonds to make all the difference in the nutritional value and physical properties of these three kinds of fatty acids.

Saturated means that no more hydrogen atoms can be bonded to any of the carbon atoms in the chain; in other words, the carbon atoms are saturated with hydrogen atoms. An example of a saturated fatty acid is stearic acid, shown in Figure 4-3. Stearic acid is an 18-carbon chain with no double bonds that is found in butter, egg yolk, chocolate, and lard.

There are two types of *unsaturated fatty acids: monounsaturated,* having one double bond in the chain; and *polyunsaturated,* having two or more double bonds in the chain. These are also shown in Figure 4-3. An example of a monounsaturated fatty acid is oleic acid, which is a chain with 18 carbons and one double bond; it is found in peanut butter, cooking oils, French dressing, lard, almonds, and olive oil. An example of polyunsaturated fatty acid is linoleic acid, a chain with 18 carbons and two double bonds. This essential fatty acid is highest in soft margarine, peanut butter, cooking oils, walnuts, and Brazil nuts.

Triglycerides
Three fatty acids attached to one molecule of glycerol; most of the fat and oil in food and in the body are triglycerides.

Degree of Saturation
Saturated means all carbon atoms have their maximum number of of hydrogen atoms; unsaturated fat has some carbons without the maximum amount of hydrogen.

Some studies show that saturated fat elevates serum cholesterol. Therefore, high intakes may be related to coronary heart disease.

Polyunsaturated fat lowered serum cholesterol in some studies.

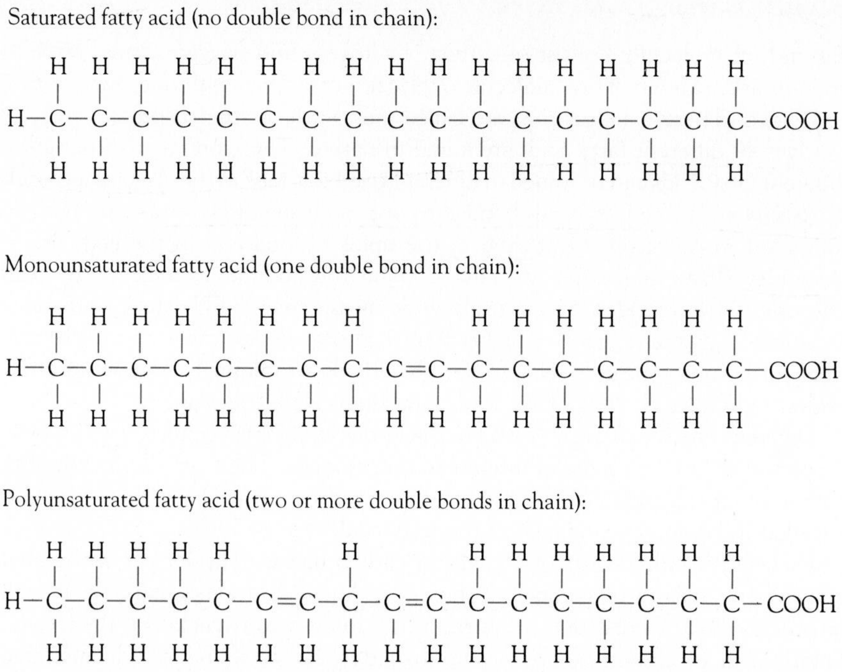

FIGURE 4-3
Three kinds of fatty acids.

Saturated fatty acid (no double bond in chain):

```
    H   H   H   H   H   H   H   H   H   H   H   H   H   H   H   H
    |   |   |   |   |   |   |   |   |   |   |   |   |   |   |   |
H—C—C—C—C—C—C—C—C—C—C—C—C—C—C—C—C—COOH
    |   |   |   |   |   |   |   |   |   |   |   |   |   |   |   |
    H   H   H   H   H   H   H   H   H   H   H   H   H   H   H   H
```

Monounsaturated fatty acid (one double bond in chain):

```
    H   H   H   H   H   H   H   H           H   H   H   H   H   H
    |   |   |   |   |   |   |   |           |   |   |   |   |   |
H—C—C—C—C—C—C—C—C—C=C—C—C—C—C—C—C—COOH
    |   |   |   |   |   |   |   |   |   |   |   |   |   |   |   |
    H   H   H   H   H   H   H   H   H   H   H   H   H   H   H   H
```

Polyunsaturated fatty acid (two or more double bonds in chain):

```
    H   H   H   H   H           H           H   H   H   H   H   H
    |   |   |   |   |           |           |   |   |   |   |   |
H—C—C—C—C—C—C=C—C—C=C—C—C—C—C—C—C—C—COOH
    |   |   |   |   |   |   |   |   |   |   |   |   |   |   |   |
    H   H   H   H   H   H   H   H   H   H   H   H   H   H   H   H
```

Most saturated fats are solids, and polyunsaturated fats are soft or liquid at room temperature. The exceptions are coconut oil and palm oil, which are highly saturated yet soft at room temperature. The greater the degree of unsaturation, the softer or more liquid the triglyceride is likely to be at room temperature. Chain length is also important. The shorter the chain length, the higher the probability the triglyceride will be a liquid at room temperature. Butterfat has many short-chain acids.

Saturated and Unsaturated Fats Have Different Food Sources

In general, the triglycerides in most foods of animal origin are saturated and those in foods of plant origin are unsaturated. However, the degree of unsaturation varies within these two groups. You can see this for yourself when, at room temperature, you squeeze fat from beef, pork, or lamb between your fingers. It is fairly firm, whereas fat from poultry is less firm. Fat from some fish is actually an oil—for example, cod liver oil. Therefore, triglycerides from some fish can be very unsaturated.

Many of the triglycerides from plants are in the form of oil, especially those from seeds. Oils rich in polyunsaturates include cottonseed, soy bean, peanut, safflower, sesame, and sunflower oil. Exceptions are cocoa butter and palm and coconut oil because they have a high degree of saturation.

You can use the above information to explain some chemical properties of margarine. It is made from vegetable oils, and is more spreadable than butter. This is in part due to a high concentration of linoleic acid. But there are differences in degree of saturation among the margarines. Tub margarine (soft) is more unsaturated than stick margarine (harder). However, note that some margarines are more spreadable because they are whipped or have added water.

Most margarines include partially hydrogenated soy bean, sunflower, or some other oil. If these oils were used in their natural state, you would have liquid margarine. Thus, the oil is hardened by *hydrogenation*—the forcing of hydrogen into polyunsaturated oils under controlled conditions, which makes the fat become more saturated. High intakes of saturated fat may be related to a higher incidence of coronary heart disease. Human beings and farm animals also hydrogenate some dietary polyunsaturated fatty acids during digestion or metabolism.

Double bonds are chemically very unstable. Oxygen in the air can react with the double bonds of fatty acids in food, producing off flavors and off odors. We say that such unpalatable food is rancid. Most likely this food will not be eaten. Rancidity is prevented by protection from air, by refrigeration, by partial hydrogenation (because the number of double bonds is reduced), or by the use of antioxidants. A natural antioxidant is vitamin E. However, it is rarely added to foods for this purpose. It is expensive, and is not as effective as synthetic antioxidants. Antioxidant food additives include BHT *(butylated hydroxytoluene)* and BHA *(butylated hydroxyanisole)*, which appear frequently on food labels. Vitamin C also prevents rancidity in foods.

Knowledge of Lipid Chemistry Has Medical Applications

"No cholesterol!" the commercials shout. "High in polyunsaturates!" Many medical experts think that high levels of cholesterol in blood increase the risk of coronary heart disease,[1] and so they advise people to reduce the amount of cholesterol in their diet. Some studies indicate that blood cholesterol is decreased by polyunsaturated fats in the diet and increased by saturated fat—hence the advertising emphasis on oils and margarines high in polyunsaturates.

Two Physical Properties of Fat Are Important in Nutrition

Fat has two physical properties that we should take notice of:

- It is insoluble in water
- It floats on water

What does this mean for your health?

Insolubility in water

Because fats are insoluble in water, they may cause problems during digestion and in the transportation of lipids in blood. Certainly you don't want lumps of fat just sitting in your intestine or floating in your blood.

A related problem is that fat-soluble substances are not excreted after they are absorbed into the body, only water-soluble substances are. In other words, you cannot urinate or sweat away fat or chemicals soluble in fat, which shows why it's difficult to lose excess fat if you're overweight. The only ways to get rid of excess body fat are to reduce the intake of kcalories, to exercise more, or, best of all, to combine both of these methods.

Food technology

Hydrogenation
Addition of hydrogen to unsaturated fat; used to harden oils in the manufacture of some foods, such as margarine.

BHT, BHA
Butylated hydroxytoluene, butylated hydroxyanisole; food additives that are antioxidants.

It is impossible to "melt away" body fat, because it cannot be excreted in urine or perspiration.

These facts about solubility also explain why you are more likely to suffer a toxic reaction from swallowing excessive amounts of fat-soluble vitamins (A, D, E, and K) than from taking in excess water-soluble vitamins (C and B-complex), which are excreted in the urine and usually don't build up to toxic levels.

The body, which is 60% to 70% water, deals with the insolubility of lipids in water in a clever way. Water-insoluble fat is attached to a protein, forming water-soluble lipoproteins. Lipoproteins are important in the transport and measurement of cholesterol in the blood.

Floating on Water

Fat floats on water, which is why you see fat-rich cream floating on the top of milk and why it can be easily skimmed off. In the same way, a fat person floats more easily in water than a muscular person of the same weight. This is the basis for one method of body fat measurement; the person is weighed under water and then out of the water; the differences in flotation are used to calculate the amount of body fat he or she has (see page 298).

(see page 298)

The fact that fat floats on water also has implications for your digestion. When you eat a meal the carbohydrates, proteins, and fats become separated in the stomach: fat floats on top, leaving carbohydrates and proteins near the bottom of the stomach, which means they will move on to the small intestine before the fat will. This explains the effect called *satiety:* if you eat a meal high in fat, the fat remaining in your stomach will make you feel "full" for a longer time than if you eat a low-fat meal.

> Lipids are fats, oils, and other chemical substances (the best known are cholesterol and lecithin) that are insoluble in water. Fats and oils contain glycerol and fatty acids. Fatty acids may be saturated (mainly in foods of animal origin), or unsaturated (mainly in oils from plants). Oils can be "hardened" by hydrogenation. Antioxidants like BHT, BHA, or vitamin E prevent rancidity in foods. About 95 percent of the lipids in our food and bodies are triglycerides. In the typical U.S. diet, saturated, monounsaturated, and polyunsaturated fatty acids amount to 37%, 41%, and 12%, respectively.

FAT: DO WE NEED IT AND CAN WE SEE IT?

By now you may think the message is strong and clear: you don't need fat in your life. But this is not quite true; you need some. However, to avoid taking in too much requires some skill, since fat is so "invisible" in the American diet. Let us consider these two aspects of fat intake.

Five Reasons You Need Some Fat in Your Diet

Source of essential fatty acid

This is the most important reason why we need fat in our diet. *Linoleic acid*—a polyunsaturated fatty acid found in highest amounts from plants—is the only

---

Margin notes:

You will feel hungry sooner after a meal high in carbohydrate or protein than after a "fatty" meal.

Linoleic Acid
Essential fatty acid, polyunsaturated; available in foods from plants.

essential fatty acid (EFA). Recent evidence suggests that other fatty acids may be essential, but it is too soon to say with certainty which ones are EFAs.[2] Deficiency symptoms of EFA include below-normal growth, scaly skin, and above-normal loss of water through the skin. The experts suggest a minimum dietary requirement for EFA of 1% of total kcalorie intake and the optimum at about 4%.[3] Translating this into practical terms, there are very few people in the population who should suffer from a dietary deficiency of EFA. We saw above that margarine, peanut butter, cooking oils, and certain nuts are rich sources. These, combined with other good plant sources, plus small amounts from foods of animal origin, provide adequate amounts of linoleic acid in our diet.

It may seem odd that progress in medical science in recent years caused most of the incidences of EFA deficiency. Total parenteral nutrition (TPN) supplies nutrient requirements through a vein to patients who cannot take food by mouth. In the early days there was very little fat in TPN solutions because of the problems of putting a water-insoluble substance directly into the blood. Some patients showed symptoms of EFA deficiency when TPN without lipids was used over a long time period. This problem has been solved now.

Medicine

Source of energy

Because 1 g of fat or oil provides 9 kcalories of energy, and 1 g of carbohydrate or protein provides only 4 kcalories, fat is 2¼ times more concentrated in energy than either carbohydrate or protein. Therefore, it is a more efficient form of energy storage in the body than the same weight of glycogen. Fat is important in special diets requiring high amounts of energy in limited volume. More attention is given to the negative aspects of high fat intakes. For many people, especially those who do not exercise a lot, the high energy content of fat may cause problems in body weight control.

Carrier of fat-soluble vitamins

The fat-soluble vitamins—A, D, E, and K—are carried in fat in plant and animal foods. Some dietary fat is needed to absorb fat-soluble vitamins.

Palatability

Palatability means taste, flavor, and juiciness, qualities that fat enhances in food.[4] Knowing this, you can see why it is so difficult to follow government guidelines about reducing fat in your diet. Hamburger, for instance, has about 30% fat when you buy it in the supermarket. You *can* buy lean ground meat with only 5% to 10% fat, but many people might find this healthy hamburger dry and tasteless.

Pure fat is almost tasteless, but it can absorb many fat-soluble flavors. Palatability is a growing area of research activity. Until recently few studies have examined taste responsiveness to a variety of fatty and creamy flavors.[4]

Sometimes the most nutritious form of a food may not be the most palatable.

Satiety Value

Lipids delay the emptying of the stomach. Therefore, a full feeling lasts longer after eating a fatty or oily meal. This may have negative effects immediately before athletic events.

TABLE 4-1 Consumption of Visible and Invisible Food Fats per Person, 1967–1981

	Pounds per Person	
	1967	1980
Visible Fat		
Butter (fat content)	4.4	3.6
Lard (direct use)	5.4	2.5
Margarine (fat content)	8.4	9.2
Shortening	16	18
Cooking and salad oils	13	21
Other oils and fats	2.4	1.5
Total Visible Fat	49.2	56.4
Invisible Fats		
Dairy products, excluding butter	16	15
Eggs	4.2	3.5
Meat, poultry, fish	47	48
Beans, nuts, soy, cocoa	6.2	5.8
Fruits, vegetables	1.1	1.1
Grain products	1.7	1.7
Total Invisible Fat	75	74
Total Visible and Invisible Fats and Oils	125	131

About Half of the Lipid in the U.S. Diet Is Invisible

An internationally known tennis player stated not long ago that she eats no fat. Could she be right? Not really; on a balanced diet, eating no fat is almost impossible because fat is present in so many foods—and much of it is invisible. What she meant, therefore, is that there is no *visible* fat in her diet. Table 4-1 shows how visible and invisible food fats are usually present in the average American's diet. Note that between 1967 and 1980, a person was more likely to put on pounds from invisible fat than from visible fat.

What we have seen is that futurists and tennis players alike may have insufficient information about fat intake. Because they are not alone in their ignorance, in 1986 the National Cancer Institute set an objective that by 1990, 70% of the population should be able to identify foods that are low in fat.[5] This means that many people in the United States simply are unaware of the triglyceride content of different foods—which is unfortunate, because low fat intake is an important means of preventing killers like coronary heart disease and some cancers.

If you really want to reduce fat in your diet, the sources of visible fat are easy to recognize, as Table 4-1 shows. Almost anything greasy contains fat. However, let us now consider some surprising sources of hidden fat (Table 4-2). We use pats

TABLE 4-2 Fat Is Hidden in Some Surprising Places

Food Name	Fat Content (Equivalence to Pats of Butter*)	Fast-food Supplier
Chicken Items		
Chicken Sandwich (on wheat bun)	2	Wendy's
Chicken Breast (Original Recipe)	2½	Kentucky Fried Chicken
Roasted Chicken Breast (no bun)	2½	Arby's
Chicken McNuggets	4	McDonald's
Chicken Fillet Sandwich	5	Hardee's
Chicken Breast Sandwich (fried)	5½	Arby's
Chicken Supreme Sandwich	7	Jack-in-the-Box
Specialty Chicken Sandwich	8½	Burger King
Extra Crispy Dark Dinner	11	Kentucky Fried Chicken
Fish Items		
Shrimp Salad (no dressing)	⅕	Jack-in-the-Box
Baked Fish (with sauce)	½	Long John Silver's
Fish (with Batter, 2 pieces)	5	Long John Silver's
Filet-O-Fish	5	McDonald's
Shrimp Salad	6	Hardee's
Potato Items		
Plain potato	0	Roy Rogers
Potato with margarine	1½	Roy Rogers
Potato with Broccoli'n Cheese	3½	Roy Rogers
Mushroom & Cheese Potato	4½	Arby's
Broccoli & Cheese Potato	4½	Arby's
Broccoli & Cheese Potato	5	Wendy's
Cheese Stuffed Potato	7	Wendy's

*Two pats of butter are equivalent to the fat content of any one of the following: 1 doughnut, 2 cookies, ½ cup of tuna salad, ⅓ avocado, or 2 small bran muffins.

of butter as an easy reference point for the amount of fat in these well-known foods. There are 90 pats of butter (a pat weighs 5 g) in a pound of butter. Each pat contains 4 g of fat, amounting to 36 kcalories. Therefore, multiply 36 kcalories by the number of pats of butter to get total kcalories from fat.

Is something advertised as "low-fat" in a fast-food outlet really low fat? Chicken, fish, and potatoes, for example, are certainly low in fat—except when cooked in oil or when they have high-fat foods added to them. And when you make yourself a sandwich or salad using mayonnaise, oil, or salad dressing, you may well be adding as many kcalories as you might get in a fast-food restaurant.

Don't be fooled by ads: many low-fat foods may be cooked by high-fat methods.

Interpreting "No Cholesterol" Ads Is a Necessary Skill

As Table 4-3 shows, cholesterol is found only in foods of animal origin. Hence, any food processors who boast that their products made entirely from plants "contain no cholesterol!" are not stating anything unusual.

Three concerns to note about cholesterol are as follows:

- Though fish oils have the highest cholesterol content per 100 g, they are not usually eaten in as large amounts as some foods of lower cholesterol content.
- Until recently people with high serum cholesterol levels were advised not to eat shellfish. Now we know that not all shellfish are very high in cholesterol. The American Medical Association states that shrimp can be included occasionally in the diets of people with high serum cholesterol levels.[6]
- There is a wide range in cholesterol content within some food groups. For example, values for finfish range from 19 to 108 mg of cholesterol per 100 g of fish. Therefore, the information in Table 4-3 is useful as a general reference. (If you must regulate your cholesterol intake closely, see the information by Hepburn and others indicated at the bottom of Table 4-3.)

Always consider the quantity of a food eaten in your normal diet in determining the significance of that food on the intake of a nutrient.

> Lipids in the diet provide the essential fatty acid, energy, transport of the fat-soluble vitamins, palatability, and satiety. About half of dietary fat is invisible in eggs, dairy products, beans, nuts, grain products, meats, and fast foods. Cholesterol is in foods of animal origin only.

FIGURE 4-4
Digestion and absorption of lipids.

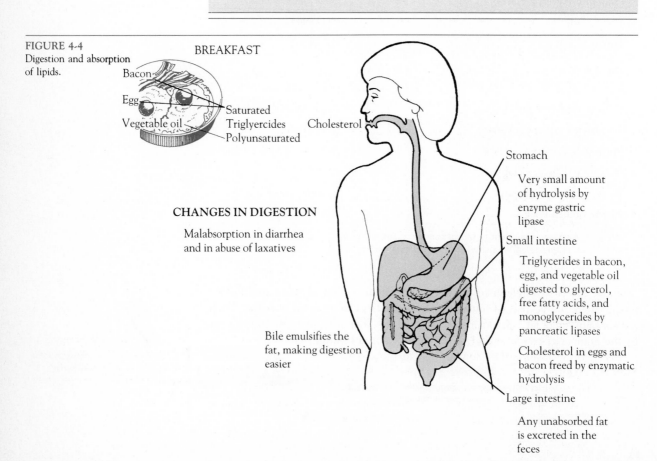

BREAKFAST

Bacon
Egg
Vegetable oil
Saturated
Triglyercides
Polyunsaturated
Cholesterol

CHANGES IN DIGESTION

Malabsorption in diarrhea and in abuse of laxatives

Bile emulsifies the fat, making digestion easier

Stomach
Very small amount of hydrolysis by enzyme gastric lipase

Small intestine
Triglycerides in bacon, egg, and vegetable oil digested to glycerol, free fatty acids, and monoglycerides by pancreatic lipases

Cholesterol in eggs and bacon freed by enzymatic hydrolysis

Large intestine
Any unabsorbed fat is excreted in the feces

TABLE 4-3 Where's the Cholesterol?

Cholesterol* (mg per 100 g, or 3½ oz)	Food Source
588 (485-766)	Fish oils
525	Whole egg
238 (219-256)	Butter, butter oil
121 (59-182)	Crab, lobster, shrimp
98 (90-105)	Cheese
95	Lard
93 (85-100)	Chicken fat, duck fat
84 (58-109)	Poultry products
84 (67-110)	Pork products
76 (60-99)	Beef
71 (71-71)	Lamb and veal
55 (30-141)	Clams, oysters, scallops
54 (19-108)	Finfish (bass, cod, herring, pike, salmon, tuna, etc)
40 (17-59)	Salad dressing (only those with cheese or eggs; for instance blue cheese or mayonnaise)
0	Cereal grains, margarine, some salad dressing, vegetable oils, fruits, legumes, nuts and seeds, vegetables

*The American Heart Association and other organizations recommend a total intake of 300 mg cholesterol per day.

HOW LIPIDS ARE DIGESTED AND ABSORBED

Most fats, whether of plant or animal origin, are digested in the body—at least in healthy people—and about 5% is eliminated with the feces. Let's examine how digestion, absorption, and transportation work.

Fat Is Digested into Free Fatty Acids, Glycerol, and Monoglycerides

Lipid molecules are too big to pass from the digestive tract to the blood. Therefore, they must be broken down to their constituents: fatty acids and glycerol. Some monoglycerides can be absorbed intact.

Figure 4-4 shows the digestion of a meal containing saturated and polyunsaturated triglycerides, cholesterol, and phospholipids. The small intestine is where most of the action in the digestion and absorption of lipids occurs. Enzymes from the pancreas attack the fat molecules. Bile emulsifies the fat globule, which makes it easier for the enzymes to do their digestive work. This emulsification can mean up to a 10,000-fold increase in surface area of the lipid. Lipids are not digested properly if the pancreas does not secrete the lipid-splitting enzymes, if bile is not

There may be adequate amounts of fat-soluble vitamins in the diet, yet the person may have a deficiency of these vitamins. This could be due to faulty fat absorption.

produced or secreted in sufficient quantities, or if there are changes in the structure of the wall of the intestine. Incomplete digestion of lipid means that other lipid-soluble substances are not absorbed either. The most notable of these are the fat-soluble vitamins. Undigested lipid and lipid-soluble substances are eliminated with the feces, giving it a soapy appearance.

Lipids Are Transported in Water-Soluble Lipoproteins

Micelles
Combinations of lipids and bile salts that bring lipids from the gastrointestinal tract into contact with the intestinal cell wall. From there the lipids are absorbed into the circulation.

Fatty acids, glycerol, some monoglycerides, and bile salts, including cholesterol, are incorporated into *micelles*, which deliver these lipids to the intestinal wall for absorption. This is where the chemical structure of the fatty acid determines which of two routes is taken to get lipids to tissues throughout the body.

Short- and medium-chain fatty acids, some preformed dietary phospholipids, and glycerol have some solubility in water. They are taken by the blood to the liver, from which they are delivered to the rest of the body.

TABLE 4-4 Lipoproteins Perform Important Functions in the Blood

	Chylomicrons	VLDL	LDL	HDL
Composition	Triglyceride	Triglyceride	Cholesterol	Cholesterol-phospholipid
Origin	Intestine	Liver and intestine	Metabolic end product of VLDL	Liver and intestine
Function	Transport dietary triglycerides	Transport dietary triglycerides	Transport cholesterol and phospholipids to cells	Believed to transport cholesterol from cells to liver

Lymphatic System
Transports some lipids, and some other nutrients after absorption from the gastrointestinal tract; it drains eventually into the blood.

Long-chain fatty acids, cholesterol, and phospholipids (found in intestinal tissues) are insoluble in water. They are made water-soluble by being surrounded by a protein to form a lipoprotein called chylomicrons. These carry the absorbed lipid through the *lymphatic system* to all parts of the body, draining eventually into the blood. Other lipoproteins important in lipid transport are HDL, LDL, and VLDL—short for high-, low-, and very low-density lipoprotein, respectively. The fact that fat floats on water is used in this classification of the lipoproteins. As Table 4-4 shows, most fat is in VLDL, less in LDL, and least in HDL. All lipoproteins have triglycerides, phospholipids, cholesterol, and protein.

> Dietary fat is digested into free fatty acids, glycerol, and monoglycerides. Lipids are transported around the body in water-soluble lipoproteins—chylomicrons, VLDL, LDL, and HDL.

THE USES OF LIPIDS IN THE BODY

Let us consider some questions and answers about fat—answers that relate to the weight-reducing diets to be discussed later in the book.

Where Does Body Fat Come From?

That lump of fatty tissue that you can pinch is the final resting place for some of the dietary fat we followed through digestion and absorption (Figure 4-4). Some of the fat in that pinch may also come from dietary carbohydrate or protein or from alcohol. Formation of fat from these sources happens when the total number of kcalories from all dietary sources is greater than the number of kcalories spent in energy. Most of these conversions take place in the liver.

What Do Fat Cells Look Like?

Fat is stored in cells called adipocytes. As the figure below shows, they are oval or round and are about 0.1 millimeter in diameter.

Cell biology

Is Fat Uniform in Various Parts of the Body?

Fat is not of uniform composition everywhere in the body. Fatty acid composition varies in *subcutaneous fat,* the fat that is nearest to the skin, from different sites within a person. Fat under the skin is more unsaturated than "deep" fat.

Fatty acid composition can vary between people not only because of diet but also because of age—a baby puts on more saturated fat than unsaturated fat during its first year. Moreover, men have more saturated fat than women do. How much

Subcutaneous Fat
Fat that is nearest to the skin.

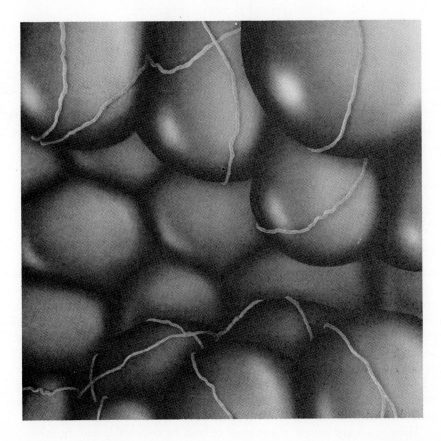

Cluster of adipocytes.
Connective tissue strands bind the cells together.

FIGURE 4-5
Body fat in men and women.

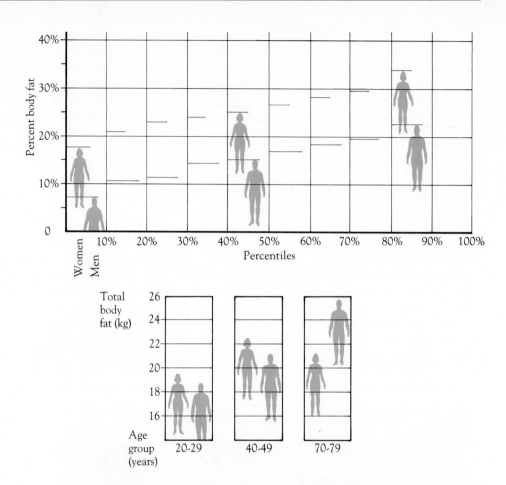

of this is due to differences in the type of diet eaten is still open to debate.[7] Even the amount of blood serving the fat depot is dependent on location in the body and the age and diet of the person.

What Are the Functions of Lipids in the Body?

Fat in the body is often criticized and seldom praised in American society, but lipids do have some useful functions. Let's discuss five functions of body fat.

Energy reserve

Up until age 70, women have greater amounts of body fat than men of the same age; this trait is illustrated in Figures 4-5. The concentrated energy in fat has played an important role in the survival of the human race. Until recent times it was not uncommon to have periods of plenty (harvest time) followed by hungry periods before the next harvest. The extra fat allowed women to survive longer than men in these times of food shortage. The same effect was observed among World War II concentration camp victims and has also been seen among survivors of famines. This protection of women is nature's way of preserving the potential to reproduce the next generation. Additional fat gained during pregnancy is an added protection against severe food shortages during pregnancy and lactation.

There is a lower limit to the amount of body fat compatible with health. Men can get by with only about 5% fat; women, however, with only 5% body fat might experience cessation of menstruation and bone loss. Five percent body fat is the amount found in the bodies of male world-class long-distance runners and of swimmers who compete over short distances. Marathon swimmers, on the other hand, tend to have over 20% body fat. The 40% to 50% found in obese people is simply unnecessary reserve energy in our affluent society.

Insulation

In order to maintain your body temperature within acceptable limits, you use a lot of kcalories. The efficiency of this process is helped by the insulating properties of fat under the skin (subcutaneous fat). This feature is helpful in cold climates but, of course, can be very uncomfortable if you live in the tropics.

Cell membranes

The movement of nutrients into cells and of the end products of metabolism out of cells requires the crossing of a barrier formed by the cell membrane. If there is a breakdown in this process, cells die from a lack of nutrients or are poisoned by a build-up of toxic end products of metabolism. Lipids in cell membranes are combined with phosphorus to form two phospholipid layers, as Figure 4-6 illustrates; notice also the presence of protein in the membrane structure. Proteins act as catalysts and help material enter and leave the cell. The proportion of different fatty acids gives membranes different degrees of fluidity. This means there are different degrees of permeability to meet the specific requirements of the cell. The fatty acid composition of the membrane is influenced by the fatty acid composition of the diet.[8] Cholesterol is also an important component of cell membranes.

Cell biology

Manufacture of prostaglandins

Prostaglandins are manufactured in the body from polyunsaturated fatty acids. Linoleic acid, the essential fatty acid, is involved in this process. The diet of most people is not deficient in these fatty acids.

Prostaglandins—misnamed because it was once believed they were produced in

---

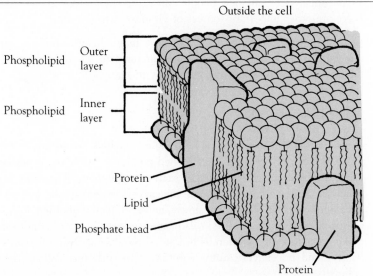

Outside the cell

Phospholipid — Outer layer

Phospholipid — Inner layer

Protein

Lipid

Phosphate head

Protein

FIGURE 4-6
Phospholipids are important in cell membranes.

Endocrinology

the prostate gland—are called "local hormones" because they are made in the tissue in which they are used. Most other hormones, by contrast, are made in one tissue but perform their function in other parts of the body. Among their many functions, prostaglandins stimulate the action of smooth muscles—for example, those involved in childbirth—reduce blood pressure, and regulate stomach secretions (important in digestion).

Protection of important body organs

In both humans and animals, fat provides a cushion around important organs. You can see examples of this in beef and pork in a butcher's meat case in the fat appearing around the kidneys, heart, and reproductive organs.

> Body fat is stored in cells called adipocytes. Diet influences their chemical composition. Body fat provides energy reserve and insulation, is part of cell membranes, is involved in making prostaglandins, and provides protection for vital body organs.

DO LIPIDS CAUSE PROBLEMS IN THE DIET?

No one likes food that is rancid—the word comes from the Latin and means "stinking"—and probably no one really wants to eat cancer-causing foods, but is there really any problem caused by lipids? Let us take a look.

Rancid Foods

The more unsaturated the fat is, the more likely it is that it will become rancid (unless an antioxidant is used). Foods most likely to go rancid are fatty fish and fish oil, deep-fried foods, and foods with a large surface area (powdered foods).

Although some chemicals produced when fat becomes rancid may be toxic and though rancidity destroys vitamin A, these scientific facts have little practical significance. After all, few people can bring themselves to eat rancid food, and there are other important sources of vitamin A in the diet.

If rancidity does not seem to be a major health problem, research still is needed on the long-term effects of what happens when people eat *mildly* rancid fats including those occurring frequently in many kitchens.[9]

Heated Cooking Oils

Fast-food restaurants use cooking oils at high temperatures while preparing foods like fried chicken or French-fried potatoes. Are toxic or potentially cancer-causing substances produced under such circumstances? This topic is controversial because some laboratory animals repeatedly fed these oils lost their appetites, developed diarrhea, grew more slowly, and even died, but others showed no harmful effects. In one study, rats fed oils heated repeatedly under conditions resembling commercial food preparation techniques showed some tissue changes—but another study found no cancer-causing substances in such oils. What, then, are we to believe?

Recently, three experts examined the most up-to-date evidence on heated fat fed to experimental animals and concluded that most of the research used unrealistic conditions.[10] Although such information may be scientifically useful, it may have little practical significance. In any case, if you are a fast-food eater, you probably have a built-in safety mechanism: food prepared with oil heated repeatedly has an unpleasant taste and odor. ◁

Take experimental results seriously if realistic conditions were used; otherwise treat them cautiously.

Trans Fatty Acids

Some polyunsaturated fatty acids are twisted into unusual shapes during hydrogenation. Enzymes involved in fat metabolism cannot act on these *trans fatty acids*.

Trans fatty acids are mentioned here for two reasons:

Trans Fatty Acids
Polyunsaturated fatty acids twisted into unusual shapes during hydrogenation. Enzymes involved in fat metabolism cannot catalyze these unusually shaped molecules.

- They illustrate how nutritional knowledge is in constant flux. Whereas 10 years ago a nutrition textbook might have mentioned the possible role of trans fatty acids in heart disease and cancer, today we can report that no reliable scientific evidence supports such a relationship. We still, however, have much to learn about the long-term effects of these substances on health.
- They illustrate how food processors respond to research. When possible adverse effects of trans fatty acids were first suggested, margarine was the food with the highest concentration of these substances, because they were produced during partial hydrogenation of the vegetable oils used in margarine manufacturing. Now food technology has reduced them to negligible amounts in most margarines.

Food technology

No health damage is likely to result from chemical changes in fat resulting from rancidity, extensive reheating of cooking oil at high temperatures, or hydrogenation causing trans fatty acids. The unpleasant odors and tastes produced are likely to warn people off.

DO LIPIDS CAUSE PROBLEMS IN THE BODY?

Although lipids may not be a threat to our health as toxic substances in the diet, there are certain lipids that seem to have connections to heart disease and cancers when they build up in the body—at least for some people. A great many reports recommend that people reduce their intakes of fat and cholesterol as a prevention against coronary heart disease and certain cancers.

Among the several august bodies in the United States that have approved this advice are: the Inter-Society Commission for Heart Disease Resources (1970), the American Heart Association (1978), the U.S. Department of Agriculture/Health and Human Services (1980), the Committee on Diet, Nutrition and Cancer of the National Academy of Sciences/National Research Council (1982), and the American Cancer Society (1984). To this list let us add the Canadian Health Protection Branch and the British Department of Health and Social Security— whose 1974 report alone took three years and ten drafts, and which has since been followed by reports in 1978, 1981, and 1984.

Because of the complex nature of coronary heart disease and cancer, however, there are differences of opinion among scientists as to the role played by dietary

Diet and heart disease. Saturated fat and cholesterol are major suspects in the killer diseases—heart disease and stroke.

Diet is only one of many factors involved in complex diseases like coronary heart disease and cancer.

and nondietary factors. Before we describe the role of lipids here, let us set down some other facts about these diseases.

Coronary Heart Disease and Cancer Are Costly Killers

Both of these classes of diseases are devastating in their effects.

Major causes of death

In the United States more people die from coronary heart disease than from any other disease. Cancer is the second most common cause of death.

The cost of heart disease

As the following figures show, the cost of coronary heart disease makes this disease an expensive killer in the United States.[11] First, the deaths and disablement:

- 550,000 deaths each year—one each minute, or one half of all deaths. Though death from heart disease has declined in recent years, this is an unacceptably high number.
- 680,000 hospitalizations
- 5.4 million people with diagnosed coronary heart disease

Then the economic costs:

- Direct health cost—$8 billion
- Total economic cost—$60 billion
- Studies of the risk factors in CHD are both large and expensive. One study lasted 10 years, cost $110 million, and involved 12,866 participants and 250 physicians, dietitians and other experts in 28 centers in the United States and Canada. Serum cholesterol and saturated fat were among the risk factors studied. Another study lasting 7½ years and costing $155 million studied the effect of a drug, cholestyramine, in lowering serum cholesterol.

When the cost of heart disease is brought down to the personal level, the dollar amounts are distressing. The high indirect costs of death are due to the significant loss of productive life years if the person dies in their mid-40's.

Equally disturbing is the increasing incidence of coronary heart disease in developing countries.[12]

Economics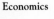

The cost of cancer

In 1986 the American Institute for Cancer Research estimated that the annual cost of cancer is $21 billion dollars.

Coronary Heart Disease and Cancer Have Many Possible Causes, Including Diet

In a review of 828 research papers from the early 1980's, 246 possible risk factors were reported in connection with coronary heart disease—an astounding number. Major risk factors included the diet—especially diets high in total fat, saturated fat, and cholesterol. However, many nondietary risk factors were also named, including heredity, age, gender, diabetes, obesity, hypertension, smoking, lack of exercise, and the use of oral contraceptives.[13]

As for risk factors related to cancer, the National Cancer Institute considers diet to be the single largest cause of cancer, as Figure 4-7 illustrates. Low fiber intakes are associated with colon and rectal cancers and, as we will see shortly, fat is considered a major factor in cancers of the breast, uterus, prostate, colon, rectum, and possibly other sites.[5]

High Lipid Intakes May Be a Major Cause of Coronary Heart Disease and Cancers

Can there be any television watcher left who has not seen or heard that previously obscure word "cholesterol"? "Networks Feed Public a Low-cholesterol Diet," headlined the *Wall Street Journal* over a story about the effects of television and magazine ads in making cholesterol appear a villain because of its possible connection with heart disease. In 1982, the Washington, D.C.–based Food Marketing Institute found that 45% of people surveyed considered cholesterol to be a serious health hazard. This was higher than the percentage concerned about salt or sugar in food, additives and preservatives, and artificial colors.

Marketing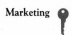

FIGURE 4-7
High dietary fat intake is associated with high death rate from breast cancer in different countries.

Age adjusted mortality per 100,000 population

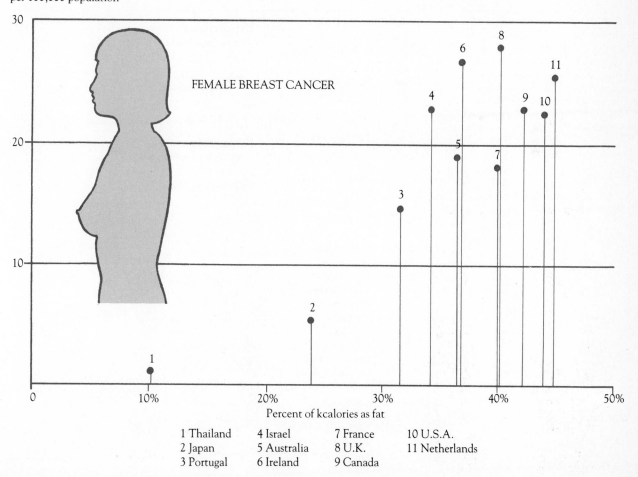

1 Thailand   4 Israel   7 France   10 U.S.A.
2 Japan   5 Australia   8 U.K.   11 Netherlands
3 Portugal   6 Ireland   9 Canada

TABLE 4-5 High-Fat Foods Are Not Necessarily High-Cholesterol Foods

	Cholesterol mg/100 g portion	Fat g/100 g portion
Ladyfingers	356	7.8
Cooked chicken liver	746	4.4
Cheddar cheese	99	32.8

The information on the cholesterol content of foods presented in Table 4-3 needs two additional qualifications:

- Some confectionary products may be high in cholesterol because of the use of eggs, milk, or butter.
- Foods high in fat are not necessarily high in cholesterol—as shown in Table 4-5.

However, cholesterol is only part of the story on lipids; there is much controversy about the relation between lipids and heart disease. Probably the majority opinion may be stated as follows: serum cholesterol is *raised* by dietary

FIGURE 4-8
Fat and blood vessels. High dietary intakes of cholesterol cause fat and cholesterol deposits in blood vessels. As fat deposits accumulate in the channels of the arteries blood flow is increasingly impaired, depriving the heart and other organs of oxygen and nutrients.

AMOUNT YIELDING 250 mg CHOLESTEROL

0-2 oz	Egg (1 large) Liver (beef)
2-5 oz	Butter Sponge cake
5-10 oz	Beef Shrimp Cheese Sardines Pie (lemon)
10-20 oz	Pork, chicken Sausage Frankfurter Tuna, herring Salad dressing Pancakes Waffles Fruit cake Pie (pumpkin) Mayonnaise
20-30 oz	Ice cream
60 oz	Milk (whole) Potatoes (au gratin)

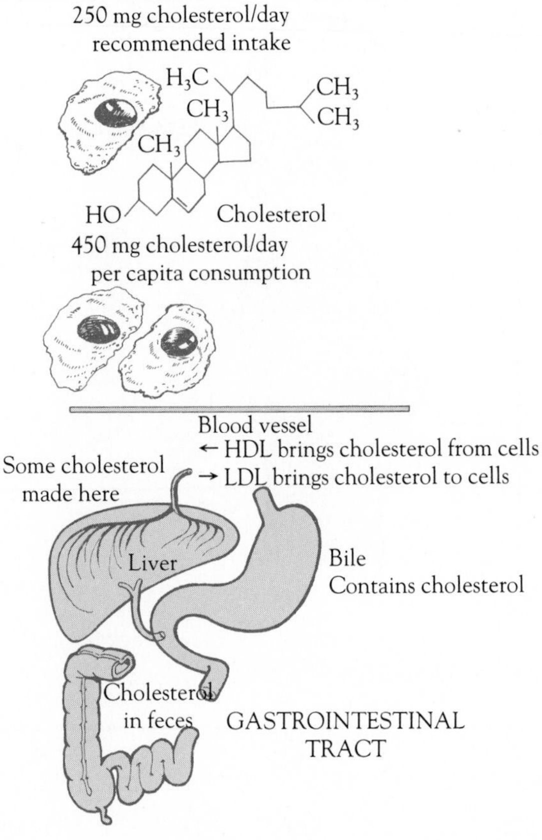

250 mg cholesterol/day recommended intake

Cholesterol

450 mg cholesterol/day per capita consumption

Blood vessel
← HDL brings cholesterol from cells
→ LDL brings cholesterol to cells

Some cholesterol made here

Liver

Bile Contains cholesterol

Cholesterol in feces

GASTROINTESTINAL TRACT

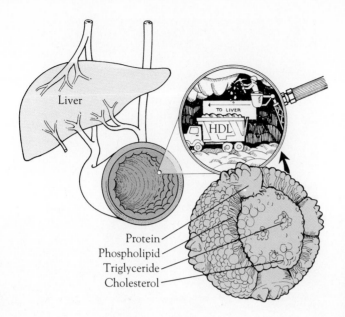

FIGURE 4-9
HDL brings cholesterol from blood vessels to the liver. HDL, considered the "good guy" in coronary heart disease, is a lipoprotein containing cholesterol, triglyceride, protein, and phospholipid.

saturated fat and cholesterol, but diet is not the only factor, for heredity and overweight may raise it also. Serum cholesterol is *lowered* by substituting polyunsaturated fatty acids for saturated fats. Recently, serum cholesterol was found to be lowered by monounsaturated fatty acids[14] and also by certain polyunsaturated fatty acids, called *omega-3 fatty acids,* found in highest amounts in cold-water fish.[15] Another method of lowering serum cholesterol is to lower the amount absorbed from the gastrointestinal system, as shown in Figure 4-8. The amount of dietary cholesterol absorbed into the body varies between 20% and 80%—one reason being the influence of some vegetable products. ⇐

Before we go on to join the chorus of abuse against lipids, however, let's examine the good aspects of cholesterol.

Omega-3 Fatty Acids
Polyunsaturated fatty acids; found in highest concentrations in fish oils.

Cholesterol Has Useful Functions in the Body

Much of the cholesterol in your body is made by your liver and intestines—which means that cholesterol is not essential in your diet.[16]

Still, cholesterol has useful functions. It has a role in the structure and function of cell membranes and it is involved in the manufacture of vitamin D, bile acids, and steroid hormones (including male and female hormones).

HDL Is Good, LDL Is Bad

Which form serum cholesterol takes is important. As we saw in Table 4-4, cholesterol is transported in lipoproteins. The HDL form is considered the "good guy," as Figure 4-9 illustrates. HDL is removed from cells and returned to the liver, where it is incorporated into bile. LDL is considered the "bad guy," because it takes cholesterol to the cells, where it builds up as *plaque*—deposits of cholesterol

Plaque
Deposits of cholesterol and calcium in the smooth muscle lining of the arteries.

Atherosclerosis is a buildup in an artery that blocks the passage of blood. The coronary artery below left shows only minor blockage. The artery below right exhibits severe atherosclerosis—much of the passage is blocked by buildup on the interior walls of the artery. The third coronary artery (top) is essentially completely blocked.

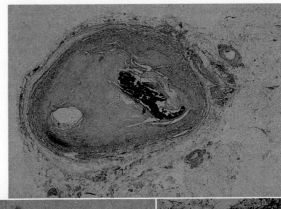

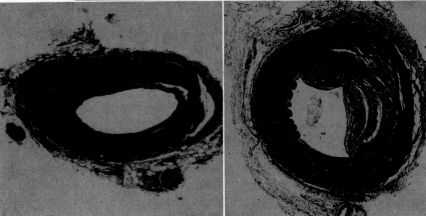

and calcium in the arteries. Over several years it causes atherosclerosis; that is, large deposits block the artery, so that the blood does not get to the heart, causing a heart attack (myocardial infarction or coronary occlusion), or to the brain, causing a stroke (cerebrovascular accident).

How Can You Avoid Building Cholesterol Deposits in the Blood Vessels?

This, like so many questions in this area, is a matter for debate. The American Heart Association has guidelines for reducing the levels of cholesterol and fat in the blood.[17] The dietary therapy has three phases, the third phase of which involves reducing your intake of certain foods (as will be described in the "Decisions" section). Specifically, phase III recommends an intake of only:

- 25% to 30% kcalories from fat—with equal amounts of saturated, mono-, and polyunsaturated fatty acids
- 60% kcalories as carbohydrate—with complex carbohydrate as the major source
- 15% kcalories as protein
- 100 to 150 mg per day of cholesterol

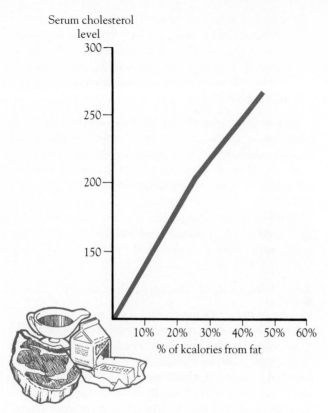

Serum cholesterol level

% of kcalories from fat

FIGURE 4-10
High fat, high cholesterol. High dietary fat intake is associated with high serum cholesterol levels. Data are from 50-year-old men.

Are These Dietary Changes Medically Justified?

Again, controversy rages. Governments in the United States and abroad recommend reductions in dietary intakes of cholesterol and fat, especially saturated fat, citing as justification the many studies showing that people with high serum cholesterol levels have high rates of coronary heart disease. They also cite indications of a direct relationship between the amount of fat in the diet and the level of cholesterol in the blood (Figure 4-10). On the other hand, an important study in the United States known as the Framingham Study found that blood cholesterol levels do *not* necessarily reflect dietary practices.[18]

Despite all these official dietary recommendations, consider these puzzles:

- The intake of dietary cholesterol has remained the same in the United States since the beginning of this century—about 500 mg per day. Recently there has been a very small drop in cholesterol intake—about 5 mg per 100 ml of blood. Yet during the same period, the death rate from heart disease has declined quite a bit—principally, it is thought, not from this small alteration in the diet but from such factors as reduced cigarette smoking, control of high blood pressure, and better hospital care of heart patients.[19]
- Laboratory animals—rats and rabbits—were fed the American diet of 1909 and of 1972 to see what would happen.[20] Rabbits fed the 1972 diet ate more fat, sugar, and calories, yet showed no difference in the severity of atherosclerosis than animals on the 1909 diet.

Contrast these fat intakes with the 42% of total kcalories from fat in the U.S. diet.

■ Two tribes in the Sahara Desert were studied by Dr. John Murray of the University of Minnesota. One tribe roamed the semi-desert for their food and 73% of their total kcalorie intake was milk, cheese, and butter. The other tribe's diet came mainly from seeds, and fat was 9% of their total kcaloric intake. However, there was no difference in the serum cholesterol of these two tribes.[21]

Are serum cholesterol levels really appropriate indicators of risk of coronary heart disease? Indeed, are there really many people walking around with high levels of serum cholesterol? In one study, only eight tenths of one percent of 480,000 men ages 35 to 59 considered to be at risk for a heart attack had two supposed "risk factors": serum cholesterol greater than 265 mg/100 ml blood and high plasma LDL.[22]

With so many distinguished scientists doubting the relevance of blood cholesterol level to heart disease, one wonders about the advisability of governments urging entire nations to change their cholesterol-related eating habits.[23]

Are These Dietary Changes Politically or Economically Justified?

Political Science ☞

"To eat or not to eat cholesterol is the question," says a U.S. Congressman, "and behind it lurks a deep and controversial political issue."[24] The issue, in other words, is not about health but about which political and economic views will prevail, since clearly a dietary change of this magnitude will have a lot of impact on people who make a living at something related to high-cholesterol foods. Those who think the government should condemn foods high in cholesterol and fat should also consider that in a free society criticism of government policy should never be suppressed: "When failure of a committee of nutritionists to conclude that the scientific evidence supports a particular public policy is taken as grounds for censure," according to proponents of this view, "we are on the road toward coercion."[25]

Actually, governments tend to formulate agricultural and food policies without much regard for nutrition considerations.[26] The reason, of course, is that important political constituencies would be affected. For instance, despite the recommendations in the British Department of Health report *Diet and Cardiovascular Disease*[27] that the European Common Agricultural Policy be changed to encourage less fat and cholesterol consumption, as long as Europe has "butter mountains" and "milk lakes" politicians won't be inclined to hurt the producers of those foods. The same line of reasoning holds for the United States and Canada.

Economics ☞

For many people, the financial stakes are high if the above dietary changes are followed.[28] Manufacturers of margarine and vegetable oils would be the winners, but the meat, egg, and dairy industries would be the losers. From a *nutrition* standpoint, however, perhaps the bottom line against government's recommending drastic cuts in the intakes of the foods high in lipids is this: these foods provide other important nutrients in the diet.

How Flexibly Can the Food Industry Respond to Dietary Changes?

Food technology ☞

So eggs are said to be high in cholesterol? The attitude of one part of the food industry was "If you can't beat 'em, join 'em"—and proceeded to market Egg Beaters, a cholesterol-free egg substitute. The main ingredients of this product were egg white, corn oil, and nonfat dry milk; nevertheless, Egg Beaters were not low in fat. In fact, whereas a natural egg had 11.4 g of fat content per 100 g, Egg Beaters had 12.5. Young rats fed the manufactured product grew more slowly than rats fed eggs, developed diarrhea within a week, and were dead within 3 to 4 weeks. Although the usefulness of this animal experiment is somewhat limited, since no human being would eat just Egg Beaters or even eggs as the only source of food, it shows that when a diet is modified to deal with one nutrition problem new nutrition problems may arise.

An offshoot of the extensive debate, widely reported in the media, about the relationship of cholesterol in eggs to coronary heart disease has been the appearance of novel claims for this or that food.[29] "Blue" eggs from the Araucana chicken, for instance, were promoted as being cholesterol-free. Actually these eggs were found to have a *higher* cholesterol content than did regular eggs.[30]

As regards the food industry's response to the cholesterol/fat controversy, the May 1986 issue of *Food Engineering* stated that reduced kcalorie or "light" foods account for more than 10 percent of the American processed food supply. From a food-processing standpoint, such foods are difficult to produce. Reducing kcalorie-rich lipids in a product does make it "lighter" in kcalories, but it also removes some physical properties unique to fat. This loss is overcome in some foods by the use of a form of cellulose as an oil replacement. We will see much more research in this area in the future.

Will People Really Buy Foods Modified to Meet Such Dietary Recommendations?

Knowing what you know so far about food and heart disease, would you eat meat produced with high polyunsaturated fat? Such meat was developed by Australian scientists and was a masterpiece of scientific achievement but a commercial disaster: it was too expensive and had unacceptable odor and flavor, consumers said.

People may be slow to modify their diets in any case. Many people, of course, simply have no way of knowing (without a physician's examination) the level of cholesterol or triglycerides in their blood. Or they are indifferent until coronary troubles develop—and only *then* are they willing to change their eating habits.

What Role Does Dietary Fat Play in Cancer?

In 1982, the National Academy of Science National Research Council concluded that of all of the dietary factors reviewed, high fat intake was considered to give the highest probability of cancer (other dietary factors will be discussed elsewhere in this book). Animal experiments showed that when total fat intake was low, polyunsaturated fats were more effective than saturated fats in reducing the risk of cancer. It is not yet known whether the same relationship applies to humans.

Recently many people have become aware of the high correlation between dietary fat intake and breast cancer in various countries (Figure 4-10). In the United States about 36,000 women die of breast cancer each year. It is calculated that if intake of dietary fat were reduced from the present intake of 40% of total kcalorie to 25%, about 9,000 lives would be saved annually.[5]

How does high dietary fat intake cause cancer? The mechanism is presently unknown—and this a great source of frustration to scientists. One difficulty comes in trying to distinguish the role of fat from that of kcalories in the process. Diets high in fat are also high in kcalories because fat contains 2¼ times more kcalories than the same amount of carbohydrate or protein. Recent evidence suggests that cancers are caused by high fat intake rather than high kcalorie intake.[31] Moreover, high fat intakes are usually associated with high protein and low carbohydrate intakes. This means that fiber intake is also low. Therefore, some cancers of the digestive system may be caused either by high fat intake or low fiber intake, or both.

An interesting new development is that rats fed high amounts of fish oils developed many fewer cancers of the pancreas than those fed corn oil,[32] possibly because of the presence of the omega-3 fatty acids. This discovery offers exciting possibilities that the omega-3 fatty acids may have beneficial effects in the prevention of cancer (and coronary heart disease also). However, as always with animal experiments, we must be careful in relating this research to cancer in human beings. Many developments are expected in this area of research within the next few years to determine the implications for people.

High fat intake is associated with coronary heart disease and certain cancers. High saturated fat and dietary cholesterol intake are related to high incidence of coronary heart disease. Poly- and (perhaps) monounsaturated fatty acids reduce serum cholesterol. Omega-3 fatty acids in fish oils may be beneficial in preventing certain cancers and coronary heart disease.

Decisions

1. How Can I Cut Down on the Amount of Fat in My Diet? Is My Fat Intake Meeting the Recommendations of the Dietary Guidelines?

First, you have to determine how much fat is in your typical diet. To do this, make a record of everything you eat and drink during a 24-hour period and determine the fat content, using the Table of Food Composition (Appendix P).

Example: You had 3 ounces of a broiled sirloin steak, and you ate the lean only. The Tables of Food Composition shows that 2 ounces has 4 grams of fat (36 kcalories). Therefore, the 3 ounces you ate had 6 grams of fat (54 kcalories).

Do similar calculations for all foods and drinks, then express the percentage of kcalories from fat as a percentage of total kcaloric intake.

Example: If your intake for 24 hours was 1,500 total kcalories and 55 grams of fat, then 495 of those 1,500 kcalories were provided by fat (55 × 9). Therefore, the percentage of kcalories from fat is

$$\frac{495 \times 100}{1,500} = 33\%$$

TABLE 4-6 When Fat Makes Up 30% to 35% of the Diet

Daily Energy Intake (kcalories)	Fat (g)
2,000	67-78
2,500	83-97
3,000	100-117

Other useful computations are shown in Table 4-6.

You can now determine whether your fat intake meets the Dietary Guidelines. The Dietary Guidelines for fat are:

- Reduce intake from present national average of 42% of total kcalories from fat to 30%.
- Saturated, mono-, and polyunsaturated fat should each provide about 10% of total kcalories in the diet.

Once you have determined the amount of fat in your diet, consider the following fifteen tips for lowering fat, saturated fat, and cholesterol[33]:

1. Steam, boil, bake or stir-fry vegetables.
2. Use herbs and spices instead of sauces, butter, or margarine to season vegetables.
3. Cut down on the amount of oil-based salad dressing, or use lemon juice.
4. To reduce saturated fat intake, use margarine instead of butter, oil instead of shortening.
5. Use whole-grain flours to reduce fat and cholesterol intake.
6. Use skim or low-fat milk instead of whole milk in puddings, soups, and baked goods.
7. Use plain low-fat yogurt, blender-whipped low-fat cottage cheese, or buttermilk in recipes that call for sour cream or mayonnaise.
8. Choose lean cuts of meat.
9. Trim fat from meat before and after cooking.
10. Roast, bake, broil, or simmer meat, poultry, or fish.
11. Remove skin from poultry before cooking.
12. Cook meat or poultry on a rack so the fat will drain off. Use a nonstick pan for cooking so that added fat is unnecessary.
13. Chill meat or poultry broth until the fat becomes solid, then spoon off the fat.
14. Limit egg yolks to one per serving when making scrambled eggs. Use additional egg whites for larger servings.
15. Substitute egg whites for whole eggs in recipes. For example, use two egg whites in place of each whole egg in muffins, cookies, and puddings.

2. If Omega-3 Fatty Acids Seem to Be So Effective in Preventing Coronary Heart Disease and Cancer, How Can I Increase My Intake of These Fatty Acids?

Fish oils seem to be the richest source of omega-3 fatty acids. Amounts of omega-3 fatty acids that significantly lowered serum cholesterol and triglycerides in men are found in the following amounts of fish:

½ to 1½ pounds of salmon, mackerel, trout

2 to 3 pounds of cod or flounder

Researchers think there may be a time/dose effect. This means that small intakes of these fish taken for a few days may have little effect.[34] Effects over longer time periods are being investigated. Many experts advise against taking omega-3 fatty acid supplements that are currently available commercially.

3. Which Tests Should I Have to Determine Blood Lipid Levels?

It's good to know your total serum cholesterol level. Improved methodologies make this possible with a small sample of blood. You should have tests done especially if one or more of the following apply:

- You are under 40 years old and have evidence of premature heart disease.
- You have a family history of heart disease.
- You have high levels of fat in the blood after a period of fasting, which can be determined only in a blood sample. Total cholesterol reflects mainly LDL cholesterol. This is considered satisfactory as an initial screening.[35]

Experts recommend that everyone have a blood cholesterol test early in life in order to establish baseline values.

4. Magazine Articles Indicate That Lecithin Helps Memory. Should I Try to Take More Lecithin into My Body?

Lecithin is produced by the liver and performs many useful functions in the body and in food. It is an emulsifying agent in bile and is added to some foods for the same purpose. It is present in high amounts in soybeans, egg yolk, liver, grains, and nuts. Most people get 500-900 mg/day, which is sufficient for all their needs. Why, then, is lecithin found in many stores?

Some early medical research suggested that lecithin might help memory and intellectual function. (Obviously, it would be a wonderful aid in studying nutrition textbooks, and could have a great humanitarian benefit for victims of Alzheimer's disease.) However, this has not been borne out; by the early 1980s, no beneficial effects on memory had been observed for increased lecithin in young or old people.[36] Lecithin has also been tried in an absolutely worthless and even dangerous weight-reducing diet. In another form of weight-reducing program, popular in the 1970s, a diet containing lecithin, kelp (from seaweed), vinegar, and vitamin B_6 was promoted; although you can lose weight on this diet, it is severely deficient in many nutrients. Finally, lecithin has been said to prevent and cure coronary heart disease because of its emulsifying properties, but there is no evidence for this.

Why, then, do people buy lecithin? Some of the reasons are highly emotionally charged since the diseases lecithin is said to help or prevent—loss of memory, coronary heart disease, obesity—are matters that evoke strong emotions.

Packagers of lecithin find it a highly profitable item to manufacture because it is simply a left-over product of soybeans after the oil is extracted. The retailers also do very well with lecithin: A recent check of the price difference between wholesale and retail prices found a mark-up in excess of 2,000%!

SUMMARY

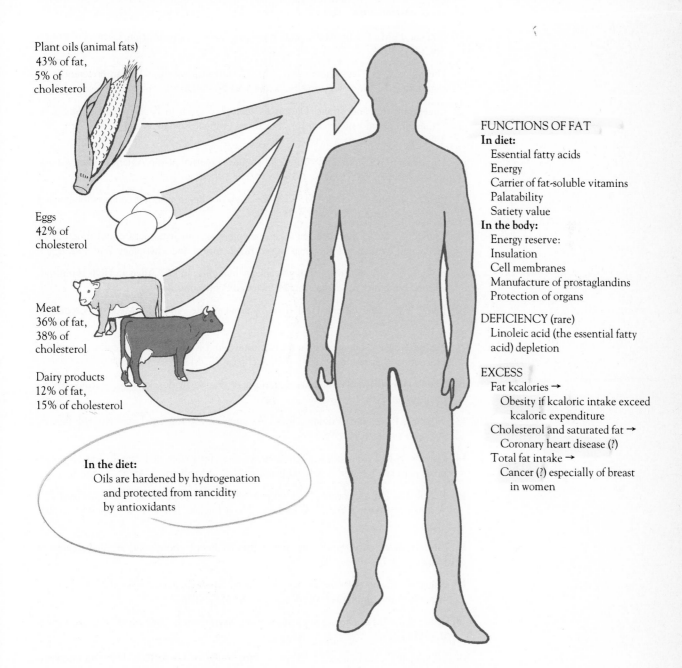

Plant oils (animal fats)
43% of fat,
5% of
cholesterol

Eggs
42% of
cholesterol

Meat
36% of fat,
38% of
cholesterol

Dairy products
12% of fat,
15% of cholesterol

In the diet:
Oils are hardened by hydrogenation
and protected from rancidity
by antioxidants

FUNCTIONS OF FAT
In diet:
Essential fatty acids
Energy
Carrier of fat-soluble vitamins
Palatability
Satiety value
In the body:
Energy reserve:
Insulation
Cell membranes
Manufacture of prostaglandins
Protection of organs

DEFICIENCY (rare)
Linoleic acid (the essential fatty
acid) depletion

EXCESS
Fat kcalories →
Obesity if kcaloric intake exceed
kcaloric expenditure
Cholesterol and saturated fat →
Coronary heart disease (?)
Total fat intake →
Cancer (?) especially of breast
in women

REFERENCES

1. Hoeg, J.M., and others: An approach to the management of hyperlipoproteinemia, Journal of the American Medical Association **255**:512, 1986.

2. Lands, W.E.M.: Renewed questions about polyunsaturated fatty acids, Nutrition Reviews **44**:189, 1986.

3. Sinclair, H.M.: Essential fatty acids in perspective, Human Nutrition: Clinical Nutrition **38C**:245, 1984.

4. Drewnowski, A., and Greenwood, M.R.C.: Cream and sugar: human preferences for high-fat foods, Physiology and Behavior **30**:629, 1983.

5. Greenwald, P., and others: Diet and chemoprevention in NCI's research strategy to achieve national cancer control objectives, Annual Review of Public Health **7**:267, 1986.

6. Mondeika, T.: Cholesterol content of shellfish, Journal of the American Medical Association **254**:2970, 1985.

7. Field, C.J., and Clandinin, M.T.: Modulation of adipose tissue fat composition by diet: a review, Nutrition Research **4**:743, 1984.

8. Clandinin, M.T., and others: Plasma membrane: can its structure and function be modulated by dietary fat? Comparative Biochemistry and Physiology **76B**:335, 1983.

9. Sanders, T.A.B.: Nutritional significance of rancidity. In J.C. Allen and R.J. Hamilton, editors: Rancidity in foods, Applied Science Publishing, London, 1983.

10. Jukes, T.H., and others: Heated fat, Journal of the American Medical Association **255**:2080, 1986.

11. National Heart, Lung, and Blood Institute: Lipid Research Clinics coronary primary prevention trial results, Nutrition Today, page 20, March/April, 1984.

12. Osuntokun, B.O.: The changing pattern of disease in developing countries, World Health Forum **6**:310, 1985.

13. Hopkins, P.N., and Williams, R.R.: A survey of 246 suggested coronary risk factors, Atherosclerosis **40**:1, 1981.

14. Grundy, S.M.: Comparison of monounsaturated fatty acids and carbohydrates for lowering plasma cholesterol, New England Journal of Medicine **314**:745, 1986.

15. Kromhout, D., and others: The inverse relation between fish consumption and 20–year mortality from coronary heart disease, New England Journal of Medicine **312**:1205, 1985.

16. Grundy, S.M.: Absorption and metabolism of dietary cholesterol, Annual Review of Nutrition **3**:71, 1983.

17. American Heart Association Special Report: Recommendations for the treatment of hyperlipidemia in adults, Arteriosclerosis **4**:445A, 1984.

18. Ahrens, Jr., E.H.: Dietary fats and coronary heart disease: Unfinished business, Lancet **ii**:1345, 1979.

19. Gillum, R.F., and others: Decline in coronary heart disease mortality: Old questions and new facts, American Journal of Medicine **76**:1055, 1984.

20. Kritchevsky, D., and others: Comparison of diets approximating American intake of 1909 and 1972: Effect on lipid metabolism in rabbits and rats, Nutrition Reports International **28**:1, 1983.

21. Murray, M.J., and others: Serum cholesterol, triglycerides and heart disease of nomadic and sedentary tribesmen consuming isoenergetic diets of high and low fat content, British Journal of Nutrition **39**:159, 1978.

22. Harper, A.E.: Diet and heart disease: Responses to the LRC-CPPT findings, Nutrition Today, 1984, p. 22, September/October.

23. Ahrens, Jr., A.E.: The diet—heart question in 1985: Has it really been settled? Lancet **i**:1085, 1985.

24. Richmond, F.: A political perspective on the diet/heart controversy, Journal of Nutrition Education **12**:186, 1980.

25. Harper, A.E.: Invited response to Congressman Richmond: Another view of the politics of cholesterol, Journal of Nutrition Education **12**:187, 1980.

26. Chafkin, S.: Nutrition policies, programs, and politics, American Journal of Agricultural Economics, p. 806, December, 1978.

27. Editorial: Food and heart disease, British Medical Journal **289**:543, 1984.

28. Marsh, J.S.: The economic implications of a health policy, Proceedings of the Nutrition Society **44**:419, 1985.

29. (Four letters to the editor), Lancet **i**:1127 and **ii**:1191, 1984.

30. Peterson, D.W., and others: Composition of and cholesterol in Araucana and commercial eggs, Journal of the American Dietetic Association **72**:45, 1978.

31. Carrol, K.K., and Reddy, B.S.: Dietary fat and cancer: Specific action or caloric effect? Journal of Nutrition **116**:1130 and 1132, 1986.

32. O'Connor, T.P., and others: Effect of dietary intake of fish oil and fish protein on the development of L-azaserine-induced preneoplastic lesions in the rat pancreas, Journal of the National Cancer Institute **75**:959, 1985.

33. Home and Garden Bulletin, Pub. No. 232–3, U.S. Department of Agriculture, Washington, D.C., 1986.

34. Harris, W.S.: Health effects of omega-3 fatty acids, Contemporary Nutrition **10**(8), 1985.

35. Marshall, W.J., and Ballantyne, F.C.: Current clinical laboratory practice: Investigation of plasma lipids—which tests and when? British Medical Journal **292**:1652, 1986.

36. Editorial: Lecithin and memory. Lancet **i**:293, 1980.

METABOLISM NOTES: *Metabolism of Lipids*

The tissues most involved in lipid metabolism are those of the liver and muscles and adipose tissue (Figure 4-11). Lipids are combined with protein, forming lipoprotein, and are released into the blood. The most important lipoproteins are the chylomicrons and VLDL because they transport lipids to the tissues, where an enzyme called lipoprotein lipase frees the lipid from the protein. Muscle is the tissue that uses the greatest amount of fatty acids for energy. The amount used varies depending on the duration and intensity of the activity. Fat not required for energy is stored in the adipose tissue.

Free fatty acids (FFA) are used by muscle during exercise. Ketones are produced between meals, but especially during fasting or during low-carbohydrate diets. The latter are a popular, but nutritionally unsound, form of weight-reducing diet. The author of one of these types of diet encourages the dieter to test his or her urine for ketone bodies. When ketones are detected in the urine, it means the dieter is in a state of ketosis—that fat is burned for energy but the metabolism is incomplete. Complete metabolism of fat produces carbon dioxide and water plus energy.

FIGURE 4-11

The metabolism of fat.

1. Importance of protein in transporting lipids in chylomicrons, in VLDL, and as albumin bound to free fatty acids in transport between adipose tissue and liver. The protein is freed from the lipid by the enzyme lipoprotein lipase.
2. Muscle is a large user of triglyceride for muscular energy.
3. Liver converts glycerol to glucose. This is a small but useful source of glucose.
4. Ketones are produced by fasting and in low-carbohydrate weight-reducing diets.

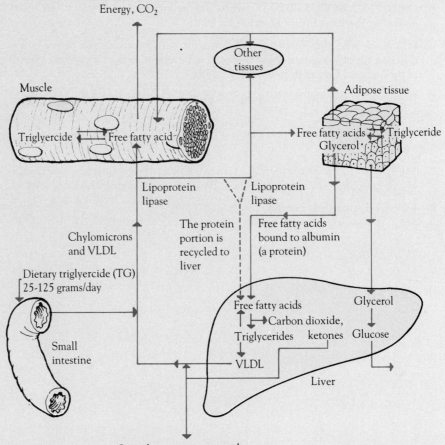

Proteins and Amino Acids 5

CONNECTIONS

Like carbohydrates and fats, proteins provide energy, but mainly for emergencies, when total energy intake is low. Proteins are found in every cell in the body, where they help growth and maintenance, regulate important body functions, and provide an ultimate source of energy.

Protein is the first nutrient we have discussed that has an RDA. During pregnancy and lactation, the demands of the fetus and the production of milk increase this RDA. Protein deficiency can be more damaging to health than carbohydrate or fat deficiencies. When high amounts of protein are ingested, they may be converted to fat. Whether cancer is associated with high intakes of protein is a subject of debate.

Protein supplements are offered for sale with a variety of health claims—such as improved athletic performance—but such claims have little scientific support. Proteins consist of combinations of 20 different amino acids, and some of these, too, are sold as supplements to cure physical and nervous disorders, but, again, there is no evidence that they work.

Proteins: many amino acids linked together
Needed for survival: body and food proteins
Dietary proteins—digested; amino acids—absorbed
Quantity and quality: why they matter
The uses of nitrogen balance studies
The effects of food processing on protein: usually insignificant
Too much protein: the health consequences
Why the fascination with high protein intakes?

"Of prime importance"—that is the meaning of the Greek word from which the word *protein* is derived.

Are proteins indeed most important? All nutrients are needed, of course, but proteins are unique because they are found everywhere in nature—in every cell in humans, animals, plants, and microorganisms. Composed of thousands of different combinations of amino acids—about 20 different building blocks in the human body—proteins are involved in:

Proteins
Complex combinations of amino acids that are essential parts of all living cells.

- Growth and maintenance
- Regulation of many of the normal workings of the cell
- Production of energy when not enough energy is available from carbohydrates and fats

Don't these seem like important matters for your survival? Clearly they are: in developing countries, children suffering from malnutrition are quite often found to have a major protein deficiency.

Foods high in protein. Combinations of different sources of food proteins are on the right. Plant foods usually have higher protein values when eaten in combination with other foods of plant or animal origin.

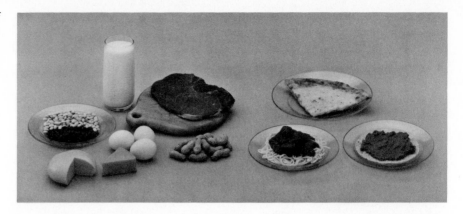

In developed countries, on the other hand, most people get sufficient protein, and the principal problem is that consumers are fed misinformation on the nutritional importance of protein. One writer gives this example:

At the local county fair, a woman stops at a booth selling herbal products. One weight-loss powder had a price tag of $30 and an accompanying brochure that reads. "This is a *high*-quality protein food. It has *all* 22 protein-building amino acids, including the 9 *essential* amino acids that your body *cannot* produce and *must* be supplied by your diet." Wow, the woman thinks, 9 *essential amino acids!* She's been meaning to go on a diet anyway, so she buys the product.[1]

Actually, the scientific information about protein and the amino acids is basically correct, although there is no magic component that increases weight loss. The problem with this kind of promotion is that it trades on consumers' misplaced reverence for the nutritional power of excess dietary protein and their ignorance of good sources of protein in the diet. There is no need for a protein supplement: a serving of meat, poultry, fish, eggs, dairy products, nuts, or a variety of cereals and vegetables will provide the same combination of amino acids at a fraction of the cost.

Protein-Energy Malnutrition
Deficiency of protein and energy; severest effects on children; one of the most common nutrition diseases in the world.

In developing countries, by contrast, getting protein-rich foods is a major problem. Every year about 10 million deaths occur, especially among young children, from *protein-energy malnutrition,* a deficiency of protein and energy that is one of the most common nutrition diseases in the world.[2]

Let us proceed, then, to examine the functions of protein in the body and the health consequences of having too much or too little protein in the diet.

PROTEINS: MANY AMINO ACIDS LINKED TOGETHER

Before you can understand the functions of protein in the body and the health consequences of having too much or too little protein in the diet, you need to know a little about the chemistry of proteins.

Amino Acids: The Links

Amino acids consist of about 20 different chemicals found in the human body and in food. These amino acids contain carbon, hydrogen, and oxygen atoms (three atoms that are part of carbohydrates and fats also) plus nitrogen. Some amino acids also contain sulfur. The chemical structure of amino acids is shown in Figure 5-1.

The NH_2, or amine group, shown at the bottom of the figure is what gives amino acids their name. We said that 20 different amino acids are in the proteins in our food and in our bodies, but some sources list as many as 22 amino acids—a matter of chemical interpretation that need not concern you. The important amino acids in nutrition are listed in Table 5-1.

Amino acids are the major source of nitrogen in the body. Small amounts of nitrogen are in nucleic acids (RNA, DNA) and in some vitamins (thiamin, riboflavin, niacin, pyridoxin, pantothenic acid, biotin, folacin, and vitamin B_{12}). Getting enough carbon, hydrogen, and oxygen to form amino acids is not much of a problem. However, obtaining enough nitrogen is the limiting factor in the formation of amino acids by plants, animals, and human beings.

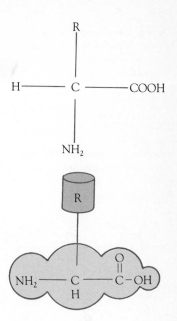

FIGURE 5-1
Chemical structure of amino acids.

TABLE 5-1 Amino Acids, Essential and Nonessential

Essential Amino Acids	Nonessential Amino Acids
Lysine	Glycine
Methionine	Tyrosine
Phenylalanine	Aspartic acid
Leucine	Glutamic acid
Isoleucine	Alanine
Valine	Serine
Tryptophan	Arginine
Threonine	Proline
Histidine	Glutamine
	Asparagine

Proteins: The Chains

Proteins are formed when amino acids are linked together. One molecule of water is lost when two amino acids (whether the same or different) are joined together:

Amino acid + Amino acid = = > Amino acid — Amino acid + water

This process may be repeated until up to several hundred amino acids are joined together.

The unique sequence of different amino acids that makes up each protein is dictated by DNA. The kind of arrangement brought about is important: If even one amino acid is missing or in the wrong sequence in a protein molecule, the consequences to the body can be serious. For instance, the disorder known as sickle cell anemia, which occurs mainly in blacks, arises because one—just one—amino acid in the normal hemoglobin molecule has been replaced by a different amino acid. This event interferes with the ability of hemoglobin to take oxygen to cells in the body. If the hemoglobin in many red blood cells is thus affected, a person becomes ill and may die.

Peptide Bond
The link between amino acids, thus allowing formation of a protein molecule.

FIGURE 5-2
Amino acid arrangements. Different amino acids have different formations. **A,** Fibrous or straight–chained protein. **B,** Coiled protein. **C,** Globular protein.

After the DNA has arranged the various amino acids that make up a protein, the result is a chain of amino acids. It may be straight-chained (fibrous), coiled, or globular, as shown in Figure 5-2. The linkage between the amino acids that makes the formation of a protein molecule possible is called the *peptide bond.* A protein may also be visualized as a necklace, with beads of amino acids strung together. We might put different colored beads in different sequences in the necklace, constructing yet another kind of necklace. In the same way, different amino acids are organized in different sequences, giving rise to the different forms of protein shown in Figure 5-2.

What difference does this change in shape make? It is the proportion of the different amino acids and their sequence in the amino acid chain that gives different

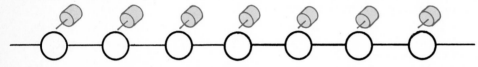

proteins their unique physical properties. For example, some proteins in blood are globular, which enables them to squeeze through narrow blood capillaries; hair proteins, by contrast, are long strands of amino acids linked together, which enables them to be rigid, a property you would expect in hair.

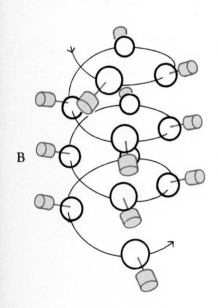

Proteins consist of amino acids joined together. Proteins are similar to carbohydrate and fat in that they contain carbon, hydrogen, and oxygen. Proteins differ from carbohydrate and fat in that they also contain nitrogen.

NEEDED FOR SURVIVAL: BODY AND FOOD PROTEINS

Some nutrients you can recognize right away: it's easy to recognize sugar as pure carbohydrate or the lump of fat on a piece of meat as fat. But where among the common foods you eat is a good example of pure protein? Because it is difficult to "see" protein in our food, we talk instead about protein-rich sources that also contain other nutrients, such as lean meat, eggs, and nuts.

In the body, tissues vary in their contribution to total body protein (Figure 5-3). But only in cases of severe protein deficiency can one see the damage to the body, the most obvious signs being muscle loss and poor quality of skin and hair. However, many other changes in the body are not visible.

To better understand what is involved, let us delineate the functions of protein in the body. As you read through the following sections, recall the three major functions of protein: growth and maintenance, regulation of body processes, and energy.

All Enzymes Are Proteins

Several thousand enzymes have been discovered, and many have been identified in pure form. They speed up chemical reactions in biological systems, usually by

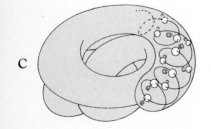

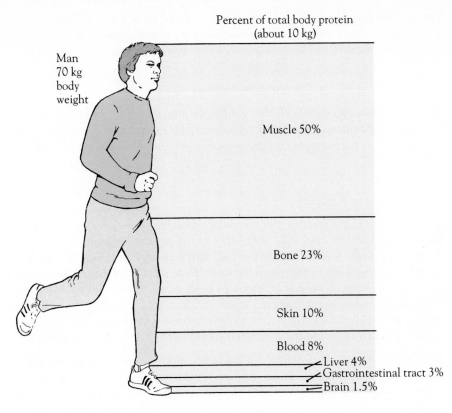

Percent of total body protein
(about 10 kg)

Man
70 kg
body
weight

Muscle 50%

Bone 23%

Skin 10%

Blood 8%

Liver 4%
Gastrointestinal tract 3%
Brain 1.5%

FIGURE 5-3
The body of an adult male contains about 10 kg of protein, the highest proportion being in muscles.

over a millionfold. This speed is useful because enzymes are involved in the build-up (anabolism) and the breakdown (catabolism) of a wide variety of chemicals in all biological systems.

All components in our body are continually being broken down and built up again. For example, the life of a red blood cell is about 120 days, whereas that of cells lining our gastrointestinal tract is 2 to 4 days. The breakdown and rebuilding of these cells requires enzymes. Catabolism therefore occurs during the normal breakdown of cells; in stresses such as starvation, illness, and various traumas; and in the breakdown of some body reserves in normal health (such as the breakdown of muscle glycogen during exercise). Anabolism occurs in growth, in recovery from illness, and in the buildup of body reserves (for example, of glycogen and fat).

Two examples of the importance of enzymes:

- As a child, you would not have been able to grow were it not for enzymes available to convert digested nutrients into body tissues.
- You might not survive a dangerous situation if you did not have enzymes, for they speedily release the energy locked up in carbohydrates, fats, and proteins.

As will be shown in Chapters 6 and 7, certain vitamins and minerals play important roles in helping enzymes work.

You may be inclined to think of proteins in terms of protein-rich foods such as milk, meat, or lima beans; however, the most abundant protein in nature—ribulose bisphosphate carboxylase/oxygenase—is an enzyme first purified from spinach leaves in 1947. This enzyme makes up most of the soluble protein in leaf extracts.

Most protein-rich foods are also rich in several vitamins and minerals.

Biochemistry

For a nutritionist, the enzyme is important because of the key role it plays in fixing carbon dioxide from the air during photosynthesis, which means that the survival of all plants, animals, and humans (who depend on plants) depends on this enzyme.

Some Hormones Are Proteins or Peptides

The hormone insulin is probably the best-known protein, but others include growth hormone, thyroxin, and adrenaline (epinephrine). Undernutrition can reduce the activity of these hormones—a major reason for the reduced growth in malnourished children.

Antibodies Are Proteins

Antibodies are blood proteins that recognize and combine with foreign substances like viruses, bacteria, and cells from other organisms and make them harmless. When the protein level in the diet is low, antibodies are not made in sufficient quantities in the body to prevent infections. If you eat a poor diet for some time you might feel run down and be prone to colds or flu. More fatal consequences occur in many developing countries where children are more prone to infections because of poor diet. Death rates from infectious diseases like measles and whooping cough are much higher in these children owing to the low level of antibodies.

IgA Antibody
A major antibody in the blood.

Early research on acquired immune deficiency syndrome (AIDS) attempted to link AIDS with undernutrition in Haiti.[3] Undernutrition is widespread in that country, where the per capita annual income is $150. Among the many consequences of low protein intake is depressed secretion of the *IgA antibody*, a major antibody in the blood. Some investigators contended that the AIDS infection in many Haitians was due to undernutrition, and that this infection was not the same type of AIDS encountered in developed countries like the United States. This proposition is unproven. It is a good example of the need for evidence before a nutritional hypothesis can be confirmed.

Some Proteins Are Important in Transport and Storage in the Body

Low dietary intake of protein can decrease the transportation of some other nutrients through the blood.

An example of transport proteins is hemoglobin, which carries oxygen in the blood to all cells. Globin is a colorless protein, and heme is a dark red chemical compound that contains iron. A related protein, myoglobin, transports oxygen in muscles. You saw in Chapter 4 how fat is transported in the blood as lipoproteins. Fat-soluble vitamins are also attached to a protein for transport in the blood. Undernourished children may suffer from deficiencies of these vitamins, especially vitamin A. One reason is the lack of transport protein to bring the vitamin from its storage site in the body to the tissue that needs it (see Chapter 6). Storage in the body of some minerals, like iron and copper, is achieved by combination with a protein.

Mechanical Support Is Given to Skin and Bone by Collagen

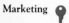
Marketing

A fibrous protein called collagen gives mechanical support to skin and bone. Because of the way the amino acids are joined together, collagen has rigidity, elasticity, and water insolubility. Collagen synthesis is adversely affected when protein intake in the diet is low. This results in poorer quality of skin and hair. Children suffering from starvation frequently have ulcers and sores on their skin, and their hair can easily be pulled out by the roots. In more prosperous societies, concerns about collagen are manifested in advertisements for hair shampoos containing proteins or for dog food that enhances the appearance of the dog's coat.

Sliding Action Between Two Protein Filaments Permits Coordinated Muscle Movement

All the coordinated movement in your muscles is made possible by the sliding action between two protein filaments, which permits muscles to contract and relax. In cases of severe undernutrition, these filaments may break, resulting in poor muscle function.

Specific Proteins Are Required for Generation and Transmission of Nerve Impulses

Some amino acids are needed as *neurotransmitters*—30 or 40 chemicals, produced in and released from nerves, that carry or transmit signals along nerves and between nerves and a target tissue. For example, the quick withdrawal of your hand when you touch a hot object occurs because the nerves respond to the pain stimulus by sending a message to muscles in the arm and hand to pull it away as fast as possible. That important junction between the nerves and the muscles is bridged by neurotransmitters.

Neurotransmitters
30-40 different chemicals that are produced in and released from nerves.

Control of Growth Requires Nucleoproteins

Nucleoproteins, of which DNA and RNA are examples, are needed to control growth. Many different proteins can be bound to DNA. These nucleoprotein fibers can be arranged structurally so that hereditary instructions can be transferred into new cells during their formation.

Proteins Help Control Water Balance in the Body

The water within the cells (intracellular fluid) and the water outside the cells (extracellular fluid) have different chemical compositions, and their unrestricted mixing can cause cells to swell and burst, thereby arresting many important chemical reactions within cells. The level of extracellular fluid is kept constant with the help of some large-molecular-weight proteins in the blood. The blood is part of the extracellular fluid. Small molecules including water can pass through the walls of blood vessels, but protein molecules are too large to penetrate. These proteins in the blood attract some fluid from the spaces between the cells and return it to the blood. In cases of severe undernutrition, the concentration of some of these proteins decreases, which in turn decreases the pull on the extracellular fluid to return to the blood vessels. As a result, an excess of fluid remains outside the cells, and it is this edema that gives the puffy appearance in the arms, legs, and stomachs of badly undernourished children. Edema is easily recognized by the imprint remaining after pressure is applied by the thumb to the swollen area.

Proteins Act as pH Buffers Against Extreme Acidity or Alkalinity

Proteins help keep most of the fluids in the body neutral or slightly alkaline, and prevent wide swings into extreme acidity or alkalinity, either of which can inactivate certain enzymes and lead to rapid death.

Proteins Provide Energy to the Body

Like carbohydrates and fats, proteins provide energy to the body—1 g of protein supplies 4 kcalories. However, proteins are not the preferred source of energy; they are to be used only in emergencies, as when a person is starving, or when one has eaten more protein than the body needs. Because only a small supply of free amino acids circulates in the blood, during starvation amino acids to be used for energy must be obtained from tissue proteins—all the body tissues except for the brain (see Figure 5-3).

The reason that starving children seem to be just "skin and bone" is that the body has to cannibalize its own tissue protein for energy. During this emergency, however, the brain remains protected. Some of the amino acids from body proteins can be converted to fat and some to glucose—the prime fuel for the brain. Only a small amount of glucose is obtained from glycerol in the breakdown of body fat. Therefore, the price that is paid to maintain brain function during starvation is the destruction of protein in other tissues.

High-protein diets present a problem in the excretion of waste nitrogen. This places extra demands on the kidneys.

When body protein is broken down for energy, there remains the problem of getting rid of the elements that make up protein molecules. Carbon and oxygen are exhaled as carbon dioxide. Waste hydrogen and oxygen are excreted as water in urine. The excretion of carbon dioxide and water is the same for protein as it is for carbohydrate and fat. However, after using protein for energy the body must also get rid of nitrogen. This nitrogen forms urea in the liver. The urea is carried by the blood to the kidneys. There nitrogen-containing compounds are filtered out of the blood and excreted in the urine. It may now be clear why high-protein weight-reducing programs require a high fluid intake: a person on such a diet needs to dilute the concentration of urea and other nitrogen-containing compounds in the urine.

Proteins Contribute to Sensory and Physical Properties of Food

Food proteins contribute such sensory and physical properties of food as color, flavor, odor, texture, thickening, and viscosity. Why is meat red? It is the result of its hemoglobin content. What determines if it is tough and chewy? It has to do with the way the muscle proteins are linked together.

> Body proteins are involved in growth and maintenance; in the regulation of body functions (enzymes, some hormones, and antibodies are proteins); in transportation and storage of some nutrients; in providing mechanical support; in the coordination of muscle and nerve function; in the control of growth; and in regulating the amount and chemical composition of cell fluid. Protein is an energy source. Proteins also affect many sensory and physical characteristics of food.

DIETARY PROTEINS—DIGESTED, AMINO ACIDS— ABSORBED

Figure 5-4 shows how a typical meal proceeds through the digestion of protein and the absorption of amino acids into the blood.

Digestion Reduces the Size of Protein Molecules

Because of their large molecular size, dietary proteins cannot squeeze between the cells lining the gastrointestinal tract and enter the blood. For this to happen, protein needs to go through the digestive process, beginning in the mouth. The act of chewing separates the food, increasing its surface area, which helps the

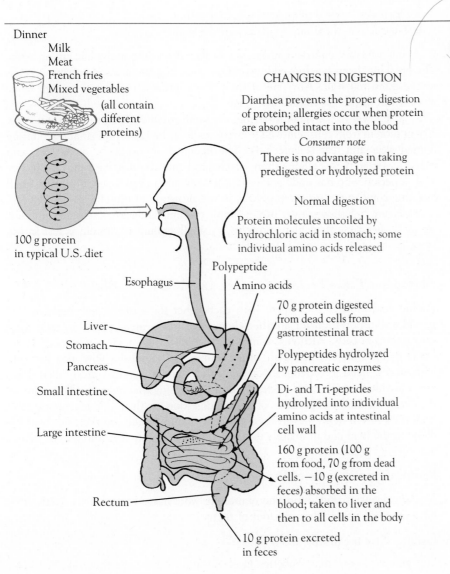

FIGURE 5-4
Normal digestion is the breaking down of proteins into individual amino acids.

Dinner
Milk
Meat
French fries
Mixed vegetables
(all contain different proteins)

100 g protein in typical U.S. diet

CHANGES IN DIGESTION

Diarrhea prevents the proper digestion of protein; allergies occur when protein are absorbed intact into the blood

Consumer note

There is no advantage in taking predigested or hydrolyzed protein

Normal digestion

Protein molecules uncoiled by hydrochloric acid in stomach; some individual amino acids released

Esophagus

Polypeptide

Amino acids

70 g protein digested from dead cells from gastrointestinal tract

Polypeptides hydrolyzed by pancreatic enzymes

Di- and Tri-peptides hydrolyzed into individual amino acids at intestinal cell wall

160 g protein (100 g from food, 70 g from dead cells. −10 g (excreted in feces) absorbed in the blood; taken to liver and then to all cells in the body

Liver

Stomach

Pancreas

Small intestine

Large intestine

Rectum

10 g protein excreted in feces

digestive enzymes in the stomach and small intestine attack the proteins. There is no digestion of dietary protein in the mouth.

Strong acid in the stomach *denatures* food proteins by changing their shapes. The denaturing uncoils the protein, opening up its structure for attack by digestive enzymes. Hydrolysis by pepsin makes proteins a little smaller in size when they leave the stomach, but they are still too large to be absorbed into the blood. Some individual amino acids may be liberated in the stomach, but the amount is of little importance. This means that people who have had part or all of their stomachs surgically removed do not have a problem with the digestion of protein.

The major breakdown of dietary protein occurs in the small intestine. Here the acid from the stomach is neutralized and the mixture of food is now slightly alkaline. Protein is broken down into three forms:

- Individual amino acids
- *Dipeptides*—two amino acids joined together
- *Tripeptides*—three amino acids joined together

About 30% of the protein molecule is broken down into individual amino acids. The breaking down is achieved by enzymes from the pancreas and enzymes in cells in the intestinal wall. Any one of these three forms is now small enough to be absorbed from the gastrointestinal tract.

A little lower in the small intestine, the same enzymes digest the approximately 70 g of protein from cells removed from the walls of the gastrointestinal tract during normal wear and tear (Figure 5-4). The liberated amino acids, dipeptides, and tripeptides from these cells are then recycled by being absorbed back into the blood. Thus a person who has undergone surgical removal of even a portion of the small intestine could suffer serious problems in the digestion of proteins.

As Figure 5-5 shows, over 80% of most proteins is digested. Animal proteins are more digestible than plant proteins. A small amount of protein is lost in the feces. Some of this protein is from bacteria.

Absorption Takes Proteins from the Intestine to the Blood

Amino acid molecules compete with each other for a *carrier*—a chemical that provides transportation for another chemical across a membrane—to take them into intestinal cells. Although transporting some amino acids across a cell membrane requires an energy input, other amino acid molecules flow into the cells without the need for energy input. Dipeptides and tripeptides are broken down into individual amino acids in the walls of cells lining the intestine. Therefore, in the blood the final end products of protein digestion are the individual amino acids from the protein molecules in the food. These amino acids are then taken in the blood to the liver and ultimately to any cell in the body that requires amino acids.

Practical Implications of Protein Digestion and Absorption

The way digestion and absorption of proteins work has led to some discoveries that have practical value. Here are four of them.

Insulin: Why it can't be taken orally

You may be aware that diabetics inject insulin. Why can't they take it orally? Insulin's unique hormonal activity is a result of the special sequence of specific

Denatures
Changes in the shape of a protein molecule. Usually produced by heat, acid, alkali, alcohol.

Dipeptides, Tripeptides
Two and three amino acids, respectively, joined by peptide bonds.

Carrier
A chemical that provides transportation for another chemical across a membrane.

PROTEIN SOURCE

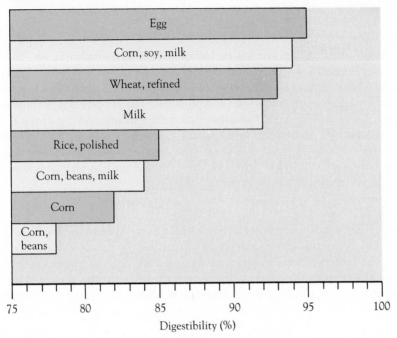

Digestibility (%)

FIGURE 5-5

Digestibility of protein. The percentage of digestibility varies among foods. These are data for children. Notice that the digestibility of some foods is increased when they are combined with other protein sources. For example, the digestibility of corn, soy, and milk taken together is higher than for corn alone. This information is important for young children on low-protein intakes. There is very little nutritional significance in this information for adults on the typical U.S. diet.

amino acids. The digestive system treats insulin taken by mouth in the same way it treats any other protein from animal or plant foods; that is, the insulin will be digested into individual amino acids, dipeptides, and tripeptides. This means that insulin has now lost all hormone activity, and the body uses these amino acids from insulin for any of the functions of proteins described above. This is why people with diabetes must inject themselves with insulin rather than take it by mouth.

Enzymes taken orally: Why they are worthless

Because all enzymes are proteins, they are digested into individual amino acids. Enzyme activity can be lost by the slightest change in enzyme structure. Therefore, when an enzyme goes through the destructive process of digestion, all enzyme activity is lost. Patients suffering from cystic fibrosis, who do not secrete certain digestive enzymes, are sometimes given enzyme preparations that are coated to protect the enzymes from the acid environment in the stomach. These enzymes can then act in digesting food in the small intestine.

    A particular kind of consumer rip-off is the business of selling enzymes purported to help digestion. Papain, for instance, comes from papayas and is used as a meat tenderizer; however, it will not cure your indigestion. Pepsin, the enzyme secreted in the stomach, is also for sale, supposedly to aid people who have had parts of their stomach surgically removed; however, the absence of pepsin is not critical because such people can still digest food protein in the small intestine. You can also buy enzymes secreted by the pancreas, which work in the slightly alkaline environment of the small intestine and are supposed to help digestion for normal people. Because such enzymes must pass through the acidic environment of the stomach before they arrive in the small intestine, some manufacturers coat these

Consumer Protection

enzymes to prevent their inactivation by stomach acids. However, there is no evidence that any enzyme preparations taken orally help digestion.

Predigested or hydrolyzed proteins: Why they are unnecessary

Proteins, carbohydrates, and fats are hydrolyzed during normal digestion. Biochemists use the term *hydrolysis* to describe a chemical reaction in which water is used as the "breaking" agent. The term has been popularized because of the use of hydrolyzed protein in some weight-loss programs. The words *predigested protein* refer to the same process but don't sound so "scientific." In any case, the idea is to make consumers think that if the manufacturer has already broken down protein beforehand, outside the body, it will save the digestive system some wear and tear. This notion is totally false. Your body can hydrolyze protein when it is required— and it will do it without additional charge.

Food sensitivities: The possible role of proteins

Food allergies and sensitivities may be caused by many different chemicals, including proteins. Some undigested protein molecules will set up an allergic reaction if absorbed into the blood intact; some of the dipeptides and tripeptides may also cause allergic reactions. Infants are particularly prone to this type of allergic reaction, but they usually outgrow the problem when the immature gastrointestinal system develops.

There is no agreement among experts on a complete list of foods responsible for allergic reactions,[4] but some common foods are (1) milk, (2) eggs, (3) fish, (4) tree nuts, (5) wheat, (6) crustacea—shrimp, crab, lobster, and (7) shellfish— clams, oysters, scallops. Diagnosis of food allergies is difficult because allergies can affect all tissues. Thus, if you are reacting negatively to certain kinds of foods, you should consult with an allergist who is working closely with a dietitian. Certainly you should avoid any attempt at diagnosis by amateurs. Food allergies are a complicated business, as the following statement by a panel of physicians makes clear:

> No estimate can be made of the prevalence of food intolerance because of a lack of adequate information. . . . A wide variety of symptoms have been incorrectly attributed to the effects of foods; even when the attribution is correct, there has been confusion between conditions caused by allergy, enzyme deficiencies, pharmacological reactions, psychological reactions and other mechanisms. Food intolerance can both mimic other conditions and be mimicked by them.[5]

Knowledge of the chemistry of protein molecules and the processes involved in protein digestion and absorption has four practical implications. Surgical removal of even a small part of the small intestine can have serious consequences in the digestion of proteins and the absorption of amino acids; removal of the stomach is less disastrous. Hormones that are proteins, like insulin, cannot be taken orally because they are digested and lose their hormone action. All enzymes are proteins and will lose their enzyme activity if taken orally; over-the-counter enzyme preparations taken orally are worthless. Many food allergies are due to the absorption of large, undigested proteins; when in the blood, these proteins set up an allergic reaction.

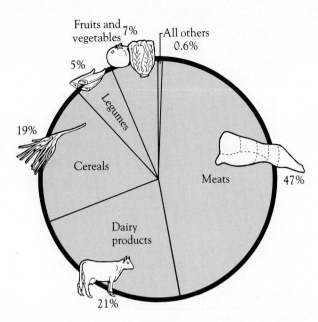

FIGURE 5-6
Percent of protein from various foods
in the United States. (Legumes are dry
beans and peas.)

QUANTITY AND QUALITY: WHY THEY MATTER

You can determine the nutritional value of protein in foods by considering what
can be called the "Two Q's"—*quantity* and *quality*. Let us analyze these.

North Americans Get More Protein from Animal Than from Plant Foods

The typical American and Canadian diet has high intakes of foods from the meat
and dairy food groups, which have a high protein content. Indeed, as Figure 5-6
illustrates, almost two thirds of the protein in the average U.S. diet comes from
foods of animal origin.

Lean Body Mass
**The soft tissue—heart, muscles, liver,
etc; excludes adipose tissue.**

There are two important points about protein in RDAs:

- Both the amount of protein and its percentages of U.S. RDA are given on
  the food product label, which was described in Chapter 2.
- The RDA for protein is higher for adults, as Figure 5-7 makes clear. However,
  as a proportion of body weight, the greatest need for protein is during the
  early years of life, the period of most rapid growth.

RDAs for adults are based on ideal body weight (see Table 9-5), and this is true
even if you are overweight or underweight. This is because the protein requirement
is based on the amount of *lean body tissue*—that is, the soft tissue of your body,
which includes the heart, muscles, and liver but excludes adipose tissues.

Here's how to calculate your own RDA for protein:

1. Convert your body weight into kilograms (pounds ÷ 2.2 = kilograms).
2. Multiply the result by 0.8. (The recommended intake for adults is 0.8 g of
   protein per kilogram of body weight per day.)
3. You can compare your answer with values described for "reference woman"
   (121 lbs or 55 kg) or "reference man" (154 lbs or 70 kg). The RDA for
   reference woman is, therefore, 44 g of protein, and 56 g of protein for
   reference man.

FIGURE 5-7
Recommended essential amino acids
and total protein. These recommendations are for children (4-6 months) and
for adult men or women. When protein RDA is expressed as total amount
of protein, it increases with age. When
protein RDA is expressed as a proportion of body weight, it is clear that
children require much more total protein and essential amino acids than do
adults.

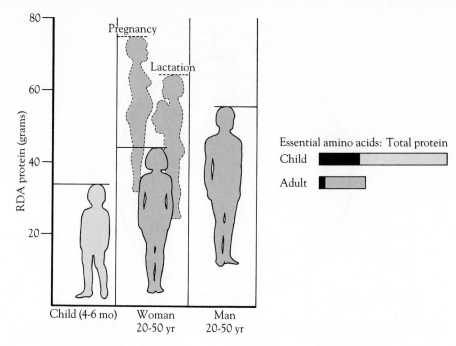

FIGURE 5-7
Recommended essential amino acids
and total protein. These recommendations are for children (4-6 months) and
for adult men or women. When protein RDA is expressed as total amount
of protein, it increases with age. When
protein RDA is expressed as a proportion of body weight, it is clear that
children require much more total protein and essential amino acids than do
adults.

The RDA of protein for pregnant women is higher because more protein is needed for the growth of the fetus and for increased blood volume and the development of the placenta in the mother. Protein RDA is higher for women during lactation because of the protein needs of milk production (see the table on the inside back cover).

Most North Americans' Protein Intake Is Well Over the RDA

A recent survey in the United States (HANES II) indicated that protein intake by men and women averaged 92 and 60 g of protein per day, respectively. These numbers are far in excess of the RDA. Research shows that most Canadians have protein intakes higher than the RDA.

The diet of a nation changes over time.

As we mentioned in an earlier chapter, people experience changing patterns of food intake over time. As you might expect, the sources of protein in your typical diet are probably different from those of your ancestors. Indeed, since the early part of this century there was a 40% increase in the consumption of protein from meat, poultry, and fish, and a 30% increase from dairy products. In the same period, the amount of protein from grain products in the U.S. diet decreased by 50%.

Protein Intake Is Expressed as a Percentage of Total Kcaloric Intake

The average consumption of protein in self-selected diets in most parts of the world is between 9% and 15% of total kcaloric intake. In the United States, however, about 12% of kcalories come from protein—and this value has been remarkably constant since the early 1900s.

Protein-Rich Foods Are Frequently High in Fat

Look at the common foods listed in Figure 5-8. It is apparent from this list that people with high protein intakes have high fat intakes as well. Therefore, their kcaloric intake is high.

Vegans and vegetarians have lower fat intakes than do nonvegetarians.

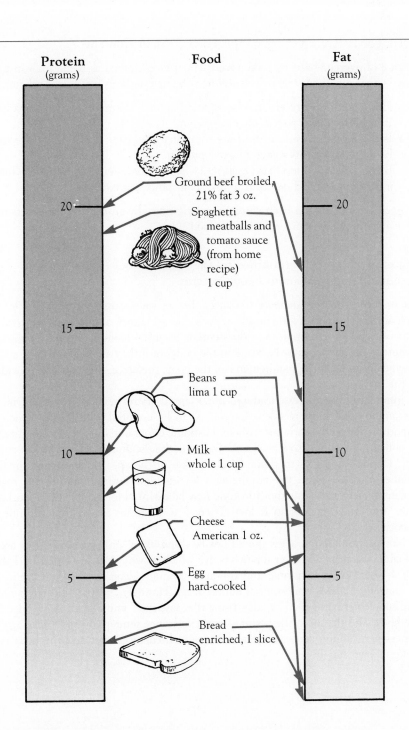

FIGURE 5-8
Many protein-rich foods are rich in fat also, unfortunately.

Protein
(grams)

Food

Fat
(grams)

Ground beef broiled, 21% fat 3 oz.

Spaghetti meatballs and tomato sauce (from home recipe) 1 cup

20

20

15

15

Beans lima 1 cup

Milk whole 1 cup

10

10

Cheese American 1 oz.

Egg hard-cooked

5

5

Bread enriched, 1 slice

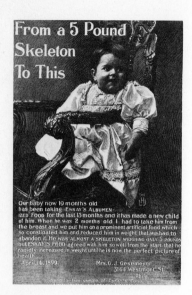

Is Eskay O.K.? Our love affair with high protein intakes is not new. Albumen referred to in this advertisement really refers to protein. Actually, the baby here looks suspiciously fat. High protein intakes are deposited as body fat.

Consumer Science

Many Protein-Rich Foods Are the Most Expensive Foods

Protein-rich foods are mostly in the meat and dairy groups. In general, these foods are more expensive than foods in the cereals and fruit and vegetable group. This is an important issue that will be explored in the "Decisions" section at the end of this chapter.

Some Foods Are Overvalued for Their Protein Content

Beware of overemphasis by food advertisers of foods touted as being high in protein—especially foods favored by children. Some questions you might ask are:

- How high is the protein in relation to other foods? Sometimes the comparison is made to a very poor source of protein.
- Is the intake of protein from the total diet adequate? If so, then there may be no need for this source of extra protein.
- Is this advertised food also high in fat, sugar, cholesterol, or sodium? This is a particularly good question to ask about processed foods.

Such advertising has been going on a long time. Even in 1899 consumers had to deal with claims about protein-rich food.

Protein Quality Is Determined by the Amount and Proportion of Essential Amino Acids in Food Proteins

Let us turn now from *quantity* to *quality*. Before we discuss specific foods, let us look at the amino acids for a moment. As Table 5-1 shows, amino acids are divided into two groups, essential and nonessential. Essential amino acids are important in nutrition. They cannot be made in the body, or if they are made, it is at a rate insufficient to meet the requirements of the body; therefore, they must be provided in the diet.

Information on the essential and nonessential amino acids is growing. One of the amino acids most recently determined to be essential is histidine, which is important during the early years of life. Histidine is found in highest concentrations in collagen in connective tissue. Collagen is the "scaffolding" supporting every cell. During rapid growth there is an increase in the size and sometimes in the number of cells. Thus, the requirement for histidine during childhood is high. Recent evidence suggests that histidine may be essential for adults also, especially when the intake of protein is low. There is a debate as to whether arginine is essential or not.

Nonessential amino acids should not be dismissed as unimportant. They are a valuable source of nitrogen for the body, which is why they are listed in Table 5-1. If your health is normal and you are eating an adequate diet, you need not be concerned about nonessential amino acids. However, people who buy amino acid supplements—gulled by advertising that says such amino acids are needed by the body, and the more the better—may experience some problems. Once again: nonessential amino acids are plentiful in a well-balanced diet and the body can make its own supply.

The Body May Not Make Proteins If Intake of Certain Essential Amino Acids Are Low

Nutritionists give most attention to the amount of the essential amino acids because these must be provided by the diet. When a person's intake of one or more of the essential amino acids is low, the proteins in the body cannot be made at optimal rates. This means that for a child such tissues as the heart, liver, and kidneys will not grow at an adequate rate and the child's overall growth will be reduced. Protein is like a house, as Figure 5-9 shows: if there are not enough bricks (amino acids), then the building (protein) cannot be completed. If certain important key foundation stones (essential amino acids) are missing, the building cannot be finished

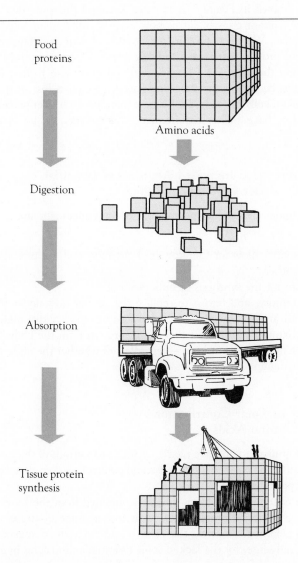

Food proteins

Amino acids

Digestion

Absorption

Tissue protein synthesis

FIGURE 5-9
Converting food proteins is like building a house. Neatly arranged stacks of amino acids are broken apart so that they are placed on a "truck" for transport to the site on which the "house" is built.

even though plenty of other bricks (nonessential amino acids) are available. Energy input is necessary to complete all buildings. Similarly, protein molecules cannot be made without expending energy. If there is not enough food energy in the diet, then protein will not be synthesized. This is why nutritionists are concerned about the energy content of the diet when they are trying to rehabilitate starving children. We will come back to the problem of protein undernutrition in a later chapter when we examine energy balance.

Infants and Adults Differ in Their Need for Essential Amino Acids

The required amount of each essential amino acid decreases as infants grow to adulthood, as shown in Figure 5-7. Having discussed the importance of essential amino acids for infant growth, let us now examine why adults need amino acids for maintenance. We need protein for growth of hair and fingernails and for replacement of protein lost from the body when cells are removed or replaced. The cells lining the digestive tract are replaced every two to four days, causing some protein to be lost in the process. Indeed, protein is lost in the breakdown and buildup of all cells in the body. Because men have a higher percentage of lean body mass, they have higher requirements than women do for essential amino acids.

The Body May Need Increased Amounts of Essential Amino Acids Under Certain Conditions

Among the circumstances that increase adult requirements for amino acids are the following:

- Pregnancy: to allow for the growth of the fetus and the reproductive organs of the mother.
- Lactation: for the synthesis of milk proteins.
- Surgery, injury, and burns: to replace the protein lost under these stresses. This is an area of active research because we know surprisingly little about the mechanisms that trigger this loss of protein from the body.[6]
- Recovery from undernutrition—regardless of whether the undernutrition was caused by famine or self-inflicted starvation.

Foods Differ in Their Contribution of Essential Amino Acids

Most foods of animal origin have nearly optimal proportions of the essential amino acids. Eggs, milk, and meat (including fish and poultry) are considered good-quality, or complete, proteins.

A notable exception is gelatin, which is obtained from the hides of cattle. A poor-quality, incomplete protein, gelatin is low in some of the essential amino acids. Eating gelatin to improve the growth and strength of fingernails does not make nutritional sense, for the lack of some essential amino acids in gelatin means that the collagen in fingernails cannot be made from it.

Plant foods are low in one or more of the essential amino acids, but there is even a gradation of protein quality within this group. Better sources include legumes—that is, beans, peas, and lentils.

Knowing Food Sources of Essential Amino Acids Is Important to People with Unusual Diets

The following groups of people may have limited intakes of essential amino acids:

- People on vegetarian diets of certain types
- Starving people with limited food sources, especially if animal foods are scarce
- People on weight-reducing diets, especially if they are teenagers.

The most vulnerable people within these groups are growing children and pregnant women.

There are different kinds of vegetarian diets, and as you read down the following list note that the amount of animal protein in the diet *increases,* which means that the problem of obtaining enough essential amino acids *decreases:*

- Fruitarians: eat only fruit, nuts, honey, olive oil
- Macrobiotic vegetarians: progress through a series of dietary stages to a very restricted diet (sometimes rice only)
- Vegans: eat foods of plant origin only
- Lactovegetarians: eat dairy foods and plant foods only
- Lactoovovegetarians: do not eat flesh but do eat dairy products and eggs
- Semivegetarians: avoid eating certain types of meat, poultry, or fish

Supplying starving people in certain parts of the world enough good-quality protein is frequently a problem in economics. Supplying vegetarians such protein, however, may often be a matter of choosing the correct plant foods.

Foods with Poor-Quality Protein Can Be Improved If Combined with the Right Other Foods

Lysine and methionine are the two essential amino acids that may be deficient in the diets of most people who do not eat foods of animal origin. Two major plant food groups are low in these amino acids. Lysine is in short supply in cereals, including rice, wheat, corn, barley, and rye. Methionine is in short supply in legumes, including soy beans, peanuts, various beans, peas, and lentils. Therefore, the protein quality of cereals and legumes is increased when cereals and legumes are combined in a meal. The low level of lysine in cereals is complemented, or mutually supplemented, by the adequate amount of lysine in legumes. *Complementary or supplementary proteins* are two or more food proteins that *together* have the proportion of essential amino acids needed by the body.

The right combination of foods from cereals and legumes can be achieved in many acceptable ways. In the typical North American diet, this combination can be found in a peanut butter sandwich, in beans combined with cornbread or toasted bread, in macaroni and cheese, and in a pizza. In Mexican cooking, the combination occurs in refried beans and rice or in beans served with corn tortillas. In Chinese and Japanese dishes, the mixture is rice and bean curd. In India, rice mixed with lentils provides the right combination. In the southern United States, the mixture is rice and black-eyed peas.[7]

Complementary or Supplementary Proteins
When two or more food proteins *together* have the proportion of essential amino acids needed by the body.

Quantity and quality of protein are important for growth and maintenance. This is not a problem for people eating the typical North American diet. More attention should be paid to quantity and quality during pregnancy, lactation, and during recovery from undernutrition, burns, injury, and surgery. Most foods of animal origin have higher protein quality than those from plants.

THE USES OF NITROGEN BALANCE STUDIES

Proteins contain nitrogen because of the nitrogen in amino acids. It is difficult to measure the amount of protein or amino acids in the diet and in the body. We learn a lot about protein in our food and in our bodies by measuring nitrogen. One of the most commonly used measurements is nitrogen balance. This measures the amount of nitrogen entering and leaving the body over a given time, usually seven days. Most of the nitrogen entering the body comes from food proteins. Nitrogen is lost from the body in the form of end products of protein metabolism in urine and sweat, in feces as unabsorbed nitrogen products and protein from dead cells in the gastrointestinal tract, in cut hair and nails, and in dead cells from the skin and elsewhere.

Nitrogen balance is changed in the following situations:

- *Positive nitrogen balance*—nitrogen intake is greater than nitrogen loss from the body. This situation occurs in all situations of growth or regrowth. It may be observed in infants and children, during pregnancy and lactation, and during recovery from starvation and severe illness.
- *Negative nitrogen balance*—nitrogen intake is less than nitrogen loss. This situation occurs with people on severe weight-loss diets, people confined to bed for long periods, or people suffering from starvation, anorexia nervosa, major traumas or burns, or some terminal cancers.
- *Nitrogen equilibrium*—nitrogen intake is the same as the amount lost from the body. This condition occurs in healthy adults eating a balanced diet.

Nitrogen balance studies tell us the protein status of a person.

THE EFFECTS OF FOOD PROCESSING ON PROTEIN: USUALLY INSIGNIFICANT

How does food processing affect protein? What happens, for example, when you cook meat?

Heat applied during commercial food processing or when food is prepared at home may destroy lysine, and thus roast meat, toasted bread, and most breakfast cereals all have reduced lysine content. However, this need concern only people eating limited food sources of protein, like infant foods. Some protein is also lost in the drippings when meat is grilled or broiled, but this, too, is of little consequence.

Heat is usually beneficial in that it opens up the structure of some food proteins, making them more digestible. It also removes an antinutritional factor in raw soybeans and prevents an antinutritional activity of eggs (raw eggs have a chemical called avidin that interferes with the activity of the B-complex vitamin, biotin). Tryptophan is destroyed during the heating process of making gelatin, but gelatin is probably not a major part of your diet.

Heat has no harmful nutritional effects on dietary proteins.

TOO MUCH PROTEIN: THE HEALTH CONSEQUENCES

Many of the important functions of protein in the body are affected when dietary intake of protein is low or high. We will examine the consequences of insufficient protein intake, as happens during famines, in a later chapter. Here let us consider what is likely to be the reverse problem for those of us living in developed countries: what happens to people with protein intakes well above the RDA for protein.

The consequences of high dietary protein intake include the following:

- Increased body fat, if total kcaloric intake is high
- High fat intake—many high-protein foods are also high in fat (as can be seen in Figure 5-8). This assumes a decreased intake in foods of plant origin and a concomitant lower intake of fiber.
- Calcium loss in the urine—when dietary protein intake is over twice the RDA, meaning over 88 g of protein for women and over 112 g for men. Calcium loss can significantly affect bone composition in older people.
- Dehydration and fluid imbalance—protein requires about seven times more water for metabolism than does either carbohydrate or fat.
- Cancer—perhaps. The relationship between protein intake and cancer has not been determined. As a 1982 report of the National Research Council on Diet, Nutrition and Cancer concluded: "Because of the relative paucity of data on protein compared to fat, and the strong correlation between the intakes of fat and protein in the U.S. diet, the committee is unable to arrive at a firm conclusion about an independent effect of protein."
- Gout—maybe. Gout has long been identified with gluttonous eating and drinking. Protein may lead to high uric acid levels in the blood, leading to deposits of uric acid crystals in the joints, causing a type of arthritis. However, high protein intake may not be responsible at all; recent evidence implicates alcohol intake as the major factor in gout.[7]

WHY THE FASCINATION WITH HIGH PROTEIN INTAKES?

In the early part of this century, nutritionists suggested that protein intake should be over 100 g per day—which is even higher than the average intake today. Over time, as scientists learned more about protein in the body, the recommended amount was lowered. Still, in developed nations, there seems to be an inordinate interest in the subject of high protein intake. Why is this? Perhaps some historical notes may explain this fascination.

Economics

Just before World War II, extensive protein deficiency was described in West Africa. In the 1950s and 1960s, this led to concerns about a shortage of dietary protein in some parts of the world. To correct the problem, nutritionists attempted to relieve poor countries' dependence on imported (and therefore expensive) protein-rich food and to substitute mixtures of local foods combined into a single manufactured food. When this experiment was tried—especially in parts of Africa and Central and South America—protein quality was high but so also, unfortunately, was the price. Some people also complained about problems with palatability. Then, in the 1960s, a revolutionary way of making protein was developed: single-cell protein (SCP) was obtained from protein-rich microorganisms. Some of the microorganisms were even grown on petroleum, yet SCP proved to have an acceptable taste.

Have you ever heard of SCP? What became of it? The answer shows some of the fascinating ways nutrition interacts with other disciplines.

Marketing

Single-cell protein (SCP) refers to single or multicellular organisms like bacteria, yeasts, fungi, algae, and perhaps protozoa. Besides protein, SCPs contain carbohydrates, fats, vitamins, minerals, and nucleic acids. Common usage of the term SCP has led to misrepresentation of its chemical composition. However, there was a marketing reason why the term *SCP* was chosen. Consider: Would you buy this product if it was called by some of its more descriptive names ("microbial protein," "bacterial protein," or "petroprotein")? Who wants to eat something associated with "diseases" (as bacteria are), or something grown on petroleum or derived from the algae slime on a pond? Quite often, the name given a food has everything to do with its being accepted.

History

In point of fact, however, SCP was hardly new; people have been eating it for thousands of years without realizing it. Brewer's yeast was used in Mesopotamia as long ago as 6000 BC; the ancient Egyptians used yeast to make bread and beer; and Hippocrates (the Greek "father of medicine") prescribed yeast for certain diseases. Indeed, a great many of today's fermented foods and drinks contain cellular organisms. Again, why the excitement about SCP and why do we no longer hear about it? The answer is threefold: SCP's chemical composition, high oil prices, and a reassessment of the significance of diet in protein deficiency.

Bacteria, and to a lesser extent yeast, could not be used as a protein source for humans because of their high nucleic acid content—which could produce a high level of uric acid and, therefore, possibly gout. In addition, some SCP products produced allergic reactions in some people. Then came the oil crisis of 1973, which made the production of SCP from petroleum uneconomic. Finally, in the mid-1970s, nutritionists began to realize that many people in the world suffered from a lack of protein *and* energy. Thus, in the space of a few years, SCP lost much of its appeal—at least for human consumption. Its promise now is as a basis for animal feeds, which the animals can then convert into protein. However, this process will not be of much help to countries with poor animal production facilities.

Economics

Another possible method of producing high-protein food, pioneered by N.W. Pirie in England, is the extracting of good-quality protein from plant leaves that would normally be thrown away after removal of the more edible plant parts. These proteins have been used successfully in increasing the protein quantity and quality of diets in India and elsewhere. Although there are problems—the high cost of the extraction equipment, difficulty in removing color and flavor from some extracts, and seasonal variation in the supply of leaves—the method holds promise of providing a good source of protein that normally would be wasted.

Acceptability of a food is important. There is little point in prolonging a discussion on the fact that many insects have the highest concentration of good quality protein! One of the best ways to increase global protein production is by genetic selection of plants and animals for greater protein quantity and quality.

DECISIONS

1. What Food is the Best Value for my "Protein Dollar"?

You can answer this question yourself by following the steps outlined below. Just be sure that you compare the cost of similar amounts of protein. The following examples do not consider the quality of the protein. These examples calculate the cost per 25 g, but it could be for any other weight also.

Loaf of Bread (85 cents)

This works out to *44 cents* for 25 g. Here's how to figure it. The food label says there are 24 servings per container, that serving size is 1 ounce (approximately 1 slice), and that there are 2 g of protein per serving. This means that there are 48 g (2 × 24) of protein in the loaf of bread. Therefore, if 48 g of protein costs 85 cents, then 25 g of protein from bread costs 44 cents (that is, 85 × 25 ÷ 48).

Hamburger from a Well-Known Fast-food Chain (69 cents)

This works out to $1.44 for 25 g. Since there is no nutrition label on the wrapper, we go to the nutrition information in Appendix P for the following information. If the hamburger weighs 102 g, it has 12 g of protein. Thus, if 12 g of protein costs 69 cents, then 25 g of the fast-food burger you bought costs $1.44.

Use the same type of calculations to see that a cheeseburger costing 79 cents from the same chain costs $1.32 for 25 g of protein. Therefore, if all you are looking for is value for protein quantity, the cheeseburger is better value than the hamburger.

A Gallon of 2% Milk for $2.49

This works out to *49 cents* for 25 g. The label says a serving size is 1 cup, there are 16 servings per container, and 8 g per serving. Therefore, total protein content in 1 gallon is 128 g (8 g protein × 16 servings), costing $2.49. Thus, 25 g of protein in milk costs 49 cents. (Remember that milk is also adequate in all other nutrients except for iron and vitamin C.)

2. Is Muscle Mass Increased and Athletic Performance Improved by Eating More Protein?

After reading some popular magazines written for athletes, you might think the answer is "yes." However, experiments with athletes with high protein intakes have not shown an improvement in performance. Many articles and advertisements advising protein supplements are based on the fact that muscle has the greatest amount of protein in the body (Figure 5-3). A theory based on "throwing dietary protein at muscle in the hope that some might cling" does not work. Evaluate some of the following reasons in coming to your decision.

Muscle mass is increased by increasing the size of cells. This is done by stressing the muscle (for instance, by lifting weights) or by taking anabolic hormones, which is ill advised. Extra dietary protein is needed in increasing muscle mass. To determine whether you need extra protein from supplements, use some of the information previously discussed. First, you know there is a limit to the size of the cell. Eating additional protein will not increase cell size, and therefore muscle size, once a certain critical point is reached. Second, protein RDA for a man is 56 g and for a woman 44 g. The average dietary intake of protein in the U.S. for males and females is 92 and 60 g, respectively. This additional protein from dietary intake is more than sufficient to meet the extra demand for additional muscle formation.

Water, not protein, has the greatest effect on athletic performance. But protein intakes in excess of protein requirements increase the amount of body water needed to excrete the end products of protein metabolism. For this reason, high protein intakes could have a harmful effect on athletic performance. Having established the scientific evidence against protein supplementation, let us look at its cost.

One protein supplement in a one-pound can sells for $7.99. There are 16 servings in the can, each containing 32 g of protein *after* one cup of milk is added. We saw above that one cup of milk has 8 g of protein. Therefore, each serving of this supplement has 24 g of protein (32 − 8). Therefore, the total amount of protein in the can is 384 g. Therefore, 25 g of protein from a supplement costs 52 cents. If it is cost you are interested in, this is certainly cheaper than the protein provided by hamburgers.

These calculations have considered protein quantity, but not protein quality.

3. Are Bee Pollen and Spirulina the Richest Sources of Protein Known to Science?

These claims are seen frequently in articles and advertisements. Let us consider bee pollen first. Carbohydrate is the nutrient in highest concentration in bee pollen.[8] Protein content varies widely because of climate and the nutritional status of the plants on which the pollen matures. Protein content can vary between 5% and 28%. Therefore, bee pollen does not compare well with soybean cake (46% protein), brewer's yeast (39%), dry pumpkin seeds (29%), and round steak (about 20%).

Spirulina is an algae. It was not discovered by Western promoters until the mid-1960s, although it was eaten for centuries in Mexico and parts of North Africa. The following *false* claims are made for spirulina in both North America and Europe[9]: it is the world's richest source of protein, it has high vitamin content (especially vitamin B_{12}), it is a helpful slimming aid, it increases defenses against sickness, and it cures all kinds of things—wrinkles, shortness of breath, hives, asthma, white hair in young people. It is also claimed that spirulina improves the quality of sex life. If these claims were true, this substance would probably be in everyone's kitchen, but alas, there is no scientific evidence to support these claims.

4. Are Amino Acid Supplements Effective?

To answer this question, one must ask *which* amino acids, and effective against what? The first fact to consider is that amino acids are chemicals and should be treated with the same caution we give to other chemicals taken orally. For example, amino acids may be toxic at high doses. These toxic effects are easiest to produce on a low-protein diet. The four amino acids most used as supplements are: tryptophan, lysine, methionine, and threonine.

Amino acid supplements are of nutritional value only if the diet is deficient in the amino acid. So why flirt with toxicity? The appeal of such products may be seen in the following extract from an advertisement for a product called Amino High, which would seem to be a pill for all ailments: "Are you nervous? Can't sleep? Bad moods? Short memory? Crave booze or sleep? Have fever blisters or herpes? Depressed? Tired? Always hungry? Have allergies? Ever heard of amino acids? Deficiencies of these 'little jewels' are directly related to the troubles listed above." Wouldn't it be terrific if this product corrected all these things?

Let us make scientific sense out of a few amino acid supplements:

Lysine

Usually sold in 500 mg capsules; the typical U.S. diet provides 6 to 7 g of lysine per day. Using 400 mg per day to treat herpes was not successful.[10] The effect of long-term lysine supplementation is not known.[11]

Tryptophan and Tyrosine

Both amino acids form part of neurotransmitters. Let us look at tryptophan first. A normal diet supplies 1 to 2 g per day. Additional intakes of 5 to 15 g of tryptophan will shorten the time required to fall asleep. Tryptophan is known in the popular literature as "nature's sleeping pill." Tryptophan is usually sold in 500 mg tablets. You would have to take 10 to 30 tablets to get to sleep faster. A summary of the latest research concludes: "In humans, tryptophan administration to normal adults or persons with medical or psychiatric problems or with severe insomnia produces inconsistent results."[12]

Tyrosine

Tyrosine has been reported to help some patients with depression or mild Parkinson's disease—a neurological disorder.[13]

A survey showed that the percentage difference between the wholesale price for large quantities and their retail price in stores was 550% for tryptophan and 525% to 875% for lysine.

5. Will Superoxide Dismutase (SOD) Taken Orally Prevent Aging?

It sure would be marvelous if it did. SOD is an enzyme that is supposed to fulfill that promise according to numerous advertisements. "Look Younger—With Incredible Youth Pill" was the headline of a story that stated: "For as little as 25 cents a day the fountain of youth can be yours—in easy-to-take pill form" (_National Enquirer_, July 28, 1981). This story is based on evidence in the scientific literature that SOD in tissues may be an important enzyme in controlling the aging process in cells in the body. The reasoning is that swallowing an extra amount of the enzyme will therefore increase the level of SOD in the tissues. Unfortunately, many people are unaware that SOD is an enzyme, and therefore a protein. SOD will be digested like any other protein into its individual amino acids. For this reason, SOD taken orally is worthless in increasing SOD levels in intestine, liver, kidney, or blood—at least in laboratory studies with mice.[14]

Summary

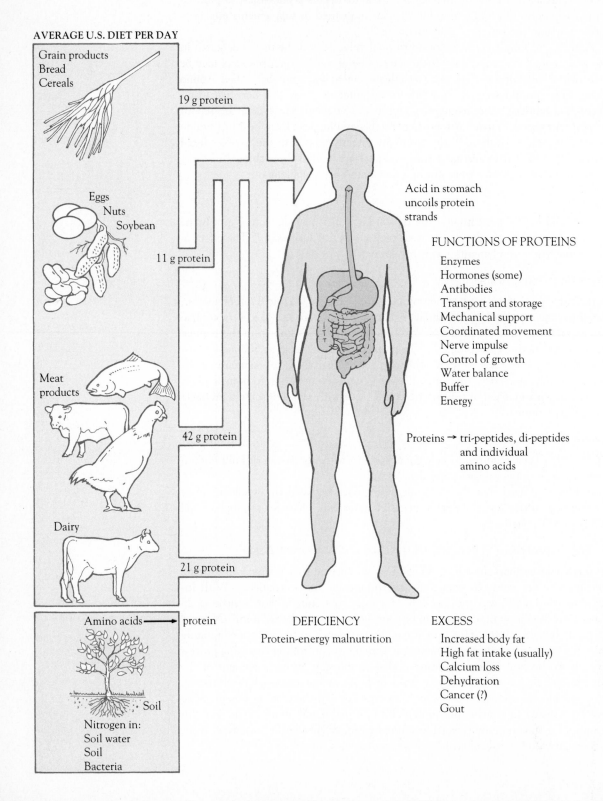

AVERAGE U.S. DIET PER DAY

Grain products
Bread
Cereals

19 g protein

Eggs
Nuts
Soybean

11 g protein

Meat
products

42 g protein

Dairy

21 g protein

Amino acids → protein

Soil

Nitrogen in:
Soil water
Soil
Bacteria

Acid in stomach
uncoils protein
strands

FUNCTIONS OF PROTEINS

Enzymes
Hormones (some)
Antibodies
Transport and storage
Mechanical support
Coordinated movement
Nerve impulse
Control of growth
Water balance
Buffer
Energy

Proteins → tri-peptides, di-peptides
and individual
amino acids

DEFICIENCY

Protein-energy malnutrition

EXCESS

Increased body fat
High fat intake (usually)
Calcium loss
Dehydration
Cancer (?)
Gout

REFERENCES

1. Ballentine, C.: The essential guide to amino acids, FDA Consumer, page 23, September, 1985.

2. Latham, M.C.: International nutrition problems and policies, In World Food Issues, 2nd edition, M. Drosdoff, editor, Cornell University Press, Ithaca, N.Y., 1984.

3. Mellors, J.W., and Barry, M.: Malnutrition or AIDS in Haiti? New England Journal of Medicine **310**:1119, 1984.

4. Institute of Food Technologists' Expert Panel on Food Safety and Nutrition: Food allergies and sensitivities, Food Technology **39**:65, September, 1985.

5. Joint Report of the Royal College of Physicians and The British Nutrition Foundation: Food intolerance and food aversion, Journal of the Royal College of Physicians of London **18**:83, 1984.

6. Rennie, M.J., and Harrison, R.: Effects of injury, disease, and malnutrition on protein metabolism in man: Unanswered questions, Lancet **i**:323, 1984.

7. Scott, J.T.: Food, drink, and gout, British Medical Journal **287**:78, 1983.

8. Larkin, T.: Bee pollen as a health food, FDA Consumer, page 21, April, 1984.

9. Bender, A.E.: Health or hoax: The truth about health food and diets, Elvendon Press, Goring-on-Thames, England, 1985.

10. DiGiovanna, J.J., and Blank, H.: Failure of lysine in frequently recurrent herpes simplex infection, Archives of Dermatology **120**:48, 1984.

11. Dubick, M.A.: Dietary supplements and health aids: a critical evaluation. II.: Macronutrients and fiber, Journal of Nutrition Education **15**:88, 1983.

12. Diet and Behavior Symposium proceedings: Summary, Nutrition Reviews, **44**(Suppl): 252, May, 1986.

13. Wurtman, R.J.: Ways that foods affect the brain, Nutrition Reviews, **44**(Suppl):2, May 1986.

14. Zidenberg-Cherr, S., and others: Dietary superoxide dismutase does not affect tissue levels, American Journal of Clinical Nutrition **37**:5, 1983.

METABOLISM NOTES: *Metabolism of Proteins and Amino Acids*

Metabolic Changes During High and Low Dietary Intake of Protein Are Important

The metabolic pathway shown in Figure 5-10 is important in *low protein intake* during starvation, severe weight-reducing diets, and anorexia nervosa, and in *high protein intake* from the regular diet or when protein supplements are taken.

A few points are important:

- The plasma amino acid pool is small. When the amino acids in the plasma are used, body protein must be broken down to replace it. This means the breaking down of tissue such as muscles, liver, and heart. There is no storage of amino acids to meet major emergencies due to a lack of dietary energy.
- In starvation, most of the amino acid supply comes from the muscles, the liver, and the gastrointestinal system.
- Deamination or the removal of the amine group ($-NH_2$) must occur if amino acids are broken down for energy, or if they are converted into fat for energy storage. Most nitrogen from the amino acid is then excreted in the urine.
- High dietary intake of protein will *not* increase protein synthesis. This fact is important in understanding what happens when protein supplements are added to a high dietary protein intake.

FIGURE 5-10
Metabolic pathway for low and high protein intakes.

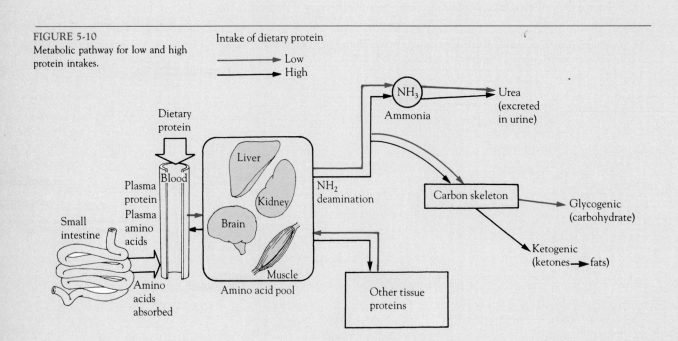

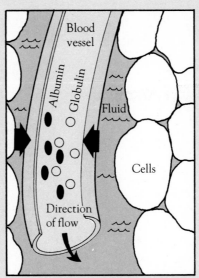

FIGURE 5-11
Influence of protein in the movement of fluid from cells.

Pull on fluid toward blood vessel

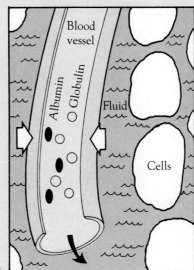

Weaker pull on fluids toward blood vessel causing an increase of extracellular fluid (edema)

Edema Is an End Result of Protein-Energy Malnutrition

Two of the many important proteins in your blood are albumin and globulin. In the healthy person, the constant level of these two proteins exerts a pull on fluid from the extracellular space, as shown in Figure 5-11.

Osmotic pressure is the "pull" that brings the fluid back to the blood vessel. It is controlled by the concentration of protein in the blood. In severe undernutrition (protein-energy malnutrition), the concentration of albumin in the blood decreases. This lowers the osmotic pressure and causes an accumulation of fluid in the extracellular space. This fluid accumulation is the edema that is observable as a puffiness of arms, legs, and so on.

FIGURE 5-12
High purine intake leads to gout.

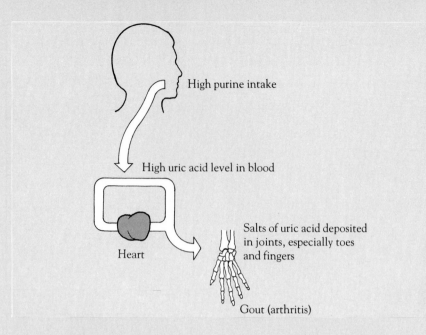

Some Supposedly "No-Aging" Diets Recommend High Purine Intakes, But You Should Consider How They Are Metabolized

This is a good example of where knowledge of metabolism is useful before starting a special diet. Chemically, purines are part of the DNA and RNA in the cell nucleus, and they contain nitrogen. Foods rich in purines are liver, kidneys, pancreas, sardines, and anchovies. Meat and fish have reasonable amounts. Only small amounts occur in vegetables and none in fruits and cereals. Unfortunately, there is no good scientific evidence to show that diets high in purines will prevent aging. Instead, what will happen is the sequence of events shown in Figure 5-12.

Gout is a painful type of arthritis. It occurs most often in middle-aged men, and in women after the menopause. Gout is rare in vegans because purine intake is low on a diet of cereals, vegetables, and fruits. Gout is curable if the sufferer does the following: reduce body weight; reduce intake of protein, purines, and alcohol; and increase fiber intake.

Vitamins

CONNECTIONS

Can a food store sell a nonprotein as a protein? No, but it can sell a nonvitamin substance as a vitamin—and such commercialism is quite common. This chapter describes what vitamins actually are—organic substances involved in much of the body's metabolism. Some are involved in releasing locked-up energy from carbohydrates, fats, and proteins, promoting bone growth, enhancing vision, making blood clotting possible, and other functions. Because vitamins are needed in only very small amounts, they are usually satisfied by a balanced diet. Will taking vitamin pills in "megadose" quantities, then, improve our health? The answer is "no." The reasons are given below.

"Every morning as the sun rises over the land," writes John Fried in *Vitamin Politics*, "between 50 and 60 million Americans rise to perform a semireligious ritual—to swallow dutifully, almost obsessively, a pill (maybe two) containing a rich allotment of vitamins and minerals."

Sound familiar? If you are a member of this large group—equivalent to twice the entire population of Canada—you are helping to stimulate a $2.6 billion industry. Many people, however, have little real knowledge about what they're buying. Indeed, although a balanced diet of common foods will provide all the vitamins you need, one out of six people does not know this, so the sale of vitamin supplements flourishes.[1] In one Canadian survey, a whopping 60% of the households studied, including people of all socioeconomic levels, used some type of vitamin supplement, and studies of other industrialized countries give similar results.[2]

How did this zeal for vitamin pills come about? And do vitamin supplements really make a difference in your health?

THE BRILLIANT HISTORY OF VITAMINS

Vitamins were always present in foods, but their existence was only learned about in the early 1900s.

Obviously, before vitamin supplements were invented, people got vitamins from where they always got them—from their food. Following the discoveries of the first vitamins in the early 1900s, and a stream of Nobel prizes for the scientists who investigated and outlined the functions of vitamins, there were spectacular advances in science and medicine, and many previously incurable vitamin-deficiency diseases began to be conquered. Poor bone formation in children, physicians realized, could be traced to vitamin D deficiency. Blindness could in some cases be traced to a shortage of vitamin A and some neurological disorders to low intakes of some B-complex vitamins. The results of these brilliant discoveries were dramatic cures and fewer deaths, and in the industrialized nations vitamin deficiencies began to disappear.

Medicine

As you might expect, with this kind of success it was only a matter of time before people began to gobble vitamins to try to boost their energy level and to help them "feel good"—and, of course, these claims are still made about vitamins today. But do vitamins really do this? The evidence is not clear. Feelings of tiredness or well-being are often difficult to measure. It is difficult to quantify the effect on energy and mood of taking large amounts of vitamins over a long time. We know approximately what kinds of doses will cure deficiency symptoms, but we don't know whether megadoses—high vitamin intake—will improve health.

Nutritionists want to quantify the effects of diet on the body. Feelings are difficult to measure.

> Nutritionists know the approximate amount of the different vitamins needed to cure deficiency symptoms, but they know little about the beneficial effects, if any, of megadoses.

VITAMINS: ONLY THIRTEEN OCCUR IN NATURE

To look in the front window of a vitamin store, you might think there are a hundred vitamins. Indeed, there *are* many substances that are advertised as vitamins to an unsuspecting public, but actually there are, like the original colonies of the United States, only thirteen vitamins. They are listed in Table 6-1. Before we describe the vitamins in detail, let us define what vitamins are.

Vitamins have three characteristics:
1. They are organic substances.
2. They are required for specific metabolic functions in the body.
3. They are needed in small amounts in the diet.

Let us consider these three qualities.

Vitamins Are Organic Substances

The term *organic substances* simply means that the substances contain the chemical element *carbon*, C, especially when bonded to hydrogen, whether derived from living organisms or not. (Note that this scientific usage of "organic" is different from the more popular usage like "organic" in organic foods meaning food produced without the use of pesticides, chemical fertilizers, or additives.) Figure 6-1 shows how carbon appears in the chemical structure of vitamins C and D. Notice that the two structures are completely different; in fact, there is no similarity in chemical structure among any of the thirteen vitamins. The only meaningful grouping of vitamins on the basis of chemical properties is that (as Table 6-1 shows) some are soluble in fat and others are soluble in water. Absorption from the diet and storage in the body are influenced by their solubility in water or fat.

Do synthetic vitamins differ in chemical structure from naturally occurring vitamins? Not at all: vitamins C and D made in a laboratory test tube look exactly the same as those shown in the figure and they have the same metabolic functions. There is no test that can distinguish synthetic from natural vitamins, and your body can't tell the difference. Thus, if you see a health food store promoting a vitamin as being "natural"—but at a higher price than a synthetic—don't be misled.

Chemistry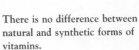

There is no difference between natural and synthetic forms of vitamins.

TABLE 6-1 The Vitamins

Common Name	Also Known As
Fat-soluble Vitamins	
Vitamin A (carotene is a precursor)	Retinol
Vitamin D (7-dehydrocholesterol is a precursor)	Cholecalciferol (D_3), ergocalciferol (D_2)
Vitamin E	Tocopherols, of which alpha-tocopherol is the most active
Vitamin K	Menadione
Water-soluble Vitamins	
Vitamin C	Ascorbic acid
B-complex vitamins	
Thiamin	Vitamin B_1
Riboflavin	Vitamin B_2
Niacin (tryptophan is a precursor)	Nicotinic acid, nicotinamide, vitamin B_3
Vitamin B_6	Pyridoxine, pyridoxamine, pyridoxal
Pantothenic acid	
Biotin	
Folacin	Folic acid, folate
Vitamin B_{12}	Cobalamin

Vitamin C

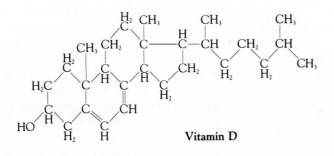

Vitamin D

FIGURE 6-1
Chemical formulas for vitamins C and D. (Compare the similarity between vitamin D and cholesterol in Figure 4-8.)

TABLE 6-2 Some Metabolic Functions of the Vitamins

Metabolic Function	Vitamins Involved
Helps in release and formation of energy in the metabolism of carbohydrates, fats, and proteins	Release: thiamin, riboflavin, niacin, vitamin B_6, biotin, pantothenic acid Formation: biotin
Blood formation	Vitamin B_{12}, folacin, vitamin B_6, vitamin C
Bone and teeth formation	Vitamins A, D, and C
Neuromuscular function	Vitamin A, thiamin, niacin, vitamin B_6, vitamin B_{12}, pantothenic acid
Maintenance of skin condition	Vitamins A, C, and B_6, riboflavin, niacin, pantothenic acid
Eye function	Vitamin A
Blood-related processes	Vitamin K (helps clotting), vitamin E (prevents red blood cells from breaking)
Reproduction	Vitamin A (sperm formation and maintenance of normal menstrual cycle), vitamin A and riboflavin (prevent birth defects)
Hormone formation	Vitamin A, pantothenic acid (steroid hormones), vitamin B_6 (norepinephrine and thyroxine)
Interaction with hormones	Vitamin D (calcium-regulating hormones)

Vitamins Are Required for Specific Metabolic Functions

Vitamins perform specific jobs in the body, as summarized in Table 6-2. For instance, vitamin A is involved in vision. Several vitamins are involved in energy release and in maintaining the skin.

If you know the normal functions for which a specific vitamin is needed, you may then have an idea of some of the disorders produced if that vitamin is in short supply. For instance, if vitamin A is needed for normal vision, then a deficiency of vitamin A will produce blindness, and you can rule out other vitamin deficiencies as a cause of this problem (Table 6-2). Not only deficiencies but oversupplies of vitamins may also cause metabolic disorders, as Table 6-3 shows. For example, whereas too little vitamin A will cause blindness, too much will cause hair loss and pain in the bones; both extremely low and extremely high intakes of vitamin A will cause death.

Fat-soluble vitamins are more likely to cause toxicity than water-soluble vitamins. The body has no mechanism for excreting fat-soluble substances through the urine or sweat. Therefore excess intakes of fat-soluble vitamins will be stored in the body and could reach toxic levels. Water-soluble vitamins, if taken in excess, are excreted in the urine. A look at Table 6-4 shows that the fat-soluble vitamins A, D, and E have a lower vitamin safety index number than most of the other

High intakes of some vitamins may damage health and may even cause death.

TABLE 6-3 Symptoms of Vitamin Deficiency and Toxicity

Vitamin	Symptoms	
	Deficiency	Toxicity
Fat-soluble Vitamins		
Vitamin A	Nightblindness, permanent blindness, skin disorders, diarrhea, respiratory infections, loss of senses of taste and smell, decreased growth, death	Growth retardation, hair loss, skin changes, pain in bones, death
Vitamin D	Poor bone formation—rickets in children, osteomalacia in adults	Growth retardation, kidney damage, calcium in soft tissue, death
Vitamin E	Anemia in premature infants because of fragile red blood cells (rare)	Inadequate evidence; (possible) severe muscle weakness, headaches, fatigue, nausea
Vitamin K	Poor blood clotting (uncommon, except in newborn babies and after long use of oral antibiotics)	Rare; impossible from dietary sources
Water-soluble Vitamins		
Vitamin C	Scurvy, delayed wound healing, poorer absorption of iron	Rebound scurvy, kidney stones, diarrhea, nausea, interferes with sugar test for diabetes
Thiamin	Beriberi—neurological changes, depression, loss of appetite	No toxicity even at high oral doses
Riboflavin	Personality changes, cracks at corners of mouth (cheilosis), tender tongue (glossitis)	Unknown
Niacin	Pellagra—diarrhea, dermatitis, depression (the three Ds), and finally death	Skin flushing, cramps, nausea, jaundice, and liver dysfunction
Vitamin B_6	A specific type of anemia (rare)	Rare, but can interact with some drugs. Sensory nerve disorders with very high doses
Pantothenic acid	Rare in humans	Minimal effects, maybe diarrhea
Biotin	Rare in humans	Never reported in humans
Folacin	Megaloblastic anemia—tired, weak. Diarrhea, loss of appetite, behavioral changes	Interferes with tests for vitamin B_{12} deficiency, fever, pain, kidney damage
Vitamin B_{12}	Pernicious anemia, nerve damage	No toxicity in humans, except rare allergic reactions

TABLE 6-4 Vitamin Safety Indexes

Vitamin	Recommended Adult Intake*	Estimated Adult Oral Minimum Toxic Dose	Vitamin Safety Index
Vitamin A	5000 IU	25,000 to 50,000 IU	5 to 10
Vitamin D	400 IU	50,000 IU	125
Vitamin E	30 IU	1200 IU	40
Vitamin C	60 mg	2000 to 5000 mg	33 to 83
Thiamin	1.5 mg	300 mg	200
Riboflavin	1.7 mg	1000 mg	588
Niacin	20 mg	1000 mg	50
Vitamin B_6	2.2 mg	2000 mg	900
Folacin	0.4 mg	400 mg	1000
Biotin	0.3 mg	50 mg	167
Pantothenic acid	10 mg	10,000 mg	1000

*The individual RDA (except those for pregnancy and lactation) or the U.S. RDA, whichever is higher.

vitamins. The safety index is the ratio of the estimated adult oral minimum toxic dose to the recommended adult intake. (Note that vitamin K is not listed—because people do not usually take vitamin K supplements, and usually you will not find them for sale in stores.) Yet this does not mean that taking large amounts of water-soluble vitamins is safe: recent evidence suggests that high intakes of these are not as safe as was once thought.

Are the adverse effects of vitamin deficiencies and toxicities, short of death, reversible? Some are and some aren't. Blindness caused by vitamin A deficiency cannot be cured. In a child, growth retardation caused by vitamin A toxicity may be reversed when the vitamin is given in normal amounts, but the child will not recapture any growth lost during the period of toxicity. Irreversible changes due to vitamin A toxicity include bone malformations and liver toxicity. Vitamin A deficiency and toxicity can produce a wide range of adverse effects, as Figure 6-2 makes clear. The levels at which deficiency- and toxicity-related disorders occur vary for different vitamins.

Some symptoms of vitamin deficiencies and toxicities are reversible. Reversible toxicity symptoms of vitamin A include dermatitis, loss of hair, and hemorrhages. Additional vitamin C will correct bleeding gums caused by scurvy, and additional vitamin K will relieve blood clotting problems caused by vitamin K deficiency. Some skin problems can be eased by alleviating some vitamin deficiencies.

It can take a long time for symptoms associated with vitamin deficiency to occur, at least for fat-soluble vitamins, because vitamins are recycled within the body after metabolic reactions take place and only small amounts are lost at each cycle. It is these small amounts that must be replaced by vitamins in the diet. Incidentally, there is a wide variation in the time required for replacement of individual vitamins because of differences in storage capacity and extent of use.

Vitamins Are Needed in Small Amounts in the Diet

No single unenriched food will provide adequate amounts of all vitamins. As Table 6-5 indicates, different food groups are sources of different vitamins. Avoiding vitamin deficiencies or toxicities, then, requires eating a wide variety of foods. However, the *amounts* of the vitamins needed are not large. Figure 6-3 shows the recommended dietary allowance (RDA) for ten vitamins. If these values are converted into the amounts recommended over one year, then less than 22 mg of vitamin C and only 1.095 mg of vitamin B_{12} are suggested. These are, indeed, very small amounts.

No doubt you have heard of people taking vitamins in huge quantities. Nobel laureate Linus Pauling has urged taking 10 vitamin C a day to fight colds. A *megadose* is defined as a vitamin intake that is more than 10 times the RDA. Since

Medicine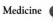

TABLE 6-5 Best Dietary Sources of Vitamins

Food Group	Good Source of
Meat, poultry, fish, beans	Thiamin, riboflavin, niacin, vitamin B_6, vitamin B_{12}, pantothenic acid, folacin
Milk, cheese	Vitamins A, D, B_6, B_{12}, riboflavin
Breads and cereals	Thiamin, riboflavin, vitamin B_6, folacin,, pantothenic acid, biotin
Fruits and vegetables	Vitamins A, C, K, riboflavin, folacin
Fats and oils	Vitamins A, E

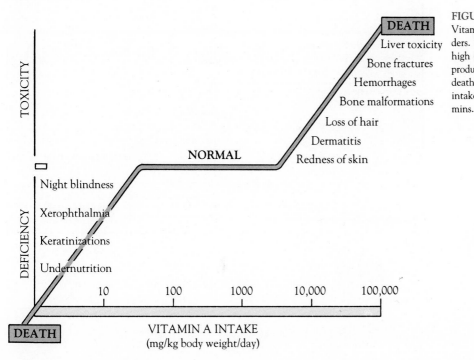

FIGURE 6-2

Vitamin A intake and range of disorders. Very low (deficiency) and very high (toxicity) vitamin A intake can produce damaging symptoms and even death. The severity of effects and the intake range vary for different vitamins.

FIGURE 6-3
RDA values for ten vitamins.

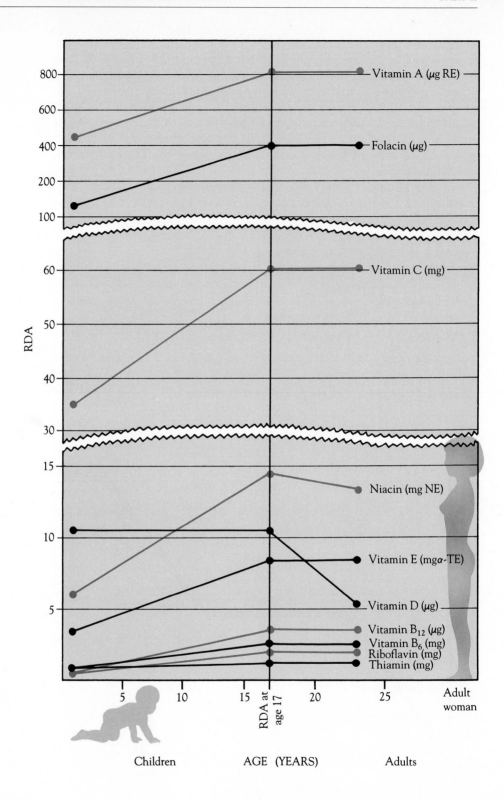

TABLE 6-6 Disorders Aggravated by Megadoses of Water-soluble Vitamins

Disorder	Vitamin
Asthma	Niacin
Diabetes mellitus	Niacin, vitamin C
Peptic ulcer disease	Niacin
Liver disease	Niacin
Gout	Niacin
Cardiac disease	Niacin
Skin disease	Niacin
Diarrhea	Niacin, vitamin C, pantothenic acid
Kidney stones	Vitamin C
Sideroblastic anemia	Vitamin C
Megaloblastic anemia	Vitamin C, folacin
Scurvy	Vitamin C
Central nervous system disorders	Vitamin B_6, thiamin, folacin
Parkinson's disease	Vitamin B_6
Sensory neuropathy	Vitamin B_6

the RDA for vitamin C is 60 mg, a megadose would be 600 mg. Table 6-6 indicates some of the disorders that may be aggravated by taking megadoses of certain water-soluble vitamins, particularly vitamin C and niacin, both of which are available without prescription and in megadose-size tablets.

Vitamins are organic substances performing specific metabolic functions in the body and are needed in small amounts in the diet.

THE VARYING VITAMINS: DIFFERENT CHARACTERISTICS

Vitamins not only have different RDAs, they have other differences as well:

- Different units of measure
- Differences in stability
- Different interactions with medications

Let us consider these.

TABLE 6-7 Different Units of Measurement for Some Vitamins

Vitamin	RDA Table	Food Composition Tables, Vitamin Supplement Labels	Conversion Factors
		Unit Used In	
A	RE (retinol equivalent)	IU	1 RE = 5 IU (This is an approximation because different forms of vitamin A differ in vitamin activity. The newer REs account for this variation; IUs do not.)
Niacin	mgNE (niacin equivalent)	mg	1 mgNE = 1 mg niacin or 60 mg tryptophan
E	mgαTE (alpha-tocopherol)	IU	No conversion factor because different forms of vitamin E are expressed in TE, only alpha-tocopherol expressed in IU

Vitamins Are Measured in Different Units

Vitamins are measured in different units, which are given in Table 6-7. The presence of vitamins is measured in *milligrams* and *micrograms,* although for vitamins A and D *International Units* (IUs) are used (a unit of measurement usually seen on commercial supplements of these vitamins). In 1980, the RDA Committee recommended that a new unit called *equivalents* be used for vitamins A and E and niacin.

Using niacin equivalents (NE) instead of milligrams (mg) is a more accurate description of the niacin content of foods. The reason is that 60 mg of the amino acid tryptophan can be converted into 1 mg of niacin. Thus, niacin equivalents take this additional source of niacin into account.

Understanding the differences in the units of measurements of vitamins is important for students of nutrition and for informed shoppers of vitamins.

Vitamins Vary in Their Stability

What is the shelf life of an average vitamin? Can you keep your multiple vitamins in a cabinet over the kitchen stove and expect them to be good after a year? No, for the following reasons.

Food preparation

Vitamins vary in their stability. Heat, light, air, moisture, and the effect of acids or alkalis can cause vitamin loss. Figure 6-4 shows which vitamins are most susceptible to heat, light, and air. It also shows how much of the vitamin is lost during cooking—for instance, all of vitamin C may be lost but only about 5% of vitamin K. Severe cooking conditions—high temperatures for a long time—will cause the most loss, but some loss also occurs during normal cooking. What's important is how much of the vitamin is left after normal food preparation: when

Vitamins unstable to:

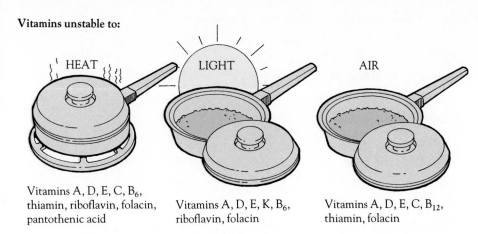

Vitamins A, D, E, C, B₆, thiamin, riboflavin, folacin, pantothenic acid

Vitamins A, D, E, K, B₆, riboflavin, folacin

Vitamins A, D, E, C, B₁₂, thiamin, folacin

FIGURE 6-4
Cooking away the vitamins. Heat, light, and air may cause severe loss of vitamins during the cooking of food, both processed food and home-prepared food.

COOKING LOSSES RANGE UP TO (%):

Vitamin A	40	Thiamin	80	Biotin	60
Vitamin D	40	Riboflavin	75	Pantothenic acid	50
Vitamin E	55	Niacin	75	Folic acid	100
Vitamin K	5	Vitamin B₆	40	Vitamin B₁₂	10
Vitamin C	100				

meat is heated, for instance, 50% of thiamin is lost, but the remaining 50% still makes meat a good source of thiamin.

Medications May Reduce Absorption

If you happen to be taking the antibiotic neomycin for intestinal upsets, it will interfere with the absorption of vitamin B₁₂ into your body. Other medications will hinder the absorption of other vitamins, as Table 6-8 shows.

TABLE 6-8 Drug Interference with the Absorption of Vitamins—Some Examples

Drug	Function	Vitamin Loss
Mineral oil	Laxative	Vitamins A, D, K, and carotene
Cholestyramine	Lowers serum cholesterol	Vitamins A, D, K, and folacin
Antacids	Neutralizes acidity	Folacin
Neomycin	Antibiotic	Vitamin B₁₂

Some vitamins are unstable in the presence of heat, light, air, and acids and alkalis. Drug-vitamin interactions are a growing area of knowledge. Megadoses of some vitamins aggravate certain disorders.

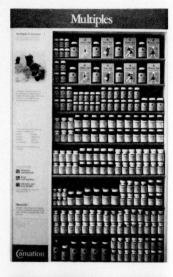

TABLE 6-9 How Expensive Is a Daily Dose of Vitamins?*

Vitamin	RDA*	Wholesale Cost (cents)†	Retail Cost (cents)‡	Percent Markup
Vitamin A	800 μg RE	0.026	0.916	3520
Vitamin D	5 μg	0.00002	not available	
Vitamin E	8 mgα-TE	0.046	0.136	300
Vitamin C	60 mg	0.06	0.598	975
Thiamin	1.0 mg	0.004	0.025	625
Riboflavin	1.2 mg	0.007	0.095	1330
Niacin	13 mgNE	0.01	0.285	285
Vitamin B_6	2.0 mg	0.008	0.076	950
Biotin	100 μg	0.055	0.647	1175
Folacin	400 μg	not available	1.106	
Vitamin B_{12}	3 μg	0.0024	0.036	1500

*100% of the RDA for a female age 23 to 50.
†Costs from Chemical Marketing Reporter, January 21, 1985.
‡Prices at a store of a national supermarket chain, Houston, Texas, January 26, 1985.

VITAMIN PILLS AND PROFITS

Vitamins are inexpensive. If you were to buy a day's worth of nine vitamins of a supermarket-label brand in bulk amounts, you would find that it costs less than 3 cents (actually 2.814 cents). A good deal, it would seem. It's also a good deal for the manufacturer and the supermarket: the wholesale price (when vitamins are sold in bulk) is only 0.218 of a cent—which means these pills have a 1290% markup! In the case of vitamin A, as Table 6-9 shows, the markup is 3520%.

Supermarket house brands of vitamins, incidentally, are less expensive than brand-name vitamins or vitamins bought in a health-food store, and there is no difference in quality.

Vitamin supplements can be inexpensive.

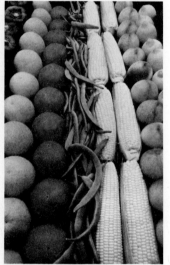

Better to get your vitamins from foods than from bottles. Foods provide minerals, protein, carbohydrates, fiber, and fat—bottled vitamins do not.

THE FAT-SOLUBLE VITAMINS: A, D, E, AND K

As you saw back at the beginning of the chapter, vitamins are either *fat-soluble* or *water-soluble*. The fat-soluble vitamins are made up of the vitamins A, D, E, and K.

Vitamin A Helps Vision

Troubled by night blindness? You could try rubbing juice from cooked liver on your eyes—that's what the ancient Greeks and Egyptians did to try to correct this disorder, which can be caused by vitamin A deficiency. Of course nowadays the intake of vitamin A can be increased in easier, more appealing ways.

Where it comes from

One active form of vitamin A known as *retinol* is found only in foods of animal origin, including liver. However, certain plants have what are known as precursors of vitamin A. A *precursor,* also sometimes called a *provitamin,* can be converted into the active form of the vitamin in the body—in this case, into retinol. In plants, the precursors of vitamin A consist of about 30 different *carotenoids*—a group of yellow and red pigments structurally related to carotene. The colorings of peaches, carrots, and many other fruits and vegetables come from carotenoids.

The most active carotenoid is beta carotene, available in carrots, sweet potatoes (white or Irish potatoes have only trace amounts), pumpkins, oranges, peaches, and dark green vegetables like spinach. It is also available in capsules in stores. In the typical North American diet, about half of the intake of vitamin A comes from beta carotene.

Beta carotene is converted into retinol in the wall of the intestine before being absorbed into the blood. The conversion is not every efficient, since the production of one retinol molecule requires six beta-carotene molecules. Retinol is absorbed from the intestine into the blood at an efficiency of between 80% and 90%.

Vitamin A in American and other diets

In the United States, vitamin A is provided principally by vegetables, meat, and dairy products, as indicated in Figure 6-5. The RDA for men is 1000 RE and for

Retinol
An active form of vitamin A found in foods of animal origin.

Precursors
Substances available in food that can be converted into the active form of the vitamin in the body. Also called provitamins.

Carotenoids
A group of yellow and red pigments structurally related to carotene. Some are converted into retinol in the body.

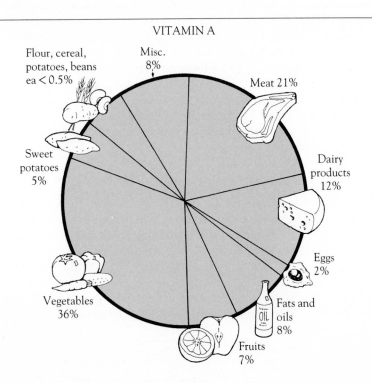

VITAMIN A

Flour, cereal, potatoes, beans ea < 0.5%
Misc. 8%
Meat 21%
Sweet potatoes 5%
Dairy products 12%
Eggs 2%
Vegetables 36%
Fats and oils 8%
Fruits 7%

FIGURE 6-5
Vitamin A in the U.S. diet.

RDA of vitamin A for adults: men 1000 RE (5000 IU), women 800 RE (4000 IU).

Nutrition education

Epithelial Cells
The cells that form the outermost part of the body (skin) and line body cavities (gastrointestinal, respiratory, genitourinary tracts).

Keratinization
A hardening of the skin caused by a lack of mucus.

Rods
Light-sensitive cells in the retina of the eye.

Xerophthalmia
Hardening of the epithelium of the eye, leading to blindness; usually due to vitamin A deficiency.

Economics

women 800 RE, or 5000 IU and 4000 IU, respectively. But the average consumed per day in the U.S. is 1640 RE (8200 IU)—considerably more than the RDA.

It is not hard to meet the RDA for vitamin A if you eat one of the small number of foods rich in that vitamin, including liver, or rich in its precursors, like dark green or dark orange vegetables, apricots, cantaloupe, and spinach. However, some diets—including those of Americans with Spanish surnames and those of children of all ethnic groups—are not high in vitamin A–rich foods, although severe disorders such as blindness are rarely caused by deficiency.

Elsewhere in the world, extreme vitamin A deficiency is an urgent matter and produces blindness in many children.[3] This disorder occurs mostly because of the lack of foods of animal origin and because so many mothers do not know how to supplement the diet of rice, wheat, and starchy foods with foods that are high in beta carotene.

As indicated in Figure 6-4, cooking losses of vitamin A can be as high as 40%. Vitamin A is also lost when fat becomes rancid, although vitamin E prevents this from occurring and is also found in many of the same foods.

What results from a deficiency of vitamin A

One of the main functions of vitamin A is to maintain the health of *epithelial cells,* which form the outermost layer of the skin; line body cavities such as the lungs and the gastrointestinal, genital, and urinary tracts; and form part of the eye's cornea (the outermost part of the eye). Deficiency of vitamin A has several effects:

- *Skin becomes hardened.* Because the epithelial cells no longer secrete sufficient mucus, they become dry and hard. The skin then becomes hardened, a condition known as *keratinization* because a protein called keratin is secreted. As a result, the epithelial cells lose their barrier effect against bacterial or viral infections.
- *Night blindness.* Rods are light-sensitive cells in the back of the eye. In normal vision, vitamin A combines with the protein opsin in the rods to form visual purple (rhodopsin); when visual purple is bleached, the eye can then see in bright light. However, with vitamin A deficiency, the time required to adapt to dim light is much longer—the condition called night blindness, which may be only embarrassing in a darkened theater but possibly fatal to a person driving a car at night.
- *Clouding of the cornea.* The hardening of the epithelium of the eye, known as the cornea, is called *xerophthalmia.* Extreme vitamin A deficiency leads to permanent blindness (see Figure 6-7).

Vitamin A deficiency in developing countries

About 40,000 deaths occur every *day* throughout the world because of vitamin A deficiency, mostly in children under age five.[3] Often the cause of death is a decreased resistance to infection. Recently there has been renewed research interest in this protective function of the vitamin.[4]

Blindness caused by lack of vitamin A affects 500,000 children every year, mostly in developing countries. In Asia alone, an estimated 5 million preschool children annually develop xerophthalmia. Fortunately, high doses of vitamin A every few months will alleviate this suffering—indeed, the supplements have been shown to decrease mortality caused by vitamin A deficiency by as much as 34%.[5] The solution is also inexpensive: 100% of a year's RDA of vitamin A for a child costs less than 5 cents wholesale.

Vitamin A deficiencies in developed countries

In Northern Ireland in the early 1980s, ten young men staging a hunger strike for political reasons were going blind after only 50 days of fasting and died not long afterward. This surprised authorities because all the men were healthy before they refused food so their reserves of vitamin A should have been sufficient to last three months to a year. Experts concluded, however, that the blindness was due to a "transportation problem": owing to a breakdown in the delivery system, vitamin A was simply not being transported from the liver, where there were sufficient reserves, to the eye.

The reason that vitamin A could not be transported was that the men consumed no protein during the 50 days. This resulted in a condition known as depressed synthesis of retinol-binding protein (RBP). RBP is a protein that turns the fat-soluble vitamin A stored in the liver into a water-soluble form, so that it can be transported to the tissues, including the eye.

In developed countries, however, the consequences of vitamin A deficiency are usually not this severe. Most forms are much milder (night blindness being the most prominent example) and are caused by low vitamin A intake or by malabsorption of fat causing malabsorption of vitamin A, as in recurrent diarrhea.

An adequate diet is required to allow transportation of some nutrients from storage sites in the body to tissues in the body.

Toxicity and fatalities

How much vitamin A is too much? As we pointed out (Table 6-4), the minimum toxic dose is 25,000 to 50,000 IU per day for an adult (5000 to 10,000 RE). But would you believe there is a case on record of a person's having taken 341,000 IU (68,200 RE) *every day?* Indeed, 25,000 IU capsules of vitamin A may be bought without prescription. There have been reports of some people buying 6 to 24 pounds of beef liver a week—and a single pound of liver, when fried, contains 240,000 IU of vitamin A.[6]

What happens when you take too much vitamin A? Early symptoms include severe headaches. They also include gouty arthritis—pain in bones and joints; such attacks often follow the consumption of alcohol, which increases the toxic effects of vitamin A.[7]

A form of toxicity occurs when chemicals closely related in chemical structure to vitamin A (like Accutane) are used for acne and other skin disorders without appropriate medical supervision. For example, it was found that women using Accutane during the first trimester of pregnancy had increased incidences of spontaneous abortions, and others gave birth to infants suffering from malformations such as defects in the face, ears, heart, nervous system, and thymus gland.[8] Check the form of vitamin A used for skin disorders because some are effective when applied to the skin, but not when taken orally.[1] Remember that these vitamin A analogs prescribed by doctors are considered to be drugs, not nutrients.

Large intakes of beta carotene are not harmful. The only ill effect is a yellowing of the skin—as has happened to people who have a passion for eating carrots—but this effect goes away when the beta carotene intake is reduced. However, eating such an unbalanced diet, in which certain nutrients are favored and others neglected, may lead to other deficiencies.

Medicine

Vitamin D, the "Sunshine Vitamin"

Vitamin D has three main functions:

- To help your body absorb calcium and phosphorus from the intestine into the blood
- To help in forming and remodeling (building up) your bones and teeth
- To help your kidney conserve minerals

Is vitamin D hard to find in food?

A healthy breakfast of cereal and fruit (although milk has vitamin D added) or even vegetables probably won't supply the RDA of vitamin D: foods of plant origin have none of the vitamin. Eggs and liver have only low amounts, and the amount of vitamin D in meat is insignificant. Some fish will provide D—provided you eat enough of it to amount to 5 μg or 200 IU (if you're an adult). In the United States, commercial cow's milk supplies the RDA, because the law requires that it have vitamin D added. Two glasses of milk or 3 ounces of canned tuna provide 5 μg or 200 IU of vitamin D. Other dairy products, like yogurt, usually are not fortified with vitamin D.

Free from the sun

Though it takes some effort to get vitamin D from food, you can get it free from the sun—or even from a sunlamp. Ultraviolet light activates a chemical called 7-dehydrocholesterol, which is present naturally in your skin. The chemical is then converted into vitamin D by your liver and kidneys.

How much sun is necessary? (After all, you wouldn't want to encourage skin cancer at the same time you're soaking up vitamin D–producing rays.) For white-skinned adults, an estimated 10 to 15 minutes exposure to the noon sun twice a week will meet vitamin D needs.[9] If the skin is dark or black, if it is a different time of day, if air pollution is present, or if you use a sun-block lotion, the amount of ultraviolet light reaching the skin is decreased.

Textiles and clothing 🔑

Some types of clothing will also reduce ultraviolet rays. Indeed, in England in the 1920s "sunshine clothing" was promoted as a way of enhancing the action of sunlight on the skin, although it has not been until recently that the correct color and tightness of knit has been developed to allow the maximum amount of ultraviolet light to penetrate a garment.[10]

"Rickety": not just old furniture

Rickets
Defective formation of bone due to vitamin D deficiency.

The word "rickety" is often used to refer to a chair or table that wobbles because of uneven legs; however, the word is taken from the form of vitamin D deficiency in children. Rickets, derived from the old English word meaning "to twist," is characterized by bowed legs and small lumps on the ribs resulting from poor bone formation.

Lifestyles are important in some nutrition problems.

Until early in this century, rickets was common in all countries. By 1966, one expert was able to say that the incidence of the disorder was reduced to that of a "medical curiosity." Unfortunately, rickets has been on the rise again—owing to such factors as premature births, prolonged breast-feeding of infants or feeding them with milk not fortified with vitamin D, lack of exposure to sunlight, and the increased interest in vegan (and therefore low–vitamin D) diets.

The problem of rickets is particularly evident among the children of Asian immigrants in Great Britain. There is an interesting conflict between cultural practice and nutritional requirements. The diet eaten by many of the Asian immigrants in Great Britain is low in vitamin D. The problem is made worse because of the cultural practice of wrapping the child in clothing during infancy. Combine the diet and clothing practice with the shortage of sunshine in the British climate, and the result is a problem with rickets in these children. However, a fabric has been developed that allows sufficient sunshine to penetrate to the skin so as to meet the infant's requirement for vitamin D.[10] In this way, cultural practices are preserved and the incidence of rickets is reduced.

Rickets is a disease of children; the equivalent deficiency in adults is called *osteomalacia,* in which weak, brittle bones, accompanied by pain, are caused by a loss of calcium. This disorder is treated with small oral doses of vitamin D.

When vitamin D is important in the life-cycle

Vitamin D intake is especially important at particular times in one's life:

- During pregnancy and lactation, because of the importance of the vitamin in bone growth in the fetus
- During infancy, childhood, and adolescence, also because of importance to bone growth
- During old age

This last deserves some explanation. Among the elderly, dietary intake of vitamin D–rich foods may be low. In addition, the elderly may get less vitamin D from exposure to sunlight, because the skin of an 80-year-old has half the capacity of that of a 20-year-old to create vitamin D. Moreover, aging kidneys are not as efficient in converting the vitamin to the active form.[10]

How much vitamin D is too much? This issue is controversial. The safety index of 125 shown in Table 6-4 suggests that vitamin D is not very toxic except at relatively high intakes for a fat-soluble vitamin. However, many experts think the gap between enough and too much is narrower.

Vitamin E is Surrounded by Myths and Controversy

Will vitamin E improve your sex life, improve the functioning of your heart and lungs, and extend your life? Since the 1920s, when it was discovered that vitamin E deficiency interfered with reproduction in rats, the marvelous, even magical, qualities attributed to this vitamin have increased. In the 1970s, Dr. Jack Bieri, an expert in vitamin E research, called it "a vitamin in search of a disease"— because there are no known deficiency diseases of vitamin E in humans. In the 1980s, vitamin E deficiency has been tentatively associated with some neurological disorders.[11] What are we to make of all this excitement?

What to eat for vitamin E

The tocopherols—"tocos" comes from the Greek word for "offspring"—are a group of eight related chemicals that are made by plants. The one with the highest biological activity in humans is alpha-tocopherol, but others of this group, especially gamma-tocopherol, are sold commercially.

The best food sources of vitamin E are plant and seed oils and margarines and shortenings made from these oils. Good sources are nuts, whole grains, leafy green vegetables, eggs, liver, and milk. All four food groups contribute reasonable

The RDA for vitamin E is easily met in vegetarian or nonvegetarian diets.

amounts of vitamin E. A bonus is that a variety of eating patterns, vegetarian or nonvegetarian, can easily provide the RDA. In the United States, for instance, the RDA for all age groups is met without difficulty in most diets: 8 to 11 mgTE (12 to 16 IU) per day.

Prevention of oxygen damage

The main function of vitamin E is to protect the fat in membranes around cells—especially the cells in nerves, muscles, the heart, and the red blood cells—from damage by oxygen. For this reason, the vitamin is called an antioxidant. Vitamin E prevents the oxidation of vitamin A. Membranes with high polyunsaturated fatty acid content are more prone to damage by oxygen, or by ozone, an atmospheric pollutant. If you eat foods high in polyunsaturated fatty acids, you are eating foods rich in vitamin E. Cigarette smokers who have adequate intakes of vitamin E are protecting their lungs from some of the damage caused by cigarette smoke; lungs have a high amount of vitamin E.

Now, as to the subject of life extension: Because of the role this vitamin plays in the protection of cells, it has been speculated that it may slow down the aging process in humans. Is this possible? The jury is still out—and probably will be for some time. How does a scientist actually *measure* aging? Moreover, how would a scientist handle the problems of measuring the effect of increased vitamin E intakes over an entire human life? Getting definitive answers from human studies would take many years.

Vitamin E has also been touted as a possible solution to some specific human disorders and diseases. Hereditary muscular dystrophy, for instance, is a genetic disorder that is still awaiting a cure. The discovery that vitamin E deficiency in experimental animals leads to a loss of muscle similar to that seen in human muscular dystrophy created much excitement for a time. Unfortunately, however, giving additional vitamin E to humans will not prevent or cure that disease in people.

New evidence suggests that vitamin E may be a remedy for fibrocystic disease, for neuromuscular disease in children, and for premenstrual syndrome (PMS), but more detailed evidence is needed.

Vitamin E deficiency and toxicity is rare

Deficiency and toxicity of vitamin E are rare in any part of the world. People who show deficiency tend to belong to one of two groups: (1) adults who have difficulty in digesting and absorbing fat, and (2) some premature infants who suffer from *hemolytic anemia*—caused by breaking down of red blood cells—as a result of their not receiving enough vitamin E from the mother before the last trimester of pregnancy.

Hemolytic Anemia
An anemia caused by the breaking down of red blood cells.

Vitamin K Stands for "Coagulation"

Discovered in the mid-1930s by Danish scientist Henrik Dam, vitamin K got its letter from *koagulation,* the Danish word for coagulation.

What it does, what it comes from

The main function of vitamin K in your body is in promoting the coagulation of blood—a process essential to stopping bleeding. Vitamin K is involved in the making of a protein in the liver that enters a series of chemical reactions in the blood that in turn lead to the formation of a blood clot that stops bleeding.

Vitamin K is found in adequate amounts in all diets, but the best sources are green, leafy plants. Good sources are fruit, cereals, dairy products, and meat. Bacteria in the large intestines synthesize the vitamin, and it is then absorbed into your blood.

Vitamin K deficiency and hemorrhaging

Vitamin K deficiency is rare in the general population. However, if there is a deficiency, it can lead to hemorrhages—because of the body's inability to form blood clots—that could cause death. When vitamin K deficiency does occur, it results either from malabsorption of fat from the intestines, or from high doses of oral antibiotics, which kill intestinal bacteria. A newborn infant may be deficient in vitamin K because the infant's intestinal system is sterile at birth; intestinal bacteria cannot supply enough of the vitamin until about seven days after birth. Thus, newborn infants are often given vitamin K immediately after birth to prevent hemorrhaging.

No known toxicity symptoms have been produced by high dietary intakes of vitamin K.

> Vitamin A is necessary mainly for good vision, vitamin D for healthy bones, vitamin E as an antioxidant, and vitamin K for blood coagulation. Most concern is for high mortality from vitamin A–poor diets in many parts of the world.

THE WATER-SOLUBLE VITAMINS: C AND B-COMPLEX

Perhaps the most important difference between the water-soluble vitamins—(C and the B-complex)—and the fat-soluble vitamins is that water-soluble vitamins are less stable. In cooking and food preparation, for instance, many water-soluble vitamins are more likely to lose potency because of long cooking times or high temperatures. Supplements of water-soluble vitamins are more likely to lose potency after being exposed to air or light, or after sitting on the shelf a long time. Although the vitamin safety index is generally higher in water-soluble vitamins, megadoses of some of them—particularly C, niacin, and B_6—can aggravate a number of medical disorders, as we have seen (Table 6-3).

The main thing the water-soluble vitamins have in common is just that—they are water-soluble. They are otherwise unrelated chemically. Still, many act together as coenzymes in important chemical reactions in your body.

Vitamin C Is Why British Sailors Were Once Called "Limeys"

How did ignorance about nutrition affect the great explorations of the world? More than half the crew of Vasco da Gama died on his two-year (1497 to 1499) trip during which he became the first European to sail around the tip of Africa and discovered the sea route to India. The cause? Scurvy, caused by a deficiency of vitamin C and marked by bleeding gums, loosening teeth, anemia, and general debility.

For years, death from scurvy was common in long sea voyages when only non-perishable foods could be carried aboard ships. Indeed, it was not until the mid-1700s that Scottish physician James Lind discovered that lemons and oranges prevented scurvy, and it took some years for his dietary recommendations to be accepted. Finally, in 1795 the British navy began to distribute regular rations of lime juice during long voyages—whence came the name *limeys* for British sailors.[12] Modern methods of transporting food have made vitamin C so regularly available to everyone that modern explorers—the astronauts—have been featured in television commercials for vitamin C–fortified drinks.

Natural versus synthetic vitamin C: no difference

Human beings, primates, and guinea pigs do not make vitamin C, but other animals—and plants—do. This "natural form" of vitamin C can be synthesized in a test tube, and your body cannot tell the difference. The chemical structure of vitamin C, which is similar to that of glucose, is illustrated in Figure 6-1.

Economics

The vitamin was first synthesized early in the 1900s. A recent commercial development is the use of bacteria to do the synthesizing, which is easier and faster than other methods. The economic implications are impressive because the market for vitamin C is $400 million a year.[13]

Where it comes from, how much is needed

As is shown in Figure 6-6, fruits and vegetables are the best sources of vitamin C, although soaking, cutting, peeling, and cooking cause some loss of the vitamin. Little vitamin C is present in foods from animal sources. What little is present in milk is lost when heat is applied during pasteurization.

The vitamin C RDA for adult men and women is 60 mg.

Any one of the following will meet the RDA for adults:

- Grapefruit: ¾ (or ¾ cup of grapefruit juice)
- Orange: 1 (or ½ cup of orange juice)
- Strawberries: ¾ cup
- Green peppers: 2 ounces

Anthropology

Today, the average American takes in about 116 mg of vitamin C per day. That is less than the 400 mg daily that prehistoric peoples ingested, according to anthropologists[14]; however, it is still more than is needed. Only 60 mg is needed to meet the adult RDA, so this is fairly easy to do. Note that the *requirement* for vitamin C is 10 mg (this means an intake of less than 10 mg per day over a few weeks should cause vitamin C deficiency signs). Therefore, if you take the amount of each food above necessary to meet the *RDA* and divide it by 6, it will indicate the small amount of each food needed to meet the *requirement* for vitamin C.

Under some conditions, however, some people require more than 60 mg. Cigarette smokers, for example, have a 50% higher requirement for vitamin C than nonsmokers do.

Women using oral contraceptives are also thought to need more. So are people who have been exposed to high or low temperatures or who have been through surgery or other trauma, although the reasons for these higher requirements are unclear.[15]

In any case, most people get enough vitamin C in their diet to meet these additional requirements.

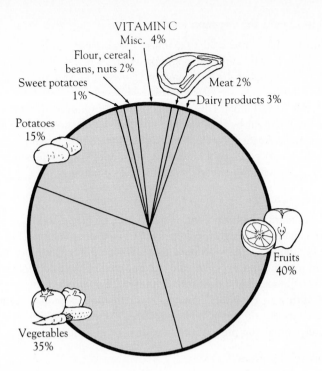

VITAMIN C

Misc. 4%

Flour, cereal, beans, nuts 2%

Sweet potatoes 1%

Meat 2%

Dairy products 3%

Potatoes 15%

Fruits 40%

Vegetables 35%

FIGURE 6-6
Sources of vitamin C. Fruits and vegetables are the best sources.

The importance of vitamin C

I mentioned that vitamin C has important influences in chemical reactions in your body, among them[15]:

- In increasing absorption of dietary iron
- In influencing cholesterol metabolism—although its influence on lowering serum cholesterol is debated[13]
- In forming antiinflammatory steroids in the adrenal gland
- In affecting the immune system
- In making leukocytes (white blood cells) function properly
- In (possibly) affecting the metabolism of drugs and toxicants by the liver
- In the synthesis of collagen

Vitamin C deficiency and scurvy

Severe vitamin C deficiency is rare in developed countries like the United States. Commercially prepared infant formulas marketed in the United States are required by law to be fortified with vitamin C. Drinks given to infants and children, like apple juice, are also fortified with vitamin C. Babies who are breast-fed receive adequate amounts of the vitamin.

In the past, the worst disorder from vitamin C deficiency was scurvy. Scurvy comes about because vitamin C is needed for the formation of collagen, a protein that provides "scaffolding" for muscles, blood vessels, bones, and cartilage. Failure to produce collagen causes weak blood vessels, muscle tissue breakdown, and an inability to produce scar tissue—thus the soft gums and bleeding blood vessels typical of scurvy. If not treated with vitamin C, scurvy leads to gangrene and death.

Does vitamin C fight the common cold?

It's almost like a bad cold that refuses to go away—the notion that huge doses of vitamin C will cure the common cold. Will it? Nobel laureate Linus Pauling says that he takes 10 g of vitamin C every day to prevent the common cold. He argues that, just as 70 kg worth of houseflies will make 10 g a day of vitamin C, so a 70 kg human (the ideal body weight of an adult male used in the RDA tables) will benefit by that amount of vitamin C.[16] However, as long ago as 1971 the American Academy of Pediatrics issued a statement warning against superdosing oneself against colds, and numerous well-controlled studies since then have confirmed that the vitamin is useless against the common cold.

Vitamin C for cancer?

More dramatic has been Pauling's advocacy of megadoses of vitamin C for treatment of cancer. Although the controversy raged since the mid-1960s, in 1985 a large, well-conducted study showed that taking 10 g a day of vitamin C was ineffective in treating cancer.[17] An editorial in a medical journal declared the study "methodologically sound and therefore definitive," but critics question the medical profession's ability to evaluate honestly novel treatments proposed for cancer.[18] The last word on the subject is one of caution: "Ascorbic acid [vitamin C] may yet have some role in the prevention or treatment of cancer."[12]

The menace of megadoses

Some beliefs about the marvels of megadoses of vitamin C have been questioned in a recent review of the literature.[12] Consider the following associations with high vitamin C intakes:

- Gout
- Destruction of vitamin B_{12} in food
- Interference with urine test for diabetes
- Hemolytic anemia among some American blacks, Sephardic Jews, and Asians

Most interestingly, high doses of vitamin C also have produced what has been called *rebound scurvy*, although the evidence is of questionable significance for human beings.[12] Here's how it is said to work: Strictly speaking, large doses of vitamin C are not toxic; however, the body has a mechanism that destroys excess amounts, a mechanism that is particularly important during pregnancy because both mother and fetus destroy the vitamin—if the intake has been in high doses—at more than *ten times the RDA*. Indeed a fetus exposed to megadoses is born with this increased destructive capacity. If it is then given human or cow's milk—neither of which is particularly high in vitamin C anyway—the infant will continue to destroy the vitamin at ten times the normal rate. The result: "rebound scurvy"—on a diet that would not normally give rise to scurvy at all.

The disorder is curable, however. It can be avoided by tapering off the megadoses during pregnancy by about 10% each day, rather than stopping them abruptly.

Vitamin C is involved in the absorption of iron, synthesis of collagen, cholesterol metabolism, and formation of antiinflammatory steroids. It affects the immune system and the metabolism of drugs and toxicants. Scurvy is the deficiency disease. Megadoses of vitamin C may be dangerous.

The B-Complex Vitamins Deal with Energy, Metabolism, and Oxygen

Let us group the B-complex vitamins according to their main functions in your body, as follows:

- *Energy release*—thiamin, riboflavin, niacin, pantothenic acid, biotin
- *Energy formation*—biotin
- *Protein and amino acid metabolism*—vitamin B_6
- *Delivery of oxygen to cells*—folacin, vitamin B_{12}

Thiamin, riboflavin, niacin, pantothenic acid, and biotin are crucial to energy release in mitochondria in cells

So many discoveries in science and medicine have come about because someone noticed that something different was happening in commonplace matters. In Southeast Asia, a new cook at a hospital switched from polished rice to whole-grain, unpolished rice. However this may have benefited the hospital's patients, Dr. Christiaan Eijkman happened to notice that chickens feeding on the leftover rice lost the weakness in their legs they had experienced with the polished rice. Eijkman's observation led to the discovery of thiamin and in 1929 the Nobel Prize.

History

Very often, disorders related to vitamin deficiencies disappear because living standards improve. In the early part of the 20th century, niacin deficiency was widespread in the southern part of the United States, resulting in 10,000 deaths in 1915 alone. The reason: a diet of grits, degerminated cornmeal, soda biscuits, corn syrup or molasses, and fatty pork—the diet of low-income people then—is a diet that is extremely low in niacin. Also, since the diet was low in protein, the intake of tryptophan was also low. (Niacin can be formed from tryptophan.) Today, however, niacin deficiency is a medical curiosity, the result not of niacin supplements, but of improved living standards and quality of diet.

Economics

Energy-releasing vitamins—intake and functions

Low dietary intakes of vitamins may interfere with their coenzyme activity. That is, all of these vitamins function as coenzymes in energy metabolism involving carbohydrates, fats, proteins, and alcohol. Thus, the RDA values for thiamin, riboflavin, and niacin are proportional to dietary energy intake, as follows:

	Men	Women
Thiamin:	1.4 mg	1.0 mg or 0.5 mg/1000 kcal
Riboflavin:	1.6 mg	1.2 mg or 0.6 mg/1000 kcal
Niacin:	18 mgNE	13 mgNE or 6.6 mgNE/1000 kcal

Recent research at Cornell University showed that exercise may increase the requirement for riboflavin. Biotin and pantothenic acid do not have RDA values. Instead, they have Estimated Safe and Adequate Daily Dietary Intakes (see Appendix F). Increasing your energy intake should have a proportional increase in intake of these vitamins to metabolize the extra energy. Fortunately, many foods that are high in energy are also high in these vitamins; the exceptions are the low-nutrient, kcalorie-dense foods—sugar, honey, fats, and oils.

FIGURE 6-7
Sources of thiamin, riboflavin, and
niacin.

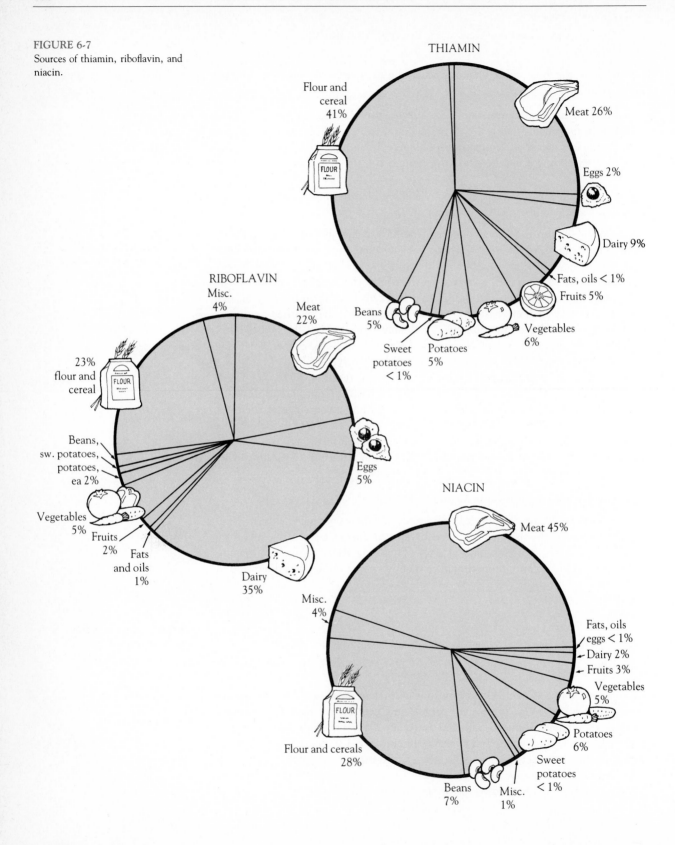

Where to find the B-complex vitamins

As Figure 6-7 indicates, the best sources of these vitamins are meats and cereals and, for thiamin and riboflavin, dairy products. Examples:

- *Thiamin*—Though all meats are good sources of thiamin, pork has about four times more thiamin than the same amount of beef.
- *Riboflavin*—If you have ever yearned for the days when milk was home-delivered, left on the doorstep in bottles, you should know this convenience had its price: much of the riboflavin in milk was lost if the bottles sat in the sun for several hours. Riboflavin is particularly sensitive to light, so the milk you pick up in a store in a cardboard or plastic container is an improvement over the old system. Because milk is such a good source of riboflavin, a deficiency of this vitamin is rare in milk-drinking countries.
- *Niacin*—Corn, or maize, is a good source of niacin, but the vitamin does not become available until the corn is treated in a certain way. In Mexico, the niacin is released when the corn is treated with lime water during the making of tortillas. In the southwestern United States, niacin becomes available when the corn is roasted in hot ashes, as practiced by the Hopi Indians.
- *Pantothenic acid*—The word *pantothenic* means "from all sides" in Greek—a clue to the source of this vitamin: it is found in adequate amounts in many foods. A deficiency of pantothenic acid has been found only in volunteers eating a specially prepared diet.
- *Biotin*—Biotin is present in many foods, especially yeast, legumes, nuts, and some vegetables. Your body also contains microorganisms in the gastrointestinal tract that provide you with some biotin; the only way to suppress this absorption is to eat raw egg whites. This is done by avidin—a protein in eggs that is inactivated when eggs are heated. In one experiment, four volunteers agreed to eat the whites of 80 raw eggs every day for 10 weeks. Yet they only suffered from excessive tiredness (biotin is involved in energy metabolism), poor appetite, muscular pain, nausea, and dry scaly skin.[19] In other words, the deprivation of biotin was not fatal.

Some traditional ways of preparing food have beneficial nutrition effects.

Deficiency in energy-release vitamins

These five vitamins—thiamin, riboflavin, niacin, pantothenic acid, and biotin—are in highest concentrations in similar foods. Thus, when people are deficient in one of these vitamins, they are usually deficient in all five, which is rare in developed countries.

Alcoholics tend to have the highest incidence of thiamin deficiency. Alcohol interferes with thiamin absorption, and prolonged deficiency may produce brain damage. Still, because white rice and white flour are enriched with thiamin, these foods have served to minimize this deficiency in developed countries.[20]

Alcohol may produce problems with thiamin deficiency.

The effects of deficiency of these vitamins are listed in Table 6-3, but two are worth noting here because they do appear in developing countries:

- *Beriberi*—The result of a thiamin deficiency, beriberi (which means "I can't, I can't") is characterized by nerve disorders such as irritability and exhaustion, possible edema, wasting of muscles (causing difficulty in walking), and heart failure.
- *Pellagra*—The result of niacin deficiency, it produces the three Ds of diarrhea, dermatitis, and dementia—and possibly the fourth D of death.

Vitamin B$_6$ Helps with Amino Acid and Protein Metabolism

How important is vitamin B$_6$? Consider this: in 1954, someone made a mistake in the manufacture of a commercial infant formula, so that it provided insufficient vitamin B$_6$. Clearly, ethical considerations would prevent this situation from ever being set up deliberately, but the result of the accident provided some important knowledge about vitamin B$_6$ functions: the infants developed convulsions. Other deficiency symptoms are depression and confusion, lowered resistance to disease, and a skin disorder.

What it does, where it comes from

Vitamin B$_6$ acts as a coenzyme in amino acid and protein metabolism. It is involved with enzymes that convert essential amino acids into nonessential amino acids. That is why the RDA for vitamin B$_6$ is related to the protein intake. It is a coenzyme for the conversion of tryptophan into niacin. It is also a coenzyme for the conversion of glycogen into glucose. In short, vitamin B$_6$ is important in metabolism because it is a coenzyme to over 60 different enzymes.

Sources of vitamin B$_6$ in the typical American diet are shown in Figure 6-8, the two principal foods being meat and dairy products. The commercially available synthetic form of vitamin B$_6$ is pyridoxine hydrochloride. Whatever the source, the RDA for adults is 2.2 mg for men and 2.0 mg for women.

When vitamin B$_6$ is deficient

Vitamin B$_6$ levels may be too low for some people. College students should know that one study found that food served in college dining halls had only 60% of the vitamin present in the precooked food, resulting in low vitamin B$_6$ intake

---

FIGURE 6-8
Sources of vitamin B$_6$.

VITAMIN B$_6$

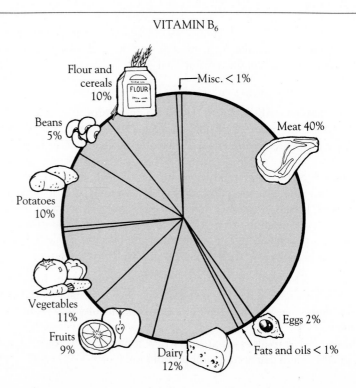

Flour and cereals 10%

Misc. < 1%

Beans 5%

Meat 40%

Potatoes 10%

Vegetables 11%

Fruits 9%

Dairy 12%

Eggs 2%

Fats and oils < 1%

for these students.[21] The intake for some teenagers may also be low; one study found inadequate intake by white and black adolescent girls in the southern United States.[22]

Several drugs interfere with vitamin B_6 and produce deficiency, among them:

- Hydralazine, used to lower high blood pressure
- Isoniazid, used to treat tuberculosis
- Penicillin
- Estrogens

Estrogens—the female sex hormones—are important because they are present in oral contraceptives. Feelings of depression can result from ingestion of oral contraceptives and may be alleviated by vitamin B_6 supplements. In addition, women who are taking estrogens for osteoporosis should be aware of possible B_6 deficiency.

Estrogens
The female sex hormones.

Can you take too much B_6?

Tablets containing 50 to 500 mg of vitamin B_6 are available in stores. Should you buy these if you feel some of the problems mentioned above? Some evidence suggests that 50 mg of vitamin B_6 per day may be beneficial in relieving premenstrual tension, but more study is needed in this area.[23]

What about larger doses? It has been known since the mid-1960s that people taking supplements of 200 mg daily become dependent on the vitamin. Adults taking 2 g per day—that's 100,000% of the RDA for a woman!—for four months experienced defects in nerve function, with unsteady walk, numbness in the feet, and clumsiness in the hands. Although they felt dramatically better after the vitamin B_6 supplements were withdrawn, they still showed residual nerve malfunctioning. Some recent evidence suggests that these effects may occur at intakes much less than 2 g of vitamin B_6.

Folacin and Vitamin B_{12} Prevent Two Types of Anemia

Folacin and vitamin B_{12} are together involved in a number of processes, including:

- Development of red and white blood cells. Improper formation causes *megaloblastic anemia*—the red blood cell is large but not fully developed. This interferes with the ability of the red blood cell to carry oxygen to all cells in the body.
- RNA and DNA formation. Folacin and vitamin B_{12} are involved in cell division during critical periods of growth.
- The metabolism of certain amino acids—that is, the interconversion of amino acids.

Megaloblastic Anemia
An anemia, or lack of oxygen-carrying capacity of the blood, due to large, irregularly shaped red blood cells.

Vitamin B_{12} is also called cobalamin, because its molecule has the trace mineral cobalt as part of its structure.

Where folacin and vitamin B_{12} come from and how much is needed

Figure 6-9 shows the principal sources of each of these vitamins. Although we have lumped the two together, note that their main food sources differ: meat and dairy products are overwhelmingly the principal food sources of vitamin B_{12}, whereas folacin is available in a variety of foods, including vegetables, fruits, and meats.

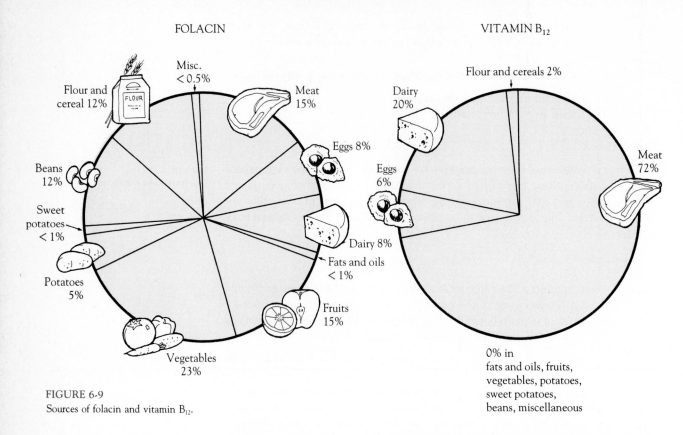

FIGURE 6-9
Sources of folacin and vitamin B$_{12}$.

Vegans—people who avoid foods of animal origins—may find vitamin B$_{12}$ in some seaweeds (although the much-promoted spirulina may be a poor source[24]); the richest sources for vegans are fermented soy and cereal products such as tofu and tempeh. Additional information on the content of folacin and vitamin B$_{12}$ is contained in Appendix K.

Much folacin may be lost during food preparation, since it is unstable in heat, light, and air. By contrast, vitamin B$_{12}$ is little affected during food preparation.

For adult men and women, the RDA for folacin is 400 μg and the RDA for vitamin B$_{12}$ is 3 μg.

The RDA for adult men *and* women for folacin is 400 μg; the RDA for vitamin B$_{12}$ is 3 μg. Over a year's time, these figures translate into only 1/190 of an ounce of folacin and only 1/25,570 of an ounce of vitamin B$_{12}$—minuscule amounts, indeed.

Nevertheless, deficiencies of these two vitamins do occur.

Folacin deficiency

A person who has a folacin deficiency may be weak, tired, pale, and forgetful. Who is at risk for folacin deficiency?

- People with low intakes of fruits and vegetables—including many teenagers and the elderly.
- Pregnant women, particularly teenagers, because pregnancy and adolescence increase folacin requirements.
- People experiencing increases in the number of red or white blood cells. One method of treating leukemia is to induce a folacin deficiency in order to slow the rate at which white blood cells multiply.
- People who use alcohol, or who take drugs to control cancer and malaria.

Vitamin B_{12} deficiency

People likely to suffer from deficiency of this vitamin include the following:

- Vegans, because they do not eat foods of animal origin. Such a deficiency is slow to develop in adults, but less slow in infants, and children of vegans may require vitamin B_{12} supplements.
- People unable to produce the intrinsic factor in the stomach that absorbs vitamin B_{12} into the lower portion of the small intestine and then into the blood. The lack of the intrinsic factor may be because of a genetic defect or because part of the stomach was surgically removed.

Because vitamin B_{12} is involved in manufacturing the sheath surrounding nerve fibers, people suffering from a deficiency of this vitamin may suffer nervous system disorders, especially in the spinal cord, which may cause interference with movement, tingling and numbness in the limbs, and possibly mental disturbance.

It has been suggested that anesthesia with nitrous oxide may precipitate nervous system disorders in people with unrecognized vitamin B_{12} deficiency. Such a disorder is represented in the handwriting of a 58-year-old patient, as shown in Figure 6–10.

Megaloblastic anemia caused by vitamin B_{12} deficiency can be corrected by giving the patient additional folacin; however, it will not repair any existing nerve damage. There is also a danger that folacin treatment may mask nerve degeneration caused by vitamin B_{12} deficiency.

Energy release is aided by thiamin, riboflavin, niacin, pantothenic acid, and biotin; energy formation by biotin; amino acid metabolism by vitamin B_6; and delivery of oxygen to cells by folacin and vitamin B_{12}. Thiamin deficiency is a problem for alcoholics, vitamin B_{12} deficiency for vegans. Folacin intake may be a problem for teenagers and the elderly.

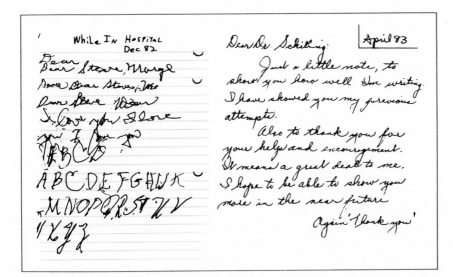

FIGURE 6-10
Nerve disorder caused by nitrous oxide anesthesia in a women deficient in vitamin B_{12}. Handwriting on the left is after an operation involving nitrous oxide anesthesia. The women was given injections of vitamin B_{12}. Four months later her handwriting is shown on the right.

Decisions

1. What Information Do I Need to Distinguish Vitamins from Nonvitamins?

There is great commercial advantage in calling a substance a vitamin. The substances in the list in Table 6-10 are commonly called vitamins despite the fact that none of them meet *all* of the criteria for a vitamin discussed earlier in the chapter.

For instance, the substances in Group A are organic substances and are required for specific metabolic functions in the body, but they are *not* needed in small amounts from the diet. Rather, they are made by the body. Two important metabolic functions worthy of attention are (1) the role of lipoic acid in the metabolism of carbohydrate, fat, and protein to produce energy and (2) the role of choline, a part of acetylcholine, in nerve function.

The two substances in Group B are more troublesome. These substances are not needed for specific metabolic functions, and are not needed in the diet. People may seek a cure by dosing themselves with these so-called vitamins instead of obtaining legitimate medical advice. Laetrile is a classical example of a confrontation between the laws of science and the laws of the land. In the 1970s many states legalized it as a vitamin because of its alleged cure for cancer. No medical evidence exists for the effectiveness of laetrile in treating cancer and it is not required by people who do not have cancer.[25]

There is no medical evidence that pangamic acid is effective against cardiovascular and rheumatic diseases. It is present in many foods containing many of the B vitamins—liver, many seeds, and yeast. Pangamic acid sales are considered illegal by the Food and Drug Administration, and the credibility of the creators of the product is questioned.

TABLE 6-10 Nonvitamins Called "Vitamins"

Nonvitamin	Also Known As
Group A	
Inositol	Myoinositol
Choline	
Lipoic acid	
Coenzyme Q	Ubiquinone
Bioflavinoids	Vitamin P, Rutin, Hisperidine
Para–aminobenzoic acid	PABA
Group B	
Pangamic acid	Vitamin B_{15}
Laetrile	Vitamin B_{17}

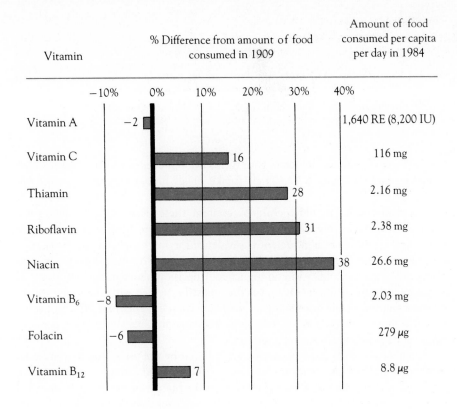

FIGURE 6-11
Then and now. Is the vitamin content available in foods the same now compared to the beginning of the century?

2. Is Vitamin D Really a Vitamin?

This seems an appropriate question since the legitimacy of other so-called vitamins was challenged above. Applying the definition of a vitamin, we see that vitamin D need not be supplied by the diet—the body can provide its own vitamin D by the effects of ultraviolet light on the skin. But the body does not have an internal, independent means of providing the vitamin. This is best seen in children of Asian immigrants in Great Britain, as mentioned previously. Because they are fed a diet low in vitamin D and deprived of sunlight, rickets is a major problem for these children. Vitamin D is sometimes classified as a hormone. It is made in one organ of the body, the skin, and acts on other organs of the body (see Metabolism Notes).

3. Is Intake of Vitamins Lower Now Than in the "Good Old Days" Because of the Processing of Food?

Not for most vitamins when U.S. Department of Agriculture data for 1909 and 1984 are compared (Figure 6-11). It is true that food processing removes some vitamins. This is especially so when cereals are refined. The reason levels of many vitamins were so high in 1984 is that vitamins are added to the refined food after final processing.

4. Are Vitamin Supplements of Value to Children?

There is no substitute for a balanced diet. A medical check-up may help in coming to a decision about vitamin supplements for children. Commercial pressure on

Vitamins in the U.S. diet for 6- to 8-year-old children (% 1980 RDA)

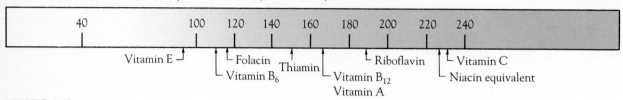

FIGURE 6-12
Vitamins in the U.S. diet for 6- to 8-year-old children.

parents to give vitamin supplements to their children does not seem to be justified from the data in Figure 6-12. Their intake of all nine vitamins measured was satisfactory.

Canadian studies in older children confirm these observations. The figures quoted are averages, but if deficiencies do occur they are usually of the mild or subclinical type. There is no scientific evidence for any beneficial effects of extra multivitamins on attention deficit disorders in children,[26] or megadoses of vitamin C on the common cold.[16] In coming to your decision about using high doses of vitamins, remember that at this level they must be treated with the same respect as other pharmacologic agents in your medicine cabinet. The toxic effects of some vitamins must be considered (Table 6-3). Yet vitamin tablets at varying concentrations are available without prescription.

Vitamins are made more attractive for children by the use of sugar or artificial sweeteners and by being made in the shape of multicolored cartoon characters from a television series. People of an older generation who missed out on such fun-filled ways of getting vitamins have their memories of foul-tasting cod-liver oil. It is possible for children to have high intakes of vitamins, not only from taking vitamin supplements or even from eating a regular diet, but also from eating breakfast cereals as a snack (especially the ones with 100% of most RDAs).

5. Do Vitamin Supplements Improve Athletic Performance?

According to one expert, "Vitamin supplements are of no further value to the athlete consuming an adequate diet and, in fact, some vitamins can be toxic when taken in large amounts."[27] The biochemical reasons are explained in the Metabolism Notes. Medical studies on commercial dietary supplements that include extra vitamins concluded that they are of no physiological value to the athlete who consumes a normal nutritionally balanced diet.[28]

Summary

FOOD SOURCES

MEAT

Thiamin, riboflavin, niacin, B_6, B_{12}, pantothenic acid, biotin

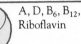
DAIRY

A, D, B_6, B_{12}, Riboflavin

BREADS/CEREAL

Thiamin, riboflavin, niacin, B_6, B_{12}, pantothenic acid, biotin

FRUITS/VEGETABLES

A, C, K, riboflavin, folacin

FATS/OILS

A, E

Developed countries (USA, Canada, Europe): Intake low for some people: vitamins A, B_6, folacin, vitamin B_{12}

Developing countries: Many people suffer from deficiencies, especially in A, D, C, thiamin, riboflavin, niacin, folacin, and vitamin B_{12}

BODY FUNCTIONS

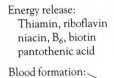

Energy release:
Thiamin, riboflavin niacin, B_6, biotin pantothenic acid

Blood formation: B_6, B_{12}, C, folacin

Blood cells: E

Blood clotting: K

Hormone formation:
Steroids
A
Pantothenic acid
Noredinephrine
Thyroxine
B_6

Reproduction:
A
Riboflavin

Eye function: A

Teeth: A, D, C

Skin:
A, C, B_6,
Niacin,
Riboflavin,
Pantothenic
acid

Neuromuscular function:
A, B_6, B_{12},
thiamin, niacin,
pantothenic acid

Bones:
A, D, C

Cell membrane:
E

Vitamins

could cause toxic symptoms → Death

Antacids, drugs, etc., → Loss of some vitamins because they are not absorbed

REFERENCES

1. Dubick, M.A., and Rucker, R.B.: Dietary supplements and health aids: A critical evaluation. I. Vitamins and minerals, Journal of Nutrition Education **15:**47, 1983.

2. Griffith, P.R., and Innes, F.C.: The relationship of socioeconomic factors to the use of vitamin supplements in the City of Windsor, Nutrition Research **3:**445, 1983.

3. Select Committee on Hunger, U.S. House of Representatives, Staff Report: Vitamin A: An urgent nutritional need for the world's children. U.S. Government Printing Office, Washington, D.C., 1985.

4. Editorial: Fall and rise of the anti–infective vitamin, Lancet **i:**1191, 1986.

5. Sommer, A., and others: Impact of vitamin A supplementation on childhood mortality, Lancet **i:**1169, 1986.

6. Selhorst, J.B., and others: Liver lover's headache: Pseudotumor cerebri and vitamin A intoxication, Journal of the American Medical Association **252:**3365, 1984.

7. Mawson, A.R.: Hypervitaminosis A toxicity and gout, Lancet **i:**1181, 1984.

8. Lammer, E.J., and others: Retinoic acid embryopathy, New England Journal of Medicine **313:**837, 1986.

9. The "right" amount of sun for making vitamin D, Tufts University Diet & Nutrition Letter, p. 7, October, 1985.

10. Hutchinson, G., and Hall, A.: The transmission of ultraviolet light through fabrics and its potential role in the cutaneous synthesis of vitamin D, Human Nutrition: Applied Nutrition **38A:**298, 1984.

11. Editorial: Vitamin E deficiency, Lancet **i:**423, 1986.

12. Levine, M.: New concepts in the biology and biochemistry of ascorbic acid, New England Journal of Medicine **314:**892, 1986.

13. Anonymous bacteria help to make vitamin C, New Scientist, p. 31, January 16, 1986.

14. Eaton, S.B., and Konner, M.: Paleolithic nutrition: A consideration of its nature and current implications, New England Journal of Medicine **312:**283, 1985.

15. Sauberlich, H.E.: Ascorbic acid. In Present knowledge in nutrition, 5th edition. The Nutrition Foundation, Inc., Washington, D.C., p. 260, 1984.

16. Anderson, T.W., and others: To dose or megadose: A debate about vitamin C, Nutrition Today, p. 6, March/April, 1978.

17. Moertel, C.G., and others: High dose vitamin C versus placebo in the treatment of patients with advanced cancer who have had no prior chemotherapy, New England Journal of Medicine **312:**137, 1985.

18. Richards, E.: Vitamin C suffers a dose of politics, New Scientist, p. 46, February 27, 1986.

19. Yudkin, J.: The penguin encyclopedia of nutrition, The Viking Press, New York, p. 52, 1985.

20. Anderson, S.H., and others: Adult thiamin requirements and the continuing need to fortify processed cereals, Lancet **ii:**85, 1986.

21. Reiter, L.A., and others: Vitamin B_6 content of selected foods served in dining halls, Journal of the American Dietetic Association **85:**1625, 1985.

22. Driskell, J.A., and others: Vitamin B_6 status of southern adolescent girls, Journal of the American Dietetic Association **85:**46, 1985.

23. Alhadeff, L., and others: Toxic effects of water-soluble vitamins, Nutrition Reviews **42:**33, 1984.

24. Herbert, V.: Vitamin B_{12}. In Present knowledge in nutrition, 5th edition. The Nutrition Foundation, Inc., Washington, D.C., 1984.

25. Jukes, T.H.: Is laetrile a vitamin? Nutrition Today, p. 12, September/October, 1977.

26. Haslam, R.H.A., and others: Effects of megavitamin therapy on children with attention deficit disorders, Pediatrics **74:**103, 1984.

27. Anonymous: Nutrition for sports success. The American Alliance for Health, Physical Education, Recreation and Dance, p. 8, 1984.

28. Barnett, D.W., and Conlee, R.K.: The effects of a commercial dietary supplement on human performance, American Journal of Clinical Nutrition **40:**586, 1984.

METABOLISM NOTES: *Vitamins Needed for Energy and Bones*

The Importance of the B-Complex Vitamins in the Liberation of Energy From Carbohydrates, Fats, and Proteins

The flow diagram in Figure 6-13 shows the major reactions (and only the major reactions); however, it is helpful in explaining the following:

- People feel tired and lack energy when they are deficient in any of these key vitamins.
- A key interaction is between pyruvate and acetyl CoA. This allows the several reactions in the Krebs or tricarboxylic acid cycle to occur. Most of the energy locked up in carbohydrates, fats, and proteins is released from this point onward. That is why thiamin deficiency leads to a lack of energy. We are lucky that pantothenic acid is so widespread in foods. A deficiency of this vitamin is rare.

FIGURE 6-13

The importance of the B-complex vitamins in the liberation of energy from carbohydrates, fats, and proteins.

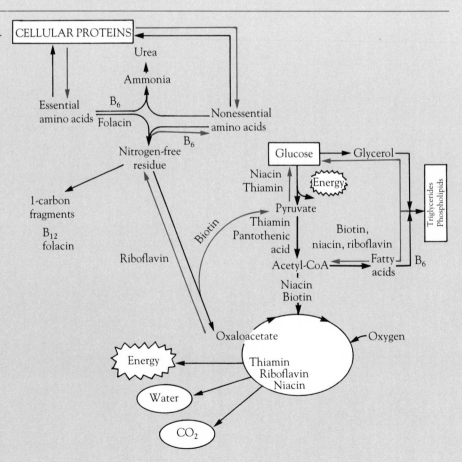

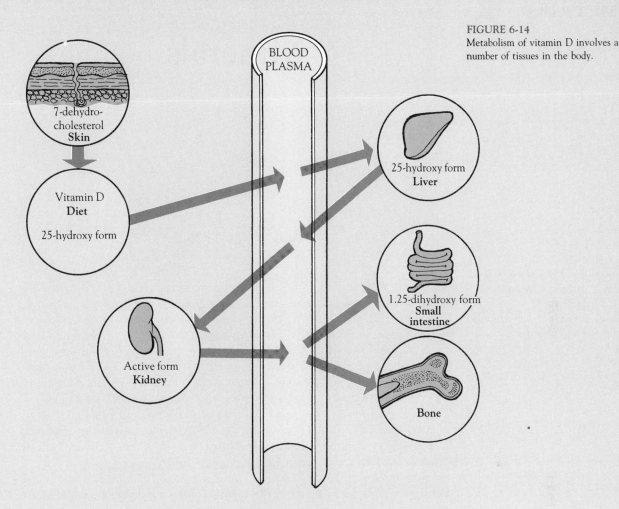

FIGURE 6-14
Metabolism of vitamin D involves a
number of tissues in the body.

- Taking vitamin supplements on top of an adequate diet will not speed up these reactions. These vitamins are needed in very small amounts for their coenzyme function, and are provided by a balanced diet.
- There is considerable interaction between carbohydrates, fats, and proteins— something to keep in mind when we look at energy balance in Chapter 9.

Metabolism of Vitamin D Involves a Number of Tissues in the Body

As Figure 6-14 illustrates, metabolism of vitamin D involves the skin, kidney, liver, small intestine, and bone. The form of vitamin D called 25-hydroxy vitamin D is the circulating form of vitamin D. The form 1,25-dihydroxy vitamin D is the active form and is produced in the kidneys only. This latter form regulates calcium metabolism (1) by aiding the absorption of calcium from the small intestine into the blood; (2) by moving calcium from bone into the blood (in the presence of parathyroid hormone); and (3) by helping phosphorus absorption.

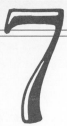

Minerals

CONNECTIONS

You may be used to hearing the phrase "vitamins and minerals" as if the two were always linked together. Indeed, minerals are tied to the metabolism and structure of vitamins but also to other nutrients previously discussed.

Minerals are of two kinds: macro and micro. Macrominerals are needed in large amounts in the body. Calcium is important in bone formation and in mitochondrial functions. Phosphorus is for storing liberated energy in phosphate compounds. Sodium, potassium, and chloride are used in nerve-muscle function. Magnesium is used in the synthesis and breakdown of energy nutrients. Sulfur gives rigidity to the structure of some proteins and is part of the structure of thiamin and biotin.

Microminerals or trace elements are needed in smaller amounts in the body, although they are just as important. Iron brings oxygen to cells to liberate energy from carbohydrates, fats, and proteins. Zinc is necessary for protein synthesis and therefore for growth. Iodine is involved in regulating metabolism. Selenium works with vitamin E as an antioxidant. Fluoride prevents tooth decay. Cobalt is part of vitamin B_{12}. Chromium is involved in glucose metabolism.

Diets that are deficient in minerals slow growth and decrease your ability to perform physical work.

Passing through rural Mississippi about 10 years ago, a writer observed two middle-aged women sitting in front-porch rocking chairs and exchanging reflections on life. "Occasionally," reported D.A. Frate, "one would reach in to the paper bag between them, grab a small handful of dirt, and eat it."

What's this? Eat dirt?

Geophagy or **Pica**
Eating clay, starch, ashes, or plaster.

Actually, these people were practicing an activity that dates back to the ancient Greeks, who ate soil for its medicinal values. In some parts of the world today girls are encouraged by a superstitious belief to eat clay at the start of menstruation. Indeed, one of the Mississippi women told Frate "It's a woman's dish. Only once did I hear of a man who consumed clay." This practice of eating clay (or ashes, plaster, or starch) in fact has a name—*geophagy* or *pica*, and nutritionists believe it is inspired by mineral deficiencies in women resulting from menstruation and pregnancy.

However strange the practice of eating dirt may seem, the minerals in our diet *do* come from the soil. But instead of eating the soil directly, we obtain minerals indirectly through food and water. In the days when people obtained food and water only from a local area, it was possible that they could be deficient in certain minerals, depending on the soil composition of their gardens or farms. Today this is not as much of a problem because soil scientists have mapped the mineral content of soils in different geographical areas and in any case the food you eat no doubt comes from many different locations.

Soil Science

MINERALS: WHAT THEY ARE, WHY WE NEED THEM

As Table 7-1 indicates, the list of essential minerals consists of *macrominerals*, which are recommended in amounts greater than 100 mg per day, and *microminerals or trace elements*, which are recommended in amounts less than 20 mg per day.

The concentration of macrominerals in foods and their role in the body are in most cases well understood. Microminerals, however, are less well understood, and experts disagree on whether other minerals should be added to the list. Perhaps this is to be expected, since such tiny amounts are being measured. Some trace elements are measured in nanograms—a nanogram is one billionth of a gram—which requires specialized instruments. Note in Table 7-1, for instance, that all the microminerals contained in the body of a person of average size weigh less than half an ounce.

Myoglobin
Transports oxygen and carbon dioxide in muscles; it gives muscle its red color.

Macromineral
Essential mineral whose RDA is over 100 mg per day.

Micromineral or **Trace Element**
Essential mineral whose RDA is less than 20 mg per day.

How do experts learn about minerals? Most answers are obtained from experiments on animals. The importance of nickel, molybdenum, and arsenic, for instance, was learned in animal research; still, experts differ on how essential these three minerals are for human beings.[1] In this chapter, however, we will try to concentrate on the established facts, all the while being mindful of the possible importance of minerals whose true significance is not known. Thirty years ago, for instance, nutritionists were not aware of the role of zinc and selenium in the diet, but they now know that zinc is needed for growth, the sense of taste, and sexual maturation and that selenium interacts positively with vitamin E and is a part of some enzymes.

The Importance of Minerals Is Not in Proportion to Their Concentration in the Diet

Minerals perform a wide variety of functions in the body, and their deficiency signs are equally varied, as Figure 7-1 indicates.

Magnesium and iron are particularly important because both are involved in two vital chemical reactions on which our very existence depends: photosynthesis and the transportation of oxygen. As we mentioned in Chapter 3, photosynthesis makes carbohydrates in plants, aided by magnesium-containing chlorophyll; plants, and therefore animals and humans, could not survive without photosynthesis. Oxygen is needed in the body to "burn" the energy locked up in carbohydrates, fats, and proteins; to transport this oxygen in the air to the tissues requires iron-containing hemoglobin in the blood.

TABLE 7-1 Minerals Contained in the Diet and Their Content in the Body of an Adult (Percentage of Total Weight)

Minerals	% of Body Weight
Macrominerals (Recommended Intake Over 100 mg/day)	
Calcium (Ca)	1.7
Phosphorus (P)	0.9
Sodium (Na)	0.14
Potassium (K)	0.21
Chloride (Cl)	0.14
Magnesium (Mg)	0.04
Sulfur (S)	0.29
Total Intake: 2433 g (87 oz)	
Microminerals or Trace Elements* (Recommended Intake Under 20 mg/day)	
Iron (Fe)	0.006
Iodine (I)	0.0002
Zinc (Zn)	0.03
Selenium (Se)	0.0003
Fluorine (F)	0.05
Copper (Cu)	0.001
Chromium (Cr)	0.00004
Cobalt (Co)	0.00002
Manganese (Mn)	0.00003
Molybdenum (Mo)	0.0002
Silicon (Si)	0.016
Nickel (Ni)	0.0001
Arsenic (As)	0.0002
Total Amount: 10.51 g (less than ½ an oz)	

* Evidence for the essentiality of vanadium (Va) is less strong. On the basis of present knowledge cadmium (Cd), lead (Pb) and probably tin (Sn) are not essential nutrients. See Nielsen, F.H. and Mertz, W.: Other trace elements. In Present knowledge in nutrition, 5th edition. The Nutrition Foundation, Washington, D.C., p. 607, 1984.

Some Minerals Are Not Friends

Environmental Health

Not all minerals are good for you. Mercury, cadmium, and lead are not nutrients; on the contrary, they are environmental toxicants that get into the food chain.[2] Mercury, which can damage the brain, is a particular problem because it shows up in fish. Cadmium, which can damage the kidney, is found in its highest concen-

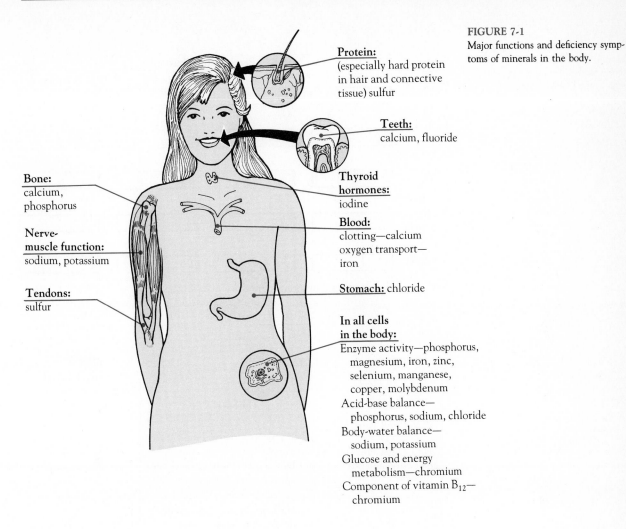

Protein:
(especially hard protein in hair and connective tissue) sulfur

Teeth:
calcium, fluoride

Bone:
calcium, phosphorus

Thyroid hormones:
iodine

Nerve-muscle function:
sodium, potassium

Blood:
clotting—calcium
oxygen transport—iron

Stomach: chloride

Tendons:
sulfur

In all cells in the body:
Enzyme activity—phosphorus, magnesium, iron, zinc, selenium, manganese, copper, molybdenum
Acid-base balance—phosphorus, sodium, chloride
Body-water balance—sodium, potassium
Glucose and energy metabolism—chromium
Component of vitamin B_{12}—chromium

trations in green leafy vegetables and in organ meats, especially kidney and liver. Lead, which can retard mental development in children, is found in food grown near lead mines and near areas exposed to heavy automobile exhaust. Indeed, some leafy vegetables grown in automobile-choked urban areas—as in gardens not far from the White House in Washington, D.C.—have been found to have high lead content.[3]

The Concentration of Minerals in Food Varies

Each mineral has different chemical properties and physiological functions in animals and plants. Therefore, the concentration of minerals in food varies. Figure 7-2 shows the contribution of various food groups in the average American diet to the intake of some important minerals, illustrating the importance of variety in the diet.

FIGURE 7-2
Minerals and food groups. This shows the contribution of food groups to the average intake of some minerals by adults in the United States.

TRACE ELEMENTS

Commodity	Percent contribution			
	Iron	Zinc	Iodine	Selenium
Dairy products	5	20	46	6
Meat, fish poultry	20	43	11	38
Grains, cereals	52	19	24	56
Fruits, vegetables	16	11	3	0.9
*Others	7	2	3	0

*Oil, fats and shortenings, sugars and adjuncts and beverages

	GI TRACT		BLOOD
	Aid	Hinder	Percent absorbed into the blood of healthy adult
CALCIUM	Lactose, Vitamin D, empty stomach (maybe)	Fiber, phytate, and oxalate; zinc supplements, laxatives, antibiotics (penicillin, tetracycline), high protein diet	Ca 30-40
IRON	Heme iron, vitamin C, alcohol, unidentified factors in milk and meat	Tannins, antibiotics (tetracycline), phosphorus (in certain forms) EDTA (food additive to prevent off-color & flavors), antacids, high pH, laxatives, fiber	Fe 7
ZINC	Protein (at high intakes)	Fiber, phytate, iron supplements, calcium supplements, copper	Zn 2-10
MAGNESIUM	Lactose	Fiber, phytate	Mg 30-40

To cells

FIGURE 7-3
Help or hindrance? Many factors aid or hinder the absorption of minerals from the gastrointestinal tract into the blood. All of the dietary factors and medications listed must be taken with the food or supplement for the effects on bioavailability to occur.

Many factors determine the amount of a mineral that finally arrives at the site of utilization in the body. _Bioavailability_ is a measure of the amount of a mineral that can be absorbed into the body and is used or is available for use. Percentage bioavailability can be expressed for all nutrients, but it is a more important gauge for minerals than for the other nutrients described in this book. Figure 7-3 shows the factors influencing the bioavailability of minerals. Note that not only do such factors differ for different minerals but that some factors assist whereas others hinder the amount of a mineral absorbed from the gastrointestinal tract. Finally, some medications influence mineral bioavailability.

Bioavailability
The amount of a nutrient that can be used by the body.

Only a Few Nutrients Are Likely to be Deficient in the North American Diet

Table 7-2 shows the average mineral intake of adult males in the United States. In general, adequate mineral intake in the United States is not a problem, although of course this is not true for everyone. The only minerals likely to be deficient in the average American diet that nutritionists are aware of are the following:

Calculation of the mineral content of your diet will not indicate what proportion of the mineral is absorbed into the blood.

- _Iron_—Intakes of iron for women of child-bearing years may be too low.
- _Calcium_—Calcium intake may be too low to prevent osteoporosis, or brittle bones, a disease occurring mainly in postmenopausal women.
- _Zinc_—Low intake, especially prevalent among people with low incomes, results in failure of sexual development.

TABLE 7-2 Average Mineral Intake of Adult Males* in the United States

Mineral	Intake (mg/day)	Percentage of RDA or ESADDI†
Macrominerals		
Calcium	1143	143
Phosphorus	1674	209
Sodium	4702	High
Potassium	3449	Adequate
Magnesium	341	97
Trace Minerals		
Iron	18.4	184
Zinc	12.8	85
Iodine	0.319	213
Copper	1.6	Low
Selenium	0.102	Adequate

*Values for women were not available from this study. Because of the higher iron RDA value for women of childbearing years, the percent RDA values would be lower.
†ESADDI, Estimated Safe and Adequate Daily Dietary Intake.

Some Mineral Deficiencies and Excesses Have Great Costs

A balanced diet will help to avoid all of the problems listed here. Taking supplements may be harmful if one is not under the supervision of a physician.

The costs of deficiencies and excesses of individual minerals may be divided into three groups: physical, psychological, and economic. Some of these factors are difficult to quantify and may differ among individuals. Moreover, some of the symptoms may also be caused by deficiencies or excesses of other nutrients. However, the point is that deficiencies and excesses of some minerals do cause a variety of problems.

The physical costs

A great deal of physical pain is brought about by certain deficiencies and excesses of specific minerals:

Neurological
Pertaining to the nervous system.

- Broken bones from calcium deficiency.
- *Neurological*, or nervous system, disturbances from magnesium deficiency.
- Heart failure from magnesium and potassium deficiency; also from excess sodium intake in some people, which causes hypertension, a factor in heart failure.
- Weakness from iron, iodine, or copper deficiency.
- Tooth decay from fluoride deficiency.
- Muscle pain from selenium deficiency.

The psychological costs

Psychology

Many of the physical costs can also have psychological consequences. Some types of psychological pain related to mineral deficiency and excess are given in the following list:

- Reduced capacity for physical activity from iron, iodine, or copper deficiency.
- Lack of sexual development from zinc deficiency.
- Impairments in mental development and physical growth from iodine deficiency. *Cretinism*, which causes dwarfism and mental retardation, occurs in infants born to mothers deficient in iodine during the first trimester of pregnancy.

Cretinism
Iodine deficiency of the mother causes the child to grow up to be a dwarf and retarded mentally.

The economic costs

Physical and psychological costs in turn have adverse economic consequences, as follows:

- Osteoporosis because of loss of calcium from bones. The National Institutes of Health Consensus Conference on Osteoporosis (1984) concluded that osteoporosis affects perhaps 15 to 20 million Americans, resulting in 1.3 million bone fractures per year in people 45 years of age and older. The cost of this disease in the U.S. has been estimated to be $3.8 billion every year.
- Iron deficiency anemia as a result of low dietary iron or from loss of iron because of blood lost during menstruation or, in tropical countries, loss of blood in parasitic infestations. Iron deficiency results in a decreased capacity for physical work, meaning lost income to those who make a living by performing physical labor.

■ Disorders from iodine deficiency. Common in parts of Africa, Latin America, and Asia, these disorders interfere with the quality of life, productivity, and education of millions of children and adults.[4]

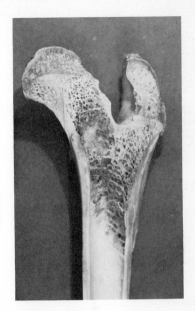

Longitudinal section of long bone showing both cancellous and compact bone.

Essential minerals assist in the transportation and formation of nutrients; become part of the structure of tissues; help muscles (including the heart), and nerves to function; and contribute to the correct chemical composition of body fluids. Mercury, cadmium, and lead are environmental toxicants that may be found in some foods and are harmful to health. Many factors influence the bioavailability of minerals. Deficiencies and excesses of some nutrients can cause physical and psychological pain and sometimes high economic costs.

MACROMINERALS

Regarding macrominerals, nutritionists show most interest in the relationship between dietary intakes of calcium and osteoporosis and of sodium and hypertension. That does not mean that phosphorus, potassium, chloride, magnesium, and sulfur are not important in nutrition.

Calcium and Phosphorus

Calcium and phosphorus are the most abundant minerals in human beings. A man has 1200 g (over 2½ lbs) of calcium and 700 g (1½ lbs) of phosphorus in his body, and a woman has about 25% less, owing to her smaller body size. More than 99% of the calcium and 85% of the phosphorus in the body are in bones and teeth. Let us look briefly at the structure of bone to understand the most important function of these two minerals.

Bone is made up of canals through which pass blood vessels that bring nutrients to the cells and nerves. *Hydroxyapatite* is the hard substance between cells in bones and teeth; it consists of a combination of calcium, phosphorus, hydrogen, and oxygen. The protein collagen is the "scaffolding" that holds hydroxyapatite in place. Bone is living tissue, increasing in length and width during growth and continually being broken down and rebuilt. Besides containing calcium and phosphorus, bone has important amounts of magnesium, iron, and zinc.

The calcium and phosphorus present in the body but not found in bone—the remaining 1% of calcium and about 15% of phosphorus—have many useful functions in the body.

Calcium has the following uses:

■ Excitation of nerves and muscles, including the heart. (Nerves become excited when a signal is passed along a nerve fiber. The signal is then transmitted to a muscle, which may then contract. If this process does not happen, then nerves and muscles cannot work.)
■ Stimulation of some hormone secretions
■ Activation of some enzymes
■ Blood coagulation

Hydroxyapatite
The hard substance between cells in bones and teeth; contains calcium, phosphorus, hydrogen, and oxygen.

Phosphorus has these functions:

- Makes up part of the nucleic acids, DNA and RNA
- Makes up part of adenosine triphosphate, necessary for energy release
- Makes up part of phospholipids in cell membranes
- Allows some vitamins to perform their coenzyme functions

With all these functions, it is clear that the quality of life, and even life itself, depends on there being an adequate supply of calcium and phosphorus.

Enough Calcium and Phosphorus Are Available for Most Functions, Except Building and Maintaining Bones

Bones are used as a reserve for calcium. The calcium level outside of bone is kept constant by a balance between two hormones. Parathyroid hormone (or para-thormone) removes calcium from storage in the bones if blood calcium is low. Calcitonin removes excess calcium from the blood and deposits it in the bones. This system of checks and balances ensures sufficient calcium is available to perform important functions in cells. The level of phosphorus in the body is not controlled by hormones. There is less likelihood of phosphorus deficiency because there are generous amounts of this mineral in a wide variety of foods.

Since the small amount of calcium not in bones (1%) is so important, should

FIGURE 7-4
Dairy products are the best dietary
source of calcium.

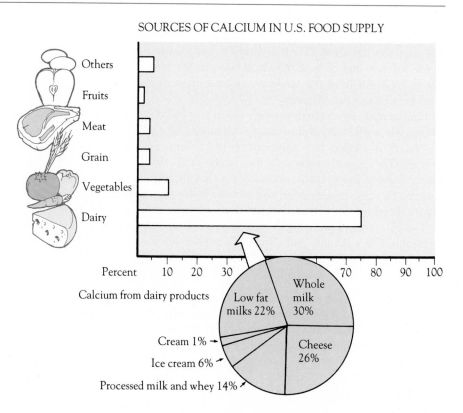

SOURCES OF CALCIUM IN U.S. FOOD SUPPLY

Others
Fruits
Meat
Grain
Vegetables
Dairy

Percent   10   20   30   70   80   90   100

Calcium from dairy products

Low fat milks 22%
Whole milk 30%
Cream 1%
Ice cream 6%
Cheese 26%
Processed milk and whey 14%

TABLE 7-3 Food Sources of the RDA of Calcium and Phosphorus for Adult Males and Females*

	Calcium	Phosphorus
Milk	2⅔ cups	3½ cups
Cheddar cheese,	4 ounces	5½ ounces
cream cheese	35 ounces	27 ounces
Yogurt	15½ ounces	20 ounces
Eggs, cooked	28 eggs	9 eggs
Beef, ground	240 ounces	13 ounces
Beef liver, fried	267 ounces	2 ounces
Sardines	6½ ounces	5½ ounces
Tuna	343 ounces	12 ounces
Peanut butter	51 ounces	7½ ounces
Beans, cooked	14½ cups	2¾ cups

*800 mg

you seek ways to increase that amount—just in case? Absolutely not. Calcium in amounts greater than 1% is a disaster because the calcium becomes insoluble in soft tissues, interfering with tissue functions like the operation of the kidney.

Food Sources Are Usually Readily Available

The dietary intake of calcium by North Americans has shown considerable variation since the beginning of the century. Today 75% of the calcium in the average U.S. diet comes from dairy products, and within that group the highest percentage of calcium is contributed by milk (Figure 7-4). The growth in popularity of low-fat milk and yogurt suggests that they will be important sources of calcium in the future.

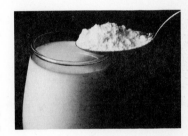

Some experts have reservations about calcium supplements. The current interest in calcium supplements to prevent osteoporosis may be ill-founded.

The RDA for both calcium and phosphorus is 800 mg in men and women. Good sources are shown in Table 7-3; any one of the foods shown there meets the RDA. Note that, except for dairy products, meeting the RDA for phosphorus requires a smaller amount of the same food than it does for meeting the RDA for calcium. Note also that the bioavailability of calcium in beans and other plant sources of calcium is low.

Americans do not take in as much calcium today as did their prehistoric ancestors: a man eats 1143 mg of calcium per day now as opposed to 1579 mg back then.[5] Many women and teenagers today have low intakes of calcium. In addition, a number of people cannot tolerate milk because of lactase deficiency, although they can increase calcium intake by eating yogurt and some cheeses (cheddar rather than cream), fish with soft bones, like sardines, tuna, and salmon, or by drinking lactose-reduced milk. This is made by adding the enzyme lactase to milk and waiting about 10 to 15 minutes for the enzyme to act.

Anthropology

FIGURE 7-5
How dietary calcium is used and excreted. The numbers refer to factors that aid or hinder the absorption and excretion of calcium. *1*, vitamin D; *2*, lactose; *3*, phosphorus; *4*, fiber; *5*, oxalate and phytate; *6*, medications; *7*, drugs; *8*, disease; *9*, alcoholism; *10*, purified protein and a variety of amino acids; *11*, caffeine; *12*, fluoride; *13*, physical activity.

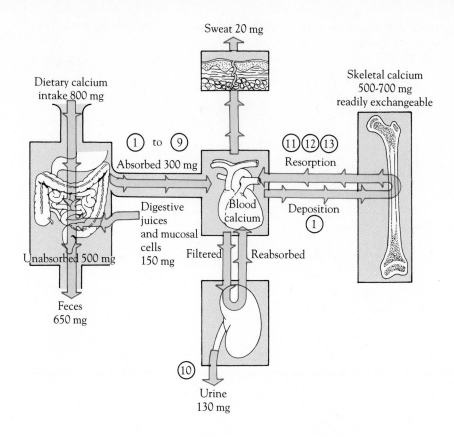

Diet, Alcohol and Caffeine Intake, Medication, and Disease and Exercise Influence How Well Calcium Is Absorbed and Utilized

Figure 7-5 shows what happens to calcium as it passes through the body and is either used or excreted. Quite a few factors affect how calcium is used, including diet, alcohol and caffeine intake, medication, and disease and physical activity. These in turn suggest whether or not a remedy lies in buying calcium supplements—and the risks and benefits of such supplements.

In general, an adequate diet will provide the amount of calcium you need for normal health. Foods supplying 100 mg of calcium are:

- Milk: ⅓ cup
- Cheese: ½ ounce
- Canned salmon or sardines (with bones): 1 ounce

The following factors help or hinder the absorption and utilization of calcium—note that the factors that hurt outnumber those that help.

Diet

Diet seems to play the biggest role in the absorption of calcium. Some food substances aid uptake and utilization:

- *Vitamin D:* This is the most important aid in calcium absorption from the intestine and calcium deposition in bone.
- *Lactose:* Lactose in milk aids calcium absorption from the gastrointestinal tract.

The following substances are thought to hinder the body's absorption and utilization of calcium.

- *Phosphorus:* When used in high amounts, this mineral is listed frequently as a cause of decreased calcium absorption. The evidence comes from animal studies where calcium and phosphorus combine in the animal's intestines to form insoluble calcium phosphate salts that cannot be absorbed. However, recent studies on humans show that high phosphorus intakes do not affect calcium absorption.[6] This observation awaits further confirmation.
- *Fiber:* In amounts greater than those found in the normal diet, fiber can hinder the absorption of calcium, which is then eliminated in the feces. Some estimates indicate that every 18 g of fiber consumed increase dietary calcium requirements by 100 mg.[7] In food terms, 18 g of fiber is provided by any one of the following foods: ½ cup of beans, 2 cups of peas, ¾ cup of All-Bran or Bran Buds.
- *Oxalate and phytate:* For a long time, it was thought that when these two substances combined with calcium in the gastrointestinal tract they made calcium unavailable for absorption into the blood. However, recent evidence suggests that they are of little importance in influencing calcium absorption in the ordinary diet.[8] Oxalates are present in high amounts in rhubarb, spinach, tea, coffee, and chocolate. Phytate is an organic compound found in high concentrations in cereals, especially bran, legumes, and some nuts.
- *Purified protein and a variety of amino acids:* These induce bone loss in people and animals.[6] Complex proteins like meat and dairy products do not cause a loss of calcium from bones.
- *Vitamin A:* Excessive intakes of vitamin A cause calcium loss from bone.

The effect of the intake of purified protein on calcium absorption is another example of the danger of taking certain supplements without complete information.

Alcohol and caffeine intake

People suffering from alcoholism show decreased intestinal absorption of calcium.

Caffeine in coffee, tea, and some soft drinks decreases calcium retention in the body.[6] Nicotine in cigarettes does the same, so more research is needed here, because people who smoke may also be heavy coffee drinkers.

Medications

Medications, including antacids and the antibiotic known as tetracycline, decrease calcium absorption. It is interesting that a popular antacid (Tums) is advertised as being high in calcium. It gives the impression that it is a good calcium supplement. However, there are questions about the bioavailability of the calcium in this antacid.

Drugs like the corticosteroids and thyroid extract cause calcium loss from the body. This is one of the long-term hazards of using steroids, whether for treatment for medical disorders or, as some athletes use them, for building muscles.

Physical Education

Fluoride lowers the incidence of osteoporosis, but such use is considered experimental now.[6]

Disease and physical activity

Some diseases, including diabetes, kidney failure, and malabsorption syndromes—especially of fat—decrease calcium absorption.

Decreased physical activity causes bone loss. This happens to patients immobilized for long periods. Zero gravity causes a loss of calcium in astronauts. Increased physical activity slows the rate of bone loss, even in the elderly.

> Dairy products and sardines are the best dietary sources of calcium and phosphorus. Meat and eggs are high in phosphorus, but not in calcium. Factors affecting calcium bioavailability include components of the diet; alcohol and caffeine intake; the use of nicotine, medications and drugs; certain diseases; and physical activity.

CALCIUM-RELATED DISORDERS: OSTEOPOROSIS, RICKETS, OSTEOMALACIA—AND HYPERTENSION

With so many factors that affect the absorption of calcium and so many people apparently affected by deficiency-related disorders (15 to 20 million Americans by osteoporosis alone), we should take a look at what the lack or excess of calcium does.

Osteoporosis Is More Common in Women Than in Men

Beginning at 30 to 40 years of age, you begin to lose bone mass. When this loss becomes so great that bone fractures occur after slight impact, it means that you have osteoporosis ("porous bones").

Osteoporosis is responsible for about 150,000 hip fractures per year in the U.S. About 12% of people with these hip fractures will die of related complications. Osteoporosis will become an even bigger problem in the future because of increased life expectancy.

White, postmenopsual women are the population at greatest risk. Osteoporosis is not as prevalent in men or in black women because they have a higher bone mass. Lower-than-normal bone density is also found in people with anorexia nervosa. Most experts agree that the greatest protection against osteoporosis is a high bone mass in the early part of life.

Predicting Osteoporosis Is Difficult

The first signs of osteoporosis are back pains, caused by a collapse of one or more vertebrae. This causes a "dowager's hump" in older women (Figure 7-6). Bones may be broken after slight impact, especially those in the spine, forearm, upper thigh, and hip. Bone loss in the jaws, called alveolar bone loss, may be an early indicator of osteoporosis, and teeth can be lost as a result. About 25 million Americans have lost all of their teeth.

Osteoporosis is called "the silent disease" because it is difficult to diagnose until it has reached an advanced stage. With increased publicity for osteoporosis comes

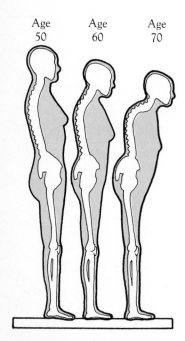

Age 50   Age 60   Age 70

FIGURE 7-6
Development of the "dowager's hump." After 50 years of age fractures of the spinal vertebrae can result in a gradual loss of height and a curvature of the spine.

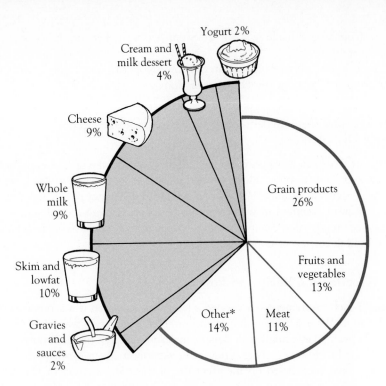

FIGURE 7-7
Women's calcium. Dairy products provide an increasingly larger share of calcium for women.

*Includes eggs, nuts, legumes, fats and oils, sugars and sweeteners, and alcoholic and nonalcoholic beverages.

increased pressure to identify people at risk. If you are in your twenties, wouldn't it be nice to have a quick, inexpensive checkup to tell you whether you will suffer from osteoporosis in later life?

Unfortunately, the tests now available require sensitive equipment and are expensive. As one observer remarks, such tests used for screening purposes are "premature, albeit profitable."[9]

Why Osteoporosis Is More Common in Women Than in Men

The possible reasons women suffer more than men from this disease follow:

- Women have lower calcium intakes than men. However, there are encouraging signs that women's dietary calcium intakes are improving (Figure 7-7).
- Bone loss is greater after menopause. This suggests hormonal factors are involved, especially the lack of estrogen.
- Pregnancy and breast feeding increase calcium requirements. This is especially critical during a teenage pregnancy because of the higher RDA value for teenagers (1200 mg).
- Weight-reducing diets, which women are more likely to try than men, are often low in calcium.
- Women live longer than men—and since osteoporosis is a disease of aging, it is seen even more often in women.

Osteoporosis is made worse if the woman is a smoker, drinks alcohol, or does not exercise.[6]

Prevention and treatment strategies for osteoporosis are controversial. We will return to this topic in the Decision section.

Rickets and Osteomalacia Are Other Calcium-Related Bone Disorders

You saw that rickets occurs in young children because of a lack of vitamin D. This deficiency leads to poor absorption and deposition of calcium in the bone. *Osteomalacia* occurs in adults as a result of a combined deficiency of calcium and vitamin D. It is most common in women whose bones are depleted of calcium because of repeated pregnancies. Symptoms are the same in rickets and osteomalacia: extreme pain and distortion of bones.

Is Hypertension Related to Low Calcium Intake?

Much excitement was created a few years ago when it was reported that low calcium intake is a cause of hypertension. This observation was made on the basis of data from a large number of Americans examined in a national nutrition survey (HANES I). However, there is now some skepticism about this hypothesis because it may have been based on incorrect use of statistical analysis of the data.[10] An editorial in an international medical journal cautions against advising the general population to increase their calcium intake to control hypertension.[11]

> Osteoporosis is more common in women than in men, is difficult to detect in its early stages, and prevention by calcium supplements is debated. There is limited evidence that low calcium intakes may be related to hypertension.

SODIUM, POTASSIUM, AND CHLORIDE: THE MAJOR ELECTROLYTES

Sodium, potassium, and chloride are three minerals that are essential to your health and are interrelated as the major electrolytes in the body. All three are involved in water balance in the body, and in acid-base balance. As shown in Figure 7-8, sodium and chloride are in highest concentration in the extracellular space—the space outside the cells. Regulation of sodium levels in the body influences the amount of fluid inside and outside the cells. If dietary sodium intake is high, it can be filtered from the blood by the kidney and excreted in the urine. Potassium appears in the intracellular fluid—the fluid within the cell. A number of factors influence the level of sodium outside the cell and potassium inside the cell. The body is particularly sensitive to any increase in sodium within the cell, and any excess is pumped back into the extracellular fluid by the sodium pump.

Sodium and potassium are necessary for the normal functioning of nerves and muscles. Both are important in carbohydrate nutrition: sodium for the absorption of glucose, potassium for the formation of glycogen. Potassium is involved also in

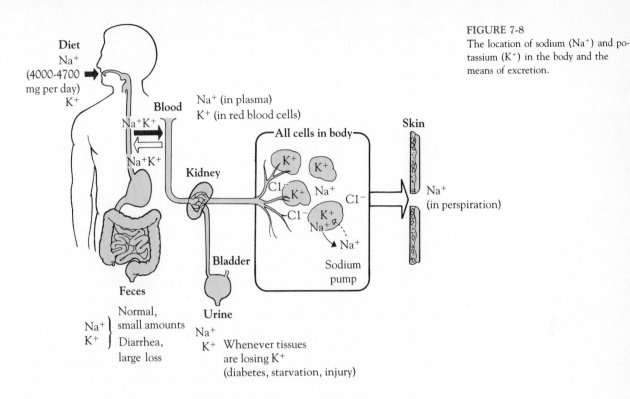

FIGURE 7-8

The location of sodium (Na^+) and potassium (K^+) in the body and the means of excretion.

protein synthesis. Chloride is combined with hydrogen to form hydrochloric acid in the stomach where it is important in digestion. Excessive loss of potassium in diarrhea can lead to death from severe dehydration and paralysis.

You are, of course, quite familiar with sodium because salt (sodium chloride, NaCl) enhances food flavor, prevents food spoilage, and influences the physical properties of some foods, including strengthening bread dough and controlling the texture of cheese. Salt is, in fact, the oldest food additive in the world. Because Roman soldiers were paid in *sal*—Latin for "salt"—the word "salary" was coined.

Needless to say, decreasing or increasing the amount of salt has a significant influence on taste preferences.[12] However, such preferences can be changed: a study of young adults who ate a low-sodium diet for five months found they came to prefer a lower level of sodium in their diet, although the initial stages of the diet were somewhat difficult. This shows that you can reduce a high-salt diet if you want to.

The Amounts of Sodium, Potassium, and Chloride Vary in the Body and in the Diet

The average adult has about 150 g of potassium and 100 g of both sodium and chloride in his or her body—equivalent to about seven tablespoonfuls (half a cup) of salt. Every day the average person in North America takes in 10 to 12 g of salt, of which 4000 to 4700 mg is sodium and the rest chloride (Figure 7-9). Not counting the salt you may add during cooking or while sitting at the table, you get most sodium from grain products, with lower and almost equal amounts from the meat, dairy, and fruit and vegetable groups. Most potassium is in fruits and vegetables

TABLE 7-4 Sodium Content of Food Varies with Method of Preparation

½ Cup of Peas	Sodium (mg)
Cooked	1
Frozen	88
Frozen, with mushrooms	240
Canned	246
Frozen in butter sauce	402
Frozen in cream sauce	534

and dairy products (Figure 7-2). Chloride is provided by processed foods and by added salt.

In recent years there has been a great deal of concern that high intake of sodium is linked to hypertension or high blood pressure in some people. (About 18% of American adults have high blood pressure.) Hypertension in turn is cited as being a risk factor in coronary heart disease, stroke, and kidney failure. As a consequence, the U.S. government has been monitoring sodium content in the diet, and food companies—amid much ballyhoo about products being "salt free"—have lowered the sodium content of many of their foods.[13] Is too much sodium clearly a threat to health? Before you decide, let us consider the sources of sodium in the diet.

Linguistics

The amount of sodium in a person's diet will vary greatly depending on the method of preparation, as is seen with the peas in Table 7-4. Clearly, then, reading the labels on foods is important. However, a variety of terms have been introduced to describe the sodium content of food. Because vague definitions of these descriptions led to abuse by some manufacturers—most particularly in the use of terms like "low sodium" and "sodium free"—and confusion among consumers, in July 1985 the Food and Drug Administration introduced the following definitions:

FIGURE 7-9
Dietary sodium comes from the sodium occurring naturally in foods, sodium added during commercial food processing, and sodium from salt added to foods by the consumer.

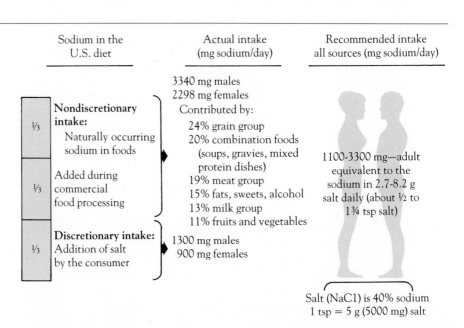

TABLE 7-5 Sources of Sodium in the Diet

One Teaspoonful of	Will Provide
Table salt	2000 mg
Onion salt	1620 mg
Garlic salt	1850 mg
Monosodium glutamate (MSG)	492 mg
Soy sauce	343 mg
Meat tenderizer	1750 mg

- *Sodium free:* less than 5 mg per serving
- *Very low sodium:* 35 mg or less
- *Low sodium:* 140 mg or less
- *Reduced sodium:* a 75% reduction in sodium content

If you add no salt to your food, then your intake of sodium occurring naturally in foods, plus the amount added during commercial food processing, would come within the limits of a *safe* intake of sodium. In the United States about one third of the sodium in the diet comes from processed foods (Figure 7-9), whereas in Canada the amount from this source is considered to be much higher.[14]

To help reduce sodium in your diet, consult Table 7-5, which shows the number of milligrams of sodium in a teaspoonful of various sodium-containing substances. Most herbs and spices, it should be noted, are *sodium free.*

Examples of sodium-containing ingredients and their uses in foods are shown in Table 7-6. From this list it is clear that there are difficulties in obtaining a low-sodium diet. Foods to avoid if you are trying to restrict your sodium intake include:

TABLE 7-6 Examples of Sodium-Containing Ingredients and Their Uses in Foods

Ingredient	Use in Food
Baking powder	Leavening agent
Baking soda	Leavening agent
Monosodium glutamate	Flavor enhancer
Sodium benzoate	Preservative
Sodium caseinate	Thickener and binder
Sodium citrate	Buffer, used to control acidity in soft drinks and fruit drinks
Sodium nitrite	Curing agent in meat; provides color, prevents botulism (a food poisoning)
Sodium phosphate	Emulsifier, stabilizer, buffer
Sodium proprionate	Mold inhibitor
Sodium saccharin	Artificial sweetener

TABLE 7-7 Commercially Prepared Condiments, Sauces, and Seasonings High in Sodium

Seasoned salt	Steak sauce
Celery salt	Barbecue sauce
Onion salt	Worcestershire sauce
Garlic salt	Chili sauce
Monosodium glutamate (MSG)	Catsup
Meat tenderizer	Mustard
Baking powder	Salad dressings
Baking soda	Pickles
Soy sauce	Relish

- *Salted snacks:* saltine crackers, pretzels, salted potato chips, nuts, and salted popcorn
- *Meat and fish that are salted or smoked:* frankfurters, ham, bacon, luncheon meat, smoked salmon, sardines, and anchovies
- *Cheese:* especially processed cheese
- *Soups:* if canned or dehydrated
- *Sauces:* for example, catsup and horseradish
- *Brine-soaked foods:* for example, pickles and olives

Be sure to look at the label on some commercially prepared condiments, sauces, and seasonings. The U.S. Department of Agriculture compiled a list of foods high in sodium as shown in Table 7-7.

There Are Both Pro and Con Arguments for Reducing Sodium Intake

Nearly one in every five adult Americans suffers from hypertension. Sodium is believed to be a contributing factor. Actually, the exact cause of hypertension is not known, but diet is not the only contributor; others include genetics, obesity, smoking, lack of exercise, and emotional stress. Should you, then, cut down on salt? Let's examine the arguments for and against reducing salt intake, based on recent research.

The arguments for reducing sodium intake

Evidence from anthropology, sociology, medicine, physiology, and epidemiology has been used to link high sodium intake to high blood pressure in people in all parts of the world.[15] (A major study called the Intersalt project is shortly expected to report on this role of salt in 58 different populations.) The sodium level of the diet of most Americans and Canadians is far in excess of the amount needed for the functions performed by sodium in the body. So why not reduce this high intake?[16] Some experts who argue for reduction say there's no way to tell who may be in the 18% of the population who will be hypertensive but that since adult hypertension may start in childhood, *no one* should go through life on a high-sodium diet—just in case he or she turns out to be among the at-risk group.

Reducing sodium in the diet may be easier than you might expect. Studies have shown that the preferences of formerly heavy users of table salt can still be satisfied with smaller amounts. Moreover, low-sodium diets need not be bland, tasteless, or expensive; herbs and spices can replace salt.

The arguments against reducing sodium intake

Although most nutritionists have no quarrel with reducing sodium intake from very high levels, some argue that, since there is no proven cause-and-effect relationship between sodium and hypertension, it is not necessary for *everyone* to lower his or her sodium intake.[17] Certainly, they say, some reduction should be done in high-sodium foods eaten in large amounts by many people, but they worry that wholesale elimination of sodium from food may actually affect its microbiological safety.[18] In addition, some nutritionists complain about the methods used to measure sodium intake.

Chloride and Potassium May Play Roles in Hypertension

There is some preliminary evidence that the chloride in sodium chloride (salt) plays a role in increasing hypertension. If these observations are confirmed, then we should speak of *sodium chloride–dependent* hypertension rather than *sodium-dependent* hypertension.

It is probably medically wise to reduce sodium intake.

Potassium may lower hypertension, but may not always be successful; moreover, excess potassium can be a health hazard.[19] Potassium chloride is not added to foods instead of salt because it has a bitter taste and because it is much more expensive than salt.

> Hypertension is a complex disease and may involve a number of different minerals in the body. Diet is only one of many risk factors. There is no nutritional justification for high dietary levels of sodium, but not everybody will get hypertension on high-sodium diets.

MAGNESIUM

Adults have about 26 g of magnesium in their bodies, 55% of it in the bones. Magnesium assists many of the enzymes involved in the synthesis and breakdown of carbohydrates, fats, and proteins and in the synthesis of DNA and RNA within the cell. It is necessary for the functioning of nerves and muscles, including the heart. Symptoms of magnesium deficiency include uncontrollable twitching of the muscles, leading to convulsions; the condition can end in death.

Magnesium intake among people in North America has not decreased during this century, with the average intake per day ranging between 180 mg and 480 mg. The RDA for adult women is 300 mg and for men 350 mg. Most people's diets are adequate in magnesium because the mineral is present in reasonable amounts in all food groups (Figure 7-2 and Table 7-8). The magnesium RDA for a woman can be met by any one of the foods listed in Table 7-8.

Magnesium deficiency occurs usually as a complication of diseases or stress. Whether stress is physical (exhausting exercise, surgery, extremes of temperature), or psychological (anger, fear, overwork), it may cause hormonal changes that can

TABLE 7-8 **Foods that Provide the RDA of Magnesium for an Adult Female***

Food	Portion
Bread, whole wheat	17 slices
Oatmeal, dry	7½ ounces
Spinach	14 ounces
Meat, poultry, fish	35 to 45 ounces
Cheese	24 ounces
Fruits and vegetables	35 to 105 ounces

*300 mg

increase magnesium loss from the body. Because everyone is vulnerable to such stresses at times, should you consider buying a magnesium supplement? Although a higher RDA is suggested in circumstances such as these,[20] if you have a varied diet, it should provide the additional magnesium needed to weather these conditions.

SULFUR

Adults have about 200 g of sulfur, most of it as part of three sulfur-containing amino acids: methionine (essential), cystine, and cysteine. Adjacent sulfur-containing amino acids can form rigid sulfur-sulfur bonds, which are important in maintaining the three-dimensional structure of proteins, especially for the proper functioning of enzymes. The more sulfur-sulfur bridges that exist, the more rigid the protein molecule is. The best examples of this are the high sulfur proteins that make up hair, nails, and skin.

Sulfur has no RDA; no sulfur deficiencies have been identified. Diets adequate in animal and plant protein are adequate in sulfur also. Two vitamins, thiamin and biotin, have sulfur as part of their molecule.

Diets in industrialized countries may be low in calcium, especially for teenagers and women, adequate in potassium, magnesium, and sulfur, and high in phosphorus, sodium, and chloride. Children suffering from protein-energy malnutrition will have low levels of potassium and magnesium in their bodies, partly because of loss of these electrolytes due to diarrhea.

MICROMINERALS OR THE TRACE ELEMENTS

Turning now from the macrominerals to the microminerals, also known as *trace elements*, we enter an area that has undergone the most rapid change in nutrition. Although the importance of iron was established in the 17th century, most discoveries about these minerals and why they are essential have been made since the 1930s, and the bioavailability of trace elements is an active area of research today.

Many fascinating factors determine the amounts of trace elements entering the body from the diet, and you may find this an exciting area for your own discovery beyond the limits of this book.[21]

Let's now examine the most important of the microminerals: iron, zinc, iodine, selenium, fluoride, and copper, plus a handful of others.

Iron Has a Higher RDA for Women Than for Men

Iron is the only nutrient that has a higher RDA for women than for men. The reason for this, as stated in a television commercial for an iron supplement, is that "America's greatest nutrition problem is iron-poor blood." Why is this peculiar to women? The answer is that iron is lost from the body during menstruation and during childbirth.

An adequate intake of dietary iron is of particular importance for women during the child-bearing years.

About three quarters of the iron in the body is in the hemoglobin molecule in the blood. Therefore, blood loss from the body will cause anemia. Many doctors cite two factors for the low body iron stores in many young women: menstrual bleeding and diets low in iron.

If an adult man is anemic, the first thing physicians suspect is a bleeding ulcer; otherwise, men do not usually suffer from a deficiency of iron. Iron deficiency anemia may occur in infants (5.7%), teenage girls (5.9%),[22] and in pregnant and lactating women.

The uses of iron: transporting oxygen and carbon dioxide

Iron is a vital part of the system that brings oxygen to every cell in the body. It performs this function as part of the hemoglobin molecule in the blood. Hemoglobin carries the oxygen from the air you breathe to every cell in your body, as Figure 7-10 indicates. After the oxygen is used to liberate the energy from carbohydrates, fats, and proteins in the cells, the carbon dioxide produced is taken by hemoglobin back to the lungs and from there is exhaled in the breath.

Muscles in particular need a lot of oxygen to quickly release the energy needed for physical work or athletic performance. Therefore, muscle has another iron-containing molecule called *myoglobin,* which picks up the oxygen from the hemoglobin in the blood (Figure 7-10). Iron is also a part of some enzymes.

Micromineral or **Trace Element**
Essential mineral whose RDA is less than 20 mg per day.

The food sources of iron

The RDA for iron is 18 mg for women and 10 mg for men. Any one of the foods shown in Table 7-9 will meet the RDA for a woman until menopause. After menopause, the RDA value decreases to 10 mg because iron is no longer lost through menstruation. For comparison purposes, the table also presents the amounts of the listed foods that fulfill a woman's RDA for zinc. The RDA for zinc is 15 mg for both women and men. The intake of both iron and zinc may be low for some people, and you may notice that in most cases the foods listed in the table are good sources for both these minerals. (An exception is the low concentration of iron in milk and other dairy products.)

An interesting source of iron, incidentally, is iron cooking utensils, which can increase significantly the iron content of food cooked in them because rust from the utensil is taken up by the food.[23]

FIGURE 7-10
Iron-containing hemoglobin helps transport oxygen to the cells and carbon dioxide away from them. Myoglobin picks up oxygen from the blood in muscles and accelerates muscular energy release.

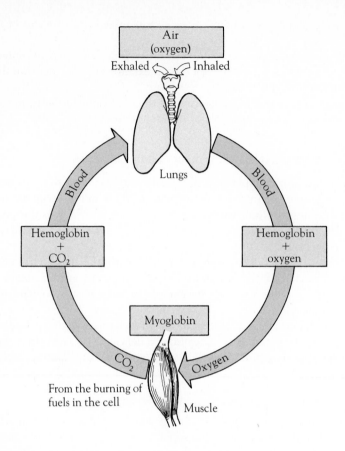

Iron absorption

People who are in iron balance absorb only about 10% of dietary iron. This increases to about 15% when the person is anemic. Many factors influence the amount of iron absorbed from the gastrointestinal tract into the blood, as Figure 7-3 indicates. You may notice that tea and coffee interfere with iron absorption from food, but not all drinks act this way. Any drink containing vitamin C, like orange juice, is valuable because vitamin C aids iron absorption. If you have a deficiency of iron, therefore, you will find a vitamin C drink like orange juice a better thirst quencher than, say, iced tea. In addition, a form of iron with high bioavailability is heme, found in meat; it is the iron-rich compound that comes from the animal's hemoglobin and myoglobin.

Iron Deficiency Severely Affects Physical Activity

Hemoglobin and myoglobin give blood and muscles their red color. People who are very pale are described as "anemic looking." Iron-deficient people cannot endure prolonged activity because of the lower amount of oxygen arriving at their muscles. This could be a particular problem for female athletes. Anemia also impairs muscle metabolism, causes cognitive disturbances in children, and reduces the absorption of sugars from the intestine.

There is one unusual problem in correcting the anemic condition in many severely undernourished people. When they are given iron supplements, they often

TABLE 7-9   Foods Required to Meet the RDA of Iron* and Zinc†
for an Adult Female

Food	Iron	Zinc
Liver	7 ounces	10 ounces
Hamburger meat, lean	18 ounces	14½ ounces
Turkey, dark meat	27 ounces	16 ounces
light meat	54 ounces	27½ ounces
Peanut butter	5½ tablespoons	7 tablespoons
Beans, cooked	3½ cups	8 cups
Egg, cooked	18 eggs	21 eggs
Bread, whole wheat	22½ slices	29½ slices
Milk, whole	180 cups	16 cups
Cheddar cheese	90 ounces	17 ounces

*18 mg

†15 mg

develop infections. This is because microorganisms causing malaria, tuberculosis, and viral diseases need iron for their growth. This odd situation occurs in parts of Africa when people are being nursed back to health. A diet adequate in iron and other nutrients makes these undernourished people more prone to malaria and the other diseases mentioned above.[24]

Attempts to increase the iron content of different foods by providing additional iron have not been a great success, except in the case of infant foods. In fact, you need to be careful about using iron supplements, for iron has one of the lowest Mineral Safety Indexes. The minimum toxic dose is 100 mg (Table 7-10). If you

TABLE 7-10   Mineral Safety Index

Mineral	RDA*	Minimum Toxic Dose (MTD)	Mineral Safety Index (MSI)
Calcium	1200 mg	12,000 mg	10
Phosphorus	1200 mg	12,000 mg	10
Magnesium	400 mg	6000 mg	15
Iron	18 mg	100 mg	5.5
Zinc	15 mg	500 mg	33
Copper	3 mg	100 mg	33
Fluoride	4 mg	20 mg	5
Iodine	0.15 mg	2 mg	13
Selenium	0.2 mg	1 mg	5

*The highest of the individual Recommended Dietary Allowance (RDA)— except those for pregnancy and lactation—or the U.S. Recommended Daily Allowance, whichever is higher.

check the label on various supplements, you will see that it is easy to exceed the toxic level. High intakes of iron lead to liver damage and heart failure.

Zinc Has Many Important Functions in the Body

Zinc is needed in over 70 enzymes in the body and is part of the insulin molecule. The effects of zinc deficiency are delayed sexual development, growth failure, loss of the sense of taste, mental lethargy, skin changes, delayed wound healing, and reduced resistance to disease. A decreased ability of the eyes to adapt to darkness is a symptom of secondary vitamin A deficiency caused by zinc deficiency. Treatment with zinc reverses all of these effects (provided they are really from a deficiency of zinc).

Zinc RDA for men and women is 15 mg, with increased amounts recommended during pregnancy and lactation. Amounts of different foods to meet the RDA for adults are given in Table 7-9. The meat group provides the most zinc (Figure 7-2). People who eat no foods of animal origin (vegans) may have a problem with receiving sufficient zinc. There are two reasons for this. First, only 30% of zinc in the typical diet of an adult American comes from grains, fruits, and vegetables (Figure 7-2). Second, zinc absorption is reduced by plant substances such as phytate and by some types of fiber. Zinc absorption is interfered with also by iron, calcium, and copper. There is a fascinating chemical tug-of-war between minerals in our digestive system after a meal. Excess zinc in food is eliminated in the feces and excreted in the urine, with only a tiny amount lost in sweat.

Deficiency of some nutrients, including zinc, may be due to factors other than diet.

Dwarfism caused by zinc deficiency has been reported in a number of countries, including the United States, China, Egypt, Morocco, and Portugal. Mild zinc deficiency is probably present in all industrialized countries.[25] People most likely to have low intakes include premature infants, children, pregnant women, adolescents, and chronic alcoholics. Many women who take oral contraceptive agents (OCAs) have lower levels of zinc in the blood, but this is not considered to be of any significance in relation to deficiency symptoms. Factors contributing to zinc deficiency include: poor diet, alcoholism, malabsorption, liver and kidney disease, and certain genetic disorders. This is yet another example of where diet is only one of many factors that can cause a deficiency of a nutrient.

Because of its many important functions in the body, zinc has become a popular addition to advertisements for nutrient supplements. Some athletes take zinc supplements in the mistaken belief that these supplements to an adequate diet will help further muscle development. Though toxic symptoms have not been reported, it is unwise to self-medicate without the guidance of a physician.[25]

Iodine Is Necessary for the Thyroid Gland

An interesting problem with iodine is summed up in an article title, "Iodine: Going from Hypo to Hyper." Let us take each in order.

Hypothyroidism and other iodine-deficiency diseases

The prefix "hypo" refers to deficiency. At one time iodine deficiency was widespread in areas located far from the sea, since most foods rich in iodine are grown in or near the ocean. In the early 1900s, many people in the upper Midwest and in central Canada were found to be suffering from goiter, the iodine-deficiency disease characterized by a swelling of the thyroid gland. In goiter, which was more prevalent in women than in men, the thyroid gland enlarges in an effort to produce more of the iodine-containing hormone, thyroxin, when the intake of iodine from the diet is low. Some drugs interfere with the incorporation of iodine into thyroxin. This can be a problem if the diet is low in iodine. Unfortunately, increasing iodine intake will not reduce the enlargement of the thyroid; this can be done only by surgery. Unfortunately also, if a woman is deficient in iodine during pregnancy the child may turn out to be a cretin—permanently retarded in its mental and physical growth.

Iodine deficiency affects millions of people in developing countries,[4] but it is now rare in developed countries. There are two reasons for this. First, you can buy salt that states on the label that it is iodized, a process begun in Michigan in 1924. Second, iodine-rich foods grown in or near the sea can now be easily transported and stored all over the country.

> A food additive (iodized salt) and improved transportation of food have all but eliminated iodine deficiency in industrialized countries.

Goitrogens are an interesting group of chemicals occurring naturally in foods like cabbage and turnips. Goitrogens interfere with the manufacture and synthesis of iodine-containing thyroxin. Since Americans do not eat large amounts of these foods on a regular basis, this is not a problem. However, in parts of Africa where millet is a staple there is a high incidence of goiter, probably caused by goitrogens in the millet.

> Certain foods have *naturally occurring* toxicants, but your intake of them has to be unnaturally high for the toxicants to affect health adversely.

Hyperthyroidism

The prefix "hyper" refers to excess. Since the 1970s concern about hyperthyroidism has risen. Hyperthyroidism causes a significant increase in basal metabolism. Drugs used to control it have some side effects. Excess iodine intake can cause thyroid enlargement (an iodine-induced goiter). Iodine intake by many people is now over five times the RDA value. A diet containing 2850 calories per day for a North American adult will contain 696 μg, compared with an RDA value of 150 μg for an adult man or woman. Dairy products supply over half, and grain and cereal products a quarter, of the iodine intake. A typical fast-food meal of hamburger, French fries, and a milkshake has three times the RDA for iodine.

> Goiter causes an enlargement of the thyroid gland because of a deficiency of iodine.

There is a general agreement that we do not need any more iodine in our diet. Iodine gets into the food supply through the use of iodine-containing chemicals that kill bacteria and fungi on dairy equipment and the iodine found in compounds used as dough conditioners in making bread.

Selenium May Help in Cancer Prevention

Might selenium prevent cancer? This nutrient has been propelled into the limelight with the news that cancer in experimental animals is reduced when they are fed additional selenium. Obviously, as this information becomes better known to the general public, you might expect to see increased commercialization of selenium supplements. However, you should treat this information with caution, for research on selenium and cancer prevention is still in the early stages. Moreover, scientists are still trying to determine which is the best chemical form of selenium for supplementation, how long high intakes are required, and what problems are associated with potentially toxic levels of intake.[26]

The minimum toxic dose for selenium is only five times in excess of its RDA (see Table 7-10). Levels of selenium given to experimental animals may be toxic in humans if taken for a long period.[27] Clinical signs of selenium toxicity are difficult to detect. Symptoms of severe selenium toxicity include liver damage and numb-

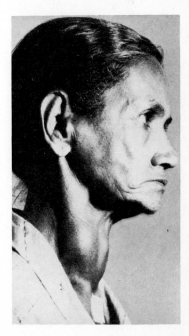

ness. Other nonspecific symptoms include nausea, vomiting, and rashes. Consequently, the experts are cautious about discussing the possible cancer prevention effects of selenium until more information is available.[26,27]

Selenium is part of one enzyme that acts as an antioxidant. Selenium interacts with vitamin E in its antioxidant activity, which prevents cell damage. The low level of selenium in parts of China causes children to develop Keshan disease, which leads to fatal heart damage. However, other factors may also be involved, since there are seasonal variations in the occurrence of the disease. A poor diet in acute alcoholism may result in selenium deficiency, which can be corrected by abstaining from alcohol and eating an adequate diet.

Plants low in protein will be low in selenium; hence, fruits and vegetables are poor sources. The best sources of selenium are meats and grains (Figure 7-2). A safe and adequate daily dietary intake for adults is 0.05 to 0.2 mg per day. Intake in the U.S. and Canada is in the range of 0.06 to 0.22 mg.

Foods grown in different parts of the United States vary in selenium content because of variation in the concentration of this mineral in the soil. Western Oregon and part of the Midwest have low soil concentrations. Parts of the Great Plains produce plants that may cause selenium toxicity in animals. New Zealand, Finland, and China have areas with low concentrations of selenium in the soil.

A recent scientific paper was titled "Growing Selenium-Enriched Tobacco." This article reports the results of increased selenium concentrations in tobacco caused by the addition of the mineral to the soil or by spraying growing tobacco plants with selenium solutions. Why do this? Apparently the incidence of lung cancer is lower in countries that produced cigarettes with three times more selenium in them than is found in American-made cigarettes. Although about 50 million Americans smoke, there are better ways to increase your selenium intake!

Fluoride Prevents Tooth Decay

The addition of fluoride to the water supply of many communities has been very successful in preventing dental caries.[28] A 1970 government report, "Fluoridation: No Better Health Investment," estimated that every dollar spent on fluoridation produced $50 in savings in dental bills.

Fluoride prevents tooth decay by strengthening hydroxyapatite crystals. This has led to some speculation that fluoride may delay the onset of osteoporosis. Further work is necessary before this can be stated with certainty.

For most people, water is the greatest source of fluoride, but tea and seafood are other good sources. Adults consume 0.9 to 2.3 mg of fluoride per day. Higher intakes cause mottling or brown spots in teeth, but mottled teeth, though cosmetically unappealing, are very strong and cavity-resistant. However, long-term intakes of water with eight times the recommended concentration of fluoride can eventually lead to severe bone and joint disorders. High use of aluminum-containing antacids causes a significant loss of fluoride from the body.

There has been a lot of political controversy about the matter of fluoridating public water supplies. It is noteworthy that fluoridation is the only public health measure that Americans vote on directly, and frequently the voting takes place in an atmosphere of misinformation or inadequate information about the health benefits of fluoride. One fear, for example, has been that fluoride causes cancer, although there is no evidence that this is so.[29]

Soil Science

Dentistry

Political Science

Copper Is Part of Many Enzymes

Copper is involved in many activities in the body. It is a part of many enzymes; it is involved in protein metabolism and iron metabolism, in the prevention of a type of emphysema, in the healing of wounds, and in the protection of nerve fibers. It works with vitamin C to help make elastin in muscles. Therefore, a deficiency of copper will cause anemia and central nervous system disorders and increase the possibility of infection.

However, though low intakes of copper have been observed (Table 7-2), copper deficiency has not been reported in the U.S. population. The suggested daily intake for adults is 2 to 3 mg. Meat, liver, sea foods, green leafy vegetables, legumes, and whole grains are the best food sources of copper.

Other Trace Elements Are Recommended in Very Small Amounts

The remaining trace elements known to be essential in nutrition are recommended in very small amounts, as shown in Table 7-11. Chromium is used for glucose metabolism. Cobalt is a part of vitamin B_{12}. Manganese helps enzymes in the metabolism of lipids and carbohydrates. Molybdenum helps the activity of a variety of enzymes. This cursory treatment of trace elements does not mean that they are unimportant, and in the future you may well be reading about many exciting discoveries regarding these minerals.

> The body needs: iron to take oxygen to the cells, zinc for growth and sexual maturation, iodine to regulate metabolic rate, selenium as a possible prevention of certain cancers, fluoride to prevent tooth decay, copper for enzyme activity, chromium for glucose metabolism, cobalt as a part of vitamin B_{12}, manganese to help enzymes in the metabolism of lipids and carbohydrates, and molybdenum for the activity of a variety of enzymes.

TABLE 7-11 Some Trace Elements

	ESADDI* (mg)	Food Sources	Functions	Severe Deficiency Symptoms
Chromium	0.05 to 0.2	Liver, meat, sea food, brewers' yeast	Needed for glucose metabolism	Altered glucose metabolism
Cobalt			Part of vitamin B_{12}	Only as vitamin B_{12} deficiency
Manganese	2.5 to 5.0	Whole grains, nuts, fruit, vegetables	Part of enzymes in lipid and carbohydrate metabolism	Defects in bones
Molybdenum	0.15 to 0.5	Cereals, legumes	Part of enzymes	Not known in humans

*Estimated safe and adequate daily dietary intake.

DECISIONS

1. Should I Take Mineral Supplements?

If you are advised by your doctor, yes. If you are eating a balanced diet, no. Check your dietary intake of minerals from the information in Appendixes J and P. Special circumstances require additional amounts of some minerals—pregnancy, lactation, recovery from surgery, and children's recovery from protein-energy malnutrition. Some women may feel the necessity for additional iron during the child-bearing years or for calcium as a protection against osteoporosis.

Decisions on the use of mineral and vitamin supplements must be made by people in the following circumstances:

- Iron—for women with excessive menstrual bleeding
- Iron, calcium, folacin—especially important for women who are pregnant or breast-feeding
- Calcium, iron, zinc, and vitamin B_{12}—some vegetarians may not have adequate intake
- Vitamin K—given to newborns under medical supervision to prevent abnormal bleeding
- All nutrients—for people on very low kcalorie intakes

The above guidelines are endorsed by The American Dietetic Association, American Institute of Nutrition, American Society for Clinical Nutrition, and the National Council Against Health Fraud. They are consistent with American Medical Association policy on nutrient supplementation. These guidelines and other recommendations on mineral and vitamin supplements were presented at a news conference in New York on April 8, 1987.

2. If I Must Take a Mineral Supplement, What Choices Must I Make?

Care must be exercised with the supplementation of any nutrient, and minerals are no exception. Check the following:

- Amount of the mineral in a typical day's food intake.
- RDA for the mineral.
- Percentage of the RDA provided by the diet and by the supplement.
- Form of the mineral. Bioavailability of ferrous iron is better than ferric iron. Selenium exists in inorganic and organic forms, each with different degrees of toxicity. Calcium supplements are sold usually as calcium carbonate.
- Minimal amount of the mineral needed to give toxic symptoms. The information in Table 7-10 is useful here.
- Severity of the symptoms caused by excessive intake. Although immediate death does not always happen, the damage can be serious. For example, high intakes of zinc interfere with copper metabolism and reduce high-density lipoprotein cholesterol (HDL). Some forms of chromium are toxic and may cause kidney damage.
- Extent of contamination of the supplement. Instead of taking calcium carbonate as a calcium supplement, you can take dolomite. This is obtained from rocks. It is a combination of calcium carbonate and magnesium carbonate. Some samples were shown to have high levels of the toxic minerals lead, mercury, and arsenic. Sea salt may be contaminated with toxic metals.

3. Am I Getting Value for Money with Mineral Supplements?

This question is best answered by looking at two examples.

Example 1: Many people use sea salt because it is considered to be healthful. There is no evidence that it is any more nutritious than ordinary table salt, but it is certainly more expensive.

Example 2: Consider the two most popular over-the-counter mineral supplements, calcium and iron.

Computing the Economic Value of Calcium

In the fall of 1986 the cost of providing the RDA for adults (800 mg) ranged from 5.2 to 17.3 cents in a random sample of eleven different calcium supplements sold in supermarkets. Let's look at the highest priced one, a $6.49 jar of sixty 500 mg tablets.

$$60 \text{ tablets} \times 500 \text{ mg per tablet} = 30,000 \text{ mg calcium}$$

Since this cost $6.49, then the cost of the RDA is

$$\left(\frac{6.49 \times 100 \times 800}{30,000} \right) \text{ cents}$$

which equals 17.3 cents per 800 mg.

An October 1986 issue of *Chemical Marketing Reporter* reported that one ton of calcium carbonate sold for $170. Since there are 1016 kg in one ton, 1 kg of calcium carbonate costs 16.73 cents ($170 \times 100/1016$). And since 1 kg is 1000 g, this 1 g costs 0.0167 cents ($16.73 \times 1/1000$). Consequently, the RDA of 800 mg of calcium at the wholesale level costs 0.0134 cents ($0.0167 \times 800/1000$).

In short, the percentage difference between 800 mg of calcium carbonate bought in bulk wholesale (0.0134 cents) and the same amount bought as a supplement in the supermarket (17.3 cents) is

$$\frac{17.3 \times 100}{0.0134}$$

which works out to 129,104%. How about *that* for a markup!

The Economics of Buying an Iron Supplement

Lest you think this huge percentage markup is unique to calcium, we can apply the same arithmetic to iron and see what happens. A $4.19 jar of iron tablets contains 30 capsules, each capsule containing 78 mg iron, which adds up to 2340 mg of iron. This means the RDA for a woman (18 mg) will cost 3.22 cents. The *Chemical Marketing Reporter* lists one pound of ferrous sulfate as costing 49 cents. This is the usual form of iron in supplements. One pound equals 455 g, so 1 g costs 0.1077 cents. Therefore, the 18 mg to meet the RDA for a woman costs only 0.00194 cents wholesale. Thus, the difference between wholesale and retail cost of an iron supplement is—ready?—165,979%.

We should, of course, take the broadminded view here. You get a 30-day supply of a calcium supplement and an iron supplement for $6.49 and $4.19, respectively, but if these supplements are beneficial in preventing the suffering and ill health caused by osteoporosis and iron deficiency anemia, they may well be worth it. Still, is it fair that such astronomically high profits are made on these supplements?

Incidentally, our knowledge of the bioavailability of mineral supplements is not adequate to predict how much of the minerals is absorbed and used. This is the ultimate test of value for money.

4. Is Calcium Supplementation the Best Way to Prevent Osteoporosis?

This idea is being increasingly questioned, and for a number of reasons.[30] Evidence suggests that estrogen treatment in postmenopausal women is better than calcium supplementation in controlling osteoporosis. Estrogen treatment has its side effects and should be used only under medical supervision. One interpretation of the present craze for calcium supplements is less than enthusiastic: "Current evidence does not support the notion that a high calcium intake, either premenopausally or postmenopausally, will prevent postmenopausal osteoporosis. Furthermore, now that thousands of women are taking more than a gram of calcium daily, one may wonder whether we can expect an epidemic of kidney stones."[30] In addition, you should not forget that exercise is an excellent way to maintain bone mass.

There are a variety of calcium supplements available today.

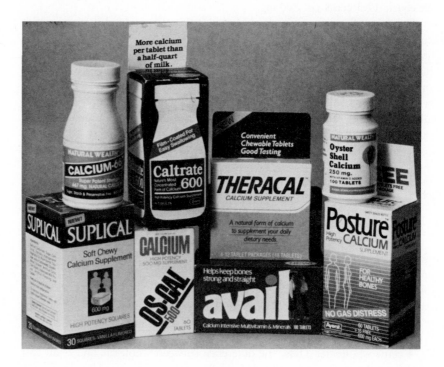

SUMMARY

FOOD SOURCES

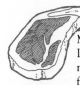

MEAT:
Iron, zinc, phosphorus, sodium (cured meats), potassium, iodine (in marine fish), selenium, copper, cobalt, chromium

DAIRY:
Calcium, phosphorus, sodium (processed cheese), potassium, iodine

BREADS/CEREALS:
Phosphorus, magnesium, potassium, iron, iodine, zinc, selenium, manganese, molybdenum

FRUITS/VEGETABLES:
Vegetables—magnesium, calcium, potassium, iron, copper, chromium, manganese, molybdenum
Fruits—potassium, manganese

FATS/OILS:
None

Most common mineral problems in North America and other industrialized countries:
iron (women), calcium, magnesium, zinc (sometimes) intake too low; sodium intake too high

DEFICIENCY SYMPTOMS

Most deficiencies of minerals cause decreased growth rates

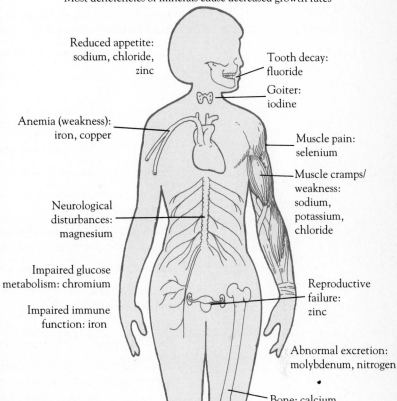

Reduced appetite:
sodium, chloride, zinc

Tooth decay:
fluoride

Goiter:
iodine

Anemia (weakness):
iron, copper

Muscle pain:
selenium

Muscle cramps/weakness:
sodium, potassium, chloride

Neurological disturbances:
magnesium

Impaired glucose metabolism: chromium

Impaired immune function: iron

Reproductive failure:
zinc

Abnormal excretion:
molybdenum, nitrogen

Bone: calcium, phosphorus, copper, manganese

REFERENCES

1. Nielsen, F.H., and Mertz, W.: Other trace elements. In Present knowledge in nutrition, 5th edition. The Nutrition Foundation, Inc., Washington, D.C., p. 607, 1984.

2. Lindsay, D.G., and Sherlock, J.C.: Environmental contaminants. In Adverse effects of foods, E.F.P. Jelliffe and D.B. Jelliffe, editor. Plenum Publishing Corp., New York, p. 85, 1982.

3. Preer, J.R., and others: Metals in downtown Washington, D.C. gardens, Biological Trace Element Research 6:79, 1984.

4. Editorial: Prevention and control of iodine deficiency disorders, Lancet ii:433, 1986.

5. Eaton, S.B., and Konner, M.: Paleolithic nutrition, New England Journal of Medicine 312:283, 1985.

6. Spencer, H., and Kramer, L.: Factors contributing to osteoporosis, Journal of Nutrition 116:316, 1986.

7. Allen, L.H.: Calcium and osteoporosis, Nutrition Today, page 6, May/June, 1986.

8. Heaney, R.P.: Calcium bioavailability, Contemporary Nutrition 11(8),1986.

9. Ott, S.: Should women get screening bone mass measurements? Annals of Internal Medicine 104:874, 1986.

10. Gruchow, H.W., and others: Alcohol, nutrient intake, and hypertension in U.S. adults, Journal of the American Medical Association 253:1567, 1985.

11. Editorial, Hypertension: Is there a place for calcium? Lancet i:359, 1986.

12. Bertino, M., and others: Increasing dietary salt alters salt taste preference, Physiology and Behavior 38:203, 1986.

13. Wolf, I.D., and others: USDA activities in relation to the sodium issue, 1981–1983, Food Technology, p. 59, September, 1983.

14. Shah, B.G., and Belonje, B.: Calculated sodium and potassium in the Canadian diet if comprised of unprocessed ingredients, Nutrition Research 3:629, 1983.

15. Blackburn, H., and Prineas, R.: Diet and hypertension: Anthropology, epidemiology, and public health implications, Progress in Biochemical Pharmacology 19:31, 1983.

16. Beevers, D.G.: Should recommendations be made to reduce dietary sodium intake: the case for recommendations, Proceedings of the Nutrition Society 45:263, 1986.

17. Lever, A.F.: Should recommendations be made to reduce sodium intake: The case against recommendations, Proceedings of the Nutrition Society 45:259, 1986.

18. Council on Scientific Affairs, American Medical Association: Sodium in processed foods, Journal of the American Medical Association 249:784, 1983.

19. Smith, S.J., and others: Moderate potassium chloride supplementation in essential hypertension: Is it additive to moderate sodium restriction? British Medical Journal 290:110, 1985.

20. Seelig, M.S.: Magnesium requirements in human nutrition, Contemporary Nutrition 7(1), 1982.

21. O'Dell, B.L.: Bioavailability of trace elements, Nutrition Research 42:301, 1984.

22. Dallman, P.R., and others: Prevalence and causes of anemia in the United States, 1976 to 1980, American Journal of Clinical Nutrition **39:**437, 1984.

23. Brittin, H.C., and Nossaman, C.E.: Iron content of food cooked in iron utensils, Journal of the American Dietetic Association **86:**897, 1986.

24. Murray, M.J., and others: Adverse effects of normal nutrients and foods on host resistance to disease. In Adverse effects of foods, E.F.P. Jelliffe and D.B. Jelliffe, editors: Plenum Publishing Corp., New York, p. 313, 1982.

25. Sandstead, H.H., and Evans, G.W.: Zinc. In Present knowledge in nutrition, 5th edition. The Nutrition Foundation, Inc., Washington, D.C., p. 479, 1984.

26. Clark, L.C., and Combs, Jr., G.F.: Selenium compounds and the prevention of cancer: Research needs and public health implications, Journal of Nutrition **116:**170, 1986.

27. Burk, R.F.: Selenium and cancer: Meaning of serum selenium levels, Journal of Nutrition **116:**1584, 1986.

28. Anonymous: Lasting benefits of short periods of fluoride ingestion, Nutrition Reviews **45:**137, 1987.

29. National Research Council: Diet, nutrition, and cancer. National Academy Press, Washington, D.C., p. 162, 1982.

30. Gordan, G.S., and Vaughan, C.: Calcium and osteoporosis, Journal of Nutrition **116:**319, 1986.

METABOLISM NOTES: *Metabolic Pathway of Minerals*

Minerals are involved in a number of ways in metabolism. Some of the enzymes involved in the digestion of food need the help of some minerals to function. Iron in hemoglobin in the blood brings oxygen to cells. This allows the release of energy in carbohydrates, fats, and proteins. We will examine this process in more detail in Chapter 8. The actual release of energy from glucose, fatty acids, and amino acids involves a large number of minerals (Figure 7-11). These help the enzymes needed to speed up the process of releasing energy. Some of the same minerals are needed for the buildup of carbohydrates, fats, and proteins in the cells.

We saw in Chapter 6 that specific vitamins play a key role in certain metabolic reactions. Two of these vitamins have a mineral as part of their structure. Thiamin has sulfur and vitamin B_{12} has cobalt.

FIGURE 7-11
Several minerals are involved in the buildup and breakdown of carbohydrates, fats, and proteins. They assist enzymes in a large number of metabolic reactions.

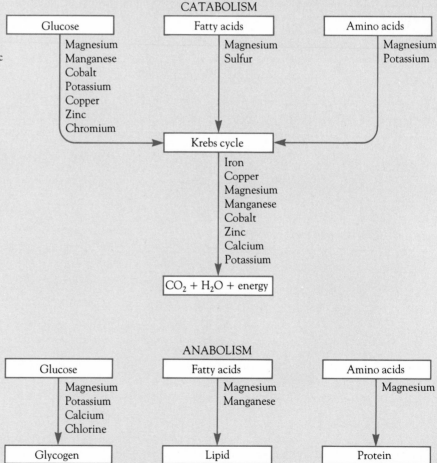

CATABOLISM

Glucose	Fatty acids	Amino acids
Magnesium	Magnesium	Magnesium
Manganese	Sulfur	Potassium
Cobalt		
Potassium		
Copper		
Zinc		
Chromium		

Krebs cycle

Iron
Copper
Magnesium
Manganese
Cobalt
Zinc
Calcium
Potassium

$CO_2 + H_2O + energy$

ANABOLISM

Glucose	Fatty acids	Amino acids
Magnesium	Magnesium	Magnesium
Potassium	Manganese	
Calcium		
Chlorine		

Glycogen	Lipid	Protein

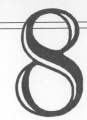

Oxygen, Water, and Other Fluids

CONNECTIONS

Energy nutrients—carbohydrates, fats, and proteins—are built up and broken down in the body with the help of vitamins and minerals, but this build-up and breakdown would not be possible without oxygen and water.

Oxygen "lights the fire" for burning carbohydrates, fats, and proteins for energy. Oxygen from the air we breathe is delivered to cells by iron-containing hemoglobin in the blood.

Water dissolves nutrients, like the water-soluble vitamins. It also helps make food palatable and allows you to digest, absorb, transport, and metabolize all the nutrients you have studied so far and to excrete and eliminate the wastes.

As you will see, you get water from food and the nutrients burned for energy and from a range of fluids: milk, juices, soft drinks, caffeine drinks, and alcohol, as well as plain old water. The quantity and quality of fluid affect how well you can perform physical activity.

The one thing you need in life—if you are to *have* a life—is oxygen: all the time, and practically every minute. You can do without almost anything else for at least 10 minutes, but not oxygen.

A substance you can do without for a few days, but that is also truly essential, is water. As one writer put it,

"While you can live without most vitamins and minerals for extended periods of time, just a few days without this nutrient will surely result in death. The nutrient, of course, is water, that colorless, calorieless compound of hydrogen and oxygen that virtually every cell in the body needs to survive."

This chapter will discuss water and other fluids at length, but first let us consider oxygen. Nutritionists are interested in oxygen for three particular reasons:

- The efficiency of its delivery to every cell in your body is influenced by many nutrients. One of the most important is the iron within red blood cells (RBCs). Oxygen is bound to iron-containing hemoglobin in each RBC. When RBCs arrive at the cells, the oxygen is released from hemoglobin.

- Cells need oxygen to liberate the energy from carbohydrate, fat, or protein—a process known as oxidation.
- Oxygen can have harmful effects in the body unless it is controlled by certain enzymes—enzymes whose activities are reduced by a diet that is deficient in such minerals as iron and selenium. Such a diet may permanently damage cells.

This last notion forms the basis for one theory about aging, an area of research being closely followed by nutritionists. As famed Nobel Prize laureate Francis Crick says about oxygen and aging,

"Molecular oxygen is a powerful but dangerous compound. It is potentially a highly toxic substance for cells, because cellular processes are liable to produce several lethal derivatives of it. . . . Many cells have special enzymes to mop up these life-threatening substances. . . ."

AIR AND WATER: THE IMPORTANCE OF QUANTITY AND QUALITY

North Americans have been in the forefront in expressing their concerns about clean air and clean water. For example, there was a 300% increase in the United States in the sale of bottled drinking water between 1975 and 1985. Indeed, Americans now drink close to $1 billion worth of bottled water each year. Let us consider both the quantity and quality of the air and water we require from a nutrition standpoint.

The Quantity of Air and Water Is Important in Nutrition

How much air and water do we really need?

Enough air

Your brain, liver, gastrointestinal tract, and muscles have a high demand for oxygen, as you can see from Table 8-1. However, during exercise, the muscles and lungs demand more oxygen, which is supplied by increasing the flow of blood to muscles and lungs and reducing the flow of blood to the gastrointestinal tract and the kidneys. In this way, the maximum amount of oxygen can be delivered to the two tissues most involved in exercise.

Inhaling too much air causes hyperventilation. This upsets blood gas levels, causing a fall in blood pressure.

Enough water

If no fluids are taken into the body, death can occur in a few days. Too little water causes dehydration and decreases physical performance in marathon running[1] and in hard physical labor. On a larger scale, too little water may even cause famine in some parts of the world. On the other hand, there is such a thing as taking in too much water, as is occasionally seen in some psychiatric patients. Drinking too much water—"water intoxication"—can cause death.

The Quality of Air and Water Is Also Important

You need not only enough air and water but also the right kind.

TABLE 8-1 Delivery and Utilization of Oxygen in Tissues in a 70 kg Man at Rest and During Light Exercise

| Tissue | Weight (kg) | Blood Flow to Tissue (ml/minute) | | Resting Oxygen Consumption (ml/minute) |
		At rest	Light Exercise	
Liver	1.7	1500		75
Skeletal muscles	20-30	1200	4500	70
Gastrointestinal tract	2.6	1400	1100	58
Brain	1.5	750	750	46
Heart	0.3	250	350	27
Kidneys	0.3	1100	900	16
Lungs	1	5000	10,000	12
Skin	4.3-9	500	1500	5

The right kind of air

Clean air *is* important. Here let's discuss just one air pollutant—lead. Nutritionists are concerned about lead entering our bodies, not only through the food chain in plants, but directly through the air from car and factory exhausts. (Some children in poor urban areas also ingest lead from eating peeling lead-based paint on old walls.) Lead produces anemia, thereby interfering with the oxygen-carrying capacity of the blood and slowing mental development. Children are more efficient than adults in absorbing lead into the blood. However, the absorption rate is slowed by a diet adequate in iron, calcium, and phosphorus.[2]

The right kind of water

Pure water is simple hydrogen plus oxygen—H_2O. However, you invariably get more than just H_2O when you drink a glass of water because the water supply in most places is not pure. The advantage of this impurity is that many minerals are dissolved in the water, some of which may be important nutrients. Often the mineral content of water depends on the mineral composition of the local soil, which explains the varying mineral content in water from different cities, as represented in Table 8-2. This variability may make a difference in a person's total intake of minerals like calcium and sodium.

Sodium intake from water may be a problem. Probably no more than 10% of your daily sodium intake should come from water,[3] but many of the nation's water supplies (about 42%) contain more sodium than they should. This is a matter of concern to dietitians in planning a diet low in sodium for people with kidney disease or for those trying to control hypertension.

Unfortunately, water may also contain toxic minerals and industrial and agricultural pollutants. Ground water pollution occurs in all parts of the United States. This pollution is a serious problem because most of these pollutants are invisible, odorless, and tasteless. Their detection is difficult and expensive.[4]

Environmental Studies

A nutritionally balanced diet helps protect against the harmful effects of air pollutants like lead.

TABLE 8-2 Water from Different Locations Can Vary Greatly in Mineral Content

| | Contribution to Intake of Minerals by 1 Liter of Water | | | | |
| | Percentage of RDA* | | Percentage of ESADDI† | | |
Source	Calcium	Iron	Sodium	Chloride	Magnesium
Atlanta	0.9	0.2	0.2	0.1	0.4
Seattle	1.4	0.4	0.4	0.2	0.1
Miami	12.0	0.7	0.8	1.6	1.2
Boston	0.5	0.6	0.2	0.2	0.1
Chicago	5.0	0.6	<0.3	0.5	3.9
Granville (Illinois)	6.3	26.5	0.5	18.8	7.5
Evian (bottled) water‡	9.7	0.5	N/A	0.1	8.0

*%RDA value for an adult woman.
†Minimum value for Estimated Safe and Adequate Daily Dietary Intake for an adult.
‡Information from the label: S.A. Evian Co., Evian-les-Bains, France.

Environmental Studies

Clean water is very important in nutrition.

Certain microorganisms in water cause cholera and typhoid, producing diarrhea and interference with normal nutrient absorption. This in turn causes nutritional deficiencies, especially in young children. Malnutrition among children in some developing countries often results from diarrhea caused by unclean water.

The sources and composition of water and the regulation of its quality are summarized in Figure 8-1.

> Oxygen from air is carried by iron-containing hemoglobin to cells to release the energy in carbohydrate, fat, and protein. A shortage of water can cause dehydration in individuals and famine in countries. The body's ability to absorb nutrients is affected by polluted air and water.

WHY WE NEED AIR AND WATER

The foregoing discussion only begins to suggest why air and water are important. Let us now take a look at the necessity for these two substances in more detail.

Oxygen Has Many Sources

Oxygen, which is vital for the development of plant and animal life, may occur either as free oxygen or in compounds in foods, in liquids, and in the body. Air, for instance, is 21% oxygen, and water is 89% oxygen. The human body, by contrast, is 65% oxygen—both free oxygen and as combined oxygen in carbon dioxide in blood, body water, protein, carbohydrate, lipids, and vitamins.

We can see the relationship between nutrition and the quality of oxygen in the

BOTTLED WATER

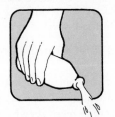

TAP WATER

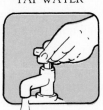

FIGURE 8-1
Main sources of water. Water quality usually refers to freedom from contamination from bacteria or environmental pollutants. Nutritionists are now paying attention to the mineral content of water also.

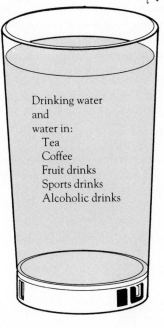

May be carbonated or natural
May have contaminants from groundwater source
Some are high in sodium

Drinking water
and
water in:
  Tea
  Coffee
  Fruit drinks
  Sports drinks
  Alcoholic drinks

Public water systems provide 90% of the U.S. population with drinking water
May be from ground (well) or surface (reservoir, rivers, and streams)
Contains:
  Added fluoride in many areas
  Varying amounts of:
    Bacteria
    Contaminants (lead, arsenic)
    Calcium and magnesium —the higher the amount, the harder the water
    Chlorine as a disinfectant

Soft water may pick up lead and cadmium from pipes
Water is cleaned of sediment by filtration; this technique is used since the ancient Egyptians

The composition of the water from your tap is regulated by the environmental protection agency (EPA) under the provisions of the Safe Water Drinking Act (1974) plus the several amendments in recent years; it prevents contamination of the water with bacteria, mercury, silver, nitrate, pesticides, radioactivity

environment simply by knowing that the availability of oxygen in lakes and rivers determines whether plants and fish will survive. The greater the amount of pollutants in a river or lake, the higher the biological oxygen demand (BOD). This means that more oxygen is needed to convert the pollutants into inorganic salts, so less oxygen is available for plants and fish, which may die. Thus, when people depend on a lake's fish supply, pollution can severely reduce their nutrient supply.

Specific details of how the body uses oxygen are given in the Metabolism section at the end of this chapter.

Water in Our Bodies: Are We "All Wet"?

An impassioned lawyer once argued for better labeling of hamburgers because he felt that, because they were 65% water when raw and 50% to 60% water when cooked, someone had been "diluting" the meat. It might have been pointed out to him that his own body is 60% water (60% of his body weight; 55% for women).

Indeed, a person's fat is 10% water, bones 30%, muscles 70%, and blood 85%. Clearly, the lawyer was "all wet"—both in his argument and in his substance.

You should note three things about water in the body:

- The high water content of blood makes it an ideal transport medium for oxygen, other nutrients, and waste.
- The moisture content of fat is low. Thus, two people may have the same body weight, but the person with more body fat will have less body water. Because women have proportionally more body fat than men, they have a lower total body water content.
- Newborn infants have a body water content of about 75% because of a higher water content in most tissues at birth. Aging from adulthood to old age decreases muscle mass, usually with an increase in fat content.

The distribution of water within the body is given in Figure 8-2. All in all, we each have approximately 12 gallons of water within us.

Water Is Necessary for Many Body Functions

How is water used within the body? The best way to understand this is to see what happens to a piece of food and a mouthful of water from the time they enter the mouth until the time of elimination.

The mouth

Saliva is about 99.5% water. In healthy individuals it makes swallowing easier by moistening food.

Digestive juices

Bile (86% water) and juices containing digestive enzymes liberate nutrients from food. Hydrolysis (breaking down substances with water) reduces large molecules of food into their smallest components: carbohydrates become monosaccharides, proteins become amino acids, and lipids become fatty acids and glycerol.

Absorption

Digestive juices form a soluble medium for the absorption of water-soluble vitamins, monosaccharides, and amino acids. Minerals are absorbed in soluble form. Some minerals, including iron, calcium, and zinc, can combine with dietary phosphorus, oxalic acid, or phytic acid in the intestinal system. These combinations are insoluble in water and are lost from the body by elimination with the feces.

The water taken with the food in this example cannot undergo further breakdown before absorption. A small amount of this water is absorbed from the stomach. Over 80% of the water is absorbed in the small intestine, the site of absorption for most nutrients. Any remaining water is absorbed from the large intestine.

Nonabsorbed material

This remains in the large intestine until it is expelled in the feces. The longer the time before defecation, the more water is removed and absorbed back into the body, increasing constipation. Chapter 3 pointed out that fiber, because it binds water, causes bulk and a resulting stimulation for defecation, and decreases intestinal transit time, can relieve constipation.

FIGURE 8-2
Fluid content of the human body.

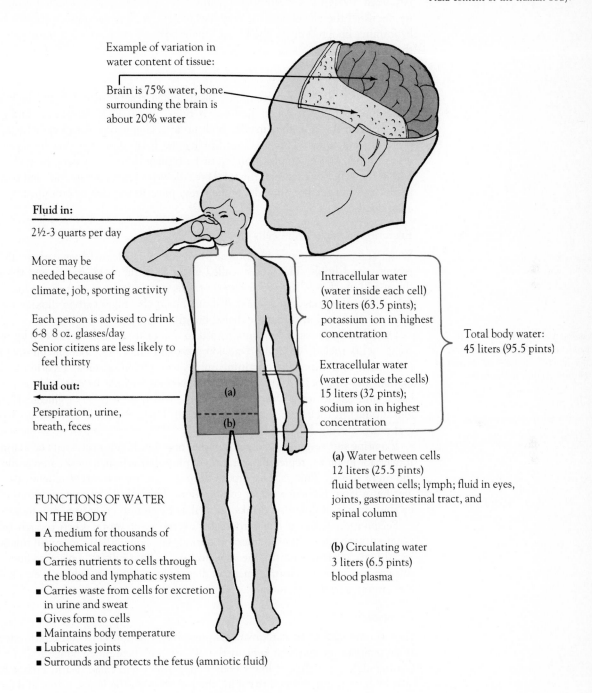

Example of variation in
water content of tissue:

Brain is 75% water, bone
surrounding the brain is
about 20% water

Fluid in:

2½-3 quarts per day

More may be
needed because of
climate, job, sporting activity

Each person is advised to drink
6-8 8 oz. glasses/day
Senior citizens are less likely to
feel thirsty

Fluid out:

Perspiration, urine,
breath, feces

Intracellular water
(water inside each cell)
30 liters (63.5 pints);
potassium ion in highest
concentration

Extracellular water
(water outside the cells)
15 liters (32 pints);
sodium ion in highest
concentration

Total body water:
45 liters (95.5 pints)

(a) Water between cells
12 liters (25.5 pints)
fluid between cells; lymph; fluid in eyes,
joints, gastrointestinal tract, and
spinal column

(b) Circulating water
3 liters (6.5 pints)
blood plasma

FUNCTIONS OF WATER IN THE BODY

- A medium for thousands of
  biochemical reactions
- Carries nutrients to cells through
  the blood and lymphatic system
- Carries waste from cells for excretion
  in urine and sweat
- Gives form to cells
- Maintains body temperature
- Lubricates joints
- Surrounds and protects the fetus (amniotic fluid)

Transport

Absorbed nutrients are transported in the blood, which is 85% water. Recall that we discussed the clever way the body has of making fatty substances water-soluble by forming lipoproteins in the blood. Some types of fatty acids are transported in the lymph.

Biochemical reactions

Water is a medium for most of the biochemical reactions within the body and sometimes a reactant. When monosaccharides, amino acids, fatty acids, and glycerol arrive in the cell, they may be built up into large molecules of carbohydrates, proteins, and lipids. This involves linking the basic units together by means of water. When these complex units must be broken down, it is done by hydrolysis within the cell. For example, the total breakdown of carbohydrate, fat, and protein produces water, carbon dioxide, and energy, plus, in the case of protein, nitrogen compounds.

Excretion of waste from cells

Water and carbon dioxide are formed when energy is released from carbohydrates, proteins, and lipids. This water, called water of metabolism, is excreted through the urine (which is 93% to 97% water) or perspiration (99% water). Some moisture is lost from the body through exhaled air; blood also takes carbon dioxide to the lungs for elimination through exhaled breath.

Testing the urine for some of these chemicals is useful in determining their intake in the diet or changes in their metabolism in the body.

Dissolved body waste amounts to 3% to 7% of total urine volume. The main components include chlorides (including sodium chloride), sodium, phosphorus, potassium, and nitrogen-containing substances including urea, creatinine, ammonia, and uric acid. Other organic compounds include ketone bodies, purine bases, and oxalic acid. Over 50% of people will have a trace of glucose (2 to 3 mg/100 ml) in their urine after a heavy meal. Diabetic people can lose up to 100 g of glucose every 24 hours.

If a urine test reveals a "cloudy" sample, one should not necessarily be alarmed. It may, for instance, represent excretion of phosphorus from a meat eaten at dinner the night before. That is the purpose of urine—to excrete excess chemicals—so diet has a large influence on its composition. The volume of urine is determined by the amount of fluid one drinks, as well as by certain environmental factors.

Perspiration is not a major route for excretion of waste. Even though sweat tastes salty, the amount of sodium lost during, say, a marathon run is well tolerated by athletes.[1] It is unwise, by the way, to take sodium pills to replace sodium lost this way, because the North American diet is already high in sodium. Perspiration also contains some potassium.

Dissipation of heat

Heat is produced when carbohydrates, proteins, and lipids are burned for energy. Body temperature must be kept in the 80° to 108° Fahrenheit range (37° to 42° Centigrade), for higher or lower body temperatures will cause death. About 85% of body heat is lost through the skin, the rest through the lungs, urine, and feces. The flow of blood to the skin during exercise (Table 8-1) or during a fever is a way of eliminating excess heat from the body. When a person is cold, the reverse occurs: less blood is circulated through the skin, reducing heat losses, which explains why your hands and legs may become pale when it is very cold. Perspiration will get rid of heat only when sweat is evaporated from the skin. Intense physical activity is dangerous in high humidity because sweat is not evaporated, causing internal body temperature to increase to dangerous levels.

Other functions of water in the body

Fluids cushion body tissues; the *amniotic fluid*, for example, surrounds and protects the fetus during pregnancy. Water also helps give cells their shape and rigidity, acts as a lubricant in tears, and provides the synovial fluid that allows bones to move freely against each other. In addition, water is the most important solvent in the body, and many substances dissolve easily in water. Note that a distinction is made between pure water and water with solutes. Because the body consists of water with solutes, it is more accurate to talk about body fluids rather than body water.

Amniotic fluid
Fluid that protects the fetus from injury, and helps maintain an even temperature in the womb.

Body fluids with a high water content that are important in nutrition include saliva, digestive juices, bile, blood, lymph, and urine. These help in the digestion or transportation of nutrients, in the excretion and elimination of waste, and in relieving excess body heat. Body fluids regulate thirst and protect vital tissues.

WATER: WHERE IT COMES FROM, WHAT IT DOES, WHERE IT GOES

We have described the sources and uses of water in general terms, but in order to appreciate its role in nutrition we need to explore some aspects of its chemistry.

How Are Ions, pH, and Buffers Involved with Body Fluids and Nutrition?

What do these have to do with body fluids and nutrition? Let us take a look.

Ions

Pure water (H_2O) consists of hydrogen ions (H^+) and hydroxyl ions (OH^-) in addition to molecules of water. Some substances dissolve in water into ions with a positive or negative charge. The best example is table salt, sodium chloride (NaCl). Dissolved salt in water breaks into (Na^+) and (Cl^-). In the human body, about 90% of the ions in the extracellular fluid are Na^+ and Cl^- ions. This is the "internal sea" referred to by physiologists. Important positively charged ions in the body include sodium and potassium. Both are involved in body water balance and in nerve and muscle function. Calcium ions help in nerve function, in blood clotting, and in the activation of some enzymes. Negative charges are carried by chloride, bicarbonate, and sulfate. "Electrolytes" is another term for ions, and it is frequently used in reference to sodium, potassium, and chloride in solution.

Physiology

pH

When dissolved in water, some substances release a hydrogen ion (H^+), making the solution acidic. The strongest acid in the body is hydrochloric acid (HCl),

FIGURE 8-3
pH values of some body fluids, foods, and drinks. Most body fluids are near neutral. One major exception is the very acidic gastric juice in the stomach.

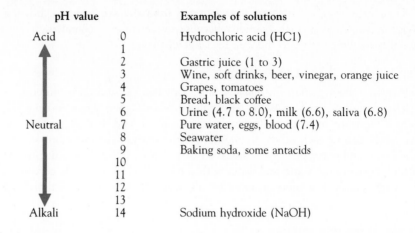

pH value		Examples of solutions
Acid	0	Hydrochloric acid (HC1)
	1	
	2	Gastric juice (1 to 3)
	3	Wine, soft drinks, beer, vinegar, orange juice
	4	Grapes, tomatoes
	5	Bread, black coffee
	6	Urine (4.7 to 8.0), milk (6.6), saliva (6.8)
Neutral	7	Pure water, eggs, blood (7.4)
	8	Seawater
	9	Baking soda, some antacids
	10	
	11	
	12	
	13	
Alkali	14	Sodium hydroxide (NaOH)

which is secreted in the stomach. More hydroxyl ions (OH^-) make the solution more alkaline or basic. There are no strong alkaline fluids in the body.

The pH scale measures the strength of an acid or base (Figure 8-3). Each enzyme works within a certain pH range. For example, enzymes in the stomach operate at low pH values (acidic); those in the small intestine need a slightly alkaline environment. If the locations of these enzymes were swapped, none of the enzymes would work in their new location. This is due to inactivation of the enzymes because they are not in the pH range in which they work. Therefore, the extraction of nutrients from food during digestion and absorption and the utilization of the nutrients (buildup and breakdown) depend on the control of pH ranges.

Buffers

You should not worry about wide fluctuations in pH in normal health. To prevent severe damage caused by large changes in pH, the body depends on buffers. These are natural components of the body, the most important being proteins and phos-

The Amount of Water in the Body Is Balanced by Many Factors

The average adult takes in and excretes about 10 cups (1 cup = ½ pint or 250 ml) of fluid per day. The sources are shown in Table 8-3.

TABLE 8-3 Sources of Water in Average Adult

Intake		Output	
Fluid	6 cups	Urine	5½ cups
Food	1¼-2 cups	Sweat	2 cups
Water of metabolism	1¼-2 cups	Breath	2 cups
		Feces	½ cup
TOTAL: *8½-10 cups (2.1-2.5 liters)*		*10 cups (2.5 liters)*	

TABLE 8-4   Water Content of Some Foods

Food	Percentage of Water by Weight
Cow's milk	87
Cheese	40
Cooked meat	
Ground beef	54-60
Steak	37-59
Chicken egg	74
Vegetables	
Baked potatoes	75
Corn	76
Tomatoes	94
Fruits (edible part)	
Apples	84
Oranges	86
Cereals	
Bread	35
Cornflakes	4

Fluids may be water, juices, milk, or broths, among other substances. The amount of water from food will vary (Table 8-4 and Appendix P). The term *sweat* needs some explaining. This refers here to the normal loss of water through the skin. Large increases in sweat volume and reduction in urine volume occur in hot climates or during prolonged strenuous exercise.

Urine volume must be maintained at a minimal level of about 2 cups (500 ml) per day. This amount is needed to excrete toxic wastes. The kidneys and other tissues may be damaged if the volume of urine is too low. Nitrogen end products of protein metabolism are best excreted in a large volume of urine so as to prevent kidney damage. This is why the authors of weight-reducing diets that recommend high intakes of dietary protein recommend that dieters drink up to eight glasses of water every day.

Urine volume can be increased by *diuretics*. Alcohol is a stronger diuretic than caffeine in the amounts commonly consumed in drinks. Diuretics, including caffeine, are used in some weight-reducing programs to give dieters an impression of rapid success in weight loss. However, this is merely body water loss. The point of body weight loss is to lose body *fat*, not body water.

Nutritionists always recommend high fluid intakes for healthy people.

Diuretics
Agents that increase the volume of urine.

Who Should Increase Their Fluid Intake?

Several groups of people should be sure to take in more fluids than usual:

- Lactating women. Lack of fluid intake may stop the production of milk.
- Infants. They need greater amounts of fluid relative to their body size than adults. Blood volume and cells are increasing in size. Cells in the growing tissues have a high water content.

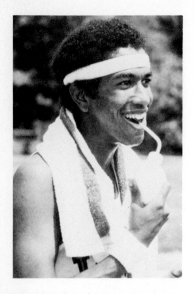

Water lost through perspiration must be replaced. Athletic performance is decreased when water losses are great.

- The elderly. Decreased sensitivity to thirst and failure to conserve water in response to the body's need for liquid may cause dehydration in the elderly.
- People with fevers. Fluids are needed to replace fluids lost through high perspiration.
- People in hot weather or high environmental temperature. Water is needed to replace lost fluids.
- People on high-protein diets. Water is needed to eliminate the nitrogen end products of metabolism. Some weight-reducing diets have high intakes of protein. Some athletic coaches incorrectly recommend high protein intakes.
- People with kidney disease. Some forms of kidney disease require a dilute urine caused by high fluid intakes. This puts less strain on the kidneys. However, people on kidney dialysis or with minimal kidney function often require measured, low-fluid intake.
- People doing hard physical work. Fluids lost through perspiration need to be replaced.

TABLE 8-5 What Every Athlete Should Know About Fluid Intake: Expected Fluid Weight Loss (in Pounds) During a 90-minute Practice for a 180 to 210 lb Athlete

Temperature (° F)	Pounds of Body Fluid Lost in 80%-100% Humidity	Pounds of Body Fluid Lost in <40% Humidity
100	7.5-8	5.5-6.5
80	5.5-6	3.5-4.5
60 or less	1-3	0-1.5

Needed to Replace These Losses	
Amount of Weight Lost	**Water Needed to Replace Loss (8-ounce glasses)**
1 lb	2
4 lb	4
8 lb	16

Dilution Factor for Fluids Used in Replacement	
Fluids	**Ratio of Parts Drink to Parts Water**
Fruit juices	1:3
Soft drinks	1:3
Gatorade	1:1
Vegetable juices	1:1
Quickick (orange flavor)	1:3
Pripps Pluss	1:3

But remember—water is the best replacement fluid.

■ People suffering from diarrhea—especially young children. Diarrhea causes dehydration.

■ Athletes. In order to prevent heat disorders, water should be drunk before, during, and after practices and competitions. The amount of body fluid lost depends on environmental temperature and humidity. The amount and type of fluid needed to replace that loss are important (Table 8-5). Most sports physiologists, incidentally, do not recommend "sports beverages." If such beverages are consumed they should be diluted with water to decrease the concentration of sugar. Sugar increases the time the fluid stays in the stomach, thereby making the fluid less effective in replacing lost body water. Some athletes are given erroneous information that drinking water during exercise will cause muscle weakness and cramps.

Composition of drinks is important during sports events.

■ Air travelers: the dry air in the cabin and the rapid circulation of the plane's ventilation system may produce large losses of water through the skin. Up to two pounds of water can be lost in a 3½-hour flight.

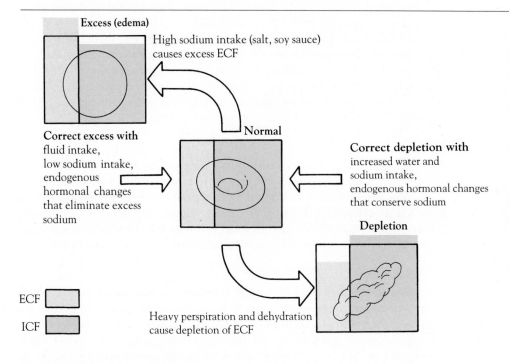

FIGURE 8-4
When sodium or water is in excess or depleted, corrections are made to restore the normal balance between the intracellular (ICF) and extracellular fluids (ECF) in the body. Sodium concentration in the ECF and total water content is maintained within narrow limits. Any change is corrected by thirst, by hormonal regulation of sodium, or by an increase in the appetite for sodium. If corrections are not made in the total fluid content of a cell, it may swell or shrink to dangerous levels.

Water Balance in the Body Is Maintained by Balancing Sodium and Potassium

The net effect of the imbalances in body fluids described above is reflected in the water balance of the billions of cells in the body. This equilibrium is maintained mainly by balancing sodium levels outside the cells and potassium levels inside the cells.

Sodium concentration in the extracellular fluid and total water content are maintained within narrow limits. Any excess or deficit is corrected by thirst, hormonal regulation of sodium, or a change in the appetite for sodium. A simple

Physiology

Physiology 🔑

way to remember how this balance works is that water will always *follow* sodium. (Artists, for example, use salt to draw water out of paints in order to create visual lined effects.) Every time sodium accumulates outside the cell, or is lost from the body, water moves in the same direction (Figure 8-4). When sweating, for example, causes a loss of sodium from its normal location, the extracellular space, water will move from the intracellular space to follow this sodium. A significant movement of water out of the cell causes cell dehydration. The reverse effect—when fluid accumulates outside the cell owing to a retention of sodium—is called edema. In this disorder, the flesh over the affected area seems puffy and spongy to the touch. Edema may occur in protein-energy malnutrition, pregnancy, heart failure, kidney disease, and during certain inflammations.

Too Little or Too Much Water Intake

Water is enormously important in nutrition, but since there are no RDA values for water how do we know how much fluid intake to recommend each day? Note that we used the word "fluid," which, of course, includes water. A reasonable guideline recommended by the National Research Council is that adults should take in 1 ml of fluid per kcalorie used for energy and infants should take in 1.5 ml per kcalorie. These apply when the person is not engaged in activities involving the loss of much body fluid. Water intake in men and women can vary from 0.26 to 2.81 liters per day, with a mean intake of 1.25 liters.[5] Information in Table 8-2 gives the concentration of minerals in 1 liter of water (slightly more than 2 pints).

Not enough water

Although fluid intake should sometimes be increased, as in the cases mentioned above, thirst is actually not a very sensitive indicator of fluid loss. Rather, body weight loss after extensive sweating is more accurate. A body weight loss of 10% to 12% after extensive sweating causes death (Figure 8-4). Physical performance is lowered at a 3% to 4% loss of body weight. It is foolish, therefore, to meet body weight limitations in events like wrestling and boxing by losing body water.

Too much water: water intoxication

Psychiatry 🔑

The effect of very high intakes of water is known as *water intoxication.* Although it cannot be stressed enough that it is better to take in too much rather than too little fluid, there are cases on record of water intoxication occurring in people with psychopathological problems like schizophrenia.[6] Early symptoms of water intoxication include headache, blurred vision, vomiting, excessive perspiration, incoordination, and excitability. In extreme cases, it includes delirium, coma, convulsions, and finally death. Some people with schizophrenia have a history of vague illnesses, neurotic traits, frequent job changes, and unsatisfactory sex adjustment.[6] However, because the signs and symptoms of water intoxication may also have other causes, water intoxication may go undetected for years.

How much intake will cause water intoxication? As we have seen, normal fluid intake is 6 cups or 1½ liters. However, our kidneys can actually cope with an intake of 80 cups (20 liters) of water a day, so it is clear that your kidneys are not working anywhere near capacity most of the time. Water intoxication occurs when large volumes of water are taken over a short time period.

Water Quality Has Many Influences on Health

Medical literature contains references to the association between water and some health problems.[5] In some cases, the association with water may be one of many factors responsible for the disease. Examples follow:

- Hypertension: If water is high in sodium or low in calcium.
- Cancer: From carcinogenic contaminants.
- Cardiovascular disease: Incidence is higher in areas with a low calcium level in the water.
- Stones in the urinary tract: May be caused by high levels of calcium in the water supply.
- Sudden infant death syndrome: High sodium levels in the water may be a factor, according to one theory.

- Legionnaires' disease[7]: Caused by presence of a particular microorganism.
- Tooth decay: Because of no water fluoridation; 40% of the U.S. water supply has no fluoride, owing to lack of funds or to fears—completely groundless— that fluoridated water will cause cancer, sickle cell anemia, or AIDS.[8] Fluoridation is recommended by the American Dental Association and the American Medical Association.   **Dentistry**
- Gastroenteritis: Causes diarrhea frequently because of contamination of the water supply by untreated sewage. This form of diarrhea is rare in developed countries today, but serious when it happens, as when untreated sewage was dumped into a river supplying the water to a Canadian town, causing diarrhea and vomiting in over half of the population.[9]   **Environmental Health**

Water Quality Is a Major Problem in Many Developing Countries

Most of us can turn on a tap in our homes and get clean water. People in many other countries are not so lucky. In parts of Africa and Asia, women and children may spend as much as 100 to 300 minutes a day obtaining water. Often water is obtained from ditches or wells, many of which are contaminated with human and animal wastes; few houses have even elementary toilet facilities.

Poor environmental sanitation causes widespread diarrhea, resulting in high infant mortality. Such mortality is reduced by clean water, as well as by improvements in literacy and socioeconomic conditions.[10] One survey of low-income women in developing countries showed that the desire for an improved water supply ranked as high as that for an adequate food supply.[11]

Infants and young children are in greatest danger of death from dehydration stemming from diarrhea. Children in many developing countries can expect to suffer from diarrhea for 30 days each year. Millions of children die because of diarrhea every year. Such horrible statistics have prompted the World Health Organization to produce *Guidelines for Drinking-Water Quality*, promoted under the slogan "Safe water supply and sanitation for all by 1990"—an optimistic goal, to say the least. The guidelines note that although drinking water may have some of 800 identified organic and inorganic chemicals, a high priority is given to microbial safety of water, since more than half the world is exposed to pathogenic organisms in the water. Such organisms, usually resulting from untreated sewage, can severely affect a child's growth, electrolyte balance, and resistance to infection.

Water is obtained from fluids, foods, and metabolism; it is excreted in urine, sweat, breath, and eliminated with the feces. Water content of different foods varies. Fluid intake should be increased at various times in the life cycle and because of various activities, diseases, and environmental temperatures. Too high or too low an intake of fluids causes death. Decreased water quality can affect health.

YOUR TASTE FOR DIFFERENT FLUIDS: HOW IT CHANGES WITH TIME

As Figure 8-5 indicates, Americans' consumption of milk and beverages has changed since the mid-1960s. Americans are replacing plain whole milk with low-fat milk, a good sign. Juice consumption has increased, also good, but so, unfortunately, has the intake of soft drinks. Tea and coffee consumption is decreasing. Per capita consumption of beer has leveled off at about 24 gallons per person per year, but consumption of wine and wine coolers is now up to nearly 2½ gallons. The annual per capita consumption of distilled spirits, such as whiskies, vodka, and gin, decreased to 2.46 gallons in 1984. Let us examine the nutritional implications of these changes.

Milk and Fruit Juices Are Nutritious Drinks

The new consumption patterns for milk and fruit juices are generally in a healthful direction.

Milk

That milk is a highly nutritious food is an undisputed fact. It is high in protein and calcium. It is a useful source of vitamins, especially of riboflavin and of vitamins A and D when the last two are added to commercial milk supplies. Drinking low-fat milk instead of whole milk reduces the butterfat intake but not the amount of solids-not-fat (protein and so forth), as Table 8-6 indicates. Some people complain that low-fat milk products lack taste and texture. Their popularity is largely due to their lower kcaloric content.

TABLE 8-6 Fat Content of Milk

Fluid Milk Products	FDA Standards* (percentage)
Butterfat	
Whole milk	3.25
Lowfat milk	0.5-2.0
Skim milk	0.5
Solids-Not-Fat	
Whole, lowfat, and skim milk	8.25

*Standards in California are higher for all categories except the butterfat content of skim milk.

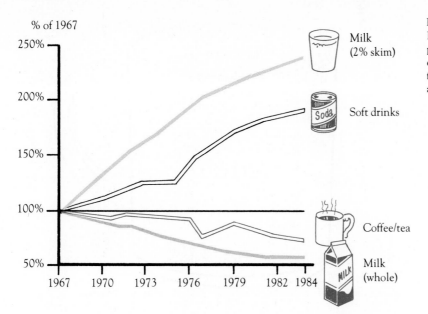

% of 1967

FIGURE 8-5
Beverage consumption patterns. Compared with 15 to 20 years ago, Americans are drinking less whole milk, coffee, and tea but more juice, soft drinks, and wine.

Cow's milk has more protein but less fat than human milk. Despite dairy industry slogans, however, cow's milk is *not* for everyone. People with allergies to milk or lactase deficiency often cannot drink or eat milk products. Milk substitutes are discussed in the Decision section of this chapter.

Fruit juices

Consumers concerned about health have also brought rapid changes to the marketing of juices. Per capita consumption of fruit juices rose 5% from 1983 to 1984: to a per capita consumption of 65.6 pints. When you buy fruit juices, however, you need to read the label to determine the nutritive value of "fruit juices" versus "fruit drinks." Fruit *drinks* usually have lower nutritive value. The label should tell you whether they contain the original juice that is diluted, or a diluted fruit flavor.

The marketing tactics for some juices and juice drinks are less than subtle. One manufacturer introduced four blended, 100% juice drinks calculated to stir mothers' guilt feelings "about giving their kids high-sugar bellywash."[12] Recently a company that purported to be selling apple juice was charged with really selling sugared water.

Citrus fruit juices provide significant amounts of vitamin C, but there is very little in apple juice unless it is fortified with vitamin C. Some fruit juices now have added calcium. Fruit juices are low in sodium and high in potassium. This makes them useful for people on low-sodium diets or those needing high potassium intakes because of treatment for hypertension or heart disease.

Soft Drinks, Caffeine Drinks, and Alcohol Are Not Very Nutritious

Whatever the good news about milk and fruit juice, it appears that Americans still have a love affair with other kinds of beverages that are not as nutritious and indeed even harmful.

Consumer Science

Beware of the manipulation of words on nutrition labels.

Some foods are good sources of water.

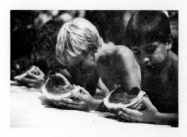

FIGURE 8-6
How much caffeine?

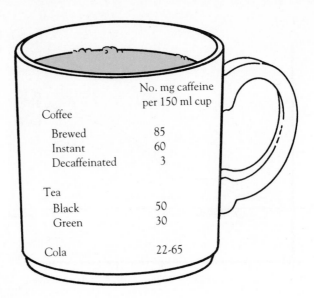

	No. mg caffeine per 150 ml cup
Coffee	
Brewed	85
Instant	60
Decaffeinated	3
Tea	
Black	50
Green	30
Cola	22-65

Soft drinks

Per capita intake of all soft drinks in the U.S. in 1984 was about 350 pints—up an incredible 16.8 pints in just one year. Cola drinks have about 63% of the market, with lime-lemon sodas at 13%, orange at 7%, and other citrus flavors at 4%. Of interest to nutritionists is the 18% to 20% increase between 1983 and 1984 in diet drink consumption. Diet drinks had about 21.5% of the market in 1984. Diet drinks taste sweet but don't have as many kcalories.

Given the importance of an adequate fluid intake, you could say soft drinks serve their purpose in encouraging fluid intake, and it is usually a losing battle to convince people to substitute water for soft drinks anyway. But soft drinks also have nutritional disadvantages. They have low nutrient density (some contain only kcalories and no nutrients), which is particularly significant during childhood and adolescence because the body in these years has high requirements for nutrients for growth. In addition, questions have been raised about the health effects of the artificial sweeteners and caffeine in some of these drinks.

Coffee, tea, and cocoa

The positive aspects of these drinks is that they offer a pleasant means of increasing fluid intake during a work break or meal. Caffeine also is a mild stimulant and diuretic. Coffee offers nutrition contributions of potassium and niacin, and tea includes a high fluoride content. Any added milk (but not cream) offers protein and sugar as a source of energy.

Tannin
Naturally occurring chemical found in tea and unripe fruits; decreases iron absorption.

Tea has a high *tannin* content, and coffee and cocoa have lower tannin concentrations. Tannin decreases iron absorption. These beverages have caffeine also, as Figure 8-6 indicates.

Pharmacologists consider a daily intake of 250 mg of caffeine "large"—about 3 cups of brewed coffee.

Caffeine is also present in many stimulants, prescription drugs, analgesics, cold preparations, and weight-control pills. Caffeine intake in excess of 250 mg is considered "large" by pharmacologists. However, a tolerance can be built up over time. This is just as well because caffeine intake by Americans is high. By the late 1970s, 160 billion cups of coffee and 40 billion cups of tea were consumed per year.

Most people are ignorant of the amount of caffeine they consume and its effects on the body.[13] This is unfortunate, because studies are now linking high caffeine intakes to certain medical problems. The March of Dimes recommends that pregnant women limit caffeine consumption to 444 mg per day, because research with experimental animals produced birth defects with high caffeine consumption. A long-term study has also shown that the risk of coronary heart disease is two to three times higher in men who are heavy coffee drinkers.[14] The National Academy of Science's Committee on Diet, Nutrition, and Cancer (1982) found no strong evidence linking coffee consumption to cancer. However, caffeine intake may be related to a higher number of nonmalignant lumps in the breasts of women (4-5 cups per day) and to cancer of the ovaries, and women with a predisposition to develop these types of cancers are urged to drink decaffeinated coffee instead. Researcher Linda Massey of Washington State University showed recently that caffeine increases the body's need for calcium.

Five cups of brewed coffee contain about 444 mg of caffeine.

Certain teas are associated with "health foods," but some of these teas are far from healthy. Ginseng abuse syndrome (GAS) produces mood alteration, anorexia, hypertension, edema, amenorrhea, diarrhea, and skin eruptions. Coca leaf tea is sold in the U.S. as "Health Inca Tea" (HIT) and as "Mate de Coca."[15] Though only decocainized coca leaf products are legal in the U.S., these teas contain some cocaine. Mild stimulation, mood elevation, and increased pulse rate occur after high intake. However, normal patterns of intake seem to produce no ill effects or abuse.[15] Coca tea was sold in Great Britain as a slimming agent until stopped by government action in 1983.

Alcoholic drinks

Alcohol intake in the United States is equivalent to more than four whisky ounce–equivalents per person per day. The amount of kcalories taken in by some drinkers can be as high as one third to one half of the total number of kcalories consumed per day.

An estimated 10.6 million Americans were alcohol dependent in 1985. About 7.3 million more had some negative experience from alcohol abuse. These included arrests, accidents, and impairment of health or job performance. Alcohol problems cost American society about $120 *billion* in 1983.

Alcohol Can Lead to Malnourishment and Cause Tissue Damage

Alcoholism is a major cause of malnutrition in industrialized countries. One gram of pure alcohol has 7 kcalories. The kcaloric content will vary between different drinks because of variation in alcohol content (Table 8-7) and content of other constituents. You can calculate the number of kcalories from alcohol in any alcoholic drink by using the formula

$$0.8 \times \text{proof} \times \text{ounces}$$

TABLE 8-7 Alcohol and Kcalorie Content of Popular Beverages and the Critical Threshold for Men and Women

Beverage	Alcohol Content (percentage of volume)	Kcalories per 1000 ml	Critical Threshold* (liters)	
			Men	Women
Beer	4	400	2	0.7
Wine	10	700-1200	0.7	0.25
Hard liquor	38	2500	0.2	0.07

*The "critical threshold" suggested for men (60 g of pure alcohol) is supplied by approximately either 4 bottles of beer, 1 bottle of wine, ½ liter of vermouth or sherry, or 5 single whiskeys. For women the critical level of 20 g of alcohol is supplied by either 1½ bottles of beer, ¼ liter of wine, 3 glasses of dessert wine, or a weak double whiskey. Beyond these critical levels, the severity of cirrhosis multiplies with increasing amounts of alcohol.

Alcohol and malnourishment

Alcoholics may be malnourished for at least three reasons.

- *Economic:* All available money may be spent on alcohol; the alcoholic may have little money for nourishing foods.
- *Empty kcalories:* Many alcoholics get from one third to one half of their total kcaloric intake from alcohol. Kcalories from alcohol are "empty" of vitamins and minerals, which means that food choices for the remaining kcalories should be made with care—something that does not usually happen with alcoholics.

Alcoholism may be the greatest cause of malnutrition in industrialized countries.

- *Negative effect on metabolism:* Alcohol has an adverse effect on the absorption, transportation, and excretion of nutrients.[16] Less of the following nutrients are absorbed by alcoholics: thiamin, folic acid, vitamin B_{12}, and glucose. Alcoholics have lower blood levels of zinc, glucose, thiamin, vitamin A, and the retinol-binding protein that transports vitamin A. Blood levels of cholesterol, phospholipids, and triglycerides are increased. Alcoholics have increased excretion of urinary zinc, magnesium, and potassium. Alcoholics have low amounts of phosphorus, vitamin B_6, and vitamin A also.

How alcohol harms the body

Alcohol has some damaging effects on the body's tissues. Indeed, the body treats alcohol as a toxic substance.[16] Its harmful effects may vary depending on the tissue, as follows:

Cirrhosis
Degenerative disease of the liver seen often in alcoholics.

- *Liver:* This is the detoxification center of the body. A fatty liver is the first sign of alcohol damage. More extensive damage causes *cirrhosis,* which can lead to liver cancer. Vitamins, protein, and other nutrient supplements will not prevent liver damage if the person still drinks alcohol.
- *Heart:* Extreme alcoholism damages the heart and causes hypertension.
- *Nervous system, including the brain:* Adverse effects here are probably due to deficiencies of thiamin, vitamin B_6, and vitamin B_{12}. These vitamins are involved in nerve function.
- *Intestinal system:* Alcohol decreases the activity of some enzymes and damages the structure of the intestine, which can cause esophageal bleeding and hemorrhoids.

- *Blood:* Anemia may arise owing to impaired iron utilization and to dietary deficiencies in iron, folic acid, copper, and protein.
- *Immune system:* The immune system is affected so that alcoholics get pneumonia and other infectious diseases more easily.[17]
- *Joints:* Gout is associated with high alcohol intake.
- *Cancer:* Cancers of the mouth, esophagus, and respiratory tract occur when high alcohol intakes and cigarette smoking are combined.

The negative effects of alcohol vary from person to person. Men, for example, have a higher critical threshold for alcohol than do women (see Table 8-7). In addition, members of some racial groups metabolize alcohol better than those of other racial groups. Orientals and American Indians have a low capacity for alcohol because of lower activity of alcohol dehydrogenase, an enzyme involved in the metabolism of alcohol in the body. Women who drink during pregnancy may be risking fetal alcohol syndrome, one of whose consequences is mental retardation in the child.

Reducing the danger of alcohol

Concerned about the negative effects of alcohol, particularly on young people and pregnant women, the American Medical Association has issued recommendations for the advertising, promotion, and consumption of alcohol.[18] **Marketing**

If you drink alcoholic beverages, it is better to sip rather than gulp drinks. In addition, alcohol absorption can be slowed by solid food or milk already in the gastrointestinal system; alcohol is not broken down into smaller parts during digestion and therefore crosses quickly from the gastrointestinal system into the blood. Finally, there are many myths about how to sober up from the effects of alcohol: coffee, cold showers, or running will not speed up the metabolism of alcohol.

Much attention has been given to the possible positive effect of moderate alcohol intake on coronary heart disease. Early studies showed that *moderate* alcohol intake increased high-density lipoprotein (HDL) in the blood. HDL is the "good guy" in protection against coronary heart disease. We know now that one form of HDL, called HDL_2, is associated with a reduction in coronary heart disease.[19] Alcohol increases HDL_3, which is not related to reduction in coronary heart disease. This is another example of refinement in scientific methods providing better understanding of biochemical mechanisms involved in disease. Consistently high amounts of alcohol produce hyperlipidemia and hypercholesterolemia, which are negative factors in coronary heart disease. **Biochemistry**

Perhaps the two principal dietary guidelines for consuming alcohol are:
1. If you drink alcoholic beverages, do so in moderation. This amounts to one or two standard-size drinks daily.
2. Abstain from alcoholic drinks during pregnancy.

Drinks high in water content can meet the body's fluid requirements. Milk is high in calcium and protein. Fruit juices are high in vitamin C and potassium. Soft drinks may be high in kcalories unless artificial sweeteners are used. Alcohol contributes kcalories and little else, and it offers the greatest health risks.

Decisions

1. How Can I Cut Down on Kcalorie Intake from Various Drinks?

The advice given by the U.S. Department of Agriculture is as follows:

- Alcoholic beverages are high in kcalories but low in nutrients.
- Fruit and vegetable juices provide you with vitamins and minerals in addition to kcalories.

The list of drinks in Table 8-8 will help you in calculating your intake of kcalories. As you examine the list pay close attention to the differences in serving size for different drinks.

2. Is the Implied Healthfulness of "Cholesterol-Free" Nondairy Creamers Real?

Beware of buzz words like "cholesterol-free" in food advertising.

There is an implied healthfulness in the use of the term *cholesterol-free.* However, that may not be strictly accurate. This is because coconut oil appears in most of 25 cholesterol-free nondairy creamers tested.[20] Coconut oil is among the highest of all dietary fats in its proportion of saturated fatty acids. Only butter approaches the degree of saturation of coconut oil. Saturated fatty acids increase serum cholesterol. A high serum cholesterol level is correlated with a higher incidence of coronary heart disease.

These nondairy creamers can add to kcaloric intake also. If you put one spoonful of cholesterol-free nondairy creamer into each of ten cups of coffee per day, it will add more than 100 kcalories of "hidden" highly saturated fat per day.[20]

Thus, in making nutrition decisions about these creamers, you should weigh their convenience against their kcalories and high saturated fat content.

3. What are the Nutrition Implications of Nonalcoholic "Beers" and "Wines"?

They have less than ½% (by volume) of alcohol compared with the much higher alcohol content of "the real thing" (Table 8-7). Moreover, the ability to get drunk on nonalcoholic drinks is overwhelmingly reduced.[21] Still, they may cause problems for an alcoholic who is trying to abstain from alcohol.

4. What Is the Best Sports Drink?

For preventing dehydration and excessive body heat, water is best. The effectiveness of carbohydrate drinks for energy depends on their composition and when they are taken in relation to the event. Taking a sugared drink, like glucose in water, 45 minutes before exercise will not have the desired result of getting glucose to the muscles quickly. In fact, it will have the reverse effect. It will produce hypoglycemia during the first 30 minutes of intensive exercise.[1] This is caused by a surge in insulin production after the sugar from the drink is absorbed. Insulin reduces blood glucose levels, so that less glucose gets to the exercising muscles by the time the event starts. Taking glucose during a marathon run is beneficial.[1] For short exercise events, it is of little value. Sugar in the water results in both the carbohydrate and the water leaving the stomach slowly. Note the importance of the time at which sugared drinks are taken.

TABLE 8-8 Kcalories Contained in Various Drinks

Drinks*	Approximate Kcalories
Beer	
Regular beer	12 fl. oz. = 150
Light beer	12 fl. oz. = 95
Liquor	(jigger = 1½ fl. oz.)
Gin, rum, vodka, and whiskey (86-proof)	jigger = 105
Vermouth, sweet	jigger = 70
Vermouth, dry	jigger = 55
Wine	
Sweet	5 fl. oz. = 200
Dry table, red	5 fl. oz. = 110
Dry table, white	5 fl. oz. = 115
Cordials and Liqueurs	jigger = 145
Carbonated Drinks	
Fruit-flavored	6 fl oz. = 90
Root beer	6 fl. oz. = 80
Cola	6 fl. oz. = 80
Ginger ale	6 fl. oz. = 55
Low-calorie soda (contains artificial sweeteners)	6 fl. oz. = 0-1
Club soda	6 fl. oz. = 0
Fruit and Vegetable Juices (unsweetened)†	
Pineapple	6 fl. oz. = 105
Orange	6 fl. oz. = 90
Grapefruit	6 fl. oz. = 75
Tomato	6 fl. oz. = 35

* If you're making a mixed drink, you have to count the kcalories in the mixer too.
† Remember: Fruit and vegetable juice provide you with vitamins and minerals in addition to kcalories. Alcohol and most carbonated beverages provide you only with kcalories.

Summary

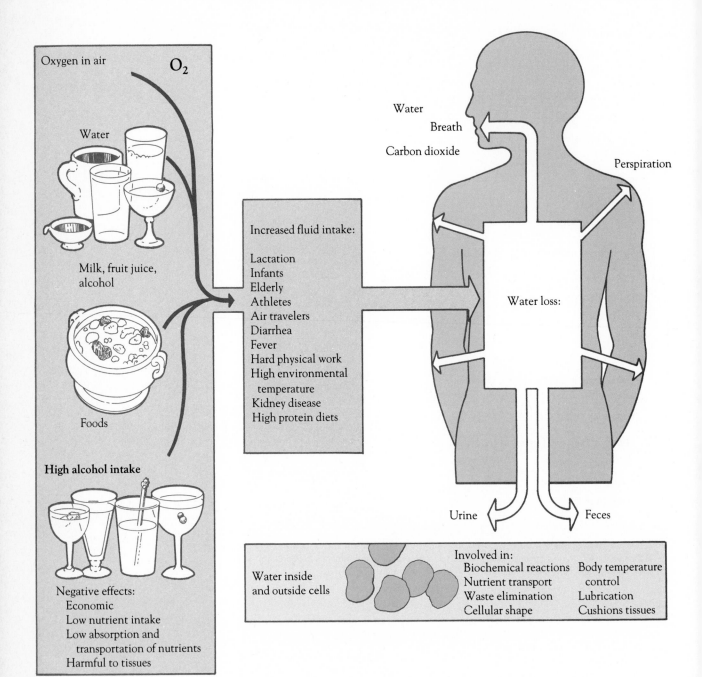

Oxygen in air   O$_2$

Water

Milk, fruit juice, alcohol

Foods

High alcohol intake

Negative effects:
  Economic
  Low nutrient intake
  Low absorption and
    transportation of nutrients
  Harmful to tissues

Increased fluid intake:

Lactation
Infants
Elderly
Athletes
Air travelers
Diarrhea
Fever
Hard physical work
High environmental
  temperature
Kidney disease
High protein diets

Water
Breath
Carbon dioxide

Perspiration

Water loss:

Urine   Feces

Water inside
and outside cells

Involved in:
  Biochemical reactions   Body temperature
  Nutrient transport   control
  Waste elimination   Lubrication
  Cellular shape   Cushions tissues

REFERENCES

1. Koivisto, V.A.: The physiology of marathon running, Science Progress **70:**109, 1986.

2. Linder, M.C.: Nutritional biochemistry and metabolism, New York, Elsevier Science Publishing Co., Inc., 1985.

3. Korch, G.C.: Sodium content of potable water: dietary significance, Journal of the American Dietetic Association **86:**80, 1986.

4. Sun, M.: Ground water ills: many diagnoses, few remedies, Science **232:**1490, 1986.

5. Gillies, M.E., and Paulin H.V.: Estimations of daily mineral intakes from drinking water, Human Nutrition: Applied Nutrition **36A:**287, 1982.

6. Singh, S., and others: Water intoxication in psychiatric patients, British Journal of Psychiatry **146:**127, 1985.

7. Shands, K.N., and others: Potable water as a source of Legionnaires disease, Journal of the American Medical Association **253:**1412, 1985.

8. Anonymous: Getting the most from the most essential nutrient, Tufts University Diet & Nutrition Letter **4**(8), October, 1986.

9. O'Neill, A.E., and others: A waterborne epidemic of acute infectious nonbacterial gastroenteritis in Alberta, Canada, Canadian Journal of Public Health **76:**199, 1985.

10. Rahman, M., and others: Impact of environmental sanitation and crowding on infant mortality in rural Bangladesh, Lancet **ii:**28, 1985.

11. Briscoe, J.: Water supply and health in developing countries: selective primary health care revisited, American Journal of Public Health **74:**1009, 1984.

12. Hannigan, K.: State of the industry: juice, soft drinks, Food Engineering, pps. 74 and 75, August, 1985.

13. Guiry, V.C., and Bisogni, C.A.: Caffeine knowledge, attitudes, and practices of young women, Journal of Nutrition Education **18:**16, 1986.

14. Lacroix, A.Z., and others: Coffee consumption and the incidence of coronary heart disease, New England Journal of Medicine **315:**977, 1986.

15. Siegel, R.K., and others: Cocaine in herbal tea, Journal of the American Medical Association **255:**40, 1986.

16. Gastineau, C.: Nutritional implications of alcohol. In Present knowlege in nutrition, 5th edition, Washington, D.C., The Nutrition Foundation, Inc., 1984.

17. MacGregor, R.R.: Alcohol and immune disease, Journal of the American Medical Association **256:**1474, 1986.

18. American Medical Association, Board of Trustees Report: Alcohol: advertising, counteradvertising, and public deception in the public media, Journal of the American Medical Association **256:**1485, 1986.

19. Lieber, C.S.: To drink (moderately) or not to drink? New England Journal of Medicine **310:**846, 1984.

20. Vannes, A.F., and McManus, B.M.: Cholesterol–free nondairy creamers: compositional conundrums and cardiovascular contradictions, New England Journal of Medicine **314:**651, 1986.

21. Miller, R.W.: Nonalcoholic "beer" and "wine": how close to the real thing? FDA Consumer, page 11, September, 1986.

METABOLISM NOTES: *Delivery and Use of Oxygen to Cells*

In this chapter you saw the importance of oxygen in the liberation of energy from carbohydrates, fats, and proteins. One of the end products of this release of energy is water of metabolism. Many nutrition factors are involved in getting oxygen to cells and where the water of metabolism is produced. We begin with air, which is 21% oxygen. Pollutants in the air hinder the delivery of oxygen to cells because they damage the lungs. Furthermore, pollutants such as ozone, nitrous oxide, and lead hinder the uptake of oxygen by hemoglobin.

Oxygen is attached to the iron-containing heme part of hemoglobin in red blood cells (RBCs) as the RBCs pass through the lungs. RBCs are formed in the bone marrow. A number of dietary components influence the production and function of RBCs. Low dietary *iron* causes a reduction in the hemoglobin level in the RBCs. A number of factors aid in increasing the bioavailability of dietary iron. These include:

- The form of the iron—ferrous iron is more bioavailable than ferric iron. That is why ferrous sulfate is the most common iron supplement available in supermarkets. The iron contained in heme in meat is the most bioavailable form of iron in foods.
- Vitamin C—helps in the conversion of ferric iron in food into the more bioavailable ferrous form. That is why iron bioavailability is usually increased when food sources high in vitamin C are contained in the meal.
- Some amino acids.
- Lactose in the diet—though milk is a poor source of iron, the amount that is present has high bioavailability because of the presence of the lactose in milk.
- Acidity in the stomach—people who secrete low amounts of hydrochloric acid in the stomach, or who abuse antacids, may have less iron absorbed into the blood.
- An increased need for iron—in deficiency and during pregnancy and lactation.

FIGURE 8-7
The role of oxygen in liberating energy from carbohydrates, fats, and proteins within cells.

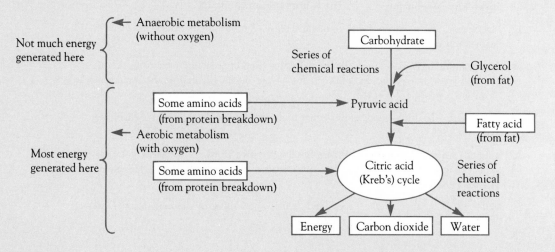

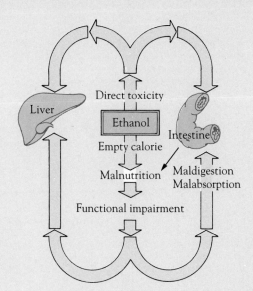

FIGURE 8-8
Why alcohol (ethanol) produces toxicity and malnutrition.

A number of factors decrease the bioavailability of iron:

- Fiber, phytic acid (in cereals), oxalic acid (spinach), and tannins (tea) can combine with dietary iron to make it unavailable for absorption.
- Diets low in protein or high in phosphorus result in low iron uptake.
- Poor fat absorption—other minerals are poorly absorbed in this situation, too.
- High iron stores in the body—this is a protective mechanism. However, if iron intake is excessively high, this protective mechanism breaks down. Iron can then accumulate to toxic levels, and death may result.

RBCs require other nutrients besides iron to allow them to carry oxygen.

- Folacin and vitamin B_{12} deficiency results in RBCs of irregular size and shape. This interferes with the oxygen-carrying capacity of the cell.
- Protein is needed to make the globin part of hemoglobin.
- Vitamin E, vitamin B_6, and copper are also necessary.

This brief review of the nutrient requirements of RBCs and of some dietary components that aid or hinder the meeting of these requirements shows the important role of diet in energy metabolism in the body.

Oxygen is taken to all cells in the body by the RBCs. The demand for the oxygen varies depending on the tissue (Table 8-1). The metabolic role of oxygen within the cell in liberating the energy from carbohydrates, fats, and proteins is shown in Figure 8-7. Most of the energy is liberated by the help of oxygen in aerobic metabolism. Notice that the end products of the breakdown of carbohydrates, fats, and proteins in the cell are energy, carbon dioxide, and water.

Why Alcohol Is So Toxic to Cells

Ethanol (alcohol) is a cause of toxicity and malnutrition, as summarized in Figure 8-8. Ethanol is toxic to all cells. The liver is the detoxification center. The enzyme alcohol dehydrogenase converts ethanol into acetaldehyde. This may be exported from the cell into the blood. The acetaldehyde is carried by the blood to the heart,

FIGURE 8-9
Pathways in liver cell. Decreased by
ethanol. These pathways are shown by
dashed lines.

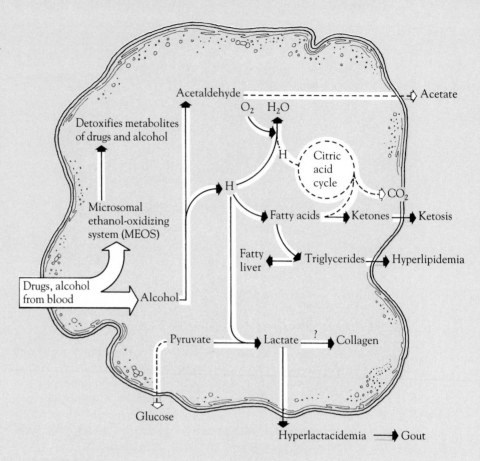

brain, and other tissues. Some of the acetaldehyde remains in the liver. In all
cases, it is harmful to cells. The ability to convert acetaldehyde to the nontoxic
acetate is reduced in the alcoholic.

Mitochondria are damaged by ethanol. Therefore, activity of the citric acid
cycle is reduced. Another outcome of ethanol metabolism is that the hydrogen
released after the conversion of ethanol into acetaldehyde is used in the formation
of fatty acids (Figure 8-9). These may be converted into ketones, causing an
increased level of ketones in the blood called ketosis. Some of these fatty acids
are synthesized into triglycerides. They are then dumped into the blood. The level
of blood lipids is now increased (hyperlipidemia). Another fate for the triglycerides
is to be deposited within the liver cells to produce a fatty liver. Finally, the hydrogen
may be involved in the formation of lactate. This is exported from the cell into
the blood, producing hyperlactacidemia, or too high a level of lactic acid in the
blood. Eventually this leads to gout, a major problem in alcoholics. Glucose production is decreased in alcoholics, partly explaining why alcoholics often have
hypoglycemia, usually after prolonged fasting after heavy drinking.

**Do not take alcohol and drugs at the
same time; they are especially
dangerous when taken together.**

Alcohol can be metabolized through another system within each liver cell. This
is the microsomal ethanol-oxidizing system (MEOS). Drugs are metabolized through
this system also. Sleeping pills, narcotics, and tranquilizers are more dangerous
when mixed with alcohol. This is due to the preferential treatment by the MEOS
in detoxifying alcohol before these other drugs are detoxified.

Energy Requirements and Energy Balance

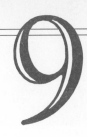

CONNECTIONS

Carbohydrates, fats, and proteins in cells in most tissues in the body produce energy to meet the body's basal energy needs, to digest and absorb food, and to accomplish physical activity. Basal energy requirements are the vital body processes that keep you alive—circulation, respiration, glandular secretion, and maintenance of body temperature and muscle tone.

Vitamins and minerals do not provide energy in the form of kcalories, although they help store and liberate energy in the body, which is why people with deficiencies of vitamins or minerals may feel tired. Increased dietary energy from food and drink is required under unusual conditions: during pregnancy and lactation, recovery from illness or starvation, or strenuous physical activity like athletics.

The concepts of energy requirements and energy balance described here will help you understand the problems of obesity, eating disorders, and starvation in the next chapter.

Even if you don't get out of bed all day—if you lie motionless, asleep—you still have energy requirements. You must draw on food and drink to provide the kcalories that "give you energy" to power each heartbeat, each breath, each metabolic activity of the cells. And, of course, if you are a marathon runner, you need considerably more in the way of kcalories for energy. Figure 9-1 presents some graphic examples of the number of kcalories required to perform certain common activities. Whatever your level of physical activity, however, you will get about 4 kcalories from a gram of carbohydrates, 4 kcalories from a gram of protein, and 9 kcalories from a gram of fat. (You will also get 7 kcalories from a gram of alcohol, which is not considered a nutrient.)

Important to the concept of energy requirements is the notion of *energy balance:* to maintain health, you must take in as much energy through kcalories in food and drink as you expend in activity. Of course, this intake and expenditure may vary from day to day, and the body is perfectly able to handle such short-term

Dietary energy intake may vary considerably from day to day.

FIGURE 9-1
"I can exercise it off." How many minutes of exercise it takes to burn up some common foods.

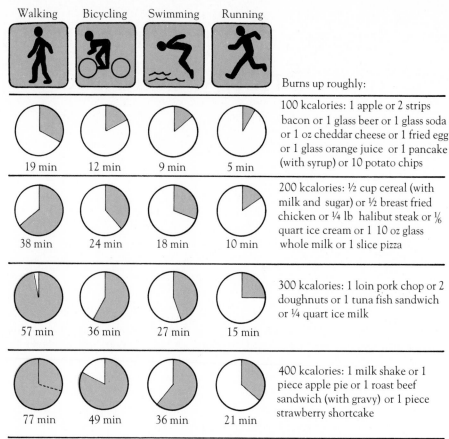

Walking   Bicycling   Swimming   Running

Burns up roughly:

Walking	Bicycling	Swimming	Running	
19 min	12 min	9 min	5 min	100 kcalories: 1 apple or 2 strips bacon or 1 glass beer or 1 glass soda or 1 oz cheddar cheese or 1 fried egg or 1 glass orange juice or 1 pancake (with syrup) or 10 potato chips
38 min	24 min	18 min	10 min	200 kcalories: ½ cup cereal (with milk and sugar) or ½ breast fried chicken or ¼ lb halibut steak or ⅙ quart ice cream or 1 10 oz glass whole milk or 1 slice pizza
57 min	36 min	27 min	15 min	300 kcalories: 1 loin pork chop or 2 doughnuts or 1 tuna fish sandwich or ¼ quart ice milk
77 min	49 min	36 min	21 min	400 kcalories: 1 milk shake or 1 piece apple pie or 1 roast beef sandwich (with gravy) or 1 piece strawberry shortcake

Kcalories expended by a 154 lb person. Walking briskly (at 3½ mph) uses up about 5 kcalories per minute; riding a bicycle, 9 kcalories per minute; swimming 11 kcalories per minute; and running, 19 kcalories per minute.

changes: you may eat enormous meals one day and light snacks the next, do only light reading beside the pool on one occasion and swim forty laps on another.

However, a lot of the human misery on this planet comes about because energy intake is, over long periods, very low or very high—in ways that are not balanced by energy expenditure. Famine, for instance, is a consequence of too little food available to provide energy and, as W. R. Akroyd writes, "essentially it means a lot of miserable people suffering from starvation, and physically and mentally damaged as a result." Overnutrition is the intake of too much food, which, as another writer states, leads to the troubles of another set of people—"those troubled by the modern American obsession with overweight and obesity." Of course, if you eat too much, the best way to establish energy balance is through exercise, which, in addition, has certain side benefits: it "may enhance the quality of life, improve the capacity for work and recreation and promote a positive mental attitude even through times of illness and permanent or temporary immobility," according to Dr. Penny Kris-Etherton.

This chapter will discuss the many factors that affect energy requirements and energy balance, giving you the background needed for studying the consequences of undereating and overeating discussed in the next chapter.

KCALORIES AND FOOD: THE SOURCES OF ENERGY

The word *kcalories* has appeared repeatedly throughout this book. Kcalorie (kilocalorie, often abbreviated kcal) is the measure used to express energy intake in the diet and energy expenditure in physical activity and other requirements of the body. One kcalorie is defined as the amount of heat required to raise the temperature of 1 kg of water 1° C. The word usually used in the media and in advertising is *calorie*, but *kcalorie* is the scientifically correct term. (Europeans count *kilojoules* instead of kilocalories; 1 kilocalorie equals 4.18 kilojoules.)

Let us now look at the kcaloric intake in our diet.

Food Is the Source of All Your Energy

Vitamins and minerals, you may recall, do not provide any energy, although they are important in liberating energy from the energy nutrients. This means that all energy in the diet is provided by carbohydrates, proteins, and fats (and alcohol).

If you know the amounts of carbohydrates, proteins, and fats in a food you can easily calculate the number of kcalories it provides and the percentage of total kcalories provided by carbohydrate, by fat, and by protein. For tomorrow, as a learning experience, try calculating your total kcaloric intake for the entire day by doing the following: keep a record of the amount of each food and drink you consume. Then calculate your total kcaloric intake by using one of the following methods.

- *Method 1:* the nutrition label on a loaf of bread, for example, says that a serving of two slices contains the following:

Protein	5 g =	20 kcals =	13% of total kcals
Carbohydrate	28 g =	112 kcals =	75% of total kcals
Fat	2 g =	18 kcals =	12% of total kcals
TOTAL		= 150 kcals =	100% of total kcals

Here is how this is calculated: the total of 150 kcals from protein, carbohydrate, and fat equals 100%; this means that

$$20 \text{ kcals from protein} = \frac{100 \times 20}{150} = 13\%$$

$$112 \text{ kcals from carbohydrate} = \frac{100 \times 112}{150} = 75\%$$

$$18 \text{ kcals from fat} = \frac{100 \times 18}{150} = 12\%$$

(Note: kcalories per serving are rounded to the nearest 10 kcalories on food labels.) Using this method, you can convert the carbohydrate, fat, and protein content of each food and drink into kcalories (see Appendix B). From this you can calculate the percent of kcalories provided by carbohydrate, fat, or protein. The kcaloric value of any alcohol consumed should be calculated also.

- *Method 2:* As a shorter method, obtain the kcaloric content of food you eat from the Table of Food Composition in Appendix P. Using bread as an example, the table shows that the kcaloric value of one slice of white bread is 70 kcalories. Therefore, two slices give 140 kcalories. This amount is similar to the kcaloric value calculated above from the amount of carbohydrate, fat, and protein on the label.

Scientists obtain very accurate measurements of the energy value of a food, or of a combination of foods, by burning the food under carefully controlled conditions in a device with the unlikely name of "bomb calorimeter." This instrument measures the amount of heat liberated from the food when it is burned to an ash. This allows the number of calories to be measured, since kcalories are units of heat. A correction must be made for any fiber in the food. Fiber is combustible so it contributes to the total kcaloric content measured by this method. However, most of the fiber in the diet is indigestible, so that energy is excreted in the feces. Therefore, the energy value of fiber should be subtracted from the total energy value if the most accurate value is required.

The Preparation Method Can Change a Food's Kcaloric Value

If you add another energy nutrient to a food during preparation—especially a high-fat ingredient like butter or cream—it will, of course, increase that food's kcaloric content. Other ingredients like sugar for sweetening or starch for thickening will do likewise. Consider the potato: are people right when they say potatoes are "fattening"? It depends on what happens to the potatoes after they leave the ground.

The addition of fat will change the kcaloric content of potatoes greatly, as shown in Table 9-1. In point of fact, potatoes are no more fattening than any other food. Indeed, it is wrong to use the term "fattening food" because there is no secret fattening factor in any food.

TABLE 9-1 Adding Fat to Potato Changes the Kcalorie Content

Method of Cooking	Kcalories per 100 g
Baked	75
Boiled	80
Mashed, milk and butter added	93
In potato salad	100
As hashed browns	223
French-fried	270
As potato chips	575

Are Your Actual and Ideal Intakes of Dietary Energy the Same?

Once you have calculated your total kcaloric intake over a 24-hour period, you can make some interesting comparisons. The percentage of total kcalories provided by carbohydrate, fat, and protein in your diet can be compared with the information given in Table 9-2.

TABLE 9-2 Comparisons of Ancient Diet and Typical American Diet of the 1980s

	Ancient Diet (%)	Typical American Diet (%)	Dietary Guidelines (%)
Protein	34	12	12
Carbohydrate	45	46	58
Fat	21	42	30

Ideally, your diet should provide the kcaloric distribution recommended in the Dietary Guidelines. However, as the table shows, the "typical American diet" differs considerably from the Dietary Guidelines and from that of your ancient ancestors, who got most of their kcalories from complex carbohydrates. Today, by contrast, in the typical North American diet too high a proportion of energy comes from fat. The Dietary Guidelines recommend that you increase your intake of kcalories from complex carbohydrates by eating more bread, pasta, and similar starchy foods. Some foods rich in complex carbohydrates, such as pasta, potatoes, rice, and whole-grain breads, are high in fiber also. If today's food has become more fatty, much of this is because fat adds flavor and juiciness—as you can see from Table 9-1.

Anthropology

To achieve the ideal diet, you must also avoid "empty-calorie" foods. Some nutritionists have objected to this term on the basis that all calories are the same. Still, it is useful because it describes foods that provide kcalories but are "empty" of other nutrients. Among the empty-calorie foods are sugar, honey, and alcohol, which contain little or no vitamins or minerals (Appendix P).

TABLE 9-3 Contribution of Food Groups to Energy Intake in 1909-1913 and 1980

Food Group	Percent of Total Energy (kcal) Intake	
	1909-1913	1980
Meat, fish, poultry	16	21
Dairy products	9	10
Fats, oils	12	18
Fruits, vegetables	4	6
Potatoes	5	3
Grain products	38	20
Sugar and other sweeteners	12	17
Other*	4	5

* Includes eggs, dry beans, peas, nuts, and soy products.

How Does Today's Dietary Energy Intake Compare with That of the Early 1900s?

As Table 9-3 demonstrates, Americans today consume about the same number of kcalories as Americans at the beginning of this century, but the sources of the kcalories differ. Today Americans consume fewer grain products and fewer potatoes. By contrast, your great-grandparents ate fewer fats and oils, meat, fish and poultry, and sugar and other sweeteners. Because life was also less convenient—there were fewer labor-saving devices and automobiles—they probably expended more kcalories of energy than you do. As a result, they had fewer problems with overweight and obesity.

The composition of today's diet is different from that of your great-grandparents.

One gram of carbohydrate or protein provides 4 kcalories, 1 g of fat provides 9 kcalories, and 1 g of alcohol provides 7 kcalories. The desirable proportion of kcalories in the diet is 58% from carbohydrates, 30% from fats, and 12% from proteins. The energy content of a food can be increased considerably by the addition of sugar, fat, oil, or other sources of kcalories.

ENERGY: THE FORCE THAT KEEPS YOU ALIVE

Whatever your age, you need energy for three important functions in your body:

- *Basal energy*—the energy needed to maintain life (basal metabolic rate [BMR])
- *Physical activity*
- *Dietary thermogenesis*—the body heat produced in the metabolism of food (dietary thermogenesis is also called the "specific dynamic effect of food").

For most people not involved in extensive physical activity, the greatest amount of energy is used for basal metabolism (Figure 9-2).

Basal Energy Is Needed To Keep You Alive

All your vital body functions require energy inputs, as the following "action words" (*-ing* words) would seem to suggest:

- *Pumping* blood around the body
- *Inflating* the lungs in breathing
- *Generating* heat in order to maintain body temperature
- *Maintaining* tension in muscles
- *Secreting* substances from glands and cells
- *Firing* nerve impulses

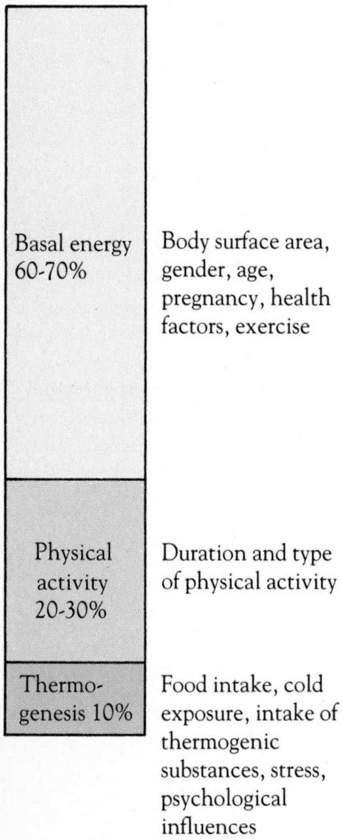

The number of kcalories you use for basal energy depends on some personal factors. Your body composition may be different from someone else's for instance, which means that you have different proportions of bone, fat, and lean tissue (muscles, liver, kidneys, etc). All tissues do not have the same metabolic activity. Muscles and other lean tissues, collectively called *lean body mass,* require more energy for metabolism than fat and bone. Basal metabolic rate is influenced by body surface area, gender, age, pregnancy, health factors, and exercise.

Body surface area

Tall, large-frame people have, of course, a large body surface area. They often also have a greater proportion of lean tissue. If so, they have a higher BMR. Body composition rather than body weight is a more important measurement in determining a person's BMR. For example, weight lifting increases body weight mainly by increasing muscle mass, which significantly raises the person's BMR. The increase in BMR will not be as great in a weight gain from increased body fat.

Basal Energy
Energy needed to maintain life.

Dietary Thermogenesis
Body heat produced in the metabolism of food.

FIGURE 9-2
Energy metabolism in sedentary people. The greatest amount of energy is used for basal metabolism in people who are not physically active.

Basal energy 60-70%	Body surface area, gender, age, pregnancy, health factors, exercise
Physical activity 20-30%	Duration and type of physical activity
Thermogenesis 10%	Food intake, cold exposure, intake of thermogenic substances, stress, psychological influences

TABLE 9-4 Proportion of Body Fat in Men and Women

	Reference Man (lb)	Reference Woman (lb)
Weight	154	124
Total fat	23 (15%)	34 (27%)
Essential fat	5 (3%)	15 (12%)
Storage fat	19 (12%)	19 (15%)
Muscle	69 (45%)	45 (36%)
Bone	23 (15%)	15 (12%)
Remainder	39 (25%)	31 (25%)
Lean Body weight	136	107

TABLE 9-5 Recommended Energy Intake—Mean Heights and Weights

Category	Age (years)	Weight (kg)	Weight (lb)	Height (cm)	Height (in)	Energy Needs (kcal)
Infants	0.0-0.5	6	13	60	24	kg × 115
	0.5-1.0	9	20	71	28	kg × 105
Children	1-3	13	29	90	35	1300
	4-6	20	44	112	44	1700
	7-10	28	62	132	52	2400
Males	11-14	45	99	157	62	2700
	15-18	66	145	176	69	2800
	19-22	70	154	177	70	2900
	23-50	70	154	178	70	2700
	51-75	70	154	178	70	2400
	76+	70	154	178	70	2050
Females	11-14	46	101	157	62	2200
	15-18	55	120	163	64	2100
	19-22	55	120	163	64	2100
	23-50	55	120	163	64	2000
	51-75	55	120	163	64	1800
	76+	55	120	163	64	1600
Pregnancy						+300
Lactation						+500

Gender

In general, men have a higher BMR than women do (Table 9-4). The principal reason is that women have a higher proportion of body fat than men do.

Age

Age affects BMR because it changes the lean body mass, especially the amount of muscle. During childhood and adolescence, when there is rapid growth, lean body mass increases, and the muscles, liver, heart, and other soft tissues increase in size. In early adulthood, loss of muscle tissue decreases BMR and is responsible in part for the "middle-age spread" at the waistline that so many people complain about. During this period of life, less dietary energy is needed to maintain metabolically active tissues, so the excess is deposited in the body as fat.

The changes in BMR at both ends of the life cycle account in part for the increasing total energy requirements during growth and decreasing requirements during late adulthood as Table 9-5 indicates. Another important factor influencing total energy requirements is the amount of exercise and physical activity.

Pregnancy

During pregnancy, the muscles in the uterus increase in size because they are needed during delivery. In addition, the tissue mass of the fetus increases during the pregnancy. These changes produce a BMR about 20% above normal during the third trimester of pregnancy.

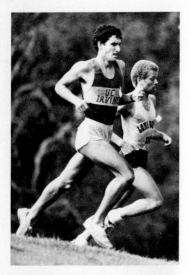

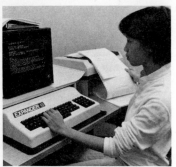

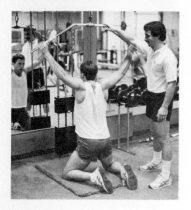

Different activities involve different energy expenditures. Sedentary occupations, and not enough physical activity, are major reasons for overweight and obesity.

Health factors

Ill health or trauma affects BMR. During starvation, injury, surgery, and severe weight-loss diets, there is a loss of some lean body mass, which decreases the BMR—actually an effective way for the body to save energy. BMR increases with recovery of lean tissues lost during the stress.

Fever increases BMR, as does an overactive thyroid gland, which produces too much of the iodine-containing hormone thyroxin. The opposite happens when the thyroid is underactive.

Exercise

Those exercises that increase muscle mass increase BMR—weight lifting is a good example. Indeed, there is some evidence that exercise slows down the natural loss of muscle mass during aging.

You Can Do a Rough Calculation of Your Own Basal Metabolic Rate

A truly accurate calculation of BMR requires elaborate procedures. However, the following formula gives an indication of the number of kcalories needed for basal metabolism. The answer is more accurate if you are of average body build. For men, the formula is:

$$1 \text{ kcalorie/kg body weight/hour}$$

For women, the formula is:

$$0.9 \text{ kcalorie/kg body weight/hour}$$

For example, if you are a young woman weighing 120 pounds, your BMR would be calculated as follows:

$$\frac{0.9 \times 120 \text{ pounds} \times 24 \text{ hours}}{2.2} = 1178 \text{ kcals}$$

Dividing by 2.2 converts pounds to kilograms (kg). Don't forget to multiply by 24 hours; you may work only an 8-hour day, but your vital body functions are working all 24 hours.

Physical Activity Is the Only Form of Energy Expenditure You Can Control

The amount of physical activity varies for different people. If you aren't very active, your physical activity may amount to only 20% to 40% of the total energy you expend.

The actual amount of physical activity expended is determined by body weight, the type and intensity of the activity, and the duration of the activity.

Body weight

You know that heavier cars use more energy (gasoline) per mile than lighter cars. The same physical principle is true of people: obese people use more energy than thin people to travel the same distance. Thus, suppose you weigh 120 lb (55 kg) and your friend weighs 200 lb (91 kg). In an hour of playing tennis, you might burn 357 kcalories and he or she would expend 595 kcalories. In an hour of aerobic dancing, you would expend 553 kcalories, but he or she would put out 922 kcalories.

Type and intensity of activity

With all the various types of physical activity available, as represented in Table 9-6, you can see that certain sports and physical tasks require much more energy than others. Obviously, an hour of cross-country running will burn off more kcalories than an hour of leisurely golf. An hour spent gently volleying a ball in a leisurely game of tennis requires fewer kcalories than an hour defending a Wimbledon championship.

TABLE 9-6　Energy Expenditure Depends on the Type and Duration of the Activity and on the Weight of the Person

| Activity | Kcaloric Expenditure (kcal) by Weight and Time | | | |
| | 120 lb (54.4 kg) | | 200 lb (90.9 kg) | |
	10 Minutes	60 Minutes	10 Minutes	60 Minutes
Running or jogging				
10 mph	137	824	229	1375
7.5 mph	105	630	175	1050
5 mph	74	442	122	736
Wrestling (practice)	110	600	180	1020
Bicycling				
12 mph	92	553	154	922
6 mph	35	210	58	349
Aerobic dancing	92	553	153	922
Dancing				
Fast	92	550	153	916
Slow	28	167	46	278
Walking				
Upstairs	79	471	131	786
4 mph	51	308	86	513
3 mph	34	206	57	344
Basketball	75	452	126	753
Football	72	432	120	720
Swimming (fast freestyle)	70	420	116	698
Skiing				
Cross-country	65	390	108	649
Downhill	50	280	78	450
Squash	60	357	99	595
Jumping rope	60	360	75	450
Hockey	60	360	75	450
Rugby	60	360	94	564
Tennis				
Singles	60	357	99	595
Doubles	35	210	58	350
Weight training	60	340	90	520
Soccer	55	330	85	512
Golf (walking and carrying bag)	46	278	77	450
Skating (ice or roller)	41	245	68	409
Calisthenics	36	216	60	360
Sailing	30	180	44	264
Volleyball	27	164	46	273
Bowling	25	150	35	210

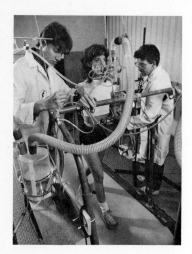

Oxygen intake and carbon dioxide output measure the energy cost of activities. This is usually done walking or running on a treadmill.

Brown Adipose Tissue (BAT)
Helps maintain body temperature so that less energy is lost in heat loss from the body.

Duration of activity

The more time you spend at an activity, of course, the more kcalories you will expend. If you spend 357 kcalories in one hour of tennis, then in two hours you will spend 714 kcalories if the game is played at the same level of intensity.

Energy Is Needed for Thermogenesis

Thermogenesis—production of body heat in the metabolism of food—is the third reason you need energy. Thermogenesis can be induced by diet, which is called *dietary thermogenesis, specific dynamic effect,* or *thermic effect of food (TEF).* Thermogenesis can also be induced by cold temperatures.

Between 5% and 10% of total energy intake is spent in digesting, absorbing, transporting, and storing food. Each one of these steps in incorporating food into your body can be related to everyday events that require energy. Digestion involves breaking large molecules into their smaller individual units. Some nutrients must be pumped across the barrier between the gastrointestinal tract and the blood. Transportation involves the energy spent by the heart in pumping the blood containing the nutrients around the body. Storage of reserves usually requires energy for synthesis, as in the combination of glycerol and fatty acids when fat is stored.

The importance of dietary thermogenesis on the overall energy balance of an individual is controversial.[1] It is not clear yet whether dietary thermogenesis is different in obese and nonobese people. It does seem that the higher the energy intake in a meal, the greater the effect on dietary thermogenesis, whereas exercise has no effect. Methodology is being improved so it can be determined if dietary thermogenesis plays any role in obesity.

Thermogenesis in *brown adipose tissue (BAT)*—which helps maintain body temperature—has in recent years surfaced in the popular press, partly because of its possible role in obesity.[2] BAT makes up only about 1% of body weight, and it is different from the white adipose tissue so many Americans struggle to control. BAT burns off excess energy as heat at a higher rate than the more common white adipose tissue. It does this through nonshivering and diet-induced thermogenesis. BAT has a high concentration of mitochondria and an excellent blood supply, which gives the tissue its brown color. BAT is important in newborn infants and in hibernating animals, which need to be able to retain adequate heat.

Why is BAT of possible significance in obesity? People with a small proportion of BAT may be more likely to become obese. They do not have the opportunity to produce a lot of heat through BAT's energy-inefficient, heat-producing metabolism. Thus, their extra dietary kcalories are stored as fat rather than burned for heat. The present conventional wisdom suggests that the contribution of BAT to metabolic rate in human beings is minor. However, researchers in obesity are still interested in BAT because of its ability to waste kcalories.[3]

Recommended Energy Intake

How much dietary energy should be consumed to meet the important energy demands of basal metabolism, physical activity, and dietary thermogenesis? The answer depends on your age, your gender, and whether you are pregnant or lactating (Table 9-5). These changes also affect recommended energy intake:

- Increased energy intake during the growing years is necessary for the synthesis of new body tissue and because of the high level of physical activity in this age group.
- Increased energy intake is recommended in pregnancy for the growth of the fetus and the body changes in the mother during pregnancy. Lactation requires extra energy for the production of milk.
- Less energy intake is required in older people because the basal metabolic rate decreases and, for most older people, the level of physical activity also drops.

This information is used in Chapter 10, when we discuss why some people are underweight and some are overweight.

> We need energy for basal metabolism, physical activity, and thermogenesis. Basal energy has the highest requirement for energy in most nonactive people. People vary in basal energy requirements because of differences in the amount of lean tissue and body fat. Recommended energy intakes depend on age, gender, and physical state (for instance, pregnancy or lactation).

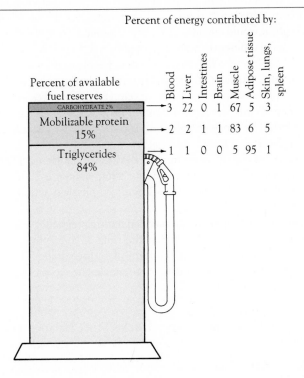

Percent of energy contributed by:

Percent of available fuel reserves

	Blood	Liver	Intestines	Brain	Muscle	Adipose tissue	Skin, lungs, spleen
CARBOHYDRATE 2%	3	22	0	1	67	5	3
Mobilizable protein 15%	2	2	1	1	83	6	5
Triglycerides 84%	1	1	0	0	5	95	1

FIGURE 9-3
Available fuel reserves in an adult man.

ENERGY STORES

The energy needed for basal energy, physical activity, and thermogenesis is provided by carbohydrates, fats, and proteins, as indicated in Figure 9-3. (See also the Metabolism Notes at the end of Chapter 8.) However, it takes time to move these

Adenosine Triphosphate (ATP)
A storage form of energy, used as an immediate source of energy.

sources of energy from their storage sites to the places of activity (usually muscles). It also takes time to liberate the energy at the activity site, for the energy nutrients must go through a series of chemical reactions. In short, your body needs to be able to store some of the energy from carbohydrates, fats, and proteins in a form that is available immediately. That energy-storage form is *adenosine triphosphate (ATP)*.

ATP contains three phosphorus atoms. (The complete chemical structure of ATP is not important here.) The energy released when ATP is broken down is used by energy-requiring cells, especially muscle cells. More ATP is produced from the energy in carbohydrates, fats, and proteins to replace what was used. As Figure 9-4 indicates, in the typical diet in industrialized countries, most of the ATP comes from carbohydrates and fat.

Most of the ATP produced from the energy nutrients is done under aerobic conditions, though some is generated anaerobically (without oxygen). This information has some practical applications. ATP helped our primitive ancestors flee from danger, but today we are more likely to use it to give us the immediate burst of energy needed to pursue a departing bus or a ball on the far side of the court.

Your Recommended Energy Intake Depends on Many Variables

How many kcalories of energy people need to take in and store depends on their basal metabolism, physical activity, and thermogenesis. If the RDAs for energy were set too high, it would encourage obesity. Therefore, scientists have established the RDA for energy differently than they established the RDAs for other nutrients. The energy RDAs represent the *average* needs of people in each age group,[4] whereas the RDAs for other nutrients represent the upper limits of variability for almost all people within the same age and sex group. Energy intakes are recommended on the basis of an average desirable weight for men of 154 lb (70 kg) and for women of 120 lb (55 kg). The range in values in Table 9-5 allows for differences in body weight and in physical activity.

RDA values for energy increase from birth through adulthood (Table 9-5). The RDA for adult men is 2700 kcalories and for adult women is 2000 kcalories. This value goes down after age 50 because of decreased physical activity and decreased basal energy requirements.

Increased energy intakes are recommended during pregnancy and lactation. The energy needs of the fetus actually start at the time of conception, but this energy comes from the mother, mainly in the form of carbohydrate. Thus, some of the increased energy RDA for pregnant women enables her to provide the necessary energy to the developing fetus.

To Keep Weight Constant, Energy Intake Must Balance Energy Expenditure

Many people in North America are overweight. This means they may need to consume *less* than the RDA intake of energy cited above.[3] On the other hand, some children and adults gain excessive amounts of body fat even though they actually are consuming an amount of energy appropriate for their body weight, gender, age, and activity, which means they should probably increase their physical activity.

FIGURE 9-4
Estimated daily production of ATP. These percentages represent the energy ingested by a person eating a North American or European diet.

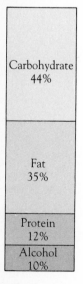

Carbohydrate 44%

Fat 35%

Protein 12%

Alcohol 10%

A few important points must be kept in mind:

- Protein synthesis requires a lot of energy intake. Especially during pregnancy, lactation, and the growing years, enough energy must be taken in to use dietary protein for growth and maintenance.
- If the energy content in a person's diet is too low (under 1200 kcalories), the diet may not provide enough minerals and vitamins. Thus, the intake of foods with low nutrient content—foods with refined sugar, fats, and alcohol—should be avoided.

It may be best to concentrate on the factor of exercise in considering energy balance. Lack of exercise may be associated with coronary heart disease, obesity, diabetes, and gallstones.

Too Much or Too Little Food or Activity May Upset Energy Storage Balance

A person's body weight will be changed by anything that upsets the balance between energy intake and energy output, whether the cause is overeating, dieting, starvation, or strenuous physical activity.

Overeating

Your weight will go up if you consume more energy in the diet than you expend in basal metabolism, physical activity, and thermogenesis. The reason is the increase in body fat. As Figure 9-3 shows, there is very little storage capacity for extra kcalories in any tissue except adipose tissue.

Dieting

Some popular weight-reducing diets require an energy intake of 600 to 800 kcalories per day. This amount is simply not adequate to meet recommended intakes of energy or the energy requirements for basal metabolism for most people. Therefore, glycogen and some amino acids are broken down into glucose to satisfy the brain's need for glucose. The amino acids come from tissue protein, especially muscle, because there is only a limited supply of free amino acids in the body (Figure 9-5). This loss of tissue protein could be harmful. Body fat is broken down to fatty acids and glycerol. Ketones are produced from fat catabolism during the advanced stage of dieting.

Starvation

Much the same series of events happens in starvation as in severe dieting. Glycogen is depleted so the body uses ketone bodies derived from fat (Figure 9-5). These are the backup sources of energy for the brain when the ability to form glucose decreases. Tissue protein continues to be broken down so that some of the amino acids can be converted into glucose. Photographs of starving people show extensive loss of muscle, because muscle protein is broken down for energy, but other tissues are also involved. The effects of starvation are seen not only in victims of famine but also in those suffering from anorexia nervosa and in some advanced stages of cancer.

Strenuous physical activity

Some athletes require enormous energy intakes, but the amounts depend on the sport or event (Table 9-6). Pole vaulters, divers, sprinters, fencers, and lighter-

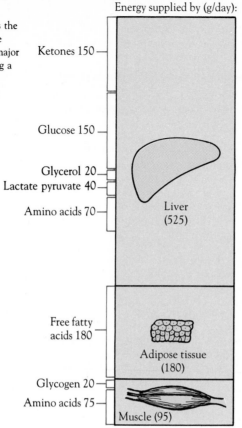

Energy supplied by (g/day):

Ketones 150

Glucose 150

Glycerol 20
Lactate pyruvate 40

Amino acids 70

Liver
(525)

Free fatty
acids 180

Adipose tissue
(180)

Glycogen 20
Amino acids 75

Muscle (95)

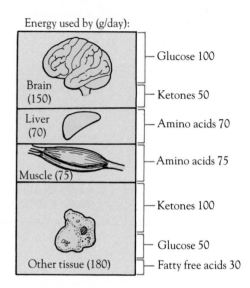

Energy used by (g/day):

Brain
(150)

Glucose 100

Ketones 50

Liver
(70)

Amino acids 70

Muscle (75)

Amino acids 75

Other tissue (180)

Ketones 100

Glucose 50
Fatty free acids 30

weight boxers may eat 4500 to 5000 kcalories a day. Long-distance runners, skiers, cyclists, and gymnasts may require 5500 to 6000 kcalories a day, as may those playing basketball, soccer, and hockey.

All of these events require a great deal of muscle work. Muscles at rest use more fat than glucose as a source of energy. This fat comes from the small amounts stored in muscle (which in raw animal meat appears as the marbling or white flecks of fat) and within the muscle fibers. ATP is the fuel that is burned to release the energy during physical activity. Because supplies of ATP are used quickly, muscle glycogen is broken down to produce more ATP. Thereafter the fuel is a mixture of carbohydrate and fat, especially during strenuous events like marathon runs.

The body needs dietary energy to meet the energy demands of basal metabolism, physical activity, and thermogenesis. Excess dietary energy is stored, mostly in the adipose tissue. Adenosine triphosphate (ATP) is the energy source available immediately on demand. Recommended dietary intake of energy depends on the body weight, age, gender, and activity pattern of a person. Body weight is lost during weight-loss dieting, starvation, or strenuous physical activity when dietary energy intake does not meet energy expenditure demands. Overeating coupled with inactivity causes body weight gains.

IN PRAISE OF EXERCISE

Exercising increases your pulse rate because the heart is working harder than usual in pumping blood to the muscles. The normal pulse rate for a person at rest is 70 to 72 beats per minute for men and 78 to 82 per minute for women. However, the optimal pulse rate during exercise varies according to one's age—and, of course, according to one's physical condition. Exercise physiologists recommend that people try to attain the "target zone" pulse rates shown in Table 9-7. The target zone is the number of heartbeats per minute sustained for 30 minutes for a person who exercises at least three times a week.

TABLE 9-7 Exercise Pulse Rates

Age	Target zone*
20	120-150
25	117-146
30	114-142
35	111-138
40	108-135
45	105-131
50	102-127
55	99-123
60	96-120
65	93-116
70	90-113

* "Target zone" is the pulse rate or heart rate in beats per minute. Exercise that sustains that target zone level for 30 minutes should be undertaken at least three times per week. Persons over 40 who have not been exercising regularly should consult a doctor before embarking on such a program.

You have been told that regular exercise throughout life has significant advantages for one's general health and well-being, as shown in Table 9-8. However, you should also note some of the disadvantages shown in the table, although most of these drawbacks occur only when the exercise is excessive and compulsive. Conditions for which exercise is said to be beneficial, both as prevention and as treatment, include obesity, cardiovascular disease, osteoporosis, diabetes, hypertension, and diseases related to impaired immunity.[5]

Fat becomes the main source of energy when the supply of muscle and liver glycogen is reduced, and this has positive effects in a weight-loss program. However, there is also a loss of muscle protein because some amino acids in muscle are sent to the liver for conversion into glucose. This loss is not a problem in well-fed people; marathon runners, for instance, have been found to have more lean tissue, including muscle, than nonmarathoners do, and they also have more bone.[6] These changes may be advantageous during the aging process.

Exercise produces no change in total cholesterol levels in the blood. However, depending on the exercise, there may be an increase in high-density lipoprotein (HDL) and a decrease in low-density lipoprotein (LDL). Casual jogging, unfortunately, does not seem to have much effect on a person's cholesterol level, but soccer and, to a lesser extent, ice hockey have a positive effect on HDL levels.[7]

Biochemistry

Be aware that different types of exercise have different effects on the body.

TABLE 9-8 Advantages and Disadvantages of Exercise During the Life Cycle

Life Stage	Benefits	Possible Adverse Consequences
Childhood	Establish lifelong exercise and health habits	Inability to meet energy needs and compromised growth and development
Adolescence	Prevent and treat obesity and eating disorders Establish lifelong exercise and health habits	Inadequate energy intake Oxidation of dietary protein for energy Irregular menstruation Negative calcium balance and reduced bone mass Sports anemia Anorexia athletica
Adulthood	Weight control Prevent and treat many diseases Promote mental health and feelings of well being	Possible increased need for riboflavin and vitamin B_6
Pregnancy	Control of excessive weight gain More favorable nutrient profile as a result of an increased energy intake Possibly less constipation and varicose veins	Low weight gain Low birth weight infant
Lactation	Promotes return to prepregnancy weight Possibly improve postpartum mental status	Excessive rate of weight loss that compromises milk production and infant growth
Elderly	Favorable effects on age-related physiological changes Prevent and treat osteoporosis Socialization	Exercise-related injuries leading to disability and other complications

If you are interested in losing weight, you may wish to know that increased physical activity is better than dieting.[8] Exercise can offer some rewards, some of which are mentioned in Table 9-8, whereas dieting can simply be frustating. On a diet, for instance, you may notice rapid weight loss at first and a slower weight loss later—the decreased rate being a result of decreased basal metabolic rate. For inactive people, BMR is the greatest user of dietary energy, and the body is quite sensitive to major changes in food intake. If a dieter switches from 3000 kcalories a day to only 600 to 800 kcalories, some scientists theorize that the body will respond as it would in a starving person: it will seek every means possible to save energy to maintain life. This means that the basal energy will be decreased. In extreme cases, all vital body processes will be affected: heart rate and breathing slow, body temperature drops, muscle tone decreases, glands slow production of secretions, and new cells are not produced. Because energy demands for all these activities are lowered, the rate of body weight loss is slowed. Possible good news, however, is that exercise during dieting will prevent this decrease in basal energy needs. Basal energy requirements remain constant; therefore, the rate of weight loss continues at a greater rate during this critical period.[9]

Nutritionists recognize the beneficial effects of exercise. It consumes excess energy eaten in the diet, increases serum HDL, and increases basal energy requirements (because of the greater proportion of muscle). The type and duration of exercise must be defined to determine the extent of the interactions with the diet.

BODY WEIGHT: CAN YOU KEEP IT CONSTANT?

Maybe weight gain (or loss) is not a problem for you, but there are certainly a number of people for whom it is. As you have seen, body weight depends on the balance of kcalories eaten and kcalories expended—and that can be finely balanced indeed.

Consider: 3500 excess kcalories will gain you one pound of body fat; a deficit of 3500 kcalories will lose you one pound. This means that if you keep your energy intake and output constant over one year, but you take half a teaspoonful of sugar (about 10 kcalories) extra in one cup of coffee every day, you will be one pound fatter at the end of the year. To remove this extra pound, a 120 lb person would have to do aerobic dancing for about five hours and a 200 lb person for about four hours. (Table 9-6 showed some other, less vigorous examples.)

Over the course of a year, meeting the daily RDA for energy requires 985,500 kcalories for men and 730,000 kcalories for women. Considered in the light of these large numbers, then, 3500 kcalories is quite small. It is a wonder, therefore, that we do not have even greater changes in body weight.

Short-term Weight Changes May Result from Water

A word about short-term changes in body weight: most of the time, they are due to increased or decreased amounts of *water* rather than changes in the amount of fat in the body. A decrease in body weight may come about because of dehydration caused by diarrhea or by diuretics, both of which are dangerous to health. An increase may occur during pregnancy, when some women retain water in the extracellular fluid, producing edema. Another reason for changes in the amount of water in the body is that some chemicals in the body combine with water; the addition of 500 g of glycogen, for example, means an extra 2.2 liters of body water.[8] The point is this: Weight changes may not be changes in body fat, only changes in water, a matter we will take up again in Chapter 10.

Alcoholics May Gain Kcalories but Lose Weight

Something does not quite add up correctly when we calculate the kcaloric contribution from alcohol into the relationship between intake and expenditure of energy in alcoholics. One gram of alcohol contains 7 kcalories (when measured in the bomb calorimeter), but alcoholics do not gain weight even though they consume a lot of these alcoholic kcalories. Although much remains to be learned about the effects of alcohol on metabolic rate, recent evidence suggests that the liver's mechanism for detoxifying alcohol and drugs increases metabolic activity.[10] As mentioned in Chapter 8 (Metabolism Notes), the microsomal ethanol oxidizing system (MEOS) involves significant increases in energy expenditure. Therefore, much of the energy from alcohol is apparently used to maintain its own detoxification system rather than being deposited as fat. This effect does not seem to occur in nonalcoholics, nor does it occur in alcoholics with liver disease, for whom the long-term effects of alcohol may have damaged the MEOS. It is estimated that there are 18 to 20 million chronic alcoholics without liver disease in the U.S.[10]

Metabolic Rate and Menstruation May Affect Body Weight in Women

New evidence suggests special considerations may be involved in calculating energy balance for women. According to the information presented in Figure 9-2, the basal metabolic rate (resting metabolic rate, RMR) accounts for about 65% to 70% of a person's daily energy expenditure. Is this really true? Some recent evidence says current available tables overestimate RMR for women by 7% to 14%.[11] This means that new equations for RMR are needed.

If you are a woman, whether nonathlete or athlete, you can calculate your own RMR using the following formulas:

For nonathlete:

$$795 + (7.18 \times \text{body weight (kg)})$$

For athlete:

$$50.4 + (21.1 \times \text{body weight (kg)})$$

As before, you find your weight in kilograms by dividing your weight in pounds by 2.2.

For example, if you are a 130 lb female *nonathlete,* your RMR will be:

$$RMR = 795 + \frac{7.18 \times 130 \text{ lb}}{2.2}$$

$$= 795 + 424 \text{ kcalories}$$

$$= 1219 \text{ kcalories}$$

If you are a 130 lb female *athlete,* your RMR will be:

$$RMR = 50.4 + \frac{21.1 \times 130 \text{ lb}}{2.2}$$

$$= 50.4 + 1247 \text{ kcalories}$$

$$= 1297.4 \text{ kcalories}$$

Even though body weights are similar, the athlete has a higher RMR, partly because she has less body fat and more muscle.

 Endocrinology

Another factor that alters energy considerations in women is menstruation. Apparently, menstruation causes about a 9% increase in 24-hour energy expenditure,[12] a matter that was confirmed when no increase in energy expenditure was observed when an oral contraceptive agent (the pill) was taken. The increase in energy expenditure is caused by progesterone, the female sex hormone, acting as a metabolic stimulant. Some women are known to increase energy intake by 500 kcalories per day in the days following ovulation.

People gain body fat slowly, yet want to lose it quickly. However, body-weight loss should be done slowly, by increasing energy expenditure or decreasing kcaloric intake. Potentially dangerous weight-reducing methods, including the use of diuretics, should be avoided. Energy in alcohol is used inefficiently by alcoholics. New information suggests attention must be given to calculating resting metabolic rate and the effect of menstruation in women.

Decisions

1. Will Light ("Lite") Beer and Food Make Me Lighter?

The light and diet food business is booming—$25.8 billion U.S. sales in 1982-1983—but what does "light" or "lite" really mean in nutrition language? You can buy so-called light versions of pancake mixes and syrups, salad dressings, pudding, cheese, gravy mixes, mayonnaise, chocolate topping, and blue cheese, and you can wash all of this down with lite beer or wine. These products may be "light" because they have less sugar, fat, or alcohol, which makes them lower in kcalories, or they may be "light" because they are light in color, taste, or texture.

Terminology is important here, and since 1980 the Food and Drug Administration has regulated the following terms:

- *Low calorie* means that a serving must have no more than 40 kcalories and no more than 0.4 kcalories per gram. Foods marketed under this term must carry a nutrition label. Foods naturally low in kcalories, such as mushrooms, cannot use the term "low calorie" before the word "mushroom," although they can be labeled "mushrooms, a low calorie food."
- *Reduced calories* means the product is at least one third lower in kcalories than a similar food in which the kcalories are not reduced. Foods marketed under this term must also carry a nutrition label.
- *Light and lite:* Light/lite food must taste and smell like the "regular" (heavy?) food. Lite beers generally have about 100 kcalories per 12 ounce serving. This gives them about one third fewer kcalories than regular beer. If the ingredients in the food are altered too much in the "lightening" of the food, then it must be labeled as "imitation" or be given a new name.

Although "light" and "lite" usually mean food that is low or reduced in kcalories, they also have other meanings. "Light cream" has at least 18% and less than 30% milk fat. Light syrup in some canned fruits has a different amount of liquid and sweeteners when compared with regular syrups. Light (lite) salt is a mixture of sodium chloride and potassium chloride. Light chocolate is paler in color than dark chocolate because it contains milk or cream. Finally, light whiskey is stored in used or uncharred oak containers. (Thanks to Louise Fenner of the Food and Drug Administration for shedding some, er, light on the subject.)

The word *balance* has been used many times in this chapter. The kcalories from light food and drink enter into the balance between energy intake and energy output. Some advertisers try to convince consumers that these kcalories are somehow "lighter" than regular kcalories, and therefore less fattening, but obviously if the total intake of kcalories is not decreased, light foods and drinks will not help anyone's weight problem.

The final word of caution. Know what the words in advertising and product descriptions really mean before making decisions about some of these so-called light foods and drinks.

Lots of foods are "light" these days. It is total kcaloric intake, and not the number of kcalories in a few "light" products, that determines whether or not a person will be obese.

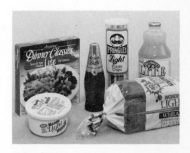

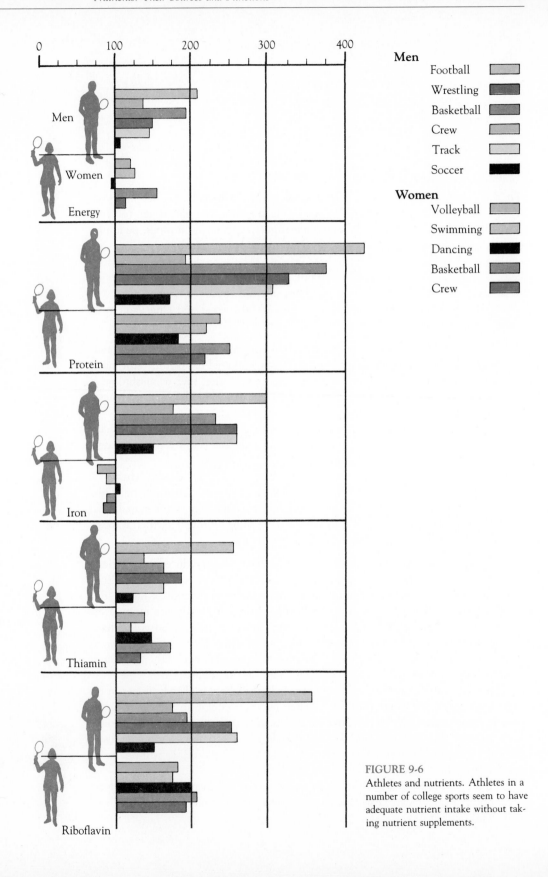

Men

Football	
Wrestling	
Basketball	
Crew	
Track	
Soccer	

Women

Volleyball	
Swimming	
Dancing	
Basketball	
Crew	

FIGURE 9-6
Athletes and nutrients. Athletes in a number of college sports seem to have adequate nutrient intake without taking nutrient supplements.

2. Will Caffeine Improve My Athletic Performance?

Caffeine has been used as a stimulant since the Stone Age,[13] and athletes have used it for years in hopes of improving performance. But does it really work? High intakes—more than 10 cups of coffee per day—can cause increased anxiety, sleeplessness, diarrhea, and altered heartbeats, so the International Olympic Committee has banned "high" intakes of caffeine. Actually, the limited evidence available suggests that caffeine has no effect anyway on energy or performance in short-term, intense exercise involving strength and power. It does, however, improve alertness in events such as shooting and archery. As for long-distance events, caffeine is thought to improve endurance by stimulating muscles to use fatty acids instead of glucose as the source of energy. This change in fuel use by the muscles is to the athlete's advantage.

3. Do Athletes Need Dietary Supplements?

The short answer is: no, athletes don't need dietary supplements—except in unusual circumstances. Most college athletes, after all, have more than adequate nutrient intakes, as Figure 9-6 makes clear. The only common nutrition problem is low dietary iron intake for female athletes; however, the extent of iron deficiency in well-trained athletes, including long-distance runners, is uncertain.[14]

Extra amounts of a nutrient will not improve performance if dietary intake is satisfactory, and most nutritionists believe that nutrient supplements are unnecessary. In ranking important factors, Peter van Handel, director of the Sports Physiology Laboratory, U.S. Olympic Committee, ranks the importance of nutrition *after* genetic potential and training.

Despite this, athletes are exposed to a lot of literature about nutrition supplements. For instance, popular magazines try to dramatize the importance of bee pollen, calling it "a vital source of energy, stamina and general good health"; "low in calories but high in energy"; "proven 100% safe in over 15,000 years of use." But how can a food be low in calories but high in energy? That doesn't make scientific sense. Bee pollen will not make you a better athlete.

Sometimes, however, even the scientific literature can contain puzzling information. A report by Russian scientists claims that a mixture of vitamins, amino acids, and minerals increased physical work capacity, the rate of muscle work, and movement coordination and reduced the time taken to make a decision or to solve mathematical problems.[15] This would be wonderful if it is true, but the paper does not state how much of each nutrient was taken and whether the subjects were deficient in these nutrients before the testing started. These scientists also had a rather poor knowledge of nutrition. Their supplement contained a substance called *rutin*, which is not a nutrient, and "organic K" and "pH salts," which are not known to nutritionists.

In summary, the promises of nutrient supplements are extravagant, and the outcome is usually disappointing.

Summary

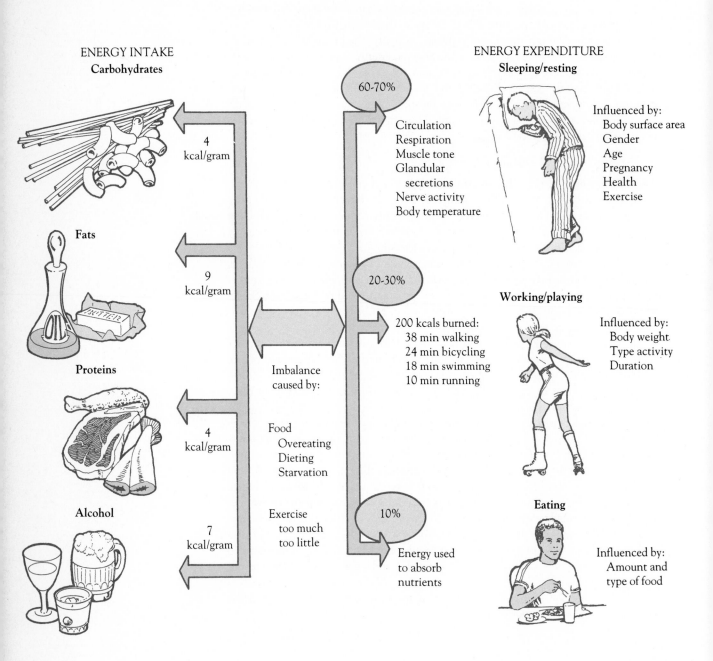

ENERGY INTAKE

Carbohydrates

4 kcal/gram

Fats

9 kcal/gram

Proteins

4 kcal/gram

Alcohol

7 kcal/gram

Imbalance
caused by:

Food
Overeating
Dieting
Starvation

Exercise
too much
too little

ENERGY EXPENDITURE

Sleeping/resting

60-70%

Circulation
Respiration
Muscle tone
Glandular
  secretions
Nerve activity
Body temperature

Influenced by:
  Body surface area
  Gender
  Age
  Pregnancy
  Health
  Exercise

20-30%

Working/playing

200 kcals burned:
  38 min walking
  24 min bicycling
  18 min swimming
  10 min running

Influenced by:
  Body weight
  Type activity
  Duration

10%

Eating

Energy used
to absorb
nutrients

Influenced by:
  Amount and
  type of food

REFERENCES

1. Belko, A.Z., and others: Effect of energy and protein intake and exercise intensity on the thermic effect of food, American Journal of Clinical Nutrition **43**:863, 1986.

2. Himms-Hagen, J.: Brown adipose tissue metabolism and thermogenesis, Annual Review of Nutrition **5**:69, 1985.

3. Schulz, L.O., Brown adipose tissue: Regulation of thermogenesis and implications for obesity, Journal of the American Dietetic Association **87**:761, 1987.

4. Committee on Dietary Allowances, Food and Nutrition Board: Recommended dietary allowances, 9th revised edition, Washington, D.C., National Academy of Sciences, 1980.

5. Kris-Etherton, P.M.: Nutrition and the exercising female, Nutrition Today, p. 6, March/April, 1986.

6. Aloia, J.F., and others: Skeletal mass and body composition in marathon runners, Metabolism **27**:1793, 1978.

7. Lehtonen, A., and Viikari, J.: Serum lipids in soccer and ice-hockey players, Metabolism **29**:36, 1980.

8. Donahoe, C.P., Jr., and others: Metabolic consequences of dieting and exercise in the treatment of obesity, Journal of Consulting and Clinical Psychology **52**:827, 1984.

9. Grand, F.: Body weight, composition and energy balance. In Present knowledge in nutrition, 5th edition, Washington, D.C., The Nutrition Foundation, Inc., p. 7, 1984.

10. Jhangiani, S.S., and others: Energy expenditure in chronic alcoholics with and without liver disease, American Journal of Clinical Nutrition **44**:323, 1986.

11. Owen, O.E., and others: A reappraisal of caloric requirements in healthy women, American Journal of Clinical Nutrition **44**:1, 1986.

12. Webb, P.: 24-hour energy expenditure and the menstrual cycle, American Journal of Clinical Nutrition **44**:614, 1986.

13. Slavin, J.L., and Joensen, D.J.: Caffeine and sports performance, Physician and Sports Medicine, May 1985, p. 191.

14. Jacobs, M.B., and Wilson, W.: Iron deficiency anemia in a vegetarian runner, Journal of the American Medical Association **252**:481, 1984.

15. Ushakov, A.S., and others: Effect of vitamin and amino acid supplements on human performance during heavy mental and physical work, Aviation, Space, and Environmental Medicine **49**:1184, 1978.

16. Koivisto, V.A.: The physiology of marathon running, Science Progress **70**:109, 1986.

METABOLISM NOTES: *Running the Marathon*

Scientists have learned much in recent years about the biochemical processes whereby energy nutrients are used for energy production in various exercises. The following is a brief sampling from a fascinating area of study.

The Nutrients Needed To Fuel a Marathon Run

Total energy consumption during a marathon run is in the 2400 to 2800 kcalorie range.[16] This is more than that consumed during 24 hours of sedentary life. When the starting gun is fired, the first fuel for energy is ATP in the muscles. Glycogen

FIGURE 9-7
Fuels used by muscles during a marathon race. When there is no more muscle glycogen the runner "hits the wall," and usually drops out of the race.

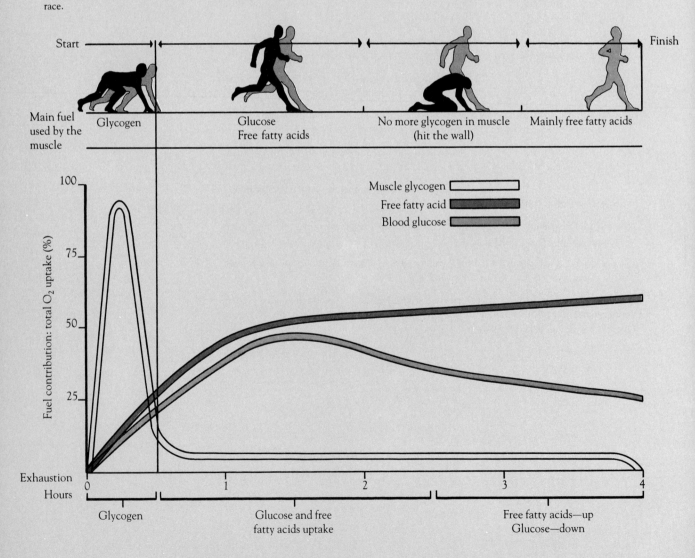

| Main fuel used by the muscle | Glycogen | Glucose Free fatty acids | No more glycogen in muscle (hit the wall) | Mainly free fatty acids |

Legend:
- Muscle glycogen
- Free fatty acid
- Blood glucose

Fuel contribution: total O₂ uptake (%)

Hours: 0, 1, 2, 3, 4 — Exhaustion

Glycogen   Glucose and free fatty acids uptake   Free fatty acids—up / Glucose—down

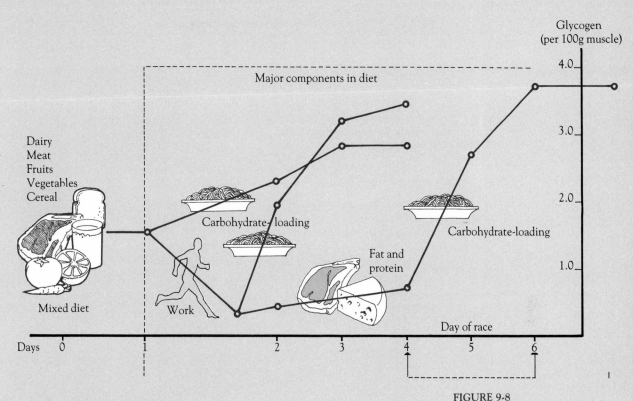

FIGURE 9-8
Carbohydrate (glycogen) loading. Exercise or hard physical work depletes muscle glycogen. Glycogen is "packed in" to the muscles by high-carbohydrate diets.

provides much of the energy during the first 20 minutes of the race (Figure 9-7). As the race progresses, the energy sources must be imported from other parts of the body. The importance of glycogen declines and that of free fatty acids and blood glucose increases. Near the end of the race, the contribution of muscle glycogen is low but nonetheless important. When the supply of muscle glycogen is exhausted, the runner is exhausted, and for him or her the race is over.

Trained Athletes Versus Untrained People: How They Metabolize Energy Nutrients Differently

Unlike most desk-bound or nonexercising people, a trained athlete uses carbohydrates less and fats more as a source of energy.[16] Most of this fat comes from adipose tissue. This helps the trained runner because the longer the athlete can use fatty acids for energy the longer it will be before the final reserves of glycogen are depleted—when he or she "hits the wall," as they say in runners' jargon, and there is no more muscle glycogen.

"Carbohydrate Loading" for Athletes: The Biochemical Explanation

Long-distance runners have become fascinated by carbohydrate (glycogen) loading in recent years. The idea is to pack as much glycogen as possible into muscles so as to delay the onset of fatigue. However, this technique should be used cautiously— certainly not by any athlete with medical problems, especially heart problems. Athletes report stiffness in muscles after carbohydrate loading, because of the accumulation of water in the muscles.

TABLE 9-9 A 3800-Kcalorie Carbohydrate-Loading Diet

	Kcalories	% Carbohydrates
8 oz orange juice	110	93
½ cup Grape-nuts	210	88
1 medium banana	140	94
8 oz low-fat milk	110	48
1 whole wheat English muffin	130	83
1 tbsp jelly	50	100
2 oz turkey, sliced	155	—
2 sl bran bread	175	74
Lettuce/tomato	25	83
8 oz apple juice	120	100
1 cup lemon sherbet	275	91
3 cup spaghetti (6 oz uncooked)	625	82
½ cup tomato sauce with mushrooms	75	64
2 tbsp Parmesan cheese	55	—
¼ loaf French bread	300	75
1 cup apple crisp with	400	82
¼ cup raisins	130	97
16 oz cranberry juice	290	100
6 fig cookies	330	80
Total kcalories =	3815	80% carbohydrate kcalories

This sample diet is not only high in carbohydrates, but also high in fiber. The competing athlete does not want to be constipated.

The supposed advantage of the technique applies only to events involving more than 90 to 120 minutes of noninterrupted activity. Forget carbohydrate loading if you are a sprinter or a football or basketball player. People practicing the technique are generally marathon runners and long-distance cross-country skiers.

The process of loading the muscles with glycogen starts about 3 to 5 days before a race (Figure 9-8) and the athlete has two choices:

- To load up the muscle with glycogen by eating a high-carbohydrate diet, such as that shown in Table 9-9.
- To do hard physical work (it can be running) about 3 to 5 days before the race in order to use up much of the stored muscle glycogen, then replace this glycogen by eating high-carbohydrate diets.

In addition, higher muscle glycogen levels are achieved if a high-fat, high-protein diet is eaten for the first 2 to 3 days *after* the exhausting work (Figure 9-8). This is followed on the third day by a diet high in carbohydrate. Notice that the muscle glycogen level is now higher than it was at the start of the carbohydrate loading exercise. This extra amount of glycogen is what is meant to make all the difference as to whether the marathon is finished or not.

When To Take Carbohydrate Drinks During a Race: The Best and Worst Times

There are biochemical reasons for the best and the worst time to take carbohydrate drinks when running a long-distance race, especially a marathon.

Don't take a glucose drink shortly before a race. This will cause a rise in blood insulin levels, and carbohydrate rather than fatty acids will now be your main energy source. Therefore, muscle glycogen is broken down at a faster rate, with the resulting earlier exhaustion. If fructose is taken instead of glucose, the insulin response does not occur. This is good for the runner because glycogen is not broken down as quickly as when glucose was the energy source in the drink.

Do take a glucose drink during the race. This is good, especially if taken in small amounts repeatedly.[16] Glucose is synthesized to glycogen, which will be used later rather than burned immediately as glucose. Studies have shown that glucose or sucrose (sugar) taken during long-distance runs and cycle races is helpful in preventing a decline in blood glucose. Glycogen breakdown is reduced by 20% in these athletes.

Note, however, that not all experts agree about taking glucose during a race. Some argue that exercise produces a decrease in the digestion and absorption of nutrients by decreasing stomach emptying. As a result, the sugar, or glucose, will sit in the stomach and will not get into the blood to be taken to the muscle. By remaining in the stomach, it can cause further trouble by having a negative effect on body fluid balance. Maintenance of proper fluid balance during endurance exercise is very important. Glucose in the right concentration when exhaustion is near may have some short-term positive effects. Clearly, this is not an area for people with little knowledge of the links between nutrition and exercise physiology.

10 Obesity, Eating Disorders, and Starvation

CONNECTIONS

What is going on in the body when food intake is too high or too low? In this chapter, you will see that a great deal of the information presented throughout the book applies here.

The problems we will discuss here are responsible for a lot of human suffering. Too high an intake of food causes obesity and bulimia, too low an intake occurs in anorexia nervosa, extreme dieting, and starvation. Anorexia nervosa, an extreme loss of appetite, and bulimia, a "binge and purge" style of eating, are called eating disorders and are found mainly among teenage girls from middle- and upper-income families.

Obesity is a problem mainly of women, quite often affecting women from lower income levels. Starvation principally occurs among very poor people, such as those suffering from famine in developing countries.

Although treatment of obesity, eating disorders, and starvation has not been very successful, success is possible, and the solutions draw on many scientific disciplines, from the social and medical sciences.

Obesity, starvation, and eating disorders are among the saddest facts of life.

How do obese people think about themselves? Here is what one woman patient told A. J. Strunkard when asked what she hoped to get out of treatment: "To become a worthwhile member of the human race. . . . I think of myself as a great mass of gray-green, amorphous material. Then at times I feel like a sloth. And just now, when I got up on the examining table, I felt like an elephant." Rarely, says Strunkard, had he heard anyone, even patients hospitalized for mental illness, condemn themselves with such intensity.

Even less fortunate, however, are people suffering from starvation. W. R. Aykroyd described victims of the 1943 famine in Bengal, India, as follows:

Many of the patients in the famine hospitals were picked up in a state of extreme weakness and collapse, often on the point of death. They were for the most part emaciated to such a degree that the description 'living skeletons' was justifiable. Many suffered from mental disorientation, showing a very marked degree of apathy and indifference to their surroundings. When taken to hospital, such patients made very little effort to help themselves and received medical attention with an indifference which sometimes amounted to passive obstruction. They did not care how dirty or naked they were.

Eating disorders, such as suppression of appetite (anorexia) and binge and purge eating (bulimia), have only come into prominence in recent years; unlike starvation and obesity, they seem to be identified with women from comfortable economic circumstances. A. H. Crisp, for example, describes a young woman from a close-knit middle-class family of three children. Her parents "attach absolute importance to academic and artistic achievement, and they maintain fitness by regular sports including jogging. Jennifer, whom the parents had expected to be a boy, kept pace with the rest of the family. . . . Tall and thin, she watched herself for any sign of flabbiness and was dismayed by evidence of her developing puberty. . . . As an aid to the maintenance of low body weight, she secretly purged herself."

Being too fat or too thin can lead to significant physical, mental, and social disturbances and even death. The reasons why a person is underweight or overweight may differ.

THE PREVALENCE OF OBESITY, EATING DISORDERS, AND HUNGER

How widespread are obesity, eating disorders such as anorexia nervosa and bulimia, and hunger and starvation?

Obesity and Overweight Are Difficult Problems to Fight

Obesity and overweight are familiar health problems in industrialized countries. People who are not obese sometimes take pains to emphasize that fact. An international medical journal recently included a photograph that featured a car in a Chicago driveway with personalized license plates that read "NOT FAT." Over 30% of adults and 15% to 20% of school-age children in the United States are overweight. The reason obesity is so widespread is simple: it is difficult to lose excess fat and to keep that excess fat off. Indeed, more than 29,000 claims, theories, and treatments have been documented for losing weight. That is not a misprint, it really is 29,000. However, fewer than 6% of these have been found to be effective, and 13% are downright hazardous. The remaining thousands of methods are so absurd or ineffective that they do not deserve mention, were it not for the fact that they help drive the multi-billion dollar weight-reducing industry.[1]

The poor success rate of methods to prevent and control obesity indicates it is a complex problem. As we will show shortly, losing weight is actually relatively easy to do. However, weight reduction can be considered successful only when the weight loss: (1) is done without harming one's health and (2) is maintained permanently. Stated another way, the problem is that:

- Fat, and not other body tissue, should be lost
- The extra pounds must be kept off permanently

Most of the popular weight-reduction methods fail on one or both counts.

> You should ask many questions about any "new" diets, but ask them of competent health professionals.

Famine and Starvation Are Still Widespread

We may be accustomed to thinking of famine and starvation as age-old problems, as indeed they are, but what we may not be aware of is the great number of famines occurring during modern times. Between 1945 and 1975, the following numbers of famines took place: Europe—1, the Middle East—4, Latin America—7, Asia—20, and Africa—23.[2] The idea of a famine in Europe may be startling; this famine was caused by World War II and was most severe in the Netherlands, the concentration camps, and vast areas of Eastern Europe and the Soviet Union.

Today there are between 460 million and 1.1 billion hungry people in the world. In the United States, there may be over 30 million going hungry.

Eating Disorders Are Mainly a Problem of Young White Women

Eating disorders refer to two disorders that are produced by obsessive desires to be thin: anorexia nervosa and bulimia, which affect an estimated 10% to 15% of adolescent girls and young women.[3]

Anorexia nervosa

History

Anorexia
Self-starvation because of a distorted body image.

The term means nervous loss of appetite. This disorder is a form of self-induced starvation. People in the advanced stage of *anorexia* have an appearance similar to that of people starving in famines. The difference is that food is available to the anorexic but is rejected, whereas in a famine the food is unavailable. Anorexia was first described in the 17th century, though it has been studied in detail only during the past 20 years.

Bulimia

Bulimia
Eating large quantities of food at one time (binging), followed by artificial elimination of the food (purging), by vomiting, laxatives, etc.

This word translates as "to eat like an ox." It is sometimes called *binge eating, stuffing,* or *binging/purging.* The enormous amount of food consumed during the binge phase is purged from the body, usually by self-induced vomiting or by using laxatives and enemas. It is difficult to determine the incidence of *bulimia.* Reports in the press speak of an "epidemic," with estimates as high as 19% among college women.[3]

Most people with eating disorders are adolescent girls and young women from white, middle-, or upper-income families. These individuals are usually ambitious but somewhat introverted. The problem is seen also in some gymnasts, ballet dancers, models, jockeys, and wrestlers. It occurs occasionally in older women and in children under 12 years of age. Only about 5% to 10% of people with anorexia nervosa are males.[4]

Mortality rates are high for very obese or very thin (starving) people though the reasons for death differ. There are hungry people in every country in the world, but the death rate from starvation is highest in developing countries. Obesity, anorexia, and bulimia occur mainly in industrialized countries. Anorexia and bulimia are due to a compulsive desire to be thin; teenage girls from middle- or upper-income families are affected most often.

IDEAL BODY WEIGHT AND AMOUNT OF FAT

Major effects on body weight are caused by overweight, obesity, anorexia, bulimia, and starvation. Also, some of the degenerative diseases such as coronary heart disease and type II diabetes are associated with excessive body weight. Before we discuss these effects, however, let us see what the ideal body weight and amount of fat is for you.

Ideal Body Weight May Be Determined from Metropolitan Height and Weight Tables

What is the ideal body weight? This is one of the most often asked questions in nutrition. It is also the most difficult to answer. It is important to deal first with reasons why it is difficult to answer.

Ideal body weights are derived from data, obtained from insurance companies, that correlate body weight with age at death. The latest version of the height and weight tables was published in 1983 by the Metropolitan Insurance Company (Table 10-1).

 Critics argue that there are a number of things wrong with using these tables:

- The population from which the numbers are obtained is not fully representative because not everybody buys life insurance. People who buy life insurance may differ from the rest of the population in all kinds of ways: economic status, age, race, health, stress levels, and personal habits (quality of diet, smoking, and exercise). Poor people, then, would be mostly excluded.
- The tables reflect the average weight for Americans in their twenties. However, these weights may be neither ideal nor desirable for adults age thirty and older. This is because of changes in body weight and body composition during the process of aging.
- Weighing scales indicate body weight but not the amount of body fat. Two people can have the same body weight but different amounts of muscle and body fat. Most health problems relate to the amount of body fat.
- The final problem is that the insurance company only knows the weight at the time of insurance. Weight may be very different at the time of death.

A little background history on the values in Table 10-1 is useful. Research and debate have been continuous over the past 150 years.[5] Even the word "ideal" in the title to this section has caused problems. Tables in 1846, 1897, 1908, and 1912 were for *average weight*; however, the 1942 version was for *ideal weight*. In 1959, the term became *desirable weight*, and finally in 1983 the tables were simply the *1983 Metropolitan Height and Weight Tables*. The removal of the words "ideal" or "desirable" from the 1983 tables was necessary because they meant different things to different people.

> Words such as "ideal" and "desirable" have different meanings for different people.

Calculations from the 1983 Metropolitan Height and Weight Tables Differ for Men and Women

There are different values in Table 10-1 for men and women because women weigh less than men of the same height and frame size. Let us show how to measure your height and weight and then make the correct interpretation.

TABLE 10-1 1983 Metropolitan Height and Weight Tables

Women					Men				
Height		Frame*			Height		Frame*		
Ft	In	Small	Medium	Large	Ft	In	Small	Medium	Large
4	10	102–111	109–121	118–131	5	2	128–134	131–141	138–150
4	11	103–113	111–123	120–134	5	3	130–136	133–143	140–153
5	0	104–115	113–126	122–137	5	4	132–138	135–145	142–156
5	1	106–118	115–129	125–140	5	5	134–140	137–148	144–160
5	2	108–121	118–132	128–143	5	6	136–142	139–151	146–164
5	3	111–124	121–135	131–147	5	7	138–145	142–154	149–168
5	4	114–127	124–138	134–151	5	8	140–148	145–157	152–172
5	5	117–130	127–141	137–155	5	9	142–151	148–160	155–176
5	6	120–133	130–144	140–159	5	10	144–154	151–163	158–180
5	7	123–136	133–147	143–163	5	11	146–157	154–166	161–184
5	8	126–139	136–150	146–167	6	0	149–160	157–170	164–188
5	9	129–142	139–153	149–170	6	1	152–164	160–174	168–192
5	10	132–145	142–156	152–173	6	2	155–168	164–178	172–197
5	11	135–148	145–159	155–176	6	3	158–172	167–182	176–202
6	0	138–151	148–162	158–179	6	4	162–176	171–187	181–207

To calculate your body frame size:

Extend your arm and bend it upwards into a 90 degree angle. Keep your fingers straight. Place your thumb and index finger of your other hand on the two bones on either side of your elbow. Measure the space between your fingers, using a tape measure or ruler (very accurate measures are done with a caliper). Compare these measurements with the "normal," or medium, values in the following chart.

Women		Men	
Height	Elbow breadth	Height	Elbow breadth
4'9"–4'10"	2¼"–2½"	5'1"–5'2"	2½"–2⅞"
4'11"–5'2"	2¼"–2½"	5'3"–5'6"	2⅝"–2⅞"
5'3"–5'6"	2⅜"–2⅝"	5'7"–5'10"	2¾"–3"
5'7"–5'10"	2⅜"–2⅝"	5'11"–6'2"	2¾"–3⅛"
5'11"	2½"–2¾"	6'3"	2⅞"–3¼"

*Body weights listed here are based on the lowest mortality in people aged 25 to 59 years. Height for both men and women includes 1-inch heel. Body weight for women includes 3 lbs for indoor clothing—for men it includes 5 lbs of indoor clothing.

Measuring height and weight

Use your height and frame size to obtain your weight in Table 10-1. Your answer will determine if you are underweight, overweight, or obese. Consider the following example.

- If you are a woman, 5 feet 6 inches tall, of medium build
- Your weight from Table 10-1 would be 130 to 144 lb
- You are *overweight* if your weight is between the weight listed in Table 10-1 and 120% of that—that is, if you weigh up to 173 lb (which is 20% in excess of 144 lb)
- You are *obese* if you weigh more than 120% of the weight in Table 10-1— that is, over 173 lb (over 20% in excess of 144 lb)

Interpreting your height and weight

Table 10-1 is useful as a guideline to what you should weigh, but if you vary considerably either way you should get medical advice. After all, not everyone who is obese is unhealthy, and a weight-reducing program could conceivably do more harm than good. On the other hand, naturally lean people perhaps should not increase their body weight.[6] Even being right in the middle offers no guarantees: there is no guarantee that the weight listed on the table is the healthiest or most attractive weight for an individual.

Ideal Weight May Also Be Determined from the Body Mass Index (BMI)

BMI is another standard of "ideal" weight used by nutritionists. To determine this figure, divide your weight in kilograms by the square of your height in meters. Here is an example:

- Suppose you are a female who weighs 185 lb, or 84.1 kg, and are 5 feet 6 inches tall, or 1.68 meters.

- Your BMI is calculated as follows: $\dfrac{84.1}{1.68^2} = \dfrac{84.1}{2.82} = 29.82$

- If you compare this with the ranges in Table 10-2, it shows that this weight is marginally obese, which agrees with the Metropolitan table.

Body Mass Index
A meaningful measure of ideal body weight that includes body weight (in kg) divided by height (in meters squared).

$$BMI = \frac{weight\ (in\ kg)}{height\ (in\ meters^2)}$$

TABLE 10-2 **Body Mass Index for Men and Women**

	Body Mass Index (BMI)	
	Women	Men
Acceptable	up to 18.5	up to 19.5
Overweight	18.5–23.5	24.5–29.5
Obese	over 29.5	over 29.5

Now use your own body weight to calculate whether you are the right weight. In interpreting the results, remember that the calculations do not indicate the relative weights of body fat and lean tissue, which is a source of concern for nutritionists.[7] After you do that, you will no doubt be interested in the next topic.

Is There a Conflict Between Ideal Body Weight for Beauty and for Health?

What, really, *is* a good-looking person? Fat used to be beautiful—look at the heavy models in the paintings of such seventeenth-century artists as Rubens and Rembrandt. Look at the fat babies in England and America around the turn of the century, whose corpulence was supposed to protect them against tuberculosis and other diseases. Look at some of today's cultures in Africa and the South Pacific, where being overweight is considered a sign of handsomeness and high social status.[8]

In most industrialized countries today, however, it is "in to be thin." A mid-1960s study of high school seniors, which is still relevant today, found that only 16% of the students were obese yet 60% of the students said that they were trying to lose weight by dieting—mostly girls who said that they were concerned about their looks.[9] Only 3% cited physical fitness as a need to lose weight. Clearly, then, dieting may be unnecessary for health reasons, and our culture's standards of appearance are a powerful motivator.

Appearance, however, is an inexact way to determine ideal body weight. You may take body weight as an indicator of how you should look, but actually it is the amount of *fat* in the body that determines whether a person is overweight or obese. Let us look at the methods used to determine the amount of body fat in an individual.

Body Fat Measurements on Individuals Can Be Accurate

You can see fat floating on top of a number of foods—oil on the top of salad dressings, for example. The fact that fat is less dense than water is used to determine a person's body fat content; in clinics with the proper equipment, a person is weighed *under water*. The more fat that is in the body, the easier it is for that person to float in water.

Calipers
An instrument with spring-loaded arms that measures folds of body fat.

The above method is accurate but expensive, and therefore is not likely to be used for a large population. When researchers are trying to measure obesity among several members of a community, they are likely to use another method—namely, that of using a *calipers*, an instrument with spring-loaded arms to determine the thickness of skin folds, which in turn can be translated into body-fat measurements. The greatest accuracy is achieved when measurements are made in a number of locations on a person's body.[10] Because fat is distributed differently in men and women, the skin-fold thickness should be measured in men in the chest near the armpit, the abdomen, and thigh. In women the measurements should be made at the triceps (at the back of the upper arm), suprailium (top of the hip), and thigh. Because some of these areas are private, researchers usually make only the triceps measurement when they are surveying a large population for obesity, although this limits the accuracy of their findings.

Ideal body weight tables are only guidelines. The amount of body fat, and its location in the body, is more important than body weight. Concerns about beauty rather than health are frequently the reasons why people go on weight-reducing diets.

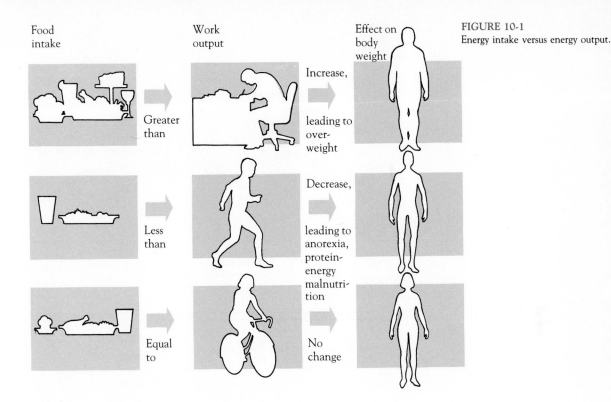

Food intake / Work output / Effect on body weight

FIGURE 10-1
Energy intake versus energy output.

Greater than → Increase, leading to overweight

Less than → Decrease, leading to anorexia, protein-energy malnutrition

Equal to → No change

FACTORS AFFECTING BODY WEIGHT

Why is your body weight what it is? The short answer lies in the balance or imbalance between energy intake (food) and energy output (work) (Figure 10-1).

Obesity Has Different Causes

Obesity is not caused *only* by an excess intake of food. Studies show that energy intake from food is the same in obese and normal-weight women. This suggests that obesity is caused by low energy expenditure. Therefore, obesity is caused by any of these factors:

- An excess intake of food
- Lower energy expenditure in basal energy
- Decreased physical activity

Several Factors Influence Body Weight

Many factors influence food intake and energy expenditure, some of which are described in Chapter 9. Note that:

- Body fat increases with age.
- Women have more fat than men do.
- Body weight is influenced by changes in basal energy requirements, physical activity, food intake, and *dietary thermogenesis*—body heat produced after food is consumed (Table 10-3).

Dietary Thermogenesis
Body heat produced after consuming food.

FIGURE 10-2
Hunger and appetite. Many factors influence the onset of hunger and appetite.

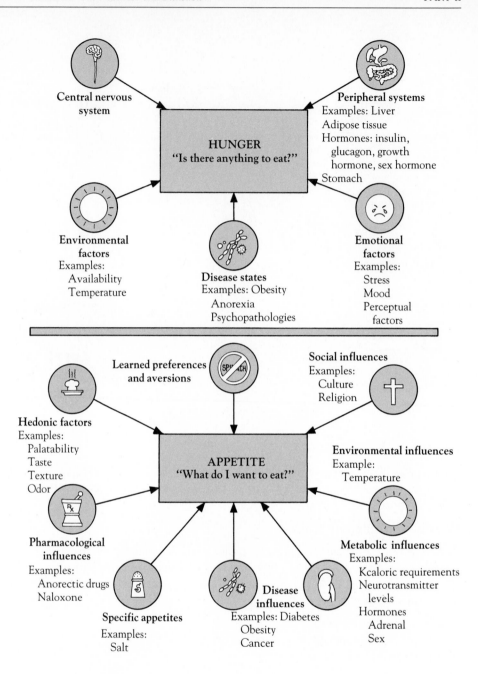

Hunger and appetite

As Figure 10-2 indicates, the amount and type of food eaten is in response to two things: hunger and appetite. These in turn are influenced by a number of psychological, environmental, and physiological factors. By controlling some of these factors, it may be possible to control *satiety*—the pleasant experience one feels when "full," a feeling most people want to repeat.[11]

Satiety tends to be produced by smaller amounts of high-fat foods, perhaps because fat moves more slowly than either carbohydrate or protein through the gastrointestinal tract. The reason you feel full for a longer time after a high-fat meal is because of a longer period of gastrointestinal distension. This is detected by nerves that send a message to the brain to stop eating. Some weight-reducing programs use this principle with nonnutritive materials ("bulking agents").

The sequence of food presentation may be important. For example, soup given prior to a meal is more effective in producing satiety than the same amount of kcalories provided by crackers, cheese, and juice.

In addition, rapid eating increases the amount of food consumed. One explanation is that time is needed before the hormones and *neurotransmitters*—the chemicals produced by the body to transmit nerve impulses between nerve cells—involved in satiety can respond to gastrointestinal distension or fullness.

Physiology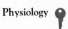

The way you eat can influence your intake of energy.

Neurotransmitters
Chemicals produced by the body to transmit nerve impulses between nerve cells.

Variety of foods

In treating people who are overweight or feeding people who are starved, serving a variety of foods is important. People will eat more if several foods are offered that differ in taste, appearance, and texture. If only one food is presented (even if that food is the person's favorite), the amount consumed is lower.

The long-term effects of a monotonous diet on weight maintenance, however, have not been fully determined.[12] Perhaps the body has a built-in mechanism that encourages the consumption of a variety of foods. Such a mechanism would make the consumption of a nutritious diet more likely. The problem of obesity, then, arises when people overeat this wide variety of food.

Still, other factors are involved. Native Americans and South Pacific islanders, for example, have a traditional diet that is low in fat and sugar and they have a low incidence of obesity. When they eat a Western-type diet, however, obesity increases.[13]

Eating practices early and later in life

Infants may get more kcalories—and hence become obese—if they are formula-fed instead of breast-fed and if they are weaned to solid food at an early age.

Pediatrics

TABLE 10-3 **Many Factors Affect Body Weight**

Basal energy requirements	Emotions
Physical activity	Socioeconomic status
Age	Culture
Sex	Dietary thermogenesis
Genetics	Food intake
Pregnancy	Type of food
Hormone levels	Meal patterns
Brain/nerve signals	Temperature
Disease	Drugs

People eating few or no foods of animal origin rarely suffer from obesity.

Eating practices later in life may also be responsible for increased fat in the body. The Dietary Guidelines described earlier in this book recommend a reduction in the intake of fat and sugar; many vegetarian diets are low in both fat and sugar, and the incidence of obesity is low among vegetarians. Further evidence for the role of fat and sugar in obesity is found by looking at animals. Wild animals, for example, do not suffer from obesity. Indeed, even laboratory rats do not become obese when given free access to a regular diet that meets all the animal's nutrient requirements. Give these same rats high-fat diets, concentrated sugar solutions, and a mixture of highly palatable human "supermarket" foods, however, and they will become obese.[14]

Meal patterns

Obesity may be influenced by meal patterns. If you'd been reprimanded for snacking when you were a child, there may be hope for you yet. When experimental animals eat snacks instead of large meals, the incidence of obesity is lower. These observations have implications for the 12 million Americans who skip breakfast and possibly for the 68 million who use low-calorie foods,[15,16] two behaviors that are often followed by the eating of large meals.

Food temperature and body temperature

Food temperature can determine energy intake. For instance, children find luke-warm food more appealing than the same food either hot or cold.

An increase in body temperature, such as in fever, will increase basal energy requirements and therefore increase energy expenditure.

Drugs

Drugs may be used to increase or decrease appetite.[17] Drugs used to treat convulsions and depression, such as Librium and Valium, increase appetite. Many patients on tranquilizers become obese because of the increased food intake. The same drugs have the opposite effect on elderly people.

Amphetamines have been used to decrease appetite, but they have dangerous side effects. They may also be ineffective for obese people who respond to the attractiveness of food rather than to appetite.

Pharmacology

Genetics

Obesity tends to run in families, as Figure 10-3 indicates. However, for many years, researchers were puzzled as to whether obesity in children of obese parents was caused by heredity or by imitating the poor eating habits of the parents. A recent study of adopted children demonstrates that genetics has a strong influence,[18] although not all experts accept this.

Pregnancy

Body fat increases during pregnancy, but much of it is lost during breast-feeding. However, if the mother gives her infant formula instead of her breast milk, she may retain much of this body fat.

Hormone levels

An underactive thyroid gland or abnormal activity of the adrenal or pituitary glands can cause obesity. However, this is not the same as the popular notion that all

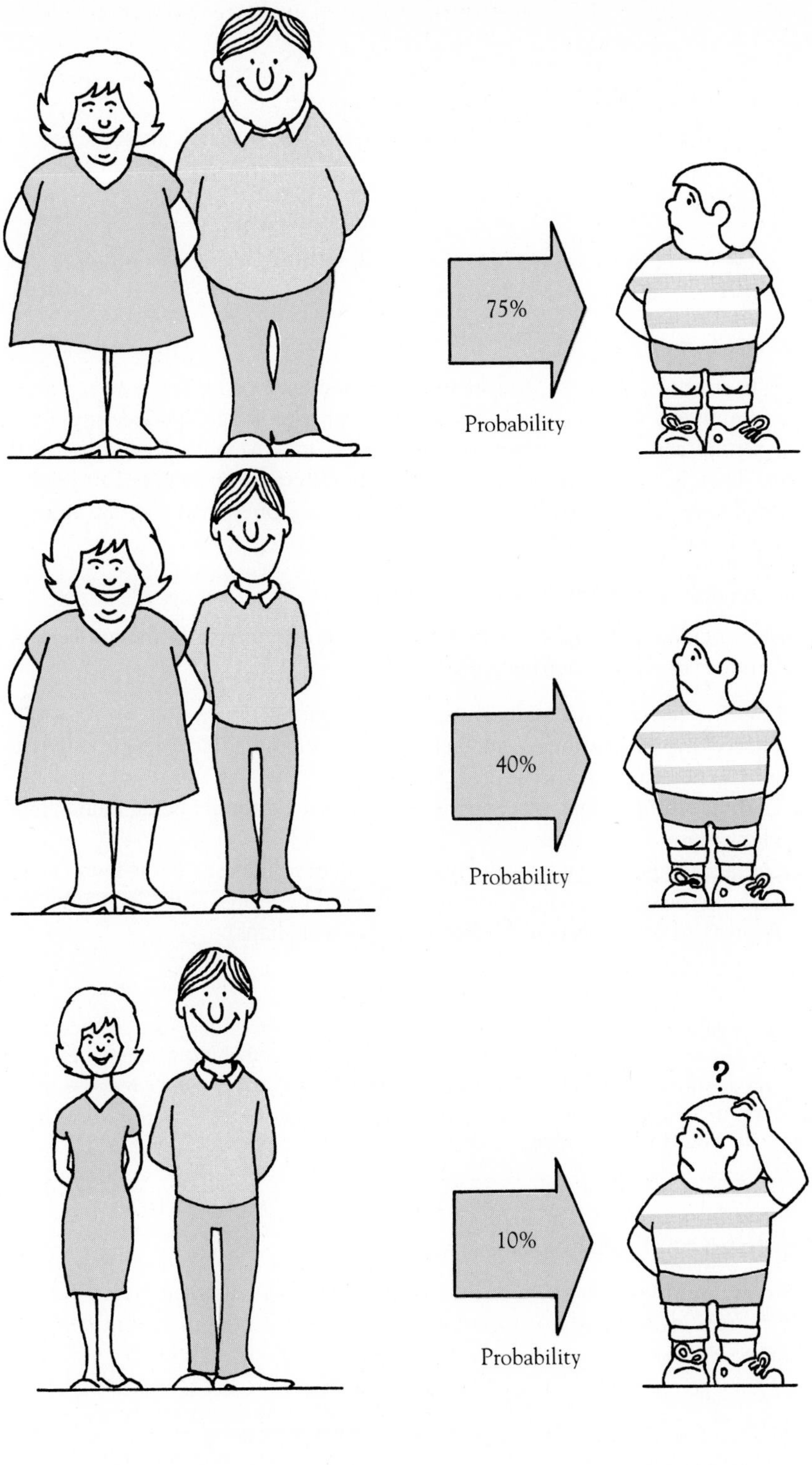

FIGURE 10-3
Obesity in families. Evidence for the
strong influence of heredity on obesity.

75%

Probability

40%

Probability

10%

Probability

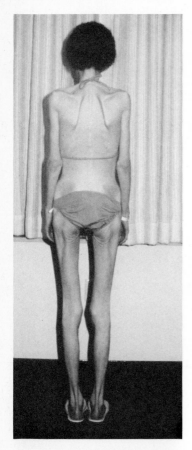

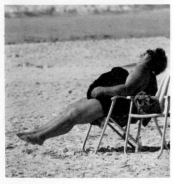

Severe nutritional problems are caused by anorexia nervosa (top) and obesity (bottom). Undereating and overeating, respectively, are the main reasons for these problems.

obesity originates in "glandular problems"; clinical evidence does not support this belief.[19]

Brain and nerve signals

Obesity can be produced by changes in brain and nerve signals caused by tumors or physical trauma affecting the hypothalamus, the appetite regulator in the brain.

Disease

Cancer and other diseases often cause a loss of appetite, thereby causing people to lose weight.

Emotional factors

Anger, frustration, boredom, and depression may affect food intake, as you doubtless know from your own experience. However, over a prolonged period, these emotional factors can make a person overweight or underweight, depending on the person. That is, people respond differently to different stresses. For example, a difficult divorce or the death of a spouse may cause one person to eat more but another person to eat less.[19]

Socioeconomic and cultural factors

A higher incidence of obesity is found among certain groups (although certainly not everyone in these groups is obese), as follows:

- Lower socioeconomic status—especially women
- Succeeding generations—first-generation immigrants have less obesity than later generations in the United States
- Certain ethnic groups—the highest prevalence of obesity being found among Hungarians and Czechs
- Certain religious groups—the highest incidence of obesity being found among Jews, followed by Roman Catholics, followed by Protestants (decreasing from Baptists to Methodists to Lutherans to Episcopalians).

> Body weight is balanced delicately between energy intake from food and energy expenditure in basal metabolism, dietary thermogenesis, and physical activity. Excess energy is stored because of a number of physiological, behavioral, and environmental factors, including diet, age, genetics, body composition, pregnancy, some diseases, lifestyle, and emotional factors.

THE RISKS OF OBESITY

Obesity is not just unattractive. It is actually a *disease*—a disease that is a potential killer.[20] Precisely because it is so serious, we need to spend a little time describing its consequences.

What Are the Health Problems Caused by Obesity?

The cause of death may be from one or more of the following health problems associated with obesity. What is frustrating, however, is that there is no *threshold* of overweight where these harmful effects begin. Thus, the experts agree that anybody with more than 20% of excess body weight should make every effort to lose weight.

- Atherosclerosis
- Diabetes—noninsulin-dependent or type II. Loss of excess weight helps control this type of diabetes.
- High blood pressure. This is reduced when weight is lost.
- Cancer—in women, obesity may lead to cancer of the breast, gall bladder, and endometrium. In men, it may lead to cancer of the colon, rectum, and prostate. The connection with obesity is less well established in other types of cancer.[20]
- Arthritis—especially in the knees and hips.
- Gallstones—especially risky for anyone who is "female, fat, and fifty," according to the slogan.
- Varicose veins—caused by the extra load on the legs.
- Gout—caused by excess intake of kcalories from protein and alcohol.
- Kidney problems.
- Breathing problems.
- More accidents.
- Increased surgical risk. Weight loss is usually recommended prior to nonemergency surgery.

The Obese Pay a High Economic and Social Price

Having to buy special clothing is only the least of the economic consequences the obese must face. The very cause of their disease is expensive—the cost of their high food intake. So are many of the weight-reducing "cures" that the obese purchase. The obese may also be unable to obtain life insurance, may have to spend more on transportation (flying first class, for example, because they need the wider seats), and may suffer job discrimination because of their appearance or the perception by prospective employers that they are greater health risks.

Economics

The obese also pay a social price for their disorder. Their loneliness and negative feelings about themselves may be reflected in less participation in sports, dancing, and other kinds of social events.

Sociology

The Location of Excess Fat in the Body May Be Related to Higher Mortality

Excess fat is not distributed evenly throughout the human body. This has obvious effects on appearance, and there are health implications also. About 30 years ago a French scientist suggested that the typical distribution of fat in males, which is mainly in the abdomen and upper body, correlates with the incidence of diabetes, atherosclerosis, and gout. The greatest amount of fat in women is on the thighs and buttocks, which has a lower association with these diseases. However, the scientist's calculations were so complex that it discouraged others from testing the hypothesis.

Recent work has confirmed that more fat in the abdomen region is associated with a greater possibility of heart disease. Another finding has shown that potbellied men and women were at greater risk of developing diabetes, hypertension, and elevated lipid levels.[21] The suspected reason is the higher metabolic activity associated with abdominal fat, which causes a higher level of fat in the blood. Another possibility is that the pot belly is due to a lack of exercise, with accompanying hypertension and high blood cholesterol. More research is needed on this subject. ⇦

Try the following to determine whether the measurements around your middle are higher than desirable.[21] The results apply to men. The pattern of fat distribution is different for women, and women do not usually suffer from pot-belly.

- The average man has a waist that is 36 inches, when measured at the navel. (This is 91.4 cm.)
- The average man's hips measure 40 inches, which gives a waist-to-hips ratio of 0.9. (Forty inches is 101.6 cm.)
- For a man "at risk," the hips will measure 40 inches or more *and* so will the waist.

In general, good health is represented by the waist-to-hips ratio of 0.9 or greater. (To find the ratio, divide your hip measurement by your waist measurement.)

Obesity may be the cause of increased health hazards including atherosclerosis, non-insulin dependent diabetes, high blood pressure, arthritis, certain cancers, gallstones, reproductive problems, and accidents. The obese are also penalized economically and socially.

TABLE 10-4 Reasons for and Methods of Body Weight Loss in Obesity, Anorexia Nervosa, and Starvation in Famines

Nutrition Problem	Body Weight Loss	
	Reasons	Methods
Obesity	Health—to reduce hypertension, serum cholesterol, risk of cancer, diabetes (type II), and to reduce the risk of complications following surgery	Increase exercise levels Diet—reduce energy intake Pharmacologic agents Surgical procedures
	Cosmetic	
Anorexia nervosa	Fear of fatness and/or fear of adulthood	Self-induced starvation Bulimia (sometimes)
Protein-energy malnutrition	Involuntary starvation	Little or no food available

THE MECHANISMS OF WEIGHT LOSS

Consider an interesting question: Are the mechanisms and consequences of weight loss in dieting, eating disorders, and starvation all the *same?*

The answer is: yes, but. Yes, many—but not all—of the physiological responses of the body are the same regardless of the reasons for low food intake. However, the reasons for the weight loss and the methods by which it is achieved differ. (See Table 10-4.)

Body weight decreases rapidly at first during dieting, eating disorders, and starvation. Of course, this may be satisfying to a person on a diet (and even temporarily satisfying to a person with an eating disorder), but it will certainly alarm a person experiencing famine. Obviously, the extent of weight loss depends on the amount of food eaten, the extent of physical activity, and whether one is eating substances that induce loss of body water rather than body fat. However, after a while, the rate of body weight loss begins to slow, even with no change in the amount of food available. The reasons for this slowing down are that:

- The basal energy requirements decrease.
- The body is lighter and so requires less energy to move.
- A person at this stage of weight loss has reduced all unnecessary movements.

Other effects of reduced food intake are seen mostly in famine victims.

As for people on voluntary weight-loss diets, why do you suppose so many people give up dieting? The answers are probably discomfort and, to some extent, vanity. People who continue dieting may find that their hair becomes dry and lusterless, their skin thin and dry, their eyes dull, their sensitivity to noise higher, and their mental alertness lower. In extreme cases they may even find themselves more susceptible to infections (such as measles and tuberculosis), to cessation of menstruation, and to personality changes.

Who Should Lose Weight?

Obviously, for all the health reasons listed above, people who are obese should lose weight. People in certain lines of work may also need to lose weight; examples are ballerinas and athletes, such as boxers and jockeys, who must maintain their body weight within certain limits. Body weight loss should not be attempted during pregnancy and lactation. Nor is it recommended for people whose only reason to lose weight is to conform to the latest clothing styles.

Weight loss is best done under medical supervision, although few people actually do this. Problems arise if considerable weight must be lost in a short time. Diuretics are a popular but dangerous means to achieve this rapid weight loss. Body fluid is removed, causing a decrease in body weight, but there is reduced physical performance.

There Are Right and Wrong Ways to Lose Body Fat Permanently

The three ways of losing body fat are by:

- Increased physical activity
- Decreased energy intake
- A combination of both

Some methods will cause the loss of body water as well as body fat, which, since most people use weighing scales as the major indicator of weight loss, can be misleading.

Increased physical activity

Physical activity has a beneficial effect on body fat by influencing both sides of the energy balance equation:

- *Energy intake:* Physical activity before a meal may cause decreased appetite, but this has not been observed in all studies.[22]
- *Energy output:* Physical activity burns kcalories. As discussed in Chapter 9, this is a slow but beneficial way to lose weight. However, you must enjoy the form the physical activity takes if the program is to succeed as a method of weight control.

Many people prefer to restrict energy intake rather than to increase energy expenditure.

Decreasing energy intake

This can be done by the following methods:

- Reducing food intake
- Varying the composition of the diet
- Using pharmacologic agents as appetite suppressants
- Having surgical treatment that enables the body to reduce the absorption of energy
- Behavior modification

In examining these methods of restricting food intake, you should consider the factors described in the next section.

There Are Four Essential Components of a Successful Weight-Reducing Diet

The keys to weight-loss success are low kcalorie consumption, palatable foods, reasonable reduction per week, and long-term change in the composition of the diet, as follows.

Low kcalories

The weight-reducing diet must be low in kcalories but adequate in all other nutrients. This cannot be achieved on an intake of less than 1000–1200 kcalories per day—more in the case of active college students. Supplements are only a partial solution for restricting the intake of a balanced diet with adequate energy level.

Palatable food

Foods in the weight-loss diet must be palatable, familiar, easily available, and economical. Some of the diets described in the next few pages fail on one or more of these counts. Many diets, for instance, are expensive, impractical for busy people on the move, and not even palatable.

Reasonable loss per week

Weight loss must not be more than 2 lb per week. This is the rate of loss recommended by the American Medical Association. Don't be seduced by promises of weight loss of 8 to 10 lb per week. Not only is such a schedule unsafe, but much of the reduction will be due to water loss and not to fat loss.

Composition of the diet

Consider the composition of the diet *after* ideal body weight is achieved. Whatever food was eaten before the weight loss, both in quantity and in type, should be avoided after the dieter has reached his or her ideal weight. Otherwise, the food that caused the obesity in the first place will probably cause it again.

Of the Many Weight-Reducing Diets Available, Many Are Unsafe or Doomed to Fail

Table 10-5 lists a few of the many, many weight-loss programs available, and you can be sure that there will be many more to come. A few of the categories of diets are examined below, but you should bear in mind two things: (1) many are unsafe, and (2) many are doomed to fail.

The principal reasons so many popular diets are failures are:

- Expense
- The food is monotonous or lacks palatability
- The rate of weight reduction feels too slow
- The diet is too inflexible for a person with a busy work or travel schedule
- Health hazards (even death)

Besides the different kinds of "fad" diets or popular diets listed in Table 10-5, there are various kinds of weight-reducing aids: pharmacologic agents, surgical treatment, and behavior modification programs. Also offered—and plainly unworkable—are all kinds of wraps, creams, and gadgets that are advertised as ways of "melting away" fat.

Pharmacologic Agents Should Be Examined with Care

Most pharmacologic agents on the market will either decrease appetite or increase water loss from the body. Although the objective of dieting is to lose body fat permanently, any of the pharmacologic methods described below will bring only a temporary decrease in body weight. Once these pharmacologic crutches are removed, people generally return to the diet that made them obese, since they have not learned anything about modifying their eating behavior.

Pharmacologic agents are classified as appetite suppressants, taste suppressants, bulking agents, food supplements, and diuretics.

Appetite suppressants

Amphetamines and some newer drugs are available by prescription; their purpose is to act on the hypothalamus to depress the appetite. However, because people may become dependent on such agents, they are not recommended by the American Medical Association.

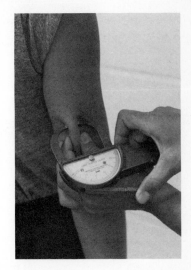

Skinfold thickness measures of body fat. Skinfold calipers measure the fat under the skin at various sites in the body—at the back of the shoulder and in the upper arm, abdomen, and thigh.

TABLE 10-5 Types of Weight-Loss Diets

Type of Diet	Composition	Adherence	Possible Health Dangers	Examples
I. Nutritionally Balanced				
1000 to 1200 kcals	High nutrient-dense foods	Good; familiar, economic, palatable food	None	Weight-Watchers diet
About 900 kcals	Formula diets	Monotonous, expensive	None, if under medical supervision	Medifast, Optifast, Nutrimed
II. Nutritionally Unbalanced (may also be calorically restricted)				
Altered portions of fat, carbohydrate, and protein	Low-carbohydrate, high-fat, high-protein	High meat intake, costly, difficult to maintain low carbohydrate intake of 20 to 50 g/day	Ketosis, fluid loss, decreased appetite, high in saturated fat and cholesterol, kidney failure or stones	Dr. Atkin's Diet Revolution, Quick Weight Loss Diet, The Complete Scarsdale Diet
	High protein	Expensive; high in fat if from high-protein foods. Vegetarian version is high in protein and carbohydrate, low in fat	High protein intake (100 g/day) May be low in vitamin B_{12}	Slendernow Diet, The Pritikin Permanent Weight-Loss Diet
Single food diets	Grapefruit, egg, rice, kelp	Poor, monotonous	Deficient in minerals and vitamins	"Fake" Mayo Diets, Beverly Hills Diet
III. Calorically Dilute Diets				
	High fiber	Poor; low fat, low in animal food	High fiber (30 to 35 g/day) reduces the absorption of some minerals	The F-Plan Diet, Dr. David Reuben's The Save Your Life Diet
IV. Fasting				
Very low calorie diets	Protein, protein/carbohydrate mixtures, 300 to 600 kcal/day	Poor; expensive	Ketosis, nausea, diarrhea, weakness, muscle cramps. Death possible from mineral imbalance	Cambridge Diet, Dr. Linn's Last Chance Diet
Total fasting	Water, vitamin and mineral supplements	Poor; person is usually hospitalized	Ketosis, nutrient deficiencies	

Most nonprescription appetite suppressants are chemically related to amphetamines. Even though they are available over the counter, they can produce nervousness, sleeping difficulties, headaches, and high blood pressure. Therefore, medical supervision is advised in their use, especially for people with hypertension or with heart, kidney, or thyroid disease.

Naloxone is a new chemical that decreases food intake by up to 25% without any increase in hunger. However, high doses may affect mood and blood pressure and so should be taken with caution.[23]

Starch blockers once held out the promise that people could eat unlimited amounts of starchy food without gaining weight. These agents consisted of an extract from kidney beans. The extract contains a natural inhibitor of the enzyme alpha-amylase that digests starch. However, a number of studies showed starch blockers were ineffective in body weight loss, and these agents are now classified as possible dangerous drugs by the Food and Drug Administration.

Taste suppressants

Candy and gum sold as taste depressants are supposed to act by anesthetizing the tongue, thereby decreasing the taste for food. However, they are not effective in long-term weight control.

Bulking agents

These agents are supposed to cause a full feeling by absorbing liquid in the stomach. Methylcellulose and glucomannan are used widely. They are not effective.

Food supplements

Spirulina, bee pollen, and certain herbal mixtures have not been approved by the Food and Drug Administration as being safe and effective in weight control.

Diuretics

These reduce body *weight* but not body *fat*, because they only increase fluid loss. In any case, they are dangerous and should not be used because they may produce dehydration and loss of electrolytes.

Various Surgical Treatments May Reduce Obesity

Very obese people who have failed to lose weight by other methods may avail themselves of certain surgical methods:

- Temporarily wiring the jaws together may reduce food intake.
- Placing a balloon in the stomach reduces the available space for food (Figure 10-4). Stapling portions of the stomach together can reduce the size of the stomach. This method reduces appetite.
- *Jejunoileal* bypass surgery removes that section of the gastrointestinal tract (the *jejunum* is the second portion of the small intestine) where absorption of kcalories is greatest. This procedure is used less frequently than in the past because it has produced complications.
- A new but unproven technique, *suction lipectomy* consists of the removal of fat cells from under the skin (Figure 10-5).[24] In the spring of 1987, some women in Houston, Texas, died following this procedure. Clearly, more information is needed about safety factors.

If you must reduce weight using pharmacologic agents, do so under medical supervision.

Biochemistry

Jejunoileal
The jejunum is the second portion and the ileum is the lower three fifths of the small intestine.

Suction Lipectomy
Removal of fat from under the skin (subcutaneous).

FIGURE 10-4
A new method for reducing weight; a balloon is placed in the stomach. There are some medical dangers.

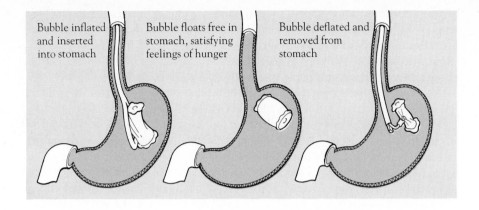

Bubble inflated and inserted into stomach

Bubble floats free in stomach, satisfying feelings of hunger

Bubble deflated and removed from stomach

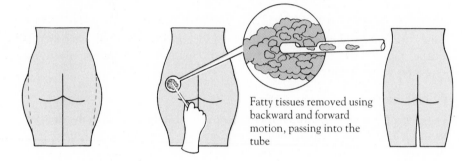

Fatty tissues removed using backward and forward motion, passing into the tube

FIGURE 10-5
Suction-assisted lipectomy. Lipectomy is a new and controversial method for removing body fat.

Surgical treatments have reduced overweight by 50% to 60%, but the price can be high. For instance, intestinal bypass surgery may produce problems from the following frightening list, ranging from minor to major disabilities: deficiency of protein, deficiency of vitamins and some minerals, chronic flatulence, dermatitis, hair loss, anemia, wound infections, muscle wasting, gallstones, arthritis, bone pain, kidney disease, and liver failure. Other problems can also arise. In one case,[25] a 37-year-old, 260 lb mother of three lost 110 lb after two rounds of surgery, an intestinal bypass and a gastric bypass. One might expect her to be uncomplaining about the cost of new clothes, but the cost of the gastric bypass alone was $4674, added to travel expenses and 4 to 6 weeks lost from work. Finally, changes in her personality and in family dynamics led to a divorce. You can see why, then, so many surgeons will not do this kind of operation.

Behavioral Modification Has Helped Many People

Psychology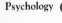

Major changes in eating and exercising are required if a person is to gain long-term control over his or her body weight. One method for achieving this control is the psychological program known as *behavior modification* or *behavior therapy*. A particular version of this therapy is presented in Table 10-6.

Behavior therapy may be practiced either through individual counseling or through self-help groups such as Overeaters Anonymous (OA), TOPS (Take Off Pounds Sensibly), and Weight Watchers. Success varies with individuals; in other words, success has been mixed.

Recent reports in the scientific literature that hypnosis produces effective weight loss remain to be confirmed.

TABLE 10-6 Outline of Behavior Therapy Program

Session Number	Topic*
1	Explanations of overweight The behavioral model The energy-balance model Calorie-counting
2	Self-monitoring of food intake and prescribed behaviors
3	Interpreting self-monitoring forms Nutrition and dieting Slowing the rate of eating
4	Hunger and signals to eat Cue control Shaping new behaviors
5	Review Diet and nutrition myths Popular diets
6	Review Diet and nutrition information
7	Controlling times, places, and activities during eating
8	Rate of weight loss Visual signals to eat Techniques for preparing meals
9	Psychology of staying thin Goal-setting Changing attitudes
10	Eating sensibly at home
11	Behavioral chains and eating Shopping for food
12	Exercise, activity, and body weight Programmed exercise and routine exercises
13	Social support from family, friends, co-workers, and others Behaviors for the family
14	Using incompatible behaviors Pre-meal monitoring
15	Eating away from home
16	Review Dealing with special occasions Planning for maintenance

Body Fat Cannot Just Be "Melted Away"

Perhaps you've seen ads that claim to simply "melt away" body fat, using wraps, sweat suits, mechanical or electrical stimulators, various creams, or chemicals in certain foods (such as grapefruit). Most of these treatments are banned by the Food and Drug Administration, and for good reason.

Before embarking on any "new" diet, check to see if it makes sense from a biochemical and physiological viewpoint.

If fat is indeed something that can be "melted," it must be removed from the body to achieve the weight loss. Since fat is not lost in sweat or urine, how is it supposedly lost? The short answer is that it is *not* lost—except by being burned for energy. Thus, if any of the "melt-away" methods actually decrease body weight, it is because of losses in body fluids. Invariably, one finds these losses are quickly replaced once the "treatment" stops.

You may also have come across ads featuring the word *cellulite*. What is cellulite? It has the same chemical properties as fat and the same appearance as less "lumpy" fat. Actually, reported the American Medical Association in a 1976 statement, "There is no medical condition known or described as cellulite in this country." Or in any other country.

Body weight loss produces mostly the same effects whether food is reduced because of dieting or eating disorders or because of famine. The initial rapid weight loss is not maintained because the body becomes more efficient in using the lower energy intake from food. This is done by lower basal energy needs, reduced physical activity, and lower energy needs to move a lighter body. In advanced stages of weight loss, there are changes in physical appearance and mental attitudes.

Body fat cannot be melted away; the body loses fat by restricting energy intake or increasing energy output. Any diet providing less than 1000 kcalories per day will cause weight loss but will not provide adequate intakes of vitamins and minerals. Weight losses of more than 2 lb per week are not recommended. Successful weight loss occurs when the desired weight is maintained permanently. Behavior modification, coupled with the correct diet, may achieve this objective.

THE EATING DISORDERS: ANOREXIA NERVOSA AND BULIMIA

People with anorexia nervosa have extreme body weight loss, a distorted image of their body, and intense fear of becoming obese. Bulimia, sometimes called bulimia nervosa, is distinct from anorexia and involves secretive binge eating episodes. These are followed by self-induced purging by means of vomiting, fasting, the use of laxatives or diuretics, or other methods (Table 10-7). The frequency of use of these methods varies also. Some people with anorexia nervosa may use bulimia as one of the ways to induce severe losses in body weight. Both disorders include a great preoccupation with body weight.[3]

Accurate Criteria for Anorexia Nervosa and Bulimia Are Difficult to Develop

Although the medical profession is seeing eating disorders in increasing frequency, physicians are still wrestling with the problems of how best to treat the medical, nutritional, and psychological problems these disorders create.[3] The first order of

TABLE 10-7   **Maximum Frequency of Bulimia-Related Behavior of 275 Women During the Course of Their Illness**
Mean age of patient = 24 years

Behavior	Several Times a Day	Once a Day	Several Times a Week	Once a Week	Less Than Once a Week	Total*
	Maximum Frequency (%)					
Binge eating	74	8	14	3	3	100
Fasting	30	13	27	14	9	92
Exercise	32	26	20	8	7	91
Vomiting	64	8	10	3	4	88
Laxatives	10	10	20	7	13	61
Diet pills	14	12	9	5	11	50
Diuretics	6	5	10	4	9	34
Saunas	2	2	2	3	4	12

*Totals may not be exact sum of each frequency because of rounding of decimal places.

business is to develop criteria for diagnosing the difference between anorexia nervosa and bulima (see Table 10-8).

Eating Disorders May Produce Weight Loss in Different Ways

Anorexia nervosa is produced by starvation and bulimia by binging and purging. Anorexia nervosa and bulimia may occur in combination.

Anorexia nervosa

Starvation among people with anorexia nervosa may come about for the following reasons:

- *Low energy intake:* This may occur either through brief fasting or through a slow eating pattern—no more than 500 to 800 kcalories per day.
- *Extensive physical activity:* Anorectic women and some male compulsive runners have similarities in family background, socioeconomic characteristics, and personality characteristics.

Bulimia

Binging and purging describes the activity whereby one eats large amounts of food (binging), then removes the food from the system (purging). You might expect bulimics to be below or at their ideal weight, but some are actually above their ideal weight. Bulimia produces negative feelings such as guilt, worry, and even a feeling of still being hungry.

The Greatest Problems with Eating Disorders Appear Among Adolescent Girls and Athletes

Over 90% of people with eating disorders are teenage girls. One survey in America found the following family characteristics of girls who were dieting and who practiced bulimia:[27]

- *Race and ethnicity:* White—80%, black—13%, Asian/Oriental—3%
- *Religion:* Roman Catholic—50%, Protestant—18%, Jewish—4%, other—28%
- *Age:* Ages 14 to 17—96% of cases
- *Parents:* Married—67%, divorced—22%, separated—5%; College educated—74% of fathers and 70% of mothers; Full-time employed—91% of fathers and 50% of mothers
- *Siblings:* No pattern in number of siblings, except that 7% of the bulimics surveyed were only children.

However, many teenagers have this family pattern and yet do not have eating disorders. Why?

TABLE 10-8 Criteria for Diagnosing Anorexia Nervosa and Bulimia

Criteria for Anorexia Nervosa

A. Intense fear of becoming obese, which does not diminish as weight loss progresses

B. Body conceptualization disturbance, e.g. claiming to "feel fat" even when emaciated

C. Refusal to maintain body weight over a minimal normal weight for age and height

D. Amenorrhea (in females)

Type I—for patients who solely restrict food intake and who do *not* binge or purge (induce vomiting or abuse laxatives or diuretics).

Type II—for patients who restrict food intake and purge but do not binge.

For patients who binge and purge and who may restrict intake as well, give additional diagnosis of bulimia nervosa.

Criteria for Bulimia

A. Recurrent episodes of binge eating (rapid consumption of a large amount of food in a discrete period of time, usually less than 2 h)

B. At least three of the following:
   1. Consumption of high-kcaloric, easily ingested food during a binge
   2. Inconspicuous eating during a binge
   3. Termination of such eating episodes by abdominal pain, sleep, social interruption, or self-induced vomiting
   4. Repeated attempts to lose weight by severely restrictive diets, self-induced vomiting, or use of cathartics or diuretics
   5. Frequent weight fluctuations greater than 10 lb due to alternating binges and fasts

C. Awareness that the eating pattern is abnormal and fear of not being able to stop eating voluntarily

D. Depressed mood and self-deprecating thoughts following eating binges

E. The bulimic episodes are not due to anorexia nervosa or any known physical disorder

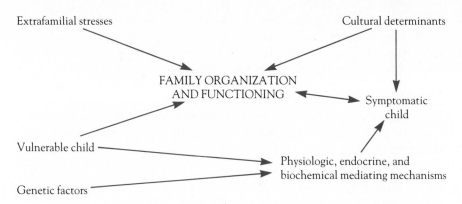

FIGURE 10-6
Model of an anorectic family.

Figure 10-6 offers a model of the anorectic's family that partly explains the problem. However, it must be emphasized that not every child in the same family will have an eating disorder. Looking at the model, let us consider some of the factors that might cause anorexia nervosa and bulimia:

- *Family organization and functioning:* Families consist of middle- or upper-income high-achievers, people who are perfectionists and who are avoiders of conflict.
- *Extrafamilial stresses:* People with eating disorders often respond to stresses from outside the family, such as the desire to be fashionable by being thin. A number of these teenagers also have alcohol and drug problems—indeed, some evidence suggests that bulimics in particular have the highest incidence of alcohol and drug abuse, as well being sexually promiscuous.[3] The small proportion of boys with eating disorders are frequently weight-conscious athletes, especially wrestlers.
- *Vulnerable child:* This term refers to "the perfect child," as the parents often describe her, who is generally a white teenager who is obedient, popular, good at academics and sports, in fact an overachiever. Male anorectics, by contrast, tend to be underachievers. Patients with anorexia nervosa bulimia have a high incidence of depression. Bulimic individuals who are not at the same time anorexic are likely to suffer from depression. Although much remains to be understood about the nature of this depression, there is evidence that it responds to antidepressant drugs.[28]
- *Physiologic, endocrine, and biochemical mediating mechanisms:* Many of these mechanisms have the effect of delaying puberty. Amenorrhea is one of the most common physiologic changes.

The process is accomplished by:

- Self-induced vomiting—in 88% of cases
- Laxative abuse—61%
- Diuretic abuse—33%
- Chewing and spitting out of food—65%

A study of thirty women who practiced bulimia showed that vomiting was a highly effective way of preventing weight gain, whereas laxative abuse was not.[26] The continued use of laxatives may cause a considerable loss of water from the body, which, as noted earlier, gives a false impression of body weight loss.

The reasons people say they indulge in binge eating are that they feel tense, anxious, and unhappy, crave certain foods, can't control their appetites, and can't sleep.[26] Most binge eating occurs in the late afternoon and early evening.

Anorexia and bulimia in combination

It is not uncommon for people who suffer from this combination to have alternating food intakes of up to 20,000 kcalories per day, followed by purging, followed by a period of fasting.

Eating Disorders Are an Old Phenomenon, but Are Becoming Increasingly Common

It might seem that anorexia nervosa and bulimia are fairly new, because the public's attention has been captured in recent years by stories of celebrities who have gone public about their experiences. However, the phenomenon of binge and purge is really age-old.

History

Over 300 years ago, a doctor described an anorexic young lady as "a skeleton only clad with skin." Today bulimia is seen mainly in economically advantaged young women who have a compulsive wish to be thin but who live in societies with a plentiful food supply. But it was not always thus. In ancient Rome, for example, people were not much concerned about weight control, but during feast times a lot of self-induced vomiting occurred because people wanted to get back to the banquet table to continue eating.

A variation today appears among the Kalahari bushmen in Africa, who binge eat every two or three days. However, the reason for their binge eating is that the food supply is very irregular in their desert environment.

Medical Problems Caused by Eating Disorders May be Life-Threatening

As Table 10-9 makes clear, many tissues in the body are affected by eating disorders. To this list must be added multiple nutrient deficiencies and disturbed sleep patterns, which occur among people with anorexia.

Education

Because some doctors may not accurately diagnose eating disorders, in 1986 the Health and Public Policy Committee of the American College of Physicians issued guidelines stressing the importance of taking a careful history for diagnosis and being sensitive to the patient's emotional insecurities and other possible medical problems during treatment. The committee emphasized the need for more education about eating disorders for both doctors and the general public.[3]

As Table 10-10 shows, extremes of weight control behavior among athletes seem to be a bigger problem among whites and Hispanics than among blacks and members of other races. Among female athletes the highest incidence of bulimia is among gymnasts and the lowest in basketball players (Table 10-11). Differences are due mainly to a sport's demand that an athlete meet specific weight qualifications in order to compete.

Some compulsive runners may be at high risk for depression and anorexia, although recent research has shown that such runners do not have the same incidence of psychiatric disorders as nonathletic anorectics.[29]

TABLE 10-9 Physical Effects of Anorexia Nervosa and Bulimia

Effect	Anorexia Nervosa	Bulimia
Endocrine system and metabolism	*Amenorrhea*	Menstrual irregularities
	Osteoporosis	
	Hypercarotenemia	
	Abnormal temperature regulation	
	Some hormonal changes	
Cardiovascular system	Slow heart rate	Poisoning from emetine (used to induce vomiting)
	Low blood pressure	
	Irregular heart rate	
Kidneys	Increased blood urea nitrogen	Hypokalemia (low blood potassium caused by excessive use of diuretics)
	Kidney stones	
	Decreased kidney function	
	Edema	
Gastrointestinal system	Constipation	Acute swelling of stomach, sometimes with rupture
	Decreased stomach emptying	Hypokalemia (laxative-induced)
	Elevated liver enzymes	Dental enamel erosion
		Inflammation of the esophagus
		Hemorrhage from the esophagus
Blood	Anemia	
	Abnormal decrease in white blood cells	
Lungs		Aspiration pneumonia (after inhaling foreign matter into the lung)

Amenorrhea
Absence or suppression of menstruation.

Hypercarotenemia
High levels of carotene (vitamin A precursor) in the blood.

TABLE 10-10 Pathologic Weight-Control Behavior in Athletes According to Race

Race	Athletes with Behavior Problems (%)
White	33
Black	18
Hispanic	33
Oriental	0
Other	33

TABLE 10-11 Pathologic Weight-Control Behavior in Female Athletes According to Sport*

Sport	Exhibited at Least One Pathogenic Weight-Control Behavior	Used Diet Pills	Self-Induced Vomiting	Used Laxatives
Basketball	8	0	8	0
Gymnastics	74	58	53	37
Swimming	11	11	11	11
Tennis	24	20	16	12
Track & field	26	22	0	22
Track (distance)	47	35	29	18
Volleyball	21	14	7	14
Golf	10	10	10	0
Field hockey	50	41	14	14
Softball	23	20	0	17

Other pathologic problems reported were excessive weight loss, binging more than twice per week, and the use of diuretics.

* As a percentage.

Treatment of Eating Disorders Requires Not Only Nutrients but Other Factors

Treatment of anorexia and bulimia is *not* for the "do-it-your-selfer." The risks are too great: although exact figures are difficult to obtain, because of the private nature of these disorders, anorexia does lead to death from starvation and bulimia can lead to suicide.

Because eating disorders involve psychology, nutrition, and medicine, professional treatment is required. The effects of starvation, for instance, mean that nutrients may have to be given intravenously. Hormonal treatment may be needed also.

In addition, the underlying psychological aspects of the family should be treated. Evidence from Canada[30] and elsewhere shows that the entire family must be involved in treatment. Parents, for instance, often feel shame and frustration about their child and attempt to keep their family problem a secret from friends. As you might expect, this leads to a high degree of tension in the family and feelings of joylessness, apathy, and fatigue.

Eating disorders are seen most often in high—achieving teenagers, usually white, and from middle- or upper-income families. The exact causes are not known, but fear of obesity and (possibly) fears of adulthood may lead to anorexia (starvation) or bulimia (binging and purging). Treatment involves the entire family, with inputs from psychology, nutrition, and medicine.

STARVATION AND HUNGER IN THE WORLD

"Give a man a fish and you feed him for a day; teach him how to fish and you feed him for life."

This Chinese proverb makes a lot of sense. Unfortunately, however, the solutions are not easy.

Ironically, today there *is* enough food in the world to actually eliminate hunger—to provide adequate amounts of nutrients to everybody. If the total amount of food on earth were equally divided, every man, woman, and child would get 2617 kcalories and 69 g of protein every day.[31] This is an adequate amount of food for everyone.

The problem, as you no doubt already suspect, is not that of enough food but of distributing the food. Food production is much better than it has been in the past, owing to better crop varieties, more irrigation, better fertilization and pest control methods, and the cultivation of more land.[32] However, present economic and distribution systems do not make this food available to everyone.

Famine and Starvation Have Agricultural, Political, and Economic Causes

Since the beginning, a sizable part of the human global family has suffered from famine. There is a difference between famine and undernutrition. *Famine* is rarely a sudden emergency, but it does not go on continually, usually lasting only a few years. Undernutrition, by contrast, is the result of ongoing starvation. (Undernutrition also does not capture as much media attention as do famines.)

Nowadays, potential famines can often be predicted. The causes of famine and starvation are as follows:

- *Drought:* Lack of rainfall may bring on drought—a problem in many African countries as of this writing.
- *Floods:* These are a less frequent cause, but they have caused problems in China and India.
- *Plant and Animal Diseases:* Earlier in the book the Irish potato famine of the 1840s was mentioned. Failure of the potato crop was caused by a disease called blight. Interestingly, the government tried to alleviate the famine by importing corn, but since the food was unfamiliar, people thought it was part of a government deception and refused to eat it.
- *War:* Perhaps the worst famines in history have been caused by war. The siege of Paris in 1871, the siege of Leningrad in Russia by the Germans in 1942, and the Germans' attempts to starve the Jews in Poland's Warsaw Ghetto during World War II are only a few of many unfortunate examples.
- *Failed economic policies:* The formation of collective farms in the Soviet Union in the 1930s was a massive failure and produced enormous food shortages.
- *Land tenure systems:* Where land is owned by many people, food production and nutritional status have been improved. However, in developing countries in which only a small number of families control most of the land, there are often food shortages.
- *Industrialization:* Industrialization in developing countries has brought loss of traditional farming practices on the one hand and growth of cities and their hungry populations on the other.
- *Income inequalities:* Needless to say, the very poor are limited in their access

Economics

Political Science

to food, as well as to education, housing, adequate sanitation, and health services. These in turn lead to low birth weight in babies, low energy and nutrient intakes among adults, poor food choices, inadequate facilities for food preparation, diarrhea and food poisoning from dirty water and food, and high mortality rates from infectious diseases such as measles.

■ *Other factors:* Corrupt politicians who use food as a political weapon, black markets, high population density in relation to available food, lack of adequate distribution facilities (roads, ports, transportation) complete this depressing list.

Lack of Education Can Produce Undernutrition and Starvation

Should an impoverished mother in a developing country breast-feed her baby or use a commercial formula instead? This is the kind of decision in which education can help prevent severe undernutrition.

A poor mother who does not breast-feed and uses a commercial formula may be giving her child a nutritionally balanced diet, but to prepare the formula she needs to have access to clean water; otherwise, the infant may suffer diarrhea, a major cause of death in developing countries. Moreover, she must be educated on how to prepare the formula so that it is not diluted.

Kwashiorkor

A deficiency disease mainly in children caused by a diet deficient in protein but adequate in energy.

Poor education may lead to the development of *kwashiorkor*, a word from the Ga language spoken by people in Ghana in West Africa, that means "the disease suffered by the displaced child." Kwashiorkor is a deficiency disease found mainly in children and is caused by a diet deficient in protein though adequate in energy.

The scenario by which kwashiorkor develops goes something like this: The mother breast-feeds her first child. This child grows normally and is healthy until she becomes pregnant with the second child. The mother thereupon looks for a replacement for her breast milk. She finds it in a watery extract from cassava, a root plant with a high carbohydrate and a low protein content. Because it is white, when mixed with water it looks like milk. Of course its nutritional value is much lower than milk. The mother forces the child to drink this unpalatable, nonnutritious drink because it is the only alternative to milk that she can find. The child does not grow well. By the time the second child is born, the first child has all of the symptoms of kwashiorkor. These include edema, poor quality of skin, discolored hair, liver malfunction, and extreme apathy.

Protein-Energy Malnutrition

Kwashiorkor and marasmus (deficiency of protein and kcalories) are classified under the term protein-energy malnutrition (PEM), formerly called protein-calorie malnutrition (PCM). Because of the emphasis on the word protein, some authors deal with PEM in a chapter on protein. But many more nutrient deficiencies besides that of protein are common in PEM. Fifteen to twenty years ago the emphasis was on protein only. Today nutritionists recognize that adequate energy and protein are necessary for an adequate diet.

A Country in Famine May Pass Through Three Stages

Would you believe that sometimes during famine food is actually *exported* while people in that country starve? This happened in Ireland during the potato famine of the 1840s. Today, exotic foods are available to tourists and wealthy residents in countries where most people are suffering from famine.

However, the hungry refugees you've seen on television clearly are not among the privileged citizens doing the exporting. Generally, a country passes through three stages when famine occurs:

- First, there is an alarm reaction, in which leading citizens and politicians search for food and relief.
- There is then a breakdown of the social order.
- Finally, there is a stage of exhaustion.

The Consequences of Starvation Are Severe Physical and Mental Retardation or Death

When a person's food intake is less than the amount needed, the following happens, the severity depending on how long the level of food intake is low:[33]

- *Tissue wasting:* This is caused by the breakdown of body tissues (especially muscle and body fat) to be burned as energy. Tissue wasting causes a "skin and bones" appearance and restricts the body's ability to do work or to participate in physical activities.
- *Susceptibility to infection:* Starvation causes a decrease in antibodies and causes decreased resistance to infections such as measles and malaria. The death rate is much higher from infectious diseases when nutrient intake is low.
- *Iron deficiency:* Resistance to infection and cognitive performance are reduced by iron deficiency. Children do not perform as well at school when they are anemic.
- *Iodine deficiency:* Goiter is rare in developed countries because of the addition of iodine to salt, and the wide distribution of food that contains iodine. However, goiter is common in Central and South America and in parts of Asia.
- *Vitamin A deficiency:* Lack of vitamin A produces blindness in many children in developing countries.

Undernutrition Has Social Costs

Undernutrition has a negative effect on national development: decreased productivity, educational achievement, well-being, and social mobility.[34] Moreover, when a country begins to rely on long-term food aid, it also begins to experience political problems. Not only is the country dependent on outside food supplies, but the food is apt to be used as a political lever. In addition, of course, the importation of food discourages incentives to produce food locally.[35]

Hunger May Occur Amid Plenty in Industrialized Countries

The United States and all other industrialized countries have hungry people. Indeed, hunger is more widespread and serious than at any time in the past 10 to 15 years.[36] The 1985 Report of the Physicians Task Force on Hunger in America considers hunger a growing epidemic.

Exactly *how many* people do not get enough food? Unfortunately, we have no way of "quantifying" the hungry feelings of a person. All that are available are physical measurements and techniques of determining nutrient deficiencies.

Whatever the number and causes, however, there are specific programs for dealing with hunger, which will be described in Chapter 15.

> There is enough food in the world to feed everybody, the problem is food distribution. Famines are caused by natural disasters, wars, and political problems. A lack of education about how to use food causes problems. Starvation causes wasting of the body, decreased resistance to infection, slowed mental development, and nutrient deficiencies. Hunger is a growing phenomenon in industrialized countries because of rising unemployment.

DECISIONS

1. Does On-Again, Off-Again Dieting Cause an Increase in Body Fat?

The answer is yes. When a person rapidly loses weight and then rapidly gains it back, it may produce a level of body fat that is actually *higher* than the amount of fat at the start of the diet. You can see this in Figure 10-7, which illustrates what happens when a healthy 23-year-old, 115 lb woman gains weight and then rapidly loses weight by dieting.

This is another example of how body weight can be misleading in the struggle against obesity. Values for percentage of body fat are important because each unsuccessful diet makes the problem of losing the extra fat more difficult.

2. How Do I Decide if a Weight-Reducing Diet is Nutritionally Sound?

Don't take anything for granted. If you can, ask the person promoting or directing the diet many questions about the ingredients and the complete nutritional profile of the diet.

Many weight-reducing diets may cause specific nutrient deficiencies if taken for several weeks without medical observation. A recent survey of 11 popular weight-reducing diets showed that *none* of them provided 100% of the U.S. RDA for the 13 vitamins and minerals studied.[37] The nutrients most often below recommended levels were thiamin, vitamin B_6, vitamin B_{12}, calcium, iron, zinc, and magnesium. Diets not providing 100% of the U.S. RDA for 13 vitamins and minerals studied:

Atkins	I Love America
Beverley Hills	I Love New York
Carbohydrate Craver's Basic	Pritikin (700 kcalories)
Carbohydrate Craver's Dense	Pritikin (1200 kcalories)
California (1200 kcalories)	Richard Simmons
California (2000 kcalories)	Scarsdale
F-Plan	Stillman

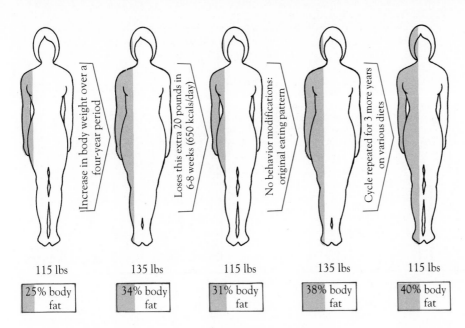

115 lbs   135 lbs   115 lbs   135 lbs   115 lbs

25% body fat   34% body fat   31% body fat   38% body fat   40% body fat

FIGURE 10-7
Effects of "yo-yo" dieting on the amount of body fat in a young woman.

3. Does Deciding on the Method of Weight Reduction Involve Consideration of the Emotional Response to the Method of Weight Loss?

Yes. Diet restriction has a significant effect on the moods of severely obese people. Depression, anxiety, irritability, and a preoccupation with food are common in many dieting people. These factors must be considered in deciding on the best diet for losing weight.

4. Can a High-Fiber Diet for Losing Body Weight Have Dangerous Effects?

Some people decide to use a high fiber intake as a means of reducing weight. The main function of the fiber is to add bulk to the contents of the gastrointestinal system and thereby reduce the desire for food (to give a "full feeling"). Glucomannan is one product that is sold for this purpose. It rapidly absorbs water and becomes so hard that it would bounce if thrown on the floor. A report from Australia tells of some unfortunate people who swallowed the dry form of glucomannan while also swallowing some water. It swelled rapidly in the esophagus to the point that it caused them to choke.[38]

5. Are There Any Inexpensive Yet Effective Weight-Loss Programs?

Weight loss competitions at your place of work are effective and cheap ways for people to lose weight.[39] Drop-outs from these programs are less than 1%. Weight loss averages 12 lb. The data in Figure 10-8 show the great advantages of these types of weight-loss programs to employer and employee.

6. Can It Be Predicted if Children Will Become Obese Adults by Examining Their Parents' Food Preferences?

It would be wonderful if nutritionists could because some early education may influence the child away from food choices that are more likely to lead to obesity.

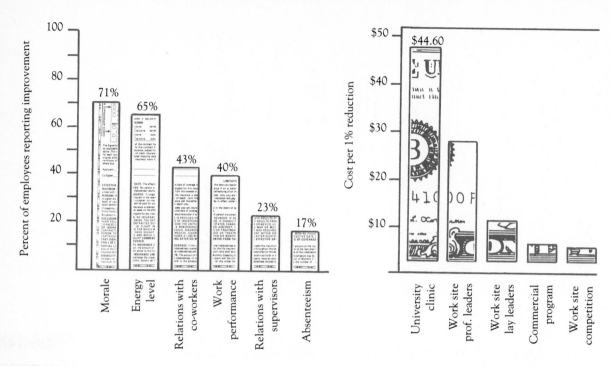

FIGURE 10-8

Weight loss at work. Weight-loss competitions at the work site have been effective at producing weight loss and improving morale, and are the most cost-effective.

However, before you decide to make major evaluations of a child's food preferences, it is important to determine whether the similarities with the parent's food preferences are due to genetic factors, environmental factors, or both. Research on preferences for actual foods has been extremely limited until recently.[40] The available evidence suggests that children's and their parents' food preferences tend to be similar. However, we must await further research before deciding upon the role of genetic and environmental influences.

7. Health Clubs and Fitness Advocates Promote the Idea That Exercise Increases the Metabolic Rate as Long as 12 to 24 Hours After the Exercise. How Can I Decide if This Happens?

It would be a marvelous way to lose some additional body fat. Just imagine: exercise itself will burn off some kcalories. And then there would be the added advantage of a type of after-exercise, additional burn-off of kcalories. This is said to occur because of an increase in basal metabolic rate.

Unfortunately, there is no "do-it-yourself" test to determine if this is happening to you. Therefore you must depend on the most recent research findings of the experts.[41] Evidence suggests that this effect on metabolic rate will not be produced by jogging for half an hour three times per week or taking several aerobics classes that each involve 20 minutes or so of vigorous exercise. It seems to work only after very intensive or very prolonged exercise. The mild activity undertaken by the average obese person is unlikely to have an effect. This does not mean that you should decide not to exercise if you are overweight. Remember, exercise itself is a way of burning kcalories.

SUMMARY

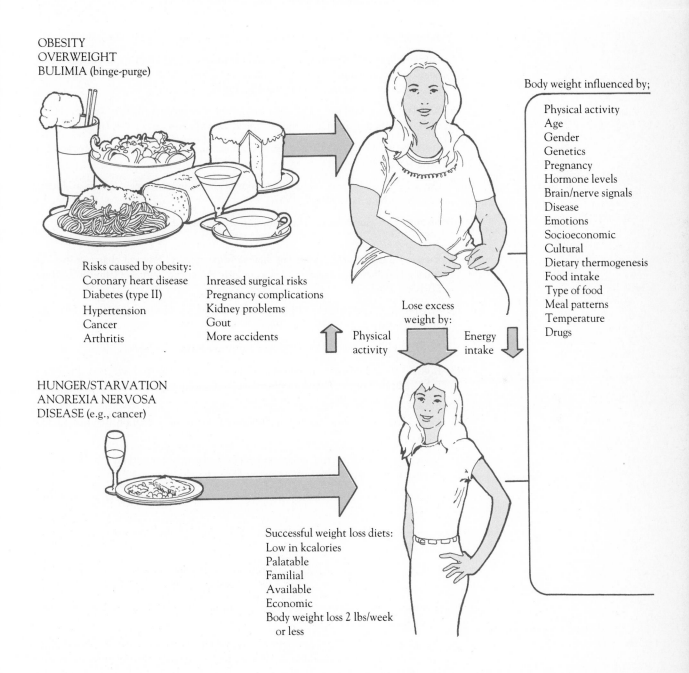

OBESITY
OVERWEIGHT
BULIMIA (binge-purge)

Risks caused by obesity:
Coronary heart disease
Diabetes (type II)
Hypertension
Cancer
Arthritis

Inreased surgical risks
Pregnancy complications
Kidney problems
Gout
More accidents

HUNGER/STARVATION
ANOREXIA NERVOSA
DISEASE (e.g., cancer)

Lose excess
weight by:

Physical
activity

Energy
intake

Body weight influenced by;

Physical activity
Age
Gender
Genetics
Pregnancy
Hormone levels
Brain/nerve signals
Disease
Emotions
Socioeconomic
Cultural
Dietary thermogenesis
Food intake
Type of food
Meal patterns
Temperature
Drugs

Successful weight loss diets:
Low in kcalories
Palatable
Familial
Available
Economic
Body weight loss 2 lbs/week
   or less

REFERENCES

1. Simonson, M.: Advances in research and treatment of obesity: an overview. Food and Nutrition News **53**(no. 4), March-April 1982.

2. Mayer, J.: Management of famine relief. Science **188**:571, 1975.

3. Health and Public Policy Committee, American College of Physicians: Eating disorders: anorexia nervosa and bulimia. Annals of Internal Medicine **105**:790, 1986.

4. Office of Research Reporting, National Institute of Child Health and Human Development: Facts about anorexia nervosa, Bethesda, Office of Research Reporting, NICHHD, National Institutes of Health, 1983.

5. Weigley, E.S.: Average? Ideal? Desirable? A brief overview of height-weight tables in the United States. Journal of the American Dietetic Association **84**:417, 1984.

6. Callaway, C.W.: Weight standards: their clinical significance. Annals of Internal Medicine **100**:296, 1984.

7. Garn, S.M., and others: Three limitations of the body mass index, American Journal of Clinical Nutrition **46**:377, 1987.

8. Bryant, C.A., and others: The cultural feast. West Publishing Co., St. Paul, p. 94, 1985.

9. Dwyer, J., and others: Adolescent dieters: who are they? Physical characteristics, attitudes, and dieting practices of adolescent girls. American Journal of Clinical Nutrition **20**:1045, 1967.

10. Jackson, A.S. and Pollock, M.L.: Practical assessment of body composition. Physician and Sportsmedicine **13**:76, May 1985.

11. Kissileff, H.R.: Satiety. Contemporary Nutrition **8**:(no. 1), January 1983.

12. Rolls, B.J., and others: The influence of variety on human food selection. In Barker, L.M., editor: The psychobiology of human food selection, AVI Publishing Co., Westport, CT, p. 101, 1982.

13. Diet change and obesity among modernizing Polynesians. Nutrition Reviews **42**:347, 1984.

14. Vasselli, J.R., and others: Obesity. In Recent knowledge in nutrition, 5th edition. The Nutrition Foundation, Inc., Washington D.C., p. 35, 1984.

15. Anonymous: Breakfast skipping: a national pastime. Food Engineering, p. 34, August 1983.

16. Anonymous: More than 68 million use low-calorie foods. Food Engineering, p. 26, May 1984.

17. Roe, D.A.: Nutrient and drug interactions. In Present knowledge in nutrition, 5th edition, The Nutrition Foundation, Inc., Washington D.C., p. 797, 1984.

18. Stunkard, A.J., and others: An adoption study of human obesity. New England Journal of Medicine **314**:193, 1986.

19. Atkinson, R.L.: Etiology, pathophysiology and treatment of obesity. In Anderson, J., editor: Dietary Excesses and Health/Disease Implications, Health Science Consortium, Inc., Chapel Hill, NC, p. 9, 1984.

20. Kolata, G.: Obesity declared a disease. Science **227**:1019, 1985.

21. Anderson, I.: Pot bellies, video displays and heart disease. New Scientist, p. 20, January 31, 1985.

22. Stern, J.S.: Is obesity a disease of inactivity? In Stunkard, A.J., and Stellar, E., editors: Eating and its disorders, Raven Press, New York, p. 131, 1984.

23. Cohen, M.R., and others: Naloxone reduces food intake in humans. Psychosomatic Medicine **47:**132, 1985.

24. Alsofrom, J.: Lipectomy: "magic bullet" for fat removal? American Medical News, p. 15, May 27, 1983.

25. Wrobel, S.B., and others: The surgical treatment of morbid obesity: economic, psychosocial, ethical, preventive, medical aspects of health care. Yale Journal of Biology and Medicine **56:**231, 1983.

26. Mitchell, J.E., and others: Characteristics of 275 patients with bulimia. American Journal of Psychiatry **142:**482, 1985.

27. Johnson, C.L., and others: A descriptive survey of dieting and bulimic behavior in a female high school population. In Understanding anorexia nervosa and bulimia. Ross Laboratories, Columbus, OH, p. 14, 1983.

28. Walsh, B.T., and others: Bulimia and depression. Psychosomatic Medicine **47:**123, 1985.

29. Blumenthal, J.A., and others: Is running an analogue to anorexia nervosa? Journal of the American Medical Association **252:**520, 1984.

30. Katz, S.: Anorexia and bulimia support group helping victims' families. Canadian Medical Association Journal **132:**1077, 1985.

31. Kazuo, H.: Economic aspects of food protein supplies in the world. Food and Nutrition Bulletin **6:**58, 1984.

32. Abelson, P.H.: World food. Science **236:**9, 1987.

33. Scrimshaw, N.S.: Consequences of hunger for individuals and societies. Federation Proceedings **45:**2421, 1986.

34. Berg, A.: Malnourished people: a policy view, The World Bank, Washington, D.C., p. 14, 1981.

35. Waterlow, J.C.: Famine relief in Africa. Lancet **i:**547, 1986.

36. Ellis, E.O.: Food for thought. Journal of the American Medical Association **253:**3299, 1985.

37. Fisher, M.C., and Lachance, P.A.: Nutrition evaluation of published weight-reducing diets. Journal of the American Dietetic Association **85:**450, 1985.

38. Henry, D.A., and others: Glucomannan and risk of oesophageal obstruction. British Medical Journal **292:**591, 1986.

39. Brownell, K.D., and others: Weight loss competitions at the work-site: impact on weight, morale and cost-effectiveness. American Journal of Public Health **74:**1283, 1984.

40. Anonymous: Similarity of children's and their parents' food preferences. Nutrition Reviews **45:**134, 1987.

41. Kolata, G.: Metabolic catch-22 of exercise regimens. Science **236:**146, 1987.

METABOLISM NOTES: *Metabolic Pathways in Obesity*

Research about and treatment for obesity involve many disciplines, among them biochemistry, physiology, genetics, neurochemistry, and psychology. The interaction of disciplines is shown in Figure 10-9, which is described below: the numbers in the text correspond to the numbers in the figure.

1. The *hypothalamus* in the brain performs many functions, one of which is to act as a hunger and satiety center. Obesity is considered to be due, in part, to a defect in these centers.

2. The enzyme *lipoprotein lipase* is believed to be a type of gatekeeper enzyme that is responsible for removing triglycerides from the blood. These are then deposited in the adipose tissue.

3. *Diet-induced thermogenesis* may be lower in some obese people. The level of thermogenesis is thought to be genetically controlled. Less energy is wasted as radiated heat by these people. The energy that is saved can be stored in adipose tissue. Lower diet-induced thermogenesis is thought to be due to a resistance to insulin in the obese person. If so, then less glucose can be stored as glycogen. The synthesis of glycogen requires an energy input.

4. Some investigators feel that obese people have a *defect in neurotransmitter function*. The brain produces a neurotransmitter called serotonin. Serotonin has a satiety-signaling effect. Therefore, high levels of serotonin will depress food intake. Serotonin production requires tryptophan, an essential amino acid. Tryptophan must be provided in the diet. Work is in progress where obese people are given 500 mg of tryptophan.

5. "Carbohydrate craving" is a phenomenon that is recognized by scientists. The craving seems to be during snacking rather than during a meal. A drug called dl-fenfluramine will increase serotonin release. When this drug is given to people there is a 40% reduction in carbohydrate snack consumption, and a 22% reduction in carbohydrates eaten in meals. People feel less depressed and fatigued, and more alert after a carbohydrate meal. Some researchers now recommend that some people take high carbohydrate intakes to alter mood in a favorable way.

6. There may be a seasonal effect on food intake. Some people become depressed during the winter, and they also overeat and crave carbohydrates.

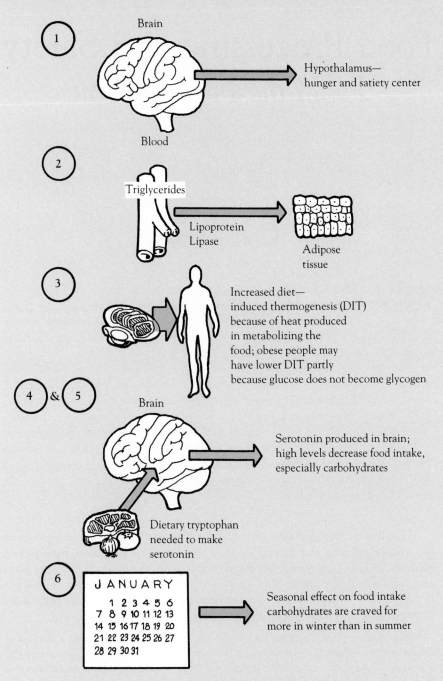

FIGURE 10-9
Summary of some recent theories of obesity.

1 Brain
Hypothalamus—
hunger and satiety center

Blood

2 Triglycerides
Lipoprotein
Lipase
Adipose
tissue

3 Increased diet—
induced thermogenesis (DIT)
because of heat produced
in metabolizing the
food; obese people may
have lower DIT partly
because glucose does not become glycogen

4 & 5 Brain
Serotonin produced in brain;
high levels decrease food intake,
especially carbohydrates

Dietary tryptophan
needed to make
serotonin

6 JANUARY
1 2 3 4 5 6
7 8 9 10 11 12 13
14 15 16 17 18 19 20
21 22 23 24 25 26 27
28 29 30 31

Seasonal effect on food intake
carbohydrates are craved for
more in winter than in summer

11

Food Processing and Safety
From the Farm to You

CONNECTIONS

Previous chapters have examined which foods have which nutrients. This chapter will describe the factors influencing the production of food, starting at the farm.

Farming is a complicated business. Farmers not only need the expertise to grow plants and care for animals but also a supportive natural environment: suitable water, land, and climate and available cheap energy.

Economic, political, and technological factors influence the amount of food that can be produced. Agricultural chemicals, for instance, can greatly increase productivity, although some people reject the use of such chemicals.

A very important technology is food preservation, which allows food to be eaten out of season and thousands of miles from the farm, although some nutrients may be lost during processing. Additives help preserve food and heighten its appeal to the senses, but some additives may be harmful to health. An understanding of such issues can enable you to have a better perspective in any debate about health, organic, and natural foods.

There is something romantically attractive about gathering fruits and berries in the wild or hunting and fishing for food. Anyone who has eaten fresh-picked blackberries or trout recently pulled from a mountain stream might envy the "savages" who used to live off the land. However, Dr. William T. Jarvis, in "The Myth of the Healthy Savage," has a different perspective. Civilized peoples have demonstrated an ability to adjust to and thrive nearly anywhere:

> Rather than envying the noble savage's health, we moderns should stand wide-eyed at the picture of civilized [people] surviving for extended periods of time on and under the sea, in arctic outposts, mountains, deserts, and even into the reaches of outer space—a tribute to the level of knowledge of nutrition science as well as our adaptive mechanisms.

But if our "adaptive mechanisms" and knowledge extend humanity's ability to survive, they also threaten it. For instance, the 1986 accident at the Chernobyl nuclear plant in the Soviet Union rendered much of the surrounding area uninhabitable and sent a cloud of radiation over Europe, which, of course, fell on many food crops. This only suggests what might happen during nuclear war. As Dr. Nevin Scrimshaw writes, "The disastrous effects of a thermonuclear exchange would not be limited to the food supply of the areas and countries directly experiencing nuclear attack; the effects on the food supply would be global."

How food is produced, and its vulnerability to war and other disasters, is important information. You will see how the nutritive value of food is influenced by how it is grown, stored, distributed, and prepared. In the following pages, therefore, we will consider farms, supermarkets, and kitchens.

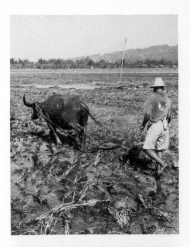

"HUNTING" FOR FOOD: THE CHANGES OF MODERN TIMES

One nutrient you get free—vitamin D from the sun. With every other nutrient, you must expend some effort—you must, in effect, "hunt" for it.

Obviously, the form of the hunt has taken a different turn since prehistoric times, when people moved from place to place in search of wild plants and animals. Although elsewhere in the world people still do this, modern agriculture provides residents of industrialized nations with a stable food supply. Clearly, agriculture has also changed. Once North America was made up of farms that grew food for the family only, a type of farming known as *subsistence agriculture*. Today agriculture is a business—*agribusiness*—whether run by a family or a giant corporation, and food is grown as a product to sell.

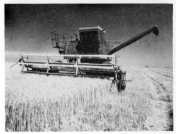

Machines produce food more efficiently than either man or beast. One major problem with machines is dependence on oil—a problem in many developing countries during the oil crisis of the 1970's.

The Quantity and Quality of Food Produced on the Farm Influences Nutrient Intake

Do you think you have what it takes to be a farmer? Success at providing enough food depends on the proper combination of skill, water, land, climate, energy inputs, use of agricultural chemicals, plant and animal genetics and pathology, and government regulation. A failure in even *one* of these areas can produce a food crisis. Let's look at each of these factors.

Skill

Farming is both a science and a business. Farmers need to know the *science* of agricultural production and the *business* of agricultural marketing. The highest yields of food are usually produced by farmers who know both, at least in North America and other advanced economies; it is not so in developing countries. In underdeveloped nations, farmers not only lack agricultural knowledge, capital, and often access to markets but even the security of owning their own land.

In controlled economies, such as those of the Soviet Union and China, farmers lack the financial incentives to produce large quantities of food. As a result, it is common in Soviet bloc countries to see long lines of people waiting to buy food. In China, however, policy makers are moving away from collective farming.

In industrialized countries—despite the fact that farmers are leaving the land in large numbers—there has been no decrease in the amount of food produced. Improvements in genetics, mechanization, and the use of fertilizers has made farming more efficient and increased food yields. However, these improvements are expensive and in the 1980s in the United States many farmers became financially overextended and there have been waves of bankruptcies and farm sales.

Many nutritionists feel strongly that having food is a human right;[1] however, food is also a commodity of commerce, and people must earn a living from its

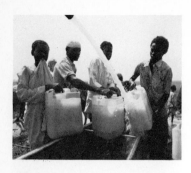

Clean water is essential for people, animals, and plants. Water is in short supply in some parts of the world.

production. When people find they can make a better living doing something else—as many farm laborers in Africa discovered when they left the land to work in the oil fields[2]—it can lead to serious problems in food production.

Water

Agricultural plants and animals, of course, need water as much as human beings do. No matter how skilled a farmer may be and how good the land, if there is no water there will be no food. Drought, in fact, has been a major cause of famine in Africa.

Indeed, it is startling to find out *how much* water it takes to produce food. The next time you eat a slice of bread, for example, try to pause and remember that producing that one slice required *35 gallons of water*—both in the growing and in the processing. Amounts of water needed to produce a pound of other kinds of foods are shown in Table 11-1.

Of course, agriculture's demand for water must compete with other demands made on water supplies—industrial, recreational, and waste-disposal, for example. The supply of water may be restricted by evaporation and pollution. Each person produces about 165 gallons of human waste (urine and feces) each year, and, according to agricultural economist Barbara Ward, it requires about *13,000* gallons of clean water to dispose of this amount.

TABLE 11-1 Amount of Water Needed for Production of Certain Foods

Food Produced (1 pound)	Pounds of Water Required
Wheat	300-500
Potatoes	600-800
Rice	1,500-2,000
Vegetables	3,000-5,000
Milk	10,000*
Meat	20,000-50,000*

*Includes water needed to produce food fed to the animal.

Land

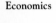

Economics

Just like everything else, land changes, and every year much agricultural land is lost. Some gives way to buildings and roads. Some deteriorates owing to soil erosion. Other land is abandoned because it is contaminated with chemicals. In the United States, some land is not cultivated at all—simply because farmers are paid not to cultivate it, in order, supposedly, to prevent overproduction of food and sustain food prices at a high level.

Climate

To appreciate that climate is important for agriculture, one need only observe what happens when the climate changes. In Africa, for example, changes in weather patterns have been one cause of famines.

Scientists debate whether the "greenhouse effect"—a global warming trend believed to result from increased levels of carbon dioxide in the atmosphere resulting from the burning of fossil fuels—will gradually increase the temperature on earth, leading to changes in the ability to grow certain crops in some parts of the world.

Air pollutants can also change climate by preventing the earth's heat from escaping into the atmosphere.

Energy

It takes energy—muscle power or machine power—to produce food. Energy for the muscle power of humans or farm animals is produced by food; energy for machines is produced by fossil fuels.

In developing countries, women do much of the planting and gathering of food. However, their productivity may be hindered by iron-deficiency anemia and by the demands of pregnancy and lactation, especially if their diet is poor.[3]

The use of petroleum-based products in agriculture also has limitations. When the price of oil goes up, so does the cost of many agricultural inputs and activities: irrigation, fertilizers, planting, harvesting, and transportation. As a result, food prices increase in industrialized countries, which may be affordable to their residents but not to those people in less-developed parts of the world who depend on imports of food from industrialized countries.

Agricultural chemicals

An estimated two-thirds of America's crop lands are treated with pesticides every year, according to the U.S. Department of Agriculture. By the early 1980s, this amounted to almost 1.2 billion lb of pesticides per year.

Agricultural chemicals pose a real quandary. On the plus side, they increase the amount of food produced, making more nutrients available at lower cost. On the minus side such chemicals may have an adverse effect on health, as first suggested in Rachel Carson's famous 1962 book, *Silent Spring*. DDT in human milk, antibiotics in cow's milk, and pesticides in foods are unacceptable hazards. Such chemicals can enter people's bodies when they are young, and their effects over a lifetime are largely unknown. Such problems must be addressed not only by the agricultural industry but also by consumers and government. Consumers in particular have expressed more concern about pesticides than about cholesterol, salt, or sugar as problems in food.[4]

Unfortunately, the consumers have no way of seeing the chemicals in food, which puts them at the mercy of the food industry. The growth of the health food business has been in part a reaction to this problem. However, as mentioned earlier, though the words "organic" and "natural" are used to describe foods that are grown without agricultural chemicals, in truth these terms have no legal meaning. In short, whatever kind of food the consumers buy, they are dependent on the truthfulness of the food producer.

Modern food production technology offers us the benefits of more abundant nutrients but presents risks from certain agricultural chemicals.

Plant and animal genetics

You might think that vitamin C content wouldn't vary much from one variety of tomato to another, but actually it can vary considerably, depending on the genetics of the particular strain. The same is true with other fruits and vegetables. Florida and California avocados have the same amount of vitamin C, but the California variety has more kcalories and fat (see Appendix P).

In animals the amount of fat in meat and milk varies, depending on the breed of the animal.

Similar foods may vary widely in nutrient content.

Harvesting and storage

When and how a crop is harvested and stored affects its nutrient content. A plant that is not yet ripe or that is overripe when harvested may have a lower vitamin content. Food can also be lost because of physical damage or inefficient harvesting techniques.

Faulty storage of food, as when a crop is stored at too high or low a temperature, may cause loss of heat-sensitive vitamins. Insects and rodents can also destroy food during harvesting and storage.

Diseases

Plants or animal diseases have often caused much loss of food, especially in many developing countries. Over a million people died in Ireland's potato famine in the mid-1840s, the failure of the potato crop due to blight.

Economics and politics

In controlled economies, government policies affect the amounts and kinds of foods produced. In so-called free economies, they reflect both the laws of supply and demand and also government intervention in the form of subsidies or taxes. Ever heard of "butter mountains" and "wine lakes"? These were food surpluses produced in the European Economic Community as a result of political decisions—government subsidies to keep the farmers happy.

Governments also use food as a weapon. In the late 1970s, for instance, the United States put an embargo on grain exported to the Soviet Union. U.S. grain production declined because this embargo artificially reduced demand.

Transportation Has Changed the Availability of Food

Trucks, trains, and planes—their cargoes often refrigerated—haul oranges from Florida, lettuce from Calfornia, and seafood from the Gulf coast to all parts of the country. Americans can now get exotic foods from far away and nearly all year round—kiwi fruit from New Zealand, for instance—and thus are able to create an exciting, varied diet less dependent on local foods.

Sophisticated transportation techniques provide nutritional benefits. Iodine deficiency, once prevalent in the upper Midwest and central Canada because of low iodine content in the soil, is no longer a problem there partly because iodine-rich food can be transported from coastal states.

Countries with poor infrastructures—transportation systems of roads, rails, and bridges—lack the means for distributing food effectively. Thus, food for famine relief has been known to rot in ships in ports because of bottlenecks in the transportation system. But the importance of transportation is also demonstrated in developed countries, when labor troubles in the transportation industry prevent food from leaving the farm gate.

The quantity of food produced depends on the farmers' skills, the quality of land and water, the use of agricultural chemicals, the genetic strains of the food plants and animals grown, the incidence of plant and animal disease, harvesting and storage techniques, and economic and political policies. Once the food is produced, the distribution of food to the population depends on the transportation system.

FOOD IN THE SUPERMARKET

Today North Americans "hunt," if that is the word for it, for food in the convenient environment of the supermarket. Your ancestors had most of their food choices dictated to them: they ate whatever plants were in season and whatever fish, fowl, or animal they were fortunate enough to catch, a tiring enterprise. You, however, may be tired for different reasons—from having to make choices from among the thousands of different processed foods available in a single store.

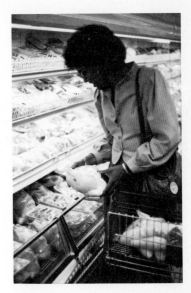

Hunting for food in supermarkets is very different from hunting for survival done by our ancestors.

Individuals Differ in Their Preferences for Various Foods

"What a strange collection of food," you may think, looking over the shopping cart of the customer ahead of you in the check-out line. Fresh, frozen, canned, pasteurized, fermented, milled, irradiated, salted, dehydrated, whatever—the foods that a person chooses represent personal preference.

Let us examine what some of the reasons for selecting a food are, whether it is from a supermarket shelf or from a restaurant menu.

Appearance

Nature and the food industry are experts in using color to make food attractive. Nature uses color to help you determine if a food is ripe or rotten. The food industry uses color—either natural (from animals, plants, or minerals) or artificial (from dyes)—to excite the eye. Studies show that foods do not taste "right" if they are not colored "right." For example, research has shown that people think a sherbet has a different flavor when the color is changed.[5]

Aroma

No doubt you've noticed how unappealing any kind of food is when you have a cold. This is testimony to the importance of food aroma and your sense of smell to the experience of taste. The human nose is usually accurate in helping one decide if a food has spoiled. Spices help make bland foods more appealing.

Texture

You may not even be consciously aware of the importance of this attribute, but it strongly affects the enjoyment of food. For instance, most people like meat tender, not tough. On the other hand, many people reject raw oysters because they are too "slimy." Similarly, the texture of liver does not appeal to some people.

Flavor

You may prefer sweet, bitter, acidic, or salty foods. You may hide flavors with spice. The attractiveness or distaste of a food's flavor is lodged in your memory.

Sound

Certain sounds are associated with certain characteristics of food—the "sizzle" sound of meat on a barbeque, for instance. Television commercials often use sounds—or words that sound like sounds, such as "snap, crackle, pop"—to evoke an impression of freshness or other pleasant characteristics of food.

Familiarity

Many people are simply not very adventurous eaters, and most prefer to stick with familiar food. Even starving people are not inclined to eat unfamiliar foods.

Culture

Because of the way different cultures treat the same basic ingredients there may be big differences in nutritive value and appearance of the resulting foods.[6] For example, wheat, corn, and oats may come to the table as bread made from refined and fortified flour or from whole-grain wheat, as sugar-laden breakfast cereals, as porridge (in Scotland), as grits (in the southern United States), as unleavened bread (in the Middle East), as tortillas (in Mexico), or as chipati (in India). Most orientals prefer rice as their main cereal food.

Recently in North America there has been a growing appreciation not only for the foods of foreign cultures—Italian, Greek, Mexican, and so on—but also for regional dishes: Creole, Cajun, New England style, and the like (see Chapter 2).[7]

Religion

Some foods are forbidden by some religions: pork for Jews and Muslims, beef for Hindus, all meat for Seventh Day Adventists, Mennonites, and Trappist (Roman Catholic) monks. These exclusions are of little nutritional significance if the rest of the diet is varied and balanced.

Religion has a positive influence on the nutritional status of some elderly people because of church dinners and picnics, assistance with shopping, invitations to share meals, and gifts of food from fellow church members.[8] Many religions teach moderation in all things, and some require abstinence from alcohol and tobacco.

Advertising

Nutritionists are concerned about some aspects of food advertising. First, foods high in kcalories and low in nutrients are advertised more often than nutritious foods. Many advertisements entice you to consume alcoholic drinks, tea and coffee, cakes and dessert mixes, breakfast cereals, sweeteners and syrups, soft drinks, and potato chips. Advertisements for vegetables, seafood, chicken, milk and other dairy products, nuts and fruits are seen less frequently. Children, the elderly, and those on medically supervised diets are vulnerable to this type of advertising.

A second concern is the "policing" of food advertisements. Certain words are often misused in food ads; "nutritious," "wholesome," and "natural" are subject to varying interpretations. The Federal Trade Commission is responsible for monitoring health care and curative claims, including information directed at diabetics and people with cholesterol or heart disease problems. The FTC is also supposed to keep an eye on claims related to low sugar, low sodium, low kcalorie, and low cholesterol intake and on claims regarding fiber content, weight loss, and nutrient comparisons. The Food and Drug Administration has control over food labels but not food advertisements.

Lifestyles

Your grandmothers may have baked cakes from scratch, your mother may have baked cakes from cake mixes, and you might buy cakes already baked and frosted. In other words, this is an era of convenience foods, whether finger foods or microwave-ready frozen dinners (see Figure 11-1).

Convenience often has a trade-off. A TV dinner is easier to prepare and it may taste good, but at 200 to 350 kcalories per meal, it may not provide enough energy, especially for many men. Protein quantity and quality may be high, but so is fat content, and so also is sodium content relative to the number of kcalories.[9] Finally, a lot of convenience food is expensive per serving.

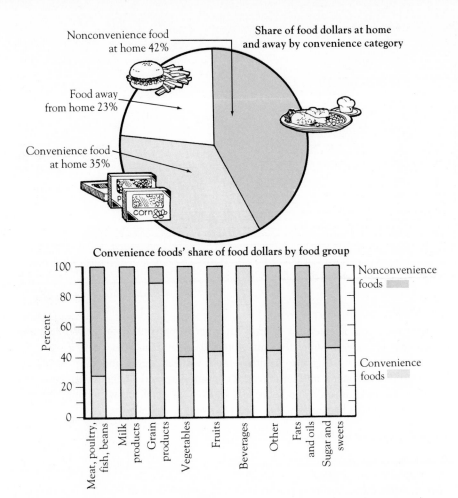

Share of food dollars at home and away by convenience category

Nonconvenience food at home 42%

Food away from home 23%

Convenience food at home 35%

Convenience foods' share of food dollars by food group

Nonconvenience foods

Convenience foods

FIGURE 11-1

Convenience foods make nutrients more accessible. The nutrient content of convenience foods may be excellent or poor depending on the food.
Pie chart: Based on 1977 data. Convenience foods: fully or partially prepared foods which transfer significant time, culinary skill, or energy from the homemaker's kitchen to commercial food processors and distributors. Nonconvenience foods: fresh or basic processed foods (such as flour) used in home recipes. *Bar graph:* Based on 1977 data. Meat group includes eggs, nuts, peanut butter. Beverages include beverage powders and mixes, ades, punches, regular soft drinks, alcoholic beverages. Other includes diet soft drinks, plain coffee, tea, cocoa. Mixtures are in group of main ingredient.

Family structure

The amount and type of food eaten may be influenced by family structure. Nearly 60% of today's infants will be living with only one parent before they are 18 years old. This may be a time of emotional and economic stress. It could have an influence on the amount and type of food eaten. However, little is known about the effects of this social problem on the nutritional status of the children. There is limited evidence from Britain that children of fatherless families are shorter.[10] Nutrition may be one factor involved if this observation is confirmed.

Status

Status seekers use food to impress others. Scarce and expensive foods have high status, but this can change with time. In London in the 1830s, salmon was a food of the common people—and, of all things, *beans* were a food desired by the affluent.

Health factors

Often people will increase their consumption of a particular food because of its health benefits. Dairy products may be eaten to increase calcium intake to prevent

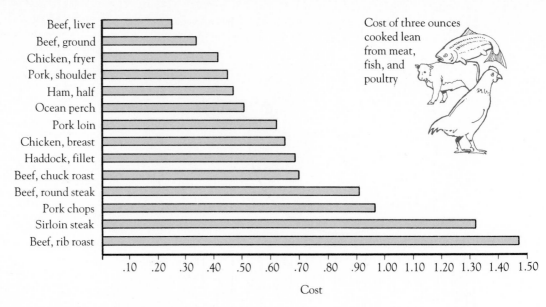

FIGURE 11-2
Meat, poultry, and fish do not differ greatly in nutritive value. Cost differences reflect differences in palatability and in consumer demand.

osteoporosis. Meat is eaten for its iron, in order to prevent anemia. Whole-grain cereals may provide the fiber that may forestall colon cancer.

Foods are also avoided for health reasons—meat, eggs, and dairy products because their cholesterol and saturated fat content may be connected with coronary heart disease, sodium-rich foods because of their association with hypertension, high kcalorie foods because they lead to overweight and obesity.

Preservatives and additives

A person's point of view about this matter will determine what he or she puts in the shopping cart. Indeed, if you feel strongly about the possible harmful effects of these substances, you may not shop in a supermarket at all but in a health-food store for additive-free, nonprocessed foods.

Food allergies

Obviously, if you are allergic to certain foods, they will not be on your shopping list. You can read more about this topic in the Decisions section at the end of the chapter.

Nutritional values

Nutritional significance of food choices may be negligible, moderate, or considerable. A choice between white and red grapes, or between Brand A and Brand B frozen beans has negligible effects. A choice between pork or beef, beans or peas has moderate effects, and a choice between fresh fruit and chocolates has considerable nutritional significance.

Cost

The most expensive foods do not always contain proportionally more nutrients. For example, there is wide variation in the cost of three ounces of different cuts of cooked meat, poultry, and fish (see Figure 11-2). There is not much difference in the concentration of most nutrients (see Table of Food Composition, Appendix

P). Part of the higher price is for guaranteed atractiveness of the meat, part is due to higher consumer demand.

> Your choice of foods is determined by your reaction to their appearance, aroma, texture, flavor, and even sound. People eat or avoid certain foods because of familiarity; for cultural and religious reasons; in response to advertising, pressure for status symbols, and convenience; or to conform to their family's diet. Certain foods may contribute to diseases such as heart disease and certain cancers, or food allergies. Presence of preservatives and additives may influence food choices. Finally, cost is important.

FOOD PRESERVATION: NUTRIENTS FOR ALL SEASONS

As people have become more accustomed to eating food that is fresh, low in fat, and sweeter, the food manufacturers have stepped forward to oblige—providing over 1600 new products in the first nine months of 1985 alone.[11] The amazing variety of foods available in the supermarket is partly due to the use of preservatives and additives. Foods may spoil because of microbiologic, physical, chemical, or enzyme-induced decay. These losses to food quality occur before and after harvesting or slaughter.[12] Without preservation many foods would be inedible before they reached the store or the kitchen. Food preservation may be:

- Chemical—adding salt or food additives, bleaching
- Physical—heating, cooling, drying
- Biological—fermentation

Let us now take a look at food preservation in more detail.

Food Preservation Has a 5000-Year History

Some of the food-preservation processes still in use today were first used more than 5000 years ago: drying, adding of sugar or salt, smoking, and fermentation. Today these are augmented by canning, pasteurization and sterilization, refrigeration and freezing, and irradiation.

Food-spoiling micro-organisms need water to survive. Ancient peoples discovered food could be preserved by drying or by adding sugar or salt to bind the water, which made it unavailable to the micro-organisms. Modern methods of food preservation involve the addition or removal of heat from food in order to retard or inactivate spoilage-causing mechanisms.

Let us look at the various food-preservation methods.

Drying

Drying is less popular today for economic reasons. Drying is expensive because of the high cost of fossil fuels, although sun-drying, an inefficient process, is still practiced in some parts of the world. More controlled but expensive methods of drying include oven drying, spray-drying (used mainly with milk products), and freeze-drying. The difficulty with drying is that it may lead to loss of heat-sensitive vitamins—losses as high as 50% (see Chapter 6).

Economics

Adding sugar

The addition of sugar, as in both commercial and home canning, certainly caters to a person's "sweet tooth," but it can also cause dental caries and dilute the nutrient content of the food.

Adding salt

The issue of the amount of salt added to manufactured food in affluent societies is a difficult one to resolve.[12] Food processors add salt to food to improve taste, flavor, consistency, appearance, and shelf-life of the food. However, the risk of high salt (sodium consumption), of course, is that it may cause hypertension in some people. It has been suggested that the most effective way to reduce salt intake in the North American diet is to change the manufacturing process, although this would involve extensive technological research. Others have argued, however, that changing the manufacturing process is a waste of time and resources because people will simply add salt to their food at home, that instead the way to reduce salt consumption is to concentrate on altering the population's taste for salt.

Smoking

The smoking process kills bacteria in food and protects the fat in meats. However, it also destroys up to 20% of some of the heat-sensitive vitamins. Little is known about its other effects on nutritional quality. Foods heavily smoked over wood the "natural" way may contain cancer-causing chemicals on the surface of the food. Much of the smoking now uses a liquid smoke extract from which the cancer-causing chemicals have been removed.

Fermentation

Yogurt, aged cheese, bread, soy products such as tofu and miso, pickles, sauerkraut, and wine and beer are produced by fermentation. Fermented foods are used to add flavor and color to a meal and even as main courses in some countries (India, Indonesia). Fermentation actually improves the nutritional value of a food. For example:

- Additional vitamin B_{12} is obtained from the micro-organisms used during fermentation.
- Protein in a food becomes more available after fermentation.
- The beany flavor is removed, thereby making the important source of nutrients in beans more acceptable.

However, the negative side of fermented foods is that they may have a high sodium content and they require adequate sanitation to prevent food poisoning.

Sales of fermented soy products such as tofu and miso are increasing in popularity in the United States, whereas they have actually declined in Japan. You will probably continue to see increased popularity of fermented foods in North America, for a number of reasons:

- Recent scientific interest in fermented foods
- Decreased likelihood of food poisoning from fermented foods
- Increased shelf-life of fermented foods
- Improvement in physical properties of fermented food
- Public interest in more natural products of plant origin
- Public interest in more healthy food

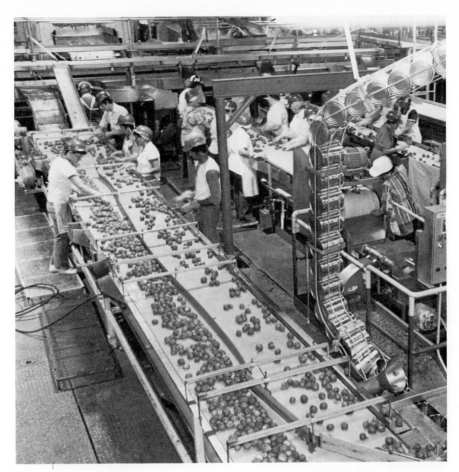

Processed foods are a major part of the diet for people in developed countries. Some advantages include increased year-round availability and safety from microbial infection. Disadvantages include loss of some nutrients due to heat or refining.

- Need for increased consumption of plant materials because of population increases
- Cultural and religious reasons

Canning

Home and commercial canning uses heat to kill harmful or spoilage-causing microorganisms; however, the heat should not be so high that it causes loss of nutrients. The trouble with canning foods is that the process causes greater losses of vitamin C, riboflavin, and niacin than either drying or freezing the food. Further losses of water-soluble nutrients occur when the food is canned in water, which consumers usually discard before eating the food.

In addition, tin from the can may accumulate in the food. This is not a problem provided the tin content does not exceed 250 ppm. Tin is an essential mineral and is relatively nontoxic, but it gives food a metallic taste.

Home canning of food must be done with care. Inadequate temperature control and improper seals on the jars permit botulism poisoning, caused by the *Clostridium botulinum* organism. Botulism is quite rare with commercially canned foods; between 1940 and 1979, over 800 billion cans of food were prepared commercially, but only five deaths from botulism related to commercially canned foods were reported. However, during the same period 700 deaths were reported from people who ate home-canned foods.[13]

Pasteurization

Exposure of food to high temperatures for short periods produces maximum destruction of disease-causing micro-organisms but keeps nutrient destruction to a minimum. Milk and fruit juices are most frequently pasteurized.

Vitamin C is again the major casualty in this heating process, causing some adverse publicity. However, it must be remembered that milk is not a large contributor of vitamin C to the diet. A similar example is that pasteurized fruit juices have less vitamin C than juice freshly squeezed from oranges or in the frozen form. However, one glass of the pasteurized orange juice will still meet 100% of the RDA for vitamin C. Also, pasteurized fruit juice sales are less than 10% of the market.

The lesson from this is twofold. First, the amount of the nutrient remaining after destruction by heat may still provide a reasonable proportion of the RDA. Second, the contribution by the food to the total intake of the nutrient may be insignificant.

Blanching

Blanching uses heat before freezing or dehydration to inactivate enzymes that cause undesirable changes in flavor, color, or nutritive value during storage. Heat-sensitive nutrients, especially heat-sensitive vitamins, are most affected by blanching with boiling water, less by steam, and least by microwaves.

Refrigeration and freezing

Refrigeration and freezing are the two best methods for maintaining the nutritive value and sensory qualities of foods.[14] One disadvantage: vitamin losses may occur in drippings when meat is thawed.

Irradiation

The negative nutritional effects of heat mentioned under the other processes do not apply here. Irradiation of food uses ionizing radiation, including X-rays. No high heat treatments are involved. The World Health Organization states that food irradiation provides two main advantages:

- It destroys certain food-borne pathogens, thus making food safer.
- It prolongs the shelf-life of food by killing pests and delaying the deterioration process.[15]

Irradiation eliminates parasites in pork and kills insects in fruits, grains, and spices. Toxins and viruses are not eliminated by irradiation. Spices especially benefit by this method because applying heat to spices changes their flavor.

Some people criticize irradiation as an untested technique that may lead to cancer and mutations, although in surveys the American public says it is willing to use irradiated foods.[16] At present, irradiation is allowed in the United States only to kill insects in wheat grains, to prevent sprouting in potatoes, and to sterilize spices. Canada and the European countries use food irradiation much more extensively.

Chemical preservatives

Some chemicals prevent the growth of food-spoiling micro-organisms. Examples of chemical preservatives are vinegar and citric acid, which lower pH in jams, relishes, and salad dressing. Calcium propionate prevents mold growth in breads. Nitrites prevent the growth of botulism-causing micro-organisms in bacon.

Chemicals also prevent nonmicrobial spoilage of food. For instance, BHT and BHA prevent foods from becoming rancid. Food that is slighly rancid loses vitamin A, and food that is very rancid is simply not eaten.

Food Preservation Developments Have Been Associated with the Military

The military has always believed that, as Napoleon said, an army travels on its stomach. Many innovations in food processing were developed to feed armies on the move. For instance, canning was invented in 1811 to help Napoleon's armies. By the mid-1800s refrigeration allowed meat to be shipped from Australia, New Zealand, and South America to Great Britain. Dehydrated foods were developed for American troops during World War II. In the Vietnam War, the traditional, heavy tin can was replaced by a flexible pouch that could be heated.

Space travel has also inspired new food-preservation techniques. Irradiated food was eaten by John Glenn in the first American manned orbit of the earth. Astronauts have dined on irradiated food in space ever since, with no apparent ill effects.

Food Preservation Has Advantages and Disadvantages for Nutrient Content in the Diet

Food preservation has one important disadvantage: some of the heat-labile nutrients are lost during processing.

However, this disadvantage is probably far outweighed by the advantages:

- Foods are available at all times of year.
- Heat increases the digestibility of cereal grains and legumes.
- A growing worldwide urban population simply cannot be given an adequate diet from fresh foods alone.
- Commercial processors are better able to control conditions such as temperature, light, air, and pH than can people preserving food at home.

Also, when a preservation method causes loss of nutrients, the contribution by the food to the total intake of the nutrient must be considered.

People have preserved foods since their earliest days. Modern food preservation methods involve chemical, physical, or biological changes in the food. Factors in the choice of method include food safety, food acceptability, nutrient losses, and cost.

FOOD ADDITIVES

Food additives, in Arnold Bender's words, "include all materials deliberately added to food to help manufacture and preserve food, improve palatability and eye-appeal." Additives, then, serve a useful purpose.

Many people, however, are concerned about the negative effects of food additives. Consider the following statement: "We have now shown that many bakers in London daily commit at least a double violation of the law, whereby they expose themselves to heavy penalties—first, in selling bread deficient of its proper weight; and secondly, in making use of the forbidden ingredient, alum."[17] Does this worry you? It needn't, for it was written in *1851.* It shows, however, that there has been concern over a long period of time about the purity of foods—in this case, bread containing alum, which causes diarrhea and nausea. (The authorities solved the problem by printing the names and addresses of the guilty bakers.) This investigation of London bakers led the British parliament in 1860 to pass the first pure-food laws. In the United States, similar laws, prompted by Upton Sinclair's novel *The Jungle,* describing filth in Chicago's meat-processing industry, were enacted in 1906.

Today's concerns about additives, however, are of a different nature. Let us explore these.

Food Additives Are Different Chemicals with Different Tasks

Between 2000 and 3900 different chemicals are classified as direct food additives. Why such a range in number? The reason is that different experts use different criteria to define a food additive.

Between now and 1995 the use of food additives is expected to increase threefold and in the United States alone additives are expected to generate $4.7 billion in sales revenues to their manufacturers. However, the cost of introducing a new food additive is high; testing alone can take 4 to 10 years at a cost of $500,000 to $10 million.[14]

Food additives are classed as intentional and incidental.

Intentional additives

These are substances added on purpose to perform specific functions. Preservation, improved flavor, taste, smell, color, texture, and/or improved nutritive value result from these additives. This group can be divided into two types:

- *Functional additives* improve the shelf-life or nutritional value of a food; they include all preservatives, including antimicrobial agents, antioxidants, nitrates, nitrites, and antibiotics. Functional additives also include nutrition supplements—minerals, vitamins, and amino acids. Finally, they include additives that influence the physical properties of food, such as anticaking agents (important in humid climates), emulsifiers, stabilizers, and humectants (which prevent loss of moisture from the food).
- *Sensory additives* make the food more appealing. They include flavoring agents (such as natural and artificial sweeteners, salt, spices, and monosodium glutamate) and food colors (natural and artificial dyes).

Incidental additives

These are additives that appear by accident because of some phase of production, processing, storage, or packaging of food. Examples are pesticides, iodine in fast foods, lead in wine (from lead bottle caps), and tin in canned food. Incidental additives may also be called contaminants.

This chapter will concentrate on intentional additives (Table 11-2).

TABLE 11-2 Food Additive Categories

Anticaking	Formulation aids:	Processing aids:
Antimicrobial	carriers, binders,	clarifying, clouding,
Antioxidants	fillers, plasticizers	catalyst, floculants,
Color, and adjuncts	Fumigants	filter aids,
Curing and pickling	Humectants	crystallization,
Dough strengtheners	Leavening	inhibitors
Drying agents	Lubricants and release	Propellants
Emulsifiers	agents	Sequestrants
Enzymes	Non-nutritive	Solvents and vehicles
Firming agents	sweeteners	Stabilizers and
Flavor enchancers	Nutritive sweeteners	thickeners
Flavoring agents	Oxidizing and reducing	Surface active agents
Flour treating	pH control	Surface finishing agents
		Synergists
		Texturizers

Additives Have Positive and Negative Nutrition Implications

The whole point of having intentional additives, of course, is to provide positive benefits. However, there are some negative aspects as well.

Positive implications

Intentional additives make foods available from any part of the world at any time of year. This enables you to have wide variations in your diet, eliminating or reducing possible nutrient deficiencies.

Such additives also lower the cost of food, because it can be produced and sold in large amounts. Lower price is particularly important, of course, for people who have low incomes, the group among whom the most nutrient deficiencies are found.

Finally, additives result in less food being wasted. Artificial sweeteners used in place of sugar also means that people may take in fewer kcalories.

Negative aspects

Two principal preservatives are sugar and salt, and these have a range of adverse health effects. Additives also permit the development of junk food—foods low in nutrients. Most serious, some food additives have been blamed for causing cancer (the sweeteners saccharin and cyclamate and the nitrite in bacon), hyperactivity in children, and problems for people on restricted diets (aspartame is harmful to people who have phenylketonuria). Evidence that additives play important roles in these problems is either tentative or nonexistent.

One great drawback is the whole matter of identifying additives. A glance at most food labels shows that you almost have to have a degree in chemistry to understand them. Indeed, many labels use the term "preservatives" or "artificial flavors" without defining which ones are in the food. And certainly many people will not understand what, say, benzoic acid is supposed to do and whether or not it is harmful. Actually, benzoic acid, used to prevent spoilage by micro-organisms, is harmless and occurs in tea, prunes, most berries, and spices such as cloves and cinnamon. Another additive, with the forbidding name erythorbic acid, has antioxidant properties and is perfectly safe, but how would a lay person know?

Safe Additives Appear on the GRAS List

An important list for anyone concerned about safety in food additives is the GRAS list. *GRAS* stands for "Generally Recognized As Safe." This list contains over 700 food additives considered safe because they have been used over a long period of time without any known ill effects. Since 1973, the compounds on the list have been periodically reviewed, and now and then a substance may be removed, as was saccharin when it became suspected of having a relationship to bladder cancer. (Saccharin was later restored to the list for use in soft drinks, provided that products containing it carry a warning to consumers about bladder cancer.)

Milling and Refining Remove Many Nutrients

Wheat, corn, rice, oats, barley, and rye are milled by removing the outer bran layers and some of the germ from the seed. Fiber and about 40 to 60 percent of the vitamin and mineral content of the grain is lost because these parts are discarded. This is why grain products must be enriched with thiamin, riboflavin, niacin, and iron to replace these losses. Calcium and vitamin D are usually added, although this is optional.[16]

Even with these government-required additives, however, the nutritive value of a slice of bread varies in different parts of the United States, owing to differences in grains, soil, and processing techniques. For example, the iron and sodium content has been found to vary considerably for the same type of bread in Los Angeles, Dallas, Chicago, and Washington, D.C.[18] Because of the importance of iron and sodium, these differences could be important for people who eat a lot of bread.

There are also considerable losses of the B-complex vitamins when whole rice is milled. Refining sugar removes all of the minerals and vitamins.

Some Nutrients Are Added to Processed Foods to Restore Nutritive Values

Vitamins, minerals, and other nutrients are added to foods and beverages after they have been lost through processing. Foods with added vitamins or minerals include margarine, pasteurized milk, enriched flour, table salt, nonfat dry milk, infant formula, and breakfast bars. The addition of nutrients is accomplished in three ways:

- *Restoration* replaces the amount of nutrients lost during processing. It is used to prevent nutrient deficiencies.
- *Fortification* consists of adding nutrients that were not present originally or were present in insufficient amounts. This technique corrects nutritional deficiencies in certain segments of the population.
- *Enrichment* is the addition of nutrients to achieve levels specified by federal standards. However, this term is often used interchangeably with restoration and fortification, although this usage is not technically correct.

The American Medical Association and the National Academy of Sciences/National Research Council approve of supplementation with nutrients if the following conditions are met[16]:

- There is a low intake of the nutrient(s) in a significant proportion of the population

- The food will be eaten in amounts large enough to make a significant contribution to the diet of the population in need
- The addition of the nutrient is not likely to cause an imbalance in other nutrients
- The nutrient added is stable under proper conditions of storage
- The body can absorb and utilize the nutrient that was added to the food
- There is reasonable assurance against excessive intake to a level of toxicity

Obviously safeguards must be met in the addition of nutrients to foods.

Advantages

Restoration, fortification, and enrichment have a number of advantages that are important in nutrition. These include:

- No changes are needed in eating, cooking, or purchasing habits
- Most added nutrients do not change the appearance, taste, or smell of the food
- The additives are usually not costly
- No special packaging, promotion, or merchandising is required
- Removal of nutrient deficiencies is quicker by fortification than by other methods
- Urban populations are reached easily

Disadvantages

The disadvantages of fortification are that:

- Only people who eat marketed processed foods will benefit. This problem is greatest in poorer countries, especially in rural areas.
- There is a certain amount of waste because people who do not need the added nutrients would get them also in the fortified food. Some breakfast cereals give 100 percent of the RDA for many vitamins. Is this really necessary if nutrient intake is adequate during the rest of the day?
- Fortification adds to the price of a food. This is not a large amount, but usually the people most in need of the extra nutrients are the least able to pay the extra price.
- Some people fear that fortification "adulterates" food. Public concern about the fluoridation of public water supplies is an example. Because many people fear food additives, they may fear even beneficial additives.
- Regulations must control the unlimited addition of nutrients to a food in the name of fortification. In the United States the FDA classifies a food as a drug if the amount of a nutrient exceeds 150 percent of the RDA per serving after fortification.
- The added nutrient may have undesirable side effects, but no reliable data are available on any harmful effects caused by the amounts allowed in food.

Fortification May or May Not Increase the Bioavailability of Nutrients

Adding nutrients to foods increases the concentration of those nutrients. It does not necessarily mean that the person will receive all or some of that added nutrient. It may combine with other nutrients or chemicals in the food or in the gastroin-

Fortification prevents some serious nutrition deficiencies.

testinal system, making it unavailable for absorption into the body. There is much to be learned in this important area.

Successful programs in which a nutrient obviously had high bioavailability were the addition of niacin to cereals in the elimination of pellagra in the southern United States, and the addition of vitamin D to margarine and milk that almost eliminated rickets in Great Britain.

Fortification Programs Offer Advantages for the Manufacturer

Fortification has improved the nutritional status of a portion of the population. However, vitamins also have a commercial application that you are not told about when their praises are sung in television commercials. Some vitamins improve product appearance and increase shelf-life.

Beta-carotene, for instance, the precursor of vitamin A, is added not so much for its vitamin A activity, or its possible cancer-blocking properties, as for its color. It gives a yellow color to popcorn, pasta, margarine, cakes, and processed cheese. Hence, it performs two functions: it replaces some food dyes, and it allows the manufacturer to make a nutritional claim about the product.

Vitamin C is an antioxidant, which prevents apple juice, apple sauce, and cut raw potatoes from darkening. A fat-soluble form of vitamin C extends the shelf-life of fast-food cooking oils. Vitamin E may help prevent the formation of nitro-samines in cooked bacon. Thiamin is a suggested flavor enhancer. All these are nice bonuses for the producer, with advantages for the consumer also.[19]

> Food additives may be intentional to improve the functional, sensory and keeping qualities of foods, or incidental from production, packaging or storage of the food. The GRAS list has over 700 additives generally recognized as safe. Addition of nutrients to foods after processing has some beneficial effects. Addition of salt and sugar as additives may have negative nutrition effects.

COOKING IN THE KITCHEN: IMPORTANT NUTRITION IMPLICATIONS

Most people do not realize that a great many nutrients can be lost during the handling and preparation of food in the kitchen. To best retain nutrients, you should attend to the following rules.

Keep Storage Time Short

The longer the storage time, the greater the loss of vitamin C, thiamin, riboflavin, and carotene.

Prevent Water from Leaching Out Nutrients

Water leaches water-soluble vitamins and minerals out of foods. Avoid this by not cutting food into small pieces and by not soaking the food for long periods. These nutrients are also lost if you discard the juice from meat or the water in which vegetables are cooked.

Prevent Heat from Destroying Vitamins

Heat destroys heat-sensitive vitamins and decreases protein quality. Least nutrition damage is done by cooking in the smallest amount of water at the optimum temperature for the shortest time. Optimum temperature is when the food is edible and all bacteria are destroyed. This is in the range of 165° to 212° Fahrenheit. The overall effect of cooking on nutrition can be summarized as follows:

- Best methods: microwave cooking, stir-frying, pressure cooking, steaming, roasting
- Moderate methods: stewing, baking, crockpot cooking
- Worst methods: boiling, braising, frying

Keeping food warm during a meal or reheating it after a meal will add to the loss of nutrients that are unstable in heat.

Positive effects of heat include the destruction of the anti-nutritional factor in raw soy beans. This factor interferes with the digestion of soy protein. Heat makes starch more digestible by opening up its structure for the digestive enzymes.

Avoid Letting Air Damage Vitamins

Oxygen in the air decreases the amount of vitamins A, B_{12}, C, D, and E, folacin, and thiamin in foods. Unsaturated fatty acids are unstable in air. It is good nutrition practice to keep food covered from air or oxygen.

Prevent Light from Damaging Vitamins

Light decreases the amount of vitamins A, B_6, B_{12}, C, D, and E, folacin, thiamin, riboflavin, and unsaturated fatty acids in foods. Milk is rich in riboflavin.

An advantage in buying your milk in a plastic or cardboard container in the supermarket, as opposed to having it delivered, as it was in the old days, is that much of the riboflavin was lost when milk was delivered in bottles and left to sit in the sun on the doorstep.

Avoid Wide Changes in pH

pH is important because vitamins A and K and folacin are unstable in an acidic environment, whereas vitamins C, D, and K, pantothenic acid, riboflavin, and thiamin are unstable in an alkaline environment.

Minimize Trimming and Peeling

Trimming and peeling should be kept to a minimum. The skin of fruits and potatoes has valuable amounts of fiber and vitamin C. The outer leaves of vegetables are valuable sources of some vitamins and minerals.

Nutrient losses are lowest if you eat the food fresh, including skin or outer leaves of fruits and vegetables. Cook uncut food in a minimum amount of water. Keep food covered, at a cool temperature, away from light, and with no wide changes in pH. Cook vegetables for as short a time as possible.

TABLE 11-3 Trends in Nutrient Consumption in the United States Since 1967

Trend	Implications
Increased Intake	
All food	Increased intake of energy and most nutrients
Animal products	Good sources of protein, iron, zinc, some vitamins
Crop products	Increased intake of fiber, unsaturated fat, some vitamins
Low-fat and skim milk	Lower fat and kcalorie intake
Poultry	Source of less saturated fat
Fruits and vegetables	Increased intake of fiber, decreased intake of fat
Vegetable oil	More polyunsaturated fat in the diet
Decreased intake	
Eggs	Less cholesterol intake
Animal fats	Less saturated fat and cholesterol
Meat	Lower intake of saturated fat, cholesterol, protein, iron, and some vitamins

SITTING DOWN TO EAT

After all of the foregoing, you are finally ready to sit down and eat. Here let us say a few words about food popularity, time of meals, and food safety and sensitivity.

The Popularity of Some Foods Changes Over the Years

Previous chapters described how much of each nutrient is required by the body. There are, however, fashions in food just like anything else. These fashions may affect nutrient consumption. In recent years, for instance, foods of plant origin and beverages have had the greatest increase in consumption (Table 11-3).

People's preferences for different foods change for a variety of reasons: price, availability, health concerns, popularity, and taste. Consumers are influenced by advertising, articles in trade journals and in the popular press, and guidelines issued by the government or groups such as national heart, cancer, or diabetes associations. Some recent positive changes include salad bars in restaurants and fast-food outlets, increased consumption of cereals such as pasta, and an increase in restaurants specializing in seafood and poultry.

A historical note shows how attitudes change. Today Americans eat about five tomatoes apiece per week, either the fruit directly or a derivative in pizza, sandwiches, soup, or catsup. In 1820, however, a person ate a tomato on the steps of the courthouse in Salem County, New Jersey, and an unbelieving crowd could not understand why he did not die from eating what was regarded as a poison.[20]

Perhaps People Should Eat When They Want To

"There appear to be no ill effects when people eat at the times they themselves prefer," says John Yudkin.

Did our ancient ancestors sit down to three square meals a day? Certainly not—they picked wild plants or hunted or fished and ate whenever they could. Today in affluent countries most people have food available from the refrigerator 24 hours a day. There is no uniform pattern of meals throughout the world. Some Europeans have four meals a day, North Americans three, some Nigerians two, and some tribes in central Africa and Brazil only a single meal, whenever the work schedule allows.[8]

Should breakfast never be missed, especially by children? Authorities in the 1940s said breakfast should not be skipped because studies showed decreased performances by school children and workers who skipped breakfast. Research since then does not, unfortunately, give a clear picture.

Is snacking harmful, especially if body weight is being held in check? People consuming the same kcaloric intake from four or five small meals did not show as high an increase in body weight or the concentration of triglycerides as when one or two big meals were eaten each day.

Food Safety May Be Judged by a Checklist

How safe is your food? Some foods contain naturally occurring toxicants. Almost every natural, unprocessed vegetable has harmful toxicants, although in small amounts.[21,22] Table 11-4 offers a short list of harmful chemicals occurring naturally in foods. This information is scientifically accurate, but because it has a high scare factor it must be emphasized that these effects happen only from excessive intake. *Normal food consumption patterns produce no known damage when the foods listed in Table 11-4 are eaten.*

TABLE 11-4 Naturally Occurring Toxicants in Foods

Food	Toxicant	Damage from Excessive Intake
Sweet potatoes	Ipomearone	Damage to liver and lungs
Nutmeg, bananas, celery	Myristin	Hallucinations, damage to fetus
Potato skins	Solanine	Death
Soybeans, beans, carrots, potatoes, cherries, plums, garlic, peanuts, wheat, rice, oats, apples, other foods[21]	Estrogen-like compounds (estrogens are female sex hormones)	Hormonal imbalances—female characteristics in men
Cabbage, cauliflower, Brussels sprouts	Goitrogens	Goiter, iodine deficiency
Spinach, lettuce, beets	Nitrite	Converted into nitrosamine by bacteria in intestine, causing carcinogens
Peanuts, corn	Aflatoxins, other molds and fungi	Produce chemicals that can cause cancer
Other Substances[22]		
	Antivitamins	Different chemicals interfere with thiamin, niacin, pyridoxine, biotin
	Chelates	Make some minerals (calcium, iron, zinc) unavailable for absorption

TABLE 11-5 Bacterial Contamination in Many Foods Can Cause Food Poisoning

Bacteria	Foods Most Frequently Affected	Clinical Features
Salmonellas	Poultry, other meats, eggs, milk, cream, chocolate, coconut, dried foods, spices	Diarrhea, vomiting, abdominal pain, fever
C. perfringens	Preheated meat (especially casseroles), canned food, meat pastes, pies, pastries	Diarrhea, abdominal pain, nausea, no fever
B. cerus	Boiled or fried rice, cereals	Diarrhea, nausea, vomiting
Staphylococci	Ham, tongue	Diarrhea, abdominal pain
C. botulinum	Canned food	Vomiting, respiratory paralysis

Food Poisoning Can Keep You From Getting All the Nutrients from Food

Food poisoning may cause diarrhea and vomiting. When this occurs, then some of the nutrients in a meal are not absorbed into the body.

Food poisoning is caused by:

- Microbiological factors—bacteria, viruses, or protozoa
  (This is the most common cause, and some of the bacteria causing the most trouble are listed in Table 11-5.)
- Solanine—in potatoes
- Chemicals in certain mushrooms and other fungi
- Certain chemicals in fish and shellfish

Unfortunately taste, smell, or appearance do not always indicate if there is a danger from food poisoning by bacteria. You can avoid the problem by:

- Keeping food either hot (over 63°C or 145°F), or cold (below 4°C or 40°F)
- Keeping food dry or otherwise preserved (frozen, pickled, fermented, or irradiated)
- Defrosting food thoroughly and heating it thoroughly
- Eating it immediately
- Not recontaminating it after cooking

Many People Have Food Sensitivity

Food sensitivity affects many people but is difficult to diagnose. According to the 1984 Joint Report of the Royal College of Physicians and the British Nutrition Foundation:

> Wide publicity is given to the unproven claim that food allergy is becoming more common, that (despite evidence to the contrary) food processing exacerbates the problem, and that the medical profession is not sufficiently well informed to deal with it. . . . There is also great uncertainty about the prevalence of this condition in the community at large, and particularly about the importance of psychological factors which may lead to food aversion.[23]

This statement applies to the problem of food allergies and sensitivities in other parts of the world as well.

Certain foods can cause one or more of the following unpleasant reactions *in some people*: asthma, sneezing, runny nose, earache, dizziness, hives, itchy skin, watery or painful eyes, itchy or swollen eye lids, increased pulse rate, irregular heartbeats, canker sores, difficulty in swallowing, cramps, diarrhea, itching or burning of the rectum, frequent and painful urination, vaginal itching and discharge, muscle weakness, muscle and joint pains, backache, headache, migraine, lethargy, tension, inability to concentrate, and stammering.

There are two important aspects to this list. First only *some* people are sensitive to a particular food. Second, these symptoms could be due to several other causes also. It is difficult sometimes to isolate the guilty food or food component from the multitude of foods eaten by most people. The most common allergenic foods are[24]: milk, eggs, tree nuts, shellfish (clams, oysters, scallops), crustacea (shrimp, crabs, lobster), legumes (peanuts, soybeans), wheat, and fish.

Because this topic is so much in the public spotlight some definitions are important[24]:

- *Individualistic adverse reactions to foods:* A collective term for both food allergies and food sensitivities
- *Food allergy:* An adverse reaction to a food or food component (often a protein) involving reactions of the body's immune system (immunological reactions)
- *Nonallergic food reactions:* Do not involve the immune system

This last category, nonallergic food reactions, includes three specific kinds of reactions:

- *Metabolic food reactions:* Also called *food intolerances;* due to a defect in metabolism—for example, the difficulty some people experience in digesting lactose in milk.
- *Anaphylactoid reactions:* From the Greek meaning "against protection"; caused by eating foods that release from the body's cellular stores the chemical triggers of allergic reactions. Foods producing this effect include strawberries, shellfish, and chocolate.
- *Food idiosyncrasies:* Adverse reaction of unknown mechanisms, including food-associated migraine headache, sulfite-induced asthma, and Chinese Restaurant Syndrome. At least one study showed that psychological reasons are not the reason for this problem.[25]

An important nutritional concern is that people who suffer from food allergies or food sensitivities must take care to maintain a balanced diet—even though they must avoid certain foods or types of foods.

The contribution of various foods to the national diet changes with time. Consuming a food in either one or several meals per day does not seem to be a problem; it is the total amount of food eaten that is important. Some foods contain naturally occurring toxicants, but they cause no known harm in a balanced diet. Food poisoning does not occur when food is handled and prepared properly. Allergic reactions to certain foods occur in some people.

Decisions

1. Which Foods Deserve the Title "Junk Food"?

One must be careful about making decisions in this area. First, foods that may taste and look like junk may not be *nutritional* junk. Second, the amount of a food eaten is important. Small amounts of some low-nutrient foods may add taste to a bland but nutritionally adequate diet. However, if such foods form a large part of the diet, then that is indeed a "junk food" diet.

The index of nutrient quality (INQ) for protein, calcium, iron, and vitamin C can help you determine the answer (Table 11-6). An INQ over 1.0 means the food has more of the nutrient (compared to the amount required) than energy (compared to the amount required). Note that, in Table 11-6, pizza is the only one of the foods listed with an INQ greater than 1.0 for all four nutrients listed. Two foods much loved by some health-food advocates, granola bars and honey, actually have low INQs for all four nutrients listed.

In summary, "junk food" is a term that nutritionists should not use.

TABLE 11-6 Index of Nutrient Quality for Some Popular Foods: A Few Surprises

Food	Index of Nutrient Quality Greater Than 1.0* (X)			
	Protein	Calcium	Iron	Vitamin C
Egg (hard cooked)	X	X	X	
Hamburger	X		X	
Cheeseburger	X	X	X	
French fries				X
Pizza	X	X	X	X
Potato chips				X
Popcorn	X		X	
Banana (without peel)			X	X
Granola bar				
Honey				

*INQ for an adult man.

2. What is the Role of Herbs in Nutrition?

Herbs are useful in making food more palatable. Some experts recommend the use of some herbs as an excellent replacement for salt, the intake of which should be reduced. However, you need to be careful about the word *herbal*. People have a kind of emotional attachment to herbs because some modern medicines were originally extracted from herbs and other plants. Use of the word "herbal" or a combination of the word "herb" and "life" exploits the attachment.

Sometimes herbs are equated with "natural" foods, or with folklore, or with drinks with no kcalories or caffeine. Ginseng is a good example.[26] In the United States, ginseng is legally considered a food supplement, which means that dose recommendations are not required. However, if the research results found in ginseng experiments in animals were repeated in experiments in humans, heavy use of the

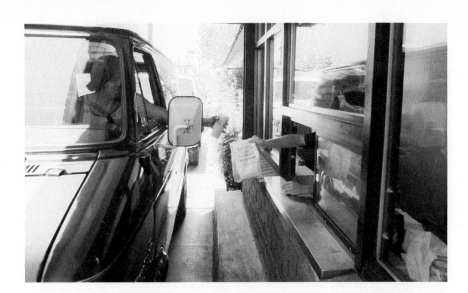

Foods commonly called "junk food" may not be *nutritional* junk. They may be high in fat and sodium.

herb might be found to lead to the development of female characteristics in men. In women, amenorrhea (cessation of menstruation) is possible. Ginseng abuse syndrome, first described in 1979, consists of mental and neurological problems, diarrhea, and skin eruptions.

Many species of ginseng are available. However, some products sold as ginseng are fake: one survey in the United States showed that seven out of twenty-four samples purchased contained no ginseng at all.

3. How Should I Interpret the Phrase on a Food Label, "Contains no. . . ."?

At present, over 40% of food advertisements state what is *not* in the food, a new trend in labeling. Usually this description is to improve the prospective buyer's attitudes toward the food.

If you examine the labels on some bottles of vitamins in a store you may find the expression "Contains no sugar, salt, milk, preservatives or chemical additives, artificial dyes, colors or flavors." This list includes just about all the nutritional villains. However, note that the same disclaimer could also be put on a bottle of any alcoholic drink.

Along this line, government regulations have been proposed to prohibit use of the statement "No cholesterol" on products such as applesauce, since no brand of applesauce contains cholesterol.

4. Is There Effective Government Regulation of the Quality of Food?

Government has played an important role in assuring the quality of food over the centuries. The Food and Drug Administration (FDA), established in 1933, has protected consumers against fraud and is now involved with food safety. Among its functions are:[27]

- Nutrition labeling—a policing role on claims, etc.
- Definition of imitation—an imitation food substitutes for a traditional food but may be nutritionally inferior
- Establishing food names—new fabricated foods must have a descriptive name, or names could promise more nutritive value than they could deliver.

By the year 2000, research will bring many changes in the way food is grown, processed, and delivered.

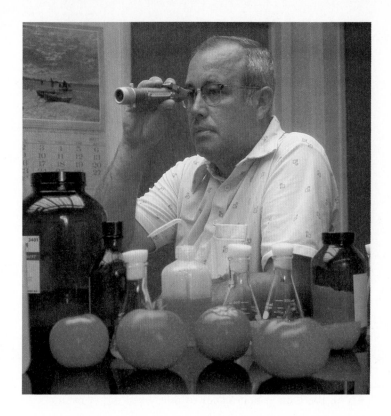

- Nutrition quality guidelines—the minimum level or range of nutrient composition appropriate for a given class of food
- Fortification guidelines—these prevent manufacturers from adding nutrients to a nutritionally poor food and making extensive claims about nutritive values
- Medical food policy—the FDA states that any reference to the control or cure of a disease by a food automatically classifies it as a drug. Recent relaxations have occurred. For example, one high-fiber breakfast cereal is advertised heavily as a means of prevention of cancer. The advertisement mentions the National Cancer Institute. This is an area requiring better control or soon every food will be promoted with unproven or exaggerated health claims.

By the year 2000 you will see many changes in how food is grown, processed, and delivered.[28] The FDA has begun seeking expert advice in universities and industry on how to monitor these changes. New methods in food processing and fabrication of food products, the role of biotechnology in food production, the effect of naturally occurring toxins, the potential for food-borne hazards of microbial origin, the monitoring of pesticides, chemical contaminants and food additives make the decisions by the FDA important to your well-being.

Although the FDA has its critics, if it did not exist there would probably be chaos in the food supply. In looking to the future, the FDA sees that it "must be in a position to deal competently and confidently with troublesome issues, i.e., on the basis of good science and in a manner which protects the public health while not ignoring possible economic and social consequences."[28]

SUMMARY

FOOD PRODUCTION

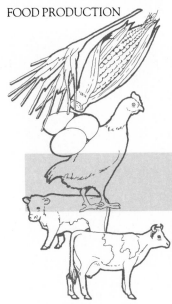

People
Water
Land
Climate
Energy
Agricultural
chemicals
Plant/animal
genetics
Harvesting
losses
Disease
Economics/
politics
Transportation

FOOD PROCESSING*

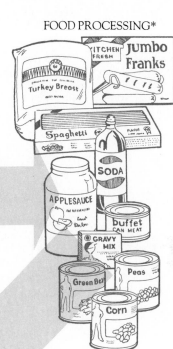

Dry
Smoke
Ferment
Add salt or
sugar
Can
Freeze
Pasteurize
Blanch
Irradiate

*Milling and
refining removes
nutrients, replaced
by enrichment and
fortification

FOOD BUYING

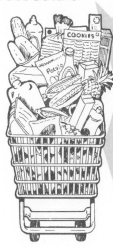

Appearance
Odor
Texture
Flavor
Sound
Familiarity
Preservatives
Additives

FOOD CHOICES

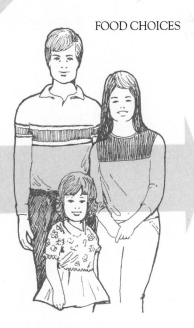

Culture
Income
Religion
Familiarity
Lifestyles
Family structure
Status
Health
Food allergies

REFERENCES

1. Eide, A., and others, editors: Food as a human right. Tokyo, The United Nations University, 1984.

2. Anonymous: West African agriculture: boom in oil, bust on the farm. The Economist, p. 85, December 5, 1981.

3. Spurr, G.B.: Physical activity, nutritional status, and physical work capacity in relation to agricultural productivity. In Energy intake and activity, Pollitt, E. and Amante, P., editors, New York, Alan R. Liss, Inc., p. 207, 1984.

4. Lecos, C.: Pesticides and food: public worry no. 1. FDA Consumer, p. 12, July-August, 1984.

5. Institute of Food Technologists, Expert Panel on Food Safety & Nutrition: Food colors. Food Technology **40**:49, 1986.

6. Wilson, C.S.: Nutritionally beneficial cultural practices. World Review of Nutrition and Dietetics **45**:68, 1985.

7. Albrecht, J.J.: Business and technology issues in U.S. food science and technology. Food Technology **40**:122, December 1986.

8. Bryant, C.A., and others: The cultural feast. St. Paul, West Publishing Co., p. 215, 1985.

9. Josephson, N.: In search of excellence . . . in TV dinners. American Health, p. 46, September 1984.

10. Jennings, A.J., and Sheldon, M.G.: Review of the health of children in one-parent families. Journal of the Royal College of General Practice, p. 478, October 1985.

11. Bunch, K.L.: Consumption trends favor fresh, lowfat, and sweet. National Food Review p. 1, Winter 1986.

12. James, W.P.T., and others: The dominance of salt in manufactured food in the sodium intake of affluent societies. Lancet **i**:426, 1987.

13. Chou, M., and Harmon D.P.: Critical food issues of the eighties. New York, Pergamon Press, Inc., 1979.

14. Levine, A.S., and others: Food technology: a primer for physicians. New England Journal of Medicine **312**:628, 1985.

15. Editorial: Food Irradiation. Lancet **i**:485, 1987.

16. Institute of Food Technologists' Expert Panel on Food Safety & Nutrition: Effects of food processing on nutritive values. Food Technology **40**:109, December 1986.

17. The Analytical Sanitary Commission: Records of the results of microscopical and chemical analyses of the solids and fluids willful addition of harmful chemicals for the commercial advantage consumed by all classes of the public. Lancet **ii**:398, 1851.

18. Ranhotra, G., and others: Minerals in selected variety breads commercially produced in four major U.S. cities. Journal of Food Science **50**:365, 1985.

19. Anonymous: Why vitamin fortification? Food Engineering, p. 96, February 1985.

20. Zamula, E.: Tale of the tomato: from "poison" to pizza. FDA Consumer, p. 24, July-August, 1984.

21. Bender, A.E.: Health or hoax? The truth about health food and diets, Goring-on-Thames, England, Elvendon Press, p. 33, 1985.

22. Hambraeus, L.: Naturally occurring toxicants in food. In Adverse effects of foods, Jelliffe, E.P.F. and Jelliffe, D.B., editors, New York, Plenum Press, p. 13, 1982.

23. Joint Report of the Royal College of Physicians and the British Nutrition Foundation: Food intolerance and food aversion. Journal of the Royal College of Physicians of London, **18:**83, 1984.

24. Institute of Food Technologists' Expert Panel on Food Safety & Nutrition: Food allergies and sensitivities. Food Technology **39:**65, September 1985.

25. Rix, K.J.B., and others: A psychiatric study of patients with supposed food allergy. British Journal of Psychiatry **145:**121, 1984.

26. Barna, P.: The case of ginseng. Lancet **ii:**548, 1985.

27. Hutt, P.B.: Government regulation of the integrity of the food supply. Annual Review of Nutrition **4:**1, 1984.

28. Miller, S.A., and others: FDA and food research: keeping pace with technological change. Food Technology p. 89, May 1987.

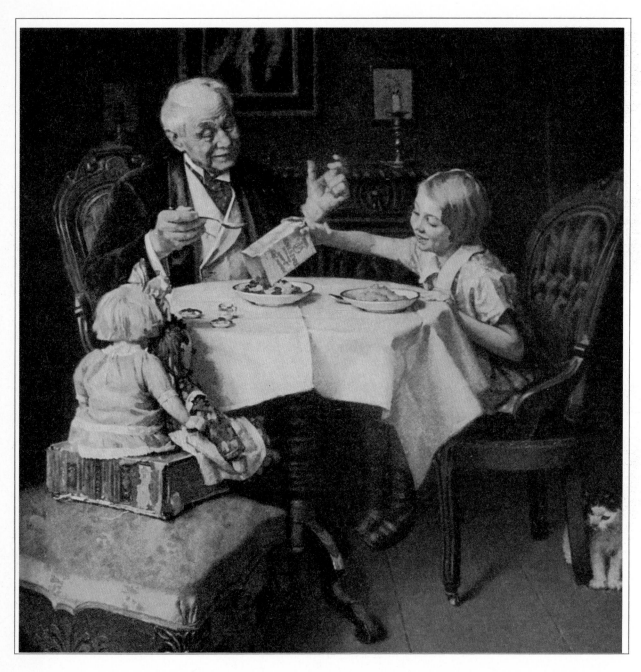

Printed by permission of Sun Diamond Growers, Pleasanton, CA
Courtesy of The Norman Rockwell Museum at Stockbridge, Stockbridge, MA

PART III

Nutrition Throughout Life

From conception to death, nutrients are essential throughout the human life-span. How we acquire those nutrients depends on many people—ourselves, parents, and friends—and many influences (available income, advertising, religion, culture, and health and disease factors).

A mother's diet and health during pregnancy and her decisions about what foods and when to feed the baby are important. Nutrient requirements are of increased concern for pregnant teenagers because they need to satisfy their own high nutrient requirements for growth. In Chapter 12 we will examine the many factors that can affect the growth of the fetus and infant, including alcohol, drugs, and smoking.

Young children may develop tastes for specific foods early in life, when they enjoy playing with food and using it to exert their independence. During the growing years, food intake is influenced by parents, culture or religion, television advertising, peer pressure and the desire to be slim or to build muscles for athletics. Eating disorders may develop in some teenagers, especially girls. Many other influences add to dietary confusion during this period, including the availability of fast foods, dieting, and snacking, which will be discussed in Chapter 13.

College students may have inadequate nutrient intake because of busy schedules, the convenience of less nutritious fast foods, or inadequate budgets. Nutrition-related concerns of adulthood include coronary heart disease, certain cancers, hypertension, obesity, diabetes, and in women, osteoporosis and anemia.

The elderly have specific nutrient requirements because of changes in lifestyle, body composition, and income. Food becomes more important as a means of social interaction for many people as they age. The possibility that nutrient supplements can slow the aging process is being investigated; however adults, both young and old, are often fooled by false nutrition claims. In Chapter 14 these nutrition-related concerns of the young and older adult will by explored.

In summary, you will learn that the quality of your diet at all periods of your life has an influence on how long you will live.

12

Pregnancy and Lactation
Nutrition for Mother and Child

CONNECTIONS

As you will see in this chapter, the mother's diet during pregnancy and lactation is important for the health of the child, because what she chooses to eat and drink affects not only herself but also the fetus and the breast-fed infant. In Chapter 1, you saw that approximately 46 essential nutrients are obtained from food and supplements taken during pregnancy and lactation (breast-feeding).

If the mother has nutrient deficiencies, they may cause deficiency symptoms in the infant (Chapters 3-8). The severity of the effects of a deficiency on the mother and infant depends on the nutrient. Those deficiencies that cause low birth weight have a higher chance of leading to infant mortality or smaller size at adulthood.

Obesity may cause problems for a pregnant woman, as we have seen in Chapter 10. Moreover, what the expectant mother ingests can cause problems for her child both before and after delivery. A woman who uses alcohol during pregnancy, for instance, may have an infant with mental retardation (as was mentioned in Chapter 8); mother's milk contaminated by alcohol, medication, or pollutants may cause problems for the breast-fed infant.

The decision to breast-feed or bottle-feed the infant is important. In less-developed countries, unclean water may contaminate infant formulas; poor sanitation may lead to diarrhea, dehydration, and high infant mortality.

All human beings were introduced to nutrients early in life in the same way— within the wombs of their mothers. It is an important beginning to our life-long association with the nutrients. "The organism uses energy from the moment it is conceived until the moment it dies," writes Elsie M. Widdowson, "First for 9 months when it is hidden out of sight in the uterus of his (her) mother."

The nutrients you received in the womb allowed you to grow from a single cell to whatever you weighed at birth, the average newborn being about 7.5 lb (3.4 kg). The rate of growth is impressive in the womb. Rapid growth continues during infancy. As Virginia Beal writes:

> During the first year the average infant triples birth weight and adds 50% to length. If this rate of growth were to continue, the child would be 96 feet tall and weigh more than 200 tons by the tenth year. Instead it will take the entire span from one to six years to increase height by 50% again, and to double the weight attained at one year.

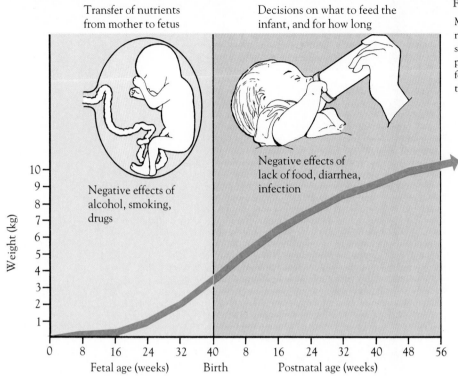

Transfer of nutrients from mother to fetus

Decisions on what to feed the infant, and for how long

Negative effects of alcohol, smoking, drugs

Negative effects of lack of food, diarrhea, infection

Weight (kg)

Fetal age (weeks)   Birth   Postnatal age (weeks)

Figure 12-1

Mother plays an important role in the nutrition of the fetus and infant. Decisions on the quality of her diet during pregnancy and the method of infant feeding have important outcomes for the child.

This chapter will examine the nutritional requirements from conception until the child's first birthday and the important role played by the mother in meeting these requirements (Figure 12-1). This is a critical period of development because the lower the body weight of infants at birth the higher the rate of infant mortality. Surviving infants with low birth weight may suffer lasting or permanent adverse effects to their physical and mental well being.

There are some critical nutritional decisions that the parents must make:

The first important matter for both mother and *fetus* is for the mother to enter pregnancy in optimal nutritional status. This means the mother must be receiving an adequate diet long *before* conception occurs. The reason, of course, is that all the nutrients the fetus receives will pass to it through the mother's placenta from nutrients in the mother's diet or from reserves in her body. In fact any nutrient deficiencies the mother may have at the start of pregnancy may worsen because of the higher nutrient demands of pregnancy. If the mother breast-feeds, she must secrete enough milk to fill the child's requirements for nutrients. Diet plays an important role in the quantity of milk produced.

If the mother decides not to breast-feed, an infant formula to replace human milk must be chosen.

The parents decide if and when to give whole cow's milk.

Finally, the parents must decide when to feed solid food to the infant, which are the best foods to give, and in what amount.

Fetus

A child in utero from the third month to birth. Until the third month it is called an embryo.

Knowledge of nutrient requirements during pregnancy and lactation are important for parents.

FIGURE 12-2

Changes in weight gain in the mother and fetus during pregnancy. Total weight change would be about half of the amount shown here if the mother is underfed.

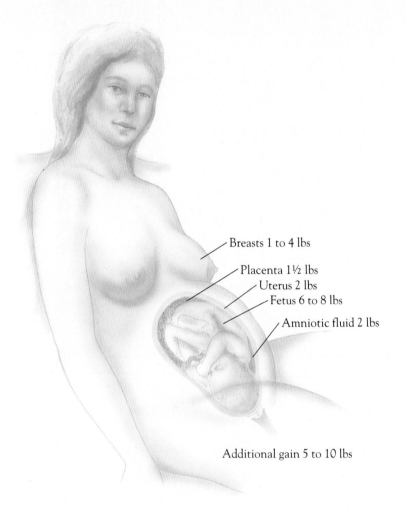

Breasts 1 to 4 lbs

Placenta 1½ lbs

Uterus 2 lbs

Fetus 6 to 8 lbs

Amniotic fluid 2 lbs

Additional gain 5 to 10 lbs

THE IMPORTANCE OF NUTRITION BEFORE PREGNANCY

Many physicians emphasize the nutrient requirements of the child from the day of birth onwards, partly because of their concerns about infant mortality, particularly in underdeveloped countries. However, optimal nutritional status is important in the woman before she becomes pregnant. As Figure 12-2 indicates, major changes in the composition of her body and in that of the fetus occur during the nine months of pregnancy.

Poor nutritional status at the start of pregnancy is a contributing factor in the greater number of complications during pregnancy in women who have had many children, or who are pregnant when they are either very young or very old. More maternal deaths occur among mothers under 15 years of age, because the high nutritional requirements of pregnancy are added to the high demands of growth in the teenager. There is a steady increase in death rate among mothers from the age of 24 years up to the over 45 year old group.[1]

In developing countries the death rate among women with low incomes (who, of course, are likely to have inadequate diets) is 100-300 deaths per 100,000 births.

These maternal death rates are similar to those in developed countries half a century ago. The current rate in the United States, in contrast, is only 7-15 maternal deaths per 100,000 births. The reasons for the decrease in developed countries such as the United States include the increased attention to a balanced diet and the success of various public health programs for expectant mothers. The causes of maternal death include hemorrhages with resulting anemia and infections caused in part by inadequate protein intakes. The lives of many pregnant women are saved by prevention of hemorrhages and by food supplements.

Severe Undernutrition Affects Reproduction

The birth weight of a baby is influenced by his or her mother's nutrition history from the time of *her own conception*. Thus, if nutrient intake was low during her fetal development and during the first few years of her life, the mother's growth was probably stunted. Consequently, the mother may have a smaller adult body size, including a smaller pelvis, and this has the effect of restricting growth of her fetus, resulting in a small baby at birth.

What kinds of nutritional factors can impede conception? Severe cases of famine, anorexia nervosa, or excessive athletic activity cause amenorrhea (absence of menstruation), which makes conception less likely to occur. This is a protective mechanism for a body unable to meet the physical and nutritional demands of pregnancy.

However, the severity of famine or anorexia nervosa required to interfere with conception is still debated.[2] Most of the data on nutrition-related infertility come from Europe during World War II, but in wartime there is separation of the sexes, which means there would be fewer opportunities for sex and conception anyway.

In any case, it seems that starvation must be severe before fertility is affected, and if conception does occur in these circumstances, it will usually result in pregnancy with a number of nutrition problems. Even if a woman recovers from any stress or starvation that caused the loss of body weight, her reserves of nutrients may be quite low as she goes into pregnancy, depending on the time interval and quality of diet during the pregnancy.

History

A healthy body is needed to meet the nutritional demands of pregnancy

Obesity May Interfere with Reproduction

Does obesity cause sterility in humans? There are mixed reports.[2] Certainly in obese animals, fertility is lower. There are no known harmful effects on conception from a woman's taking an excess of any nutrients.

Contraception May Affect Nutrition

Contraception can have positive and negative effects on nutritional status. Contraception is sometimes used to postpone a woman's pregnancy until she can recover from undernutrition or until she is past adolescence, thereby improving the chances for herself and her offspring.

On the negative side, intrauterine devices (IUDs) cause increased loss of menstrual blood, which in turn can cause iron deficiency anemia. Oral contraceptives can decrease the level of iron, folacin, and vitamin B_6 in the blood.[3] Women with deficient levels of vitamin B_6 in the blood occasionally experience depression (although they may respond to daily doses of 20 to 40 mg pyridoxine hydrochloride).

It may be dangerous to rely on the effectiveness of hormonal contraceptives when a woman is undernourished. Evidence from India suggests that orally administered hormonal contraceptives are not as effective in undernourished women.[3]

> To prepare for pregnancy, a woman should eat a balanced diet, should not be undernourished, and should control her obesity. Prolonged use of oral contraceptives reduces the levels of iron, folacin, and vitamin B_6 in the body.

WHAT NUTRITIONAL FACTORS AFFECT MATERNAL AND FETAL HEALTH?

A pregnant woman should take care to avoid a number of risks that will affect both her own health and that of the fetus, according to the American College of Obstetrics and Gynecology, the American Dietetic Association (1978), and the National Research Council (1981). They are described below.

The Mother Must Avoid Nutritional Risks at the Beginning of Pregnancy

There are eight conditions that contribute to nutritional risk in the beginning of pregnancy.

TABLE 12-1 Infant Mortality and Percentage of Mothers Younger than 20 Years of Age

Country*	Infant Mortality Rate	Percentage of All Births to Women less than 20 Years of Age
Japan	6.0	1.2
Sweden	6.4	3.8
Canada	**8.1**	**7.8**
Netherlands	8.4	2.7
Australia	9.2	6.9
United Kingdom	9.6	8.6
Ireland	10.1	4.4
United States	**10.7**	**13.7**
Israel	12.8	5.1
Czechoslovakia	15.3	11.8

*Only selected countries are chosen here for comparative purposes. Infant mortality rates are for 1984.

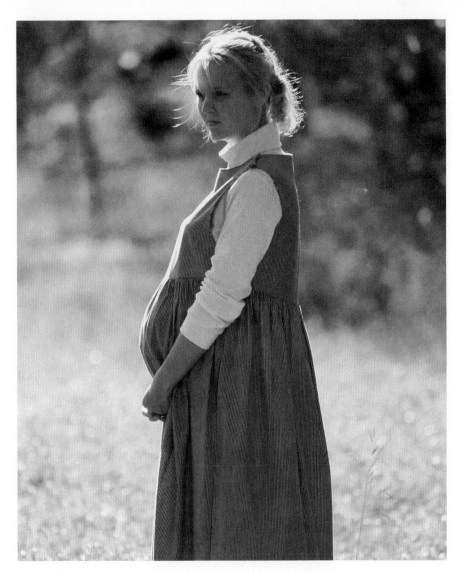

Nutrient requirements for pregnant teenagers are a concern because they need to satisfy their own nutrient requirements for growth.

Underweight or overweight

On her first prenatal visit to the doctor, if the woman has a body weight that is less than 85% or more than 120% of her standard weight, she may be at risk. Standard weights are discussed in Chapter 10.

Weight-reducing diets should *never* be undertaken during pregnancy.

Youth

A pregnant woman who is 15 years old or younger will require more nutrients than will a pregnant woman who is older. This is because she is still growing.

The proportion of teenage pregnancies is higher in the United States than in any other industrialized country, as Table 12-1 shows. This is a major reason why infant mortality is higher than in other industrialized countries. According to the statistics from one American city, Houston, Texas, preteenagers are also having babies (Table 12-2), and some 18- and 19-year-olds are having their second and third babies. Nutritional status of both young mother and baby can vary widely, depending on economic and family circumstances.

Many, closely spaced pregnancies

Pregnancy creates high demand for additional amounts of nutrients for the growth demands of the fetus and the mother's tissues (see Figure 12-2). If a woman has had three or more pregnancies within three years, she may have dangerously reduced reserves of nutrients, particularly if she is a teenager. In 1984 in the United States, it was reported that four girls under age 15 had their *fourth* child in that year.[4]

Poor obstetric history

If a woman has a history of poor obstetric or fetal health—such as miscarriages or stillbirths—this may influence her nutrient needs during later pregnancies.

Low income

Economics

Highly nutritious foods that meet the added demands for nutrients during pregnancy tend to be expensive, hence unaffordable to low-income women. Education in nutritious food choices and in economic meal planning is important.

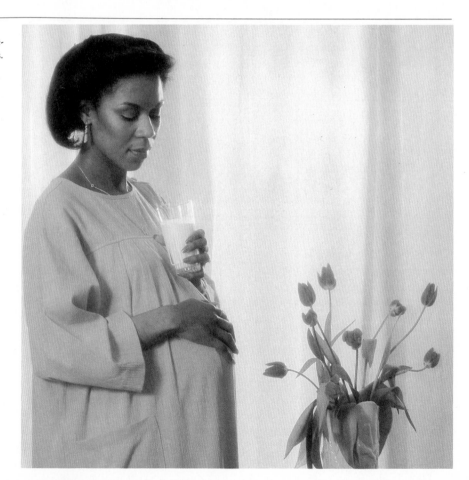

During pregnancy, it is important for women of all ages to meet the requirements for calcium and other nutrients.

TABLE 12-2 Number of Infants Born to Teenagers in Houston, Texas

	Age of Mother			
	10-14	**15-17**	**18-19**	**Total Births**
Black teenagers	83 (45%)	955 (41%)	1311 (36%)	2349
Hispanic teenagers	77 (42%)	875 (38%)	1331 (36%)	2283
White and Asian teenagers	24 (13%)	476 (21%)	1043 (28%)	1543
Total for all teenagers	184	2306	3685	6175

Vegetarianism

If a prospective mother is a follower of certain specialized diets, it is possible the diet may be unbalanced and lack important nutrients. Vegans, for example, consume no foods of animal origins, and they must therefore take great care to select foods to provide enough energy, protein, calcium, vitamin B_{12}, iron, and zinc. Vegans may overcome some of the problems by obtaining calcium-fortified soy milk, other soy products, whole grains, nuts, and seeds, as well as a wide choice in fruits and vegetables. Nutrient supplements may be required. The problem with calcium is not as severe for vegetarians who exclude only meat but continue to eat dairy products and other foods. If the pregnant woman is on some extreme, "fad" diet then the nutritional consequences to herself and to the infant may be more severe.

Modified therapeutic diets

If a prospective mother is on a therapeutic diet for a chronic systemic disease, like those for diabetes, coronary heart disease, or hypertension, she may also be deprived of nutrients essential to her pregnancy. These diets are usually adequate for the nonpregnant woman. A dietitian or physician should be consulted to determine if the therapeutic diet meets the increased nutrient demand caused by pregnancy.

Medicine

Smoking, drinking, and drug abuse

Cigarette smoking reduces appetite, thereby reducing nutrient intake. Alcohol provides kcalories but no nutrients. Women who spend a lot of money on alcohol and drugs may not have enough to spend on an adequate diet before or during pregnancy.

Nutrition Risks During Pregnancy Can Affect Both Mother and Fetus

There are five common nutrition-related health problems that might affect the mother and her child.

Low hemoglobin levels

If the woman's hemoglobin level is under 11 g, it will reduce the amount of oxygen reaching her tissues. This reduces her body's capacity to use nutrients for energy.

FIGURE 12-3
RDAs are higher for all nutrients during pregnancy and lactation. Note the difference between American and Canadian recommendations for some nutrients.

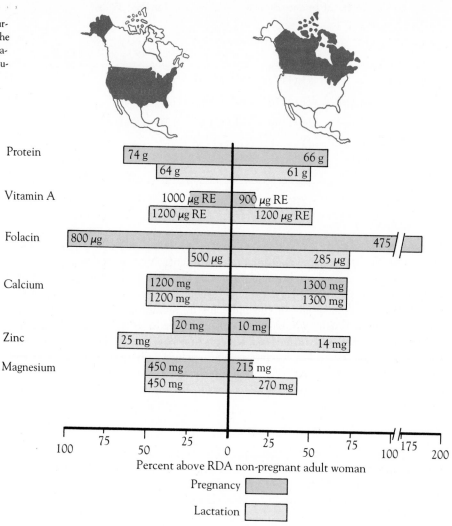

Inadequate weight gain

Inadequate weight gain is most often the result of inadequate nutrient intake, which means the fetus may not be receiving enough nutrients for normal development. Once upon a time, there was a view that the fetus was a "parasite"— that it would always get an optimal supply of nutrients at the expense of nutrient reserves in the mother's body. However, this idea is no longer accepted. In any case, the mother should not deplete her store of nutrients during pregnancy because she will also need them during the nutritionally demanding period of breast-feeding, as Figure 12-3 indicates.

Excessive weight gain

Expectant mothers who put on more than 2 lb a week should in no event convince themselves that they are "overweight" and try to go on a weight-reducing diet. No dieting should ever be done during pregnancy. It is bad from a physiological, nutritional, and emotional point of view.

Toxemia

Toxemia during pregnancy is common, especially in lower socioeconomic groups. Toxemia causes high blood pressure, excessive weight gain because of fluid retention, and a loss of protein in the urine.[5] Although its cause is still unknown, if toxemia is left untreated, the disorder will lead to coma, convulsions, and even death.

Toxemia
The condition caused by the presence of toxic substances in the blood. Symptoms include edema and hypertension during pregnancy.

Diabetes

Diabetes during pregnancy is something to be concerned about, but it is certainly manageable. Diabetes in pregnancy may be insulin-dependent diabetes mellitus (IDDM or type I), noninsulin-dependent diabetes mellitus (NIDDM or type II), or gestational diabetes. The latter form begins or is recognized during pregnancy. Whether nondiabetic or diabetic, a pregnant woman should take in the same amount of dietary energy—about 36 kcalories per kilogram of body weight per day. Protein intake should be about 1.2 to 1.5 g per kilogram of body weight per day. Carbohydrate should provide the bulk of the energy intake. Fat intake should provide no more than 35% of total kcalories.

The Optimum Weight Gain During Pregnancy is 24 to 28 Pounds

The weight gain of a woman during her pregnancy actually is an inexact measure of her nutritional status. Because of differences in fluid retention, for instance, her body weight can vary considerably. However, normal, adult, pregnant women should gain 24-28 lb, or the approximately 12 kg shown in Figure 12-2. In women, the tissues associated with pregnancy are affected severely by undernutrition.

What about women who are facing unusual circumstances? The following are some guidelines:

- *Adolescents* should gain about 35 lb.
- *Underweight adult women* have best pregnancy outcomes on a weight gain of 30 lb.
- *Obese adult women* should gain 10 to 20 lb during pregnancy.[6] Obesity causes increased pregnancy risks. These include difficulties at delivery, diabetes, hypertension, higher risks if anesthesia and surgery must be performed, blood clots, wound infections, hemorrhaging after delivery, and a higher probability of producing twins or abnormally large infants.

Recommendations for weight change during pregnancy have changed repeatedly since the early 1900s. In the 1950s and 1960s, for instance, weight gains of only 15 lb were recommended by some doctors. This was to produce an easier, less traumatic birth. However, this low weight gain is thought to have contributed to low birth weight babies, many with neurological disorders.[7]

During Pregnancy, a Nutritious Diet Should Be Adequate and Balanced

As well as being adequate and balanced, the pregnant woman's diet should also be economical, palatable, and adaptable, if possible—in other words, no different from a woman's usual dietary intake of the four food groups except that, as Figure 12-3 shows, the level of intake is higher.

TABLE 12-3 Daily Food Plan for Pregnancy and Lactation

Food	Nonpregnant Woman	Pregnancy	Lactation
Milk (skimmed or buttermilk), cheese, ice cream (food made with milk can supply part of requirement)	2 cups	3-4 cups	4-5 cups
Meat (lean meat, fish, poultry, cheese, occasional dried beans or peas)	1 serving (3-4 oz)	2 servings (6-8 oz); include liver frequently	2½ servings (8 oz)
Eggs	1	1-2	1-2
Vegetable* (dark green or deep yellow)	1 serving	1 serving	1-2 servings
Vitamin C–rich food* Good source: citrus fruit, berries, cantaloupe Fair source: tomatoes, cabbage, greens, potatoes in skin	1 good source or 2 fair sources	1 good source and 1 fair source or 2 good sources	1 good source and 1 fair source or 2 good sources
Other vegetables, fruits, juices	2 servings	4-6 servings	4-6 servings
Bread† and cereals (enriched or whole grain)	6 servings	10 servings	10 servings
Butter or fortified margarine	Moderate amount	Moderate amount	Moderate amount

*Use some raw daily
†One slice of bread or ½ cup starch (grains or vegetables) equals 1 serving.

Table 12-3 shows a daily food plan for pregnancy and lactation. During pregnancy, the fetus needs the approximately 46 essential nutrients for protein synthesis in all tissues; calcium is needed for bone growth; thiamin, riboflavin, and niacin for energy metabolism; iron and vitamin B_{12} for blood formation; vitamin A for the formation of healthy epithelial cells lining the developing respiratory, gastrointestinal, and genito-urinary tracts and for bone growth; and vitamin C for the formation of collagen, the framework for all cells. All other nutrients also play individual roles during this period of explosive growth.

In a multiracial society, like that of the United States, the kinds of foods eaten will vary. The so-called orthodox middle-class American diet of many whites in this country is not the diet of many blacks, Hispanics, and Asians, as the Committee on Nutrition of the Mother and Pre-school Child of the National Research Council has pointed out.[8] For instance, consumption of milk and cheese is low in these minority groups because many people have lactase deficiency. Some typical foods eaten by blacks and Mexican-Americans are listed by food group in Table 12-4.

Cultural practice may have a strong influence on dietary practices during pregnancy.

Should Pregnant Women Take Any Supplements, Such as Iron and Folacin?

With two exceptions, there seems to be no need to take nutrient supplements during pregnancy.[9] Rather, dietary education seems to be the best alternative, so that pregnant women are eating from all four food groups. However, the exceptions are iron and folic acid.

Iron

During pregnancy iron requirements are high. Iron is needed for hemoglobin in the increasing amount of blood in the fetus and in the maternal tissues. Because the RDA for iron during pregnancy cannot be met by the typical American diet,[5] a supplement of 30 to 60 mg of iron per day is recommended, especially during the last trimester.

TABLE 12-4 Some Characteristic Ethnic Food Choices

Protein Foods	Milk and Milk Products	Grain Products	Vegetables	Fruits	Other
Black American					
Meat	Milk	Rice	Broccoli	Apple	Salt pork
Beef	Fluid	Cornbread	Cabbage	Banana	(fat back)
Pork, ham	Evaporated in	Hominy grits	Carrots	Grapefruit	Carbonated
Sausage	coffee	Biscuits	Corn	Grapes	beverages
Pig's feet, ears, etc.	Buttermilk	Muffins	Green beans	Nectarine	Fruit drinks
Bacon	Cheese	White bread	Greens	Orange	Gravies
Luncheon meats	Cheddar	Dry cereal	Mustard	Plums	Coffee
Organ meats	Cottage	Cooked cereal	Collard	Tangerine	Iced tea
Poultry	Ice cream	Macaroni	Kale	Watermelon	
Chicken		Spaghetti	Spinach		
Turkey		Crackers	Turnip		
Fish			Lima beans		
Catfish			Okra		
Perch			Peas		
Red snapper			Potato		
Tuna			Pumpkin		
Salmon			Sweet potato		
Sardines			Tomato		
Shrimp			Yam		
Eggs					
Legumes					
Kidney beans					
Red beans					
Pinto beans					
Black-eyed peas					
Nuts					
Peanuts					
Peanut butter					

Continued.

TABLE 12-4 Some Characteristic Ethnic Food Choices—cont'd

Protein Foods	Milk and Milk Products	Grain Products	Vegetables	Fruits	Other
Mexican-American					
Meat	Milk	Rice	Avocado	Apple	Salsa (tomato-
Beef	Fluid	Tortillas	Cabbage	Apricots	pepper-onion
Pork	Flavored	Corn	Carrots	Banana	relish)
Lamb	Evaporated	Flour	Chilies	Guava	Chili sauce
Tripe	Condensed	Oatmeal	Corn	Lemon	Guacamole
Sausage (chorizo)	Cheese	Dry cereals	Green beans	Mango	Lard (man-
Bologna	American	Cornflakes	Lettuce	Melons	teca)
Bacon	Monterey Jack	Sugared	Onion	Orange	Pork crack-
	Hoop	Noodles	Peas	Peach	lings
Poultry	Ice Cream	Spaghetti	Potato	Pear	Fruit drinks
Chicken		White bread	Prickly pear	Prickly pear	Kool-aid
		Sweet bread	cactus leaf	cactus fruit	Carbonated
Eggs		(pan dulce)	(nopales)	(tuna)	beverages
			Spinach	Zapote (sapote)	Beer
Legumes			Sweet po-		Coffee
Pinto beans			tato		
Pink beans			Tomato		
Garbanzo beans			Zucchini		
Lentils					
Nuts					
Peanuts					
Peanut butter					

Folacin

Nutrient supplements during pregnancy should be taken under medical supervision.

⟵ A large increase in folacin intake is also recommended during pregnancy. Rich sources of folacin, green leafy vegetables, are not popular foods in the diets of some teenagers and adults. In addition, steroid contraceptives may interfere with the absorption and metabolism of this vitamin,[10] producing low levels of serum folicin as the woman enters pregnancy. The effects of low levels of folate on mother and infant are not clear. Some evidence points to a relationship between spontaneous abortions, fetal malformations, and subnormal infant development and low folacin levels. However, there is not unanimous agreement on their relationships to folacin deficiency. On this basis the National Research Council recommends an oral supplement of 400 μg per day of folacin. ⟶

Diet May Be Related to Discomforts Associated with Pregnancy

Certain complaints seem to be associated with pregnancy—morning sickness, heartburn, constipation, and various cravings and aversions. Could they be related to (or alleviated by) nutrition? Let us take a look at these.

Morning Sickness

⟵ Despite the word "morning," morning sickness—nausea—can actually occur at any time of day. A number of causes have been suggested, but scientists are still in the dark ages with regard to an explanation for morning sickness. One theory is that it is caused by a low blood glucose level; in this case, a dry biscuit or a light snack in the morning may help.[11] Another theory relates the problem to low levels of vitamin B_6 in the blood, which is why vitamin B_6 is included in antinausea prescription drugs to treat morning sickness. However, recent evidence finds no relationship between vitamin B_6 status and the incidence or degree of morning sickness.[12] Other suggestions are that the cause is hormonal or that it represents a problem of adaptation to the presence of foreign material because half of the genes in the fetus come from the father.

Heartburn

Caused by pressure from the fetus on the stomach, heartburn produces a "full" feeling and makes it difficult to eat—it has nothing to do with the heart. The burning sensation is produced by a mixture of food and acidic gastric secretions pushed back up the esophagus. To prevent heartburn, a pregnant woman should try eating smaller meals four, five, or six times throughout the day, avoiding foods that cause indigestion, wearing loose-fitting clothes, and remaining upright after eating.

Cravings and aversions

Cravings may occur for sweet foods, such as fruit or chocolate ice cream, and there may even be unusual cravings; yearnings for coal, soap, and soil have been reported.[11] A pregnant woman may also find that she dislikes food she once liked, such as meat, coffee, and fried food.

Constipation

Constipation and also hemorrhoids are common in pregnancy. They may be prevented by a diet high in fiber. In addition, a pregnant woman should eat more wholemeal bread, bran, and fruits and vegetables high in fiber.

> Factors important before pregnancy that can have some influence on nutritional status during pregnancy include the woman's age, the number of previous pregnancies, her income, eating habits, smoking, consumption of alcohol and drugs, the presence of diseases like diabetes and hypertension, and large changes in body weight. Risks to the mother during pregnancy include low hemoglobin levels, either too low or too high a weight gain, toxemia, and diabetes. Increased intake of food is required during pregnancy, and supplementation with iron and folacin is suggested.

NEW LIFE: NUTRITION FOR ZYGOTE, EMBRYO, AND FETUS

The differences between a *zygote* and a fetus are considerable, but what are these differences?

Zygote
A fertilized ovum (egg).

Growth of the Fetus Causes Changes in Body Composition

In the last trimester, the fetus not only undergoes rapid growth but also undergoes changes in its body composition. This is expressed in Table 12-5, which compares

TABLE 12-5 Composition of the Body of a Fetus at 6 Months Gestation and of a Baby at Term

	Percentage of Total Weight	
	6-Month Fetus	Full-Term Baby
Water	88	70
Fat	2	15
Nitrogen	1.4	2
Sodium	0.20	0.16
Potassium	0.15	0.18
Chloride	0.22	0.17
Calcium	0.59	0.82
Phosphorus	0.36	0.48
Iron	0.006	0.008
Weight	1000 g	3500 g

Placenta
The part of the uterus through which the fetus receives its nutrients.

the body composition of a six-month-old fetus with that of a full-term baby (a newborn). As you look at this, consider the nutrition implications of a premature birth. When this happens, the infant must receive the nutrients that would have been provided through the *placenta*.

There are several reasons for the changes in body composition during the last trimester, as explained below. This information is used to make up baby formulas to meet the special nutrient requirements of babies born prematurely. As a result of these special formulas—and because premature babies are kept in the hospital at a high environmental temperature—the death rate of "preemies" has been dramatically reduced.

Water

The amount of water in the fetal tissues decreases during the third trimester because cellular material increases.

Fat

The amount of fetal body fat must increase because the infant needs reserve energy and insulation. The low level of fat in the six-month fetus is a reason why environmental temperature must be kept high for a premature infant. The fetus gains much fat during the last three months of pregnancy. The amount of fat in the milk of different species is related to the amount of body fat at birth. Human milk is low in fat. This accumulation of body fat in the last trimester is important for the health of the infant during the lactation period.

Nitrogen

The amount of nitrogen in the fetal tissue increases because the protein involved in cell structure and enzymes rapidly increases.

Sodium and chloride

The concentration of sodium and chloride in fetal tissues decreases during the third trimester. Sodium and chloride ions are constituents of extracellular fluid; as the size of cells increases as tissues grow, the amount of extracellular fluid decreases, thereby decreasing the percentage of sodium and chloride in fetal tissue.

Potassium

The concentration of potassium in fetal tissue increases during the third trimester because it is the major ion in the intracellular fluid. The number and size of cells increases rapidly during pregnancy.

Calcium and phosphorus

The concentrations of calcium and phosphorus increase with the increases in bone mass.

Iron

Iron content of fetal tissue increases during the third trimester. There is an increased amount of hemoglobin in an expanding blood volume.

Certain Drugs and Food Patterns Are Hazardous to Fetal Health

Mothers-to-be certainly need to behave responsibly. Whatever tobacco, alcohol, caffeine, nonprescription drugs, megavitamins, and special foods they consume can have important consequences for their offspring. Here is how a special committee of the National Research Council described these hazards affecting the fetus.[13]

Tobacco

Smoking is one of the most important *preventable* determinants of low birth weight. Babies born to smokers are on average 200 g (7 oz) lighter than babies born to nonsmokers.[14] The reason is that the combination of nicotine and carbon monoxide deprives the fetus of oxygen. Even if the mother smokes less than one pack of cigarettes per day, it may cause a 25% increase in the incidence of vaginal bleeding, and over a pack a day pushes this figure to 92%.

⇨ It is also possible that a pregnant woman's simply being *around* smokers may harm the fetus. Disturbing new evidence shows that if nonsmoking mothers are exposed to cigarette smoke there is a higher probability of delivery of a low birth weight baby.[14] ⇦

Alcohol

Women who consume alcohol during pregnancy run high risks of causing *fetal alcohol syndrome* (FAS) in their babies (Figure 12-4). Among the awful symptoms resulting from FAS are abnormal facial appearance, delayed development, and mental retardation. For ten of the eleven children first diagnosed with FAS in 1973—all offspring of severely alcoholic mothers—life has not been pleasant.[15] One child was lost to follow-up, but of the rest, two are dead and eight are growth-retarded and deformed. Four were of borderline intelligence; the other four were severely handicapped intellectually and need complete supervision outside the home.

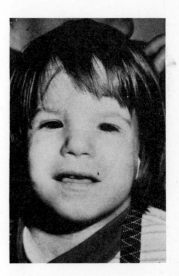

Fetal Alcohol Syndrome
Abnormalities in newborns born to alcoholic mothers. Child illustrated below has facial symptoms of fetal alcohol syndrome.

FIGURE 12-4
Fetal alcohol syndrome (FAS) causes
facial disfigurement and mental retardation. Alcohol intake during the first
three months of pregnancy is the greatest cause of FAS.

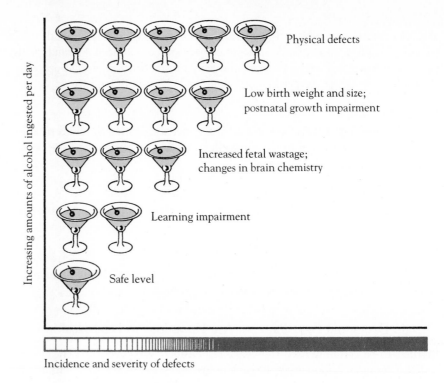

Physical defects

Low birth weight and size;
postnatal growth impairment

Increased fetal wastage;
changes in brain chemistry

Learning impairment

Safe level

(y-axis) Increasing amounts of alcohol ingested per day

Incidence and severity of defects

Caffeine

When given to experimental laboratory animals in high doses, equivalent to 12
to 40 cups of coffee per day for human beings, caffeine has been found to cause
birth defects; no such evidence has been reported for humans, however. Because
high caffeine consumption is frequently accompanied by heavy smoking or alcohol
consumption, it is difficult to pinpoint the harmful effects of caffeine by itself.
Still, the recommendation of the National Research Council is for "moderation
in caffeine intake during pregnancy."[13]

Over-the-counter drugs

Caution is advised in the use of all over-the-counter drugs. As with caffeine, it
has been found that aspirin and other nonprescription pain-killing drugs cause birth
defects in laboratory animals, although no such evidence exists for humans. However, pregnant women are advised not to use such drugs unnecessarily.

Vitamin megadoses

Reports in the scientific literature show associations between large doses of some
vitamins and abnormalities in offspring.[9] Some of these observations were made
on very few subjects. Nevertheless, the message is the same: there is nothing to
gain and much to lose by self-prescribing high doses of vitamins.

    An excess of vitamin A may lead to kidney problems and central nervous sys-
tem abnormalities in the fetus. Too much vitamin D may cause mental retar-

dation. Women with higher serum alpha-tocopherol who took megadoses of vitamin E had a higher proportion of spontaneous abortions. Megadoses of vitamin C produced "conditioned scurvy" during the first four weeks after birth. (No effects on the fetus or infant have been reported from taking high levels of thiamin, riboflavin, niacin, vitamin B_6, biotin, pantothenic acid, folacin, and vitamin B_{12}.)

Vegetarian and vegan diets

Pregnant women who eliminate meat from their diets experience no difficulties, either in themselves or their offspring—provided all the other foods they ate were varied and balanced in nutrients. Still, elimination of *all* foods of animal origin from the diet poses a higher risk of the mother delivering abnormally small infants, because of nutrient deficiencies. Iron, calcium, and vitamin B_{12} levels are difficult to maintain on vegan diets.

Pica

Pica, the practice of eating clay or laundry starch, may leave little room for consumption of nutritious foods. Cases of constipation, hypertension, and toxemia in women who practice pica have been reported.

Major changes in the composition of the fetus occur during its growth. Factors that interfere with normal growth include smoking, alcohol, caffeine, over-the-counter medicines, megadoses of vitamins, vegan diets, and pica.

BREAST-FEEDING: ADVANTAGES FOR THE MOTHER

There are important nutrition, economic, and psychological advantages of breast-feeding for the mother. Once out of fashion, breast-feeding is now "in" again, and the percentage of breast-fed babies in the United States is probably 40% to 60%. The reasons for the revival in popularity are:

- Mothers have been educated about the benefits of breast-feeding
- Better facilities for breast-feeding are now available in hospitals
- Organizations such as La Leche League have offered advice and support
- As "natural foods" became popular in supermarkets during the 1970s and '80s, it became more popular to use the most natural food in the world to feed babies

Adolescents were found to be most likely to breast-feed if they saw benefit from it, if they wanted more information about it, if they themselves had been breast-fed, if the social environment was supportive of the practice, and if they saw few barriers to breast-feeding.[16]

Factors Influencing the Preference for Breast-feeding

What determines whether a newborn baby receives human milk, cow's milk, or commercially prepared "infant formula"? The following factors seem to influence the parents' decision.

Race

Forty-four percent of Anglo-American mothers were breast-feeding their infants by the time they left the hospital, according to one study, compared to 23% of Mexican-American mothers, and 9% of black mothers. The factors that influenced a woman to breast-feed were: for Anglo-Americans—the support of the male partner; for Mexican-Americans—support of the woman's mother; for blacks—influence of close friends.[17]

Education and income

Economics

The higher the level of the mother's education and income, the more likely she is to breast-feed.

Employment status

An employed mother is less likely to breast-feed than an unemployed mother—no doubt the result of the inconvenience of having to breast-feed a baby while at work. However, many union contracts now contain a pregnancy relief clause.

Birth order

First-born children are more likely to be breast-fed than later children.

Geographical region

Geography

Breast-feeding is least popular in hospitals in the East-South-Central portion of the United States. It is most popular in the Mountain states. In Canada, the highest rate of breast-feeding is in British Columbia and Alberta, and the lowest is in the Atlantic provinces.[9]

Breast-feeding Benefits the Mother

Breast-feeding is advocated by the Surgeon General of the United States, not just for its benefits to the infant (discussed later in the chapter) but also for its benefits to the mother.

Loss of fat tissue

Breast-feeding brings about a more rapid loss of the fat tissue that accumulated in the mother's body during her pregnancy.

Birth control

Believe it or not, breast-feeding is a form of birth control. Mothers who have a complete and unrestricted breast-feeding schedule usually do not ovulate or menstruate for at least 10 weeks after delivery. However, it is not a very reliable contraceptive method because it is not certain when fertility returns.[9]

Emotional satisfaction

Bonding
The formation of a close relationship between infant and parents.

One cannot overlook the important aspect of *bonding* between mother and child.

Convenience

No preparation required. No waste. Baby receives milk under sanitary conditions. It's even becoming acceptable to do it (discretely) in public, at least in many places.

If a mother cannot breast-feed her child at work, she can pump the milk from her breasts before going to work, leave the milk refrigerated and allow another person to feed it to the baby. Of course, the baby may also be given infant formula in addition to human milk.

Research in England and Australia indicates that the output of milk is very variable among mothers. However, it is concluded that exclusive breast-feeding by well-nourished mothers can be adequate for periods from 2 to 15 months.[18]

Economics

Breast-feeding is more economical than other kinds of infant feeding, costing (in 1983) only 73 cents a day for the extra food required to meet the additional nutrient requirements of lactation. The cost of prepared formulas plus basic equipment, bottles, nipples, disposable holders and liners, was $1.49 to 1.88 per day.[9] Even allowing for inflation since 1983, breast-feeding is still very economical.

Employer benefits

One aspect of interest to employers of new mothers is that breast-fed infants are healthier than bottle-fed infants, thus reducing absenteeism of mothers staying home to care for sick children.

Breast-feeding Puts Some Extra Nutritional Demands on the Mother

A woman contemplating breast-feeding should be aware that she must eat a good diet.

In particular, she must be sure to increase her nutrient intake to meet the demands of producing 700 to 750 ml of milk each day for the first four months of lactation (Figure 12-3). Some experts are now disputing the high amount of energy recommended for lactation. Some women can produce the required amount of milk while gradually losing body weight on an intake of 2100 kcalories per day.

In addition, of course, a new mother must take care in her choice of diet, because an inadequate diet reduces the quantity, but not the nutrient quality, of breast milk.

> Breast-feeding offers the mother important nutritional, economic, and psychological advantages.

HUMAN MILK, COW'S MILK, OR FORMULA: EFFECTS ON THE INFANT

Infant feeding is an art that is based partly on tradition. In the 19th century, it became a science as a result of research on the composition of milk. This led to the use of cow's milk and recently to the development of infant formulas as alternatives to human milk.

But these are only part of the major dietary changes occurring at this critical period of life. The fetus has obtained nutrients from the mother through the placenta and from the amniotic fluid that it swallows. Then suddenly the baby is born into a different environment. Human milk, or a substitute, is now its diet. The newborn's intestinal system must deal with nutrients it has never digested before. These include milk proteins, fat, lactose. The baby's survival depends on the speed at which the gastrointestinal tract can adapt to these sudden changes. Another extensive change occurs at weaning.

Decisions About Lactation Critically Affect a Child's Development

Pediatricians now make routine checks to see if an infant's digestive system is able to cope with nutrients. One such test is made for phenylketonuria (PKU), a genetic defect that causes a failure to metabolize the essential amino acid phenylalanine. PKU occurs once in about every 40,000 births and in equal proportion between males and females. If it is untreated, it results in mental retardation, an abnormally small head, and congenital heart disease. Protein intake must be restricted to reduce the intake of phenylalanine. Older children can take special foods free of phenylalanine. Other diseases with nutrition implications for the infant include cystic fibrosis, celiac disease (person is intolerant to gluten in cereals), multiple sclerosis, and juvenile diabetes (type I).

Once considerations about PKU are out of the way, some other decisions may be made about different practices in infant feeding.

Breast Milk Is the Most Important First Food for Life

Colostrum
Breast milk secreted during the first 2 or 3 days after delivery of the infant.

During the first few weeks of life, breast milk contributes important nutrients and chemicals. *Colostrum* is particularly important because it provides high concentrations of nutrients immediately after birth (Table 12-6).

Scientists are only now learning about the nutritional significance of breast-feeding during the first five days of life. There is a huge increase in the intake of various nutrients (Figure 12-5). Iron, zinc, and copper are in forms that are more easily absorbed into the blood from human than from cow's milk. Over 20 different enzymes are present in milk, of which lipase is the most important. This aids in the digestion of fat in the infant's stomach. Many hormones are in milk, but their function is unknown.[19] Colostrum also is an important source of antibodies. These protect the infant from infections in the digestive tract caused by bacteria and viruses.

Breast milk and undernutrition

Severe undernutrition reduces the amount of breast milk produced. Infants born to undernourished mothers get a smaller amount of milk. However, with the

TABLE 12-6 The Composition of Milk

	Protein (g/100 ml)	Fat (g/100 ml)	Lactose (g/100 ml)
Human			
Colostrum	12.0	2.9	5.3
Milk	1.1	3.8	7.6
Cow			
Colostrum	14.2	3.6	3.1
Milk	3.3	3.7	4.8

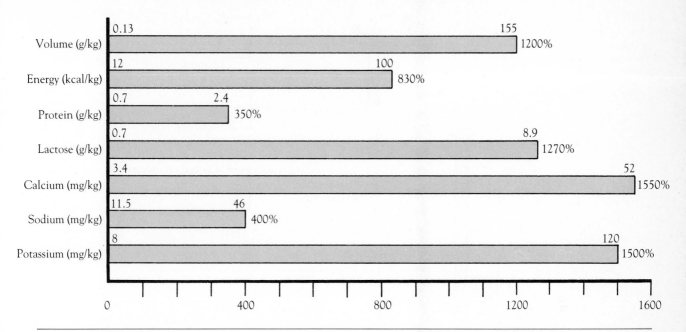

FIGURE 12-5
Huge increases in nutrient intake by the infant during the first 5 days of life. Energy is needed for growth of all tissues, protein and potassium for the growth of cells, and calcium for bone growth.

exception of some vitamins, the nutrient content of an undernourished woman's milk is similar to the milk produced by a well-nourished woman. Numerous observations from different parts of the world show that the growth rate of children breast-fed by undernourished mothers is surprisingly good.

Changes in breast milk

Breast milk changes in composition during lactation. Regardless of the nutritional status of the mother, the composition of milk changes the longer breast-feeding continues. After three months of breast-feeding, there is a decline in the concentration of protein, sodium, phosphorus, and zinc, but no change in the concentration of fat, energy, and calcium.[20] Despite these changes, it is recommended that mother's milk is the appropriate food for the first six months of life. Extra amounts of vitamin D and iron should be given to the infant to supplement the low levels of these two nutrients in milk.

Lifestyles and environment

The composition of breast milk can be affected by lifestyles and environment; the mother of an infant can only try to do her best to be sure the quality of her milk is the best possible.

Consider the transfer of toxic substances into breast milk. A new mother should give some thought to limiting her consumption of alcohol, cigarettes, oral contraceptives, and other medications, and she should be aware that if she lives in an area high in environmental pollutants—for example PCBs (polychlorinated biphenyls, an industrial chemical) or DDT, a now-banned agricultural chemical—they may find their way into her milk.

In another environmental matter, vegetarians need to consider how to breast-feed their infants adequately. In one vegan religious community, several nutritional

Toxicology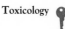

FIGURE 12-6
Failure to thrive in breast-fed infants could be due to a number of reasons. The infants should be examined by a physician.

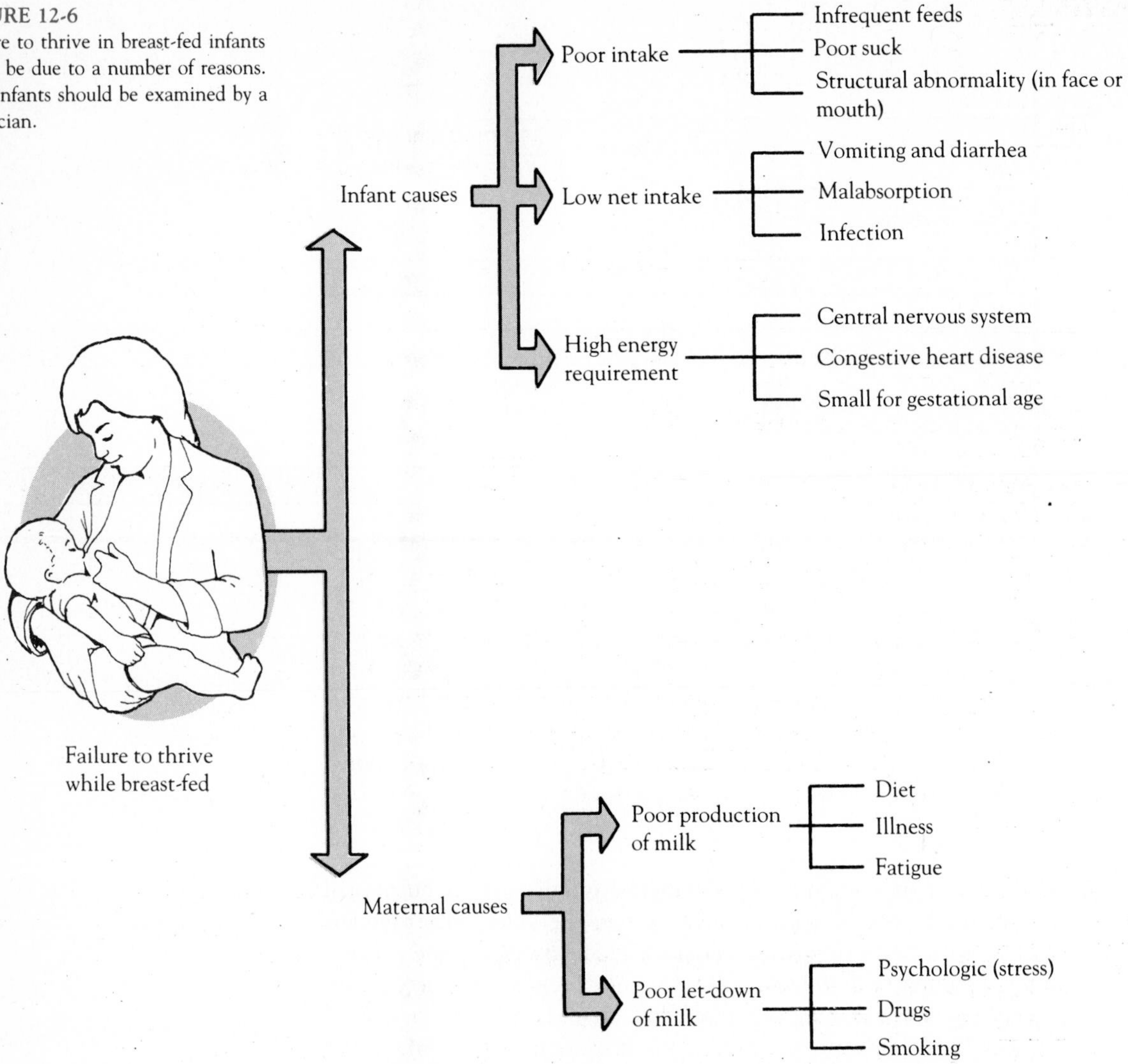

Failure to thrive while breast-fed

Infant causes
- Poor intake
  - Infrequent feeds
  - Poor suck
  - Structural abnormality (in face or mouth)
- Low net intake
  - Vomiting and diarrhea
  - Malabsorption
  - Infection
- High energy requirement
  - Central nervous system
  - Congestive heart disease
  - Small for gestational age

Maternal causes
- Poor production of milk
  - Diet
  - Illness
  - Fatigue
- Poor let-down of milk
  - Psychologic (stress)
  - Drugs
  - Smoking

deficiencies developed in infants breast-fed for three months.[21] The deficiencies were not caused by the breast-feeding, however. The mothers supplemented and in some cases replaced breast-milk with foods with very low kcaloric density, and it was this practice that resulted in the deficiencies. As a result, one baby died, and the remaining three studied had extreme protein-calorie malnutrition, severe rickets, osteoporosis, vitamin B_{12} deficiency, and other deficiencies.

Adverse reactions to breast milk

Mothers may be concerned by some reports that breast-feeding causes some infants to get eczema, a type of dermatitis. However, the evidence is far from conclusive.[22] The problem seems to be greatest when breast-feeding combined with other foods is continued beyond 12 weeks of age. However, dermatitis can also occur in some infants when cow's milk is fed.

Some babies do not thrive when breast-fed, making a mother worry about her ability to breast-feed or to give up breast-feeding early. However, a number of causes may be responsible (Figure 12-7) and should be identified by a physician.

Whether and When to Feed Infants Cow's Milk Is Controversial

The American Academy of Pediatrics recommends breast-feeding during the first 6 to 12 months of life.[23] Regarding cow's milk they state: "The appropriate age at which unheated whole cow's milk (WCM) can be safely introduced into the infant diet is unknown and remains an area of controversy."[23]

Still, on the basis of present evidence, there is no convincing reason to declare whole cow's milk harmful after 6 months provided the baby receives adequate supplementary feedings. Some nutritionists feel that whole cow's milk should not be given before 12 months of age. If breast-feeding is stopped at 6 months of age, then the Academy sees no problem in introducing whole cow's milk provided that the infants get one third of their kcalories from a balanced mixture of cereals, vegetables, fruits, and other foods. These supplements are important to make sure the infant gets enough vitamin C and iron.

No more than 1 liter per day of whole cow's milk should be given to infants. Babies fed skim milk have lower growth rates and lower fat stores, and they may be deficient in the essential fatty acids.[23]

Low-fat milk is fine for adults but not for babies.

British nutritionists give the following advice about feeding milk to infants and young children.[24] The same advice applies to infants in North America and throughout the world.

Early infancy: Exclusive breast-feeding is best; formula should be continued for six months if used; solids may be introduced from four months; soy-based formula may be used if cow's milk formula is unsuitable.

Late infancy: After 6 months of age the following are suitable—human milk, infant formulas, whole pasteurized cow's milk. Skimmed and semiskimmed milks are not recommended because of their lower energy content.

Milk for young children: Whole cow's milk should be a staple item for preschool children. Semiskimmed milk may be used from two years if the overall diet is adequate, but wholly skimmed milk is not recommended below five years.

Why some infants develop allergic reactions to cow's milk is not fully understood. Only a small proportion of the infant population (0.4% to 7.5%) is allergic to milk during the first two years of life. Heating milk does not remove the cause of the allergy, but it will reduce the amount of some heat-sensitive nutrients.

Commercial Infant Formulas Have the Composition of Breast Milk

Commercially prepared infant formulas—which come in powder, liquid concentrate, or ready-to-serve liquid form—try to replicate the composition of human breast milk, and may be used as alternatives or supplements to human milk. The American Academy of Pediatrics has set standards by which the nutrient contents of infant formulas are as near as possible to those in human milk, especially if they are iron-fortified. Therefore, there is no need for a baby to take supplements of vitamins or minerals in addition to the formula though there is still debate on the bioavailability of iron in the formulas. Cost differences between infant formulas are more for convenience value than for nutritional value.

The protein source in formulas is either cow's milk or soy. Because soy is a plant protein, the biological value of this protein is a little less than that of cow's milk; therefore, the protein content of soy-based formulas is higher. Fat is provided by vegetable oils, which are high in polyunsaturated fatty acids; these are absorbed better than saturated fatty acids. Carbohydrates are sucrose, lactose, or corn syrup. The advantage of lactose is that it helps in the absorption of calcium.

A major disadvantage of formulas is that they do not provide the antibodies contained in human milk. Moreover, allergies may not be avoided because the milk and soy proteins in formulas are capable of causing allergic reactions. Finally, formula feeding seems to cause greater deposits of subcutaneous fat.

Overall, Breast-feeding Has Advantages for the Infant

All in all, breast-feeding seems to have the most advantages for the infant, compared to cow's milk and commercial formulas:

- Breast milk is the most nutritious first food for life.
- Breast milk is the least likely to be contaminated by harmful micro-organisms.
- Antibodies in breast milk help prevent infections.
- It is least likely to cause allergic reactions.
- Its nutrients are more bioavailable—that is, a higher proportion of all nutrients in breast milk are absorbed and used by the body for the important functions they perform during this rapid period of growth.
- Colostrum protects against infections, especially in the gastrointestinal sytem, during the critical first few days after the infant is born.
- Breast-feeding helps the infant develop its jaws by suckling.
- Breast-feeding is beneficial in reducing the incidence of infantile obesity, respiratory infection, and diarrhea; it also has growth-promoting substances in the colostrum that are not in cow's milk or formula.
- Breast-feeding improves the bonding between mother and infant.

Recent evidence gives some interesting information concerning the style of breast-feeding and the possible development of obesity in later years.[25] Fewer but longer feeds and a higher sucking pressure were associated with a greater amount of adipose tissue accumulation. It seems that a vigorous infant feeding style consisting of sucking more rapidly, at higher pressure, and with a shorter interval between bursts of sucking is associated with higher kcaloric intake and greater deposition of adipose tissue. In the infants studied it was found that breast-feeding protected against the early deposition of adipose tissue only to the age of 6 months.

Breast-feeding has many advantages for the infant. It is nutritious and safe, helps to prevent infections, helps to develop the jaws, and promotes bonding between infant and mother. Whole cow's milk is a satisfactory food after the infant is 6 months old. Commercial infant formulas are nutritious and convenient, but they must be prepared properly.

LIFE THREATS TO THE INFANT: PREMATURITY, SEVERE UNDERNUTRITION, AND FIRST-YEAR MALNUTRITION

Nutrition is of great importance to an infant's survival. Let us look at the dangers of premature birth, severe undernutrition, and nutrition during the first year of life.

An Infant Born Prematurely Must Receive the Kind of Nutrients He or She Would Have Received as a Fetus

Not long ago the death rate in premature infants was high, mostly because of respiratory difficulties. Although these problems are mostly solved and death rates are now much lower, remaining problems associated with premature births can involve nutrition.

As Table 12-5 shows, there is a large flow of nutrients from the mother to the fetus during the last three months of pregnancy. When the infant is born 3 months premature, then these nutrients must be provided by the diet. Milk from mothers with preterm babies is adequate in protein, sodium, potassium, and chloride. It is not adequate in calcium, phosphorus, iron, zinc, and copper. Even so, mothers should be encouraged to breast-feed premature babies because of the better digestibility and immunological properties of their milk compared with formulas or with term milk drawn from a *milk bank.*[19]

Milk Bank
Expressed human milk saved for future use.

There is no agreement on the amount of supplementation for preterm infants' diets. If the premature infant's own mother's milk is not available, formulas designed for preterm infants are preferred over pooled milk bank samples. This is because the pooled milk bank samples have a nutrient content adequate for full-term infants. They are low in protein, energy, and several minerals.

Severe Undernutrition Is a Major Problem for Infants in Underdeveloped Countries

High infant mortality rates occur in less-developed countries especially during the first three months of life. The main causes are low birth weight and diarrhea.[26] Low birth weight in infants as a result of undernutrition also occurs in the United States. A recent study showed that 9% of white and Hispanic infants and 13% of black infants weighed less than 2500 grams (about 5.5 pounds) at birth.[27] Let us look at the problems contributing to undernutrition in infants.

Water quality and sanitation

The major cause of infant death from diarrhea is unclean drinking water or unclean water used to prepare food. Indeed, unclean water figured in a controversy several years ago regarding the use of infant formulas in less-developed countries. Although the formulas themselves were satisfactory in nutritive value, they needed to be prepared with clean water in clean utensils; these were unavailable to some people who used the formula.

Clean water is essential in preparing infant formula.

However, there have been success stories in saving children from the *dehydration* caused by diarrhea. Oral rehydration solutions containing glucose, potassium, sodium, and chloride (from a pinch of salt) are now available. (Honey is effective

TABLE 12-7 Suggested Times for Feeding Infant Semisolid Foods and Table Foods

| Food | Age (months) | | |
	4 to 6	6 to 8	9 to 12
Iron-fortified cereals for infants	Add		
Vegetables		Add strained	Gradually delete strained foods, introduce table foods
Fruits		Add strained	Gradually delete strained foods, introduce chopped well-cooked or canned foods
Meats		Add strained or finely chopped table meats	Decrease the use of strained meats, increase the varieties of table meats
Finger foods such as arrowroot biscuits, oven-dried toast		Add those that can be secured with a palmar grasp	Increase the use of small-sized finger foods as the pincer grasp develops
Well-cooked mashed or chopped table foods, prepared without added salt or sugar			Add
Juice by cup			Add

as a substitute only if glucose is unavailable in these oral rehydration solutions.[28])
These preparations can be made in the home with a teaspoon of sugar and a pinch
of salt. They are effective, safe, and inexpensive.

Infectious diseases

Measles, whooping cough, and other childhood diseases cause major wastage of
nutrients. Improvement in the diet, especially in protein content, decreases this
problem.

Poor maternal habits

Poor food habits, food preparation, and personal hygiene in the home lead to poor
nutrition and to infections in infants.

Lack of family planning

Insufficient spacing of births and poor maternal nutrition also contribute to severe
undernutrition in infants.

Poor agricultural production

Farming that produces low amounts of food and that wastes food contributes to
undernutrition in infants.

Nutrition During the First Year of Life Is Important

The tissue with which a baby is born must not only be maintained but must be added to during the first twelve months of life. Indeed, during this year, body weight is supposed to increase by 150%, and it is normally supposed to be done by higher recommended intakes for most nutrients (see the RDA table on the inside back cover).

The requirements for thiamin, riboflavin, and niacin are related to energy needs, and vitamin B_6 to amino acid and protein synthesis. The need for iron during the first few months of life is fairly small, since the infant has reserves it received from the mother *in utero*. However, after four months, increased amounts of tissues and blood require more iron in the diet.

Infants born to mothers who took megavitamin doses of vitamin C during pregnancy may have higher requirements for vitamin C. It is suggested that these infants be given 25 to 50 mg vitamin C per day.[29]

Extra vitamin D may be necessary for infants born in the northern United States and Canada. The reason is that breast milk may not contain adequate amounts of vitamin D.[29] As was mentioned in Chapter 6, deficiency of vitamin D was a big problem in Great Britain among the children of immigrants from India and Pakistan, for a combination of dietary and cultural reasons.

When Should a Baby Be Weaned?

When should a baby be fed semisolid and table foods? The approximate ages for introducing various foods are given in Table 12-7. Although the reasons for these time periods have social and psychological reasons, let us consider only the nutritional ones.

By the age of one year, the infant's intestinal and kidney functions have become capable of handling a great variety of foods. However, if weaning starts too early, the infant will usually become sick and have diarrhea.

What kinds of foods should be used in weaning? Although the choice varies

---

TABLE 12-8 How To Prepare Infant Foods in the Home

- Use fresh, high-quality fruits, vegetables, and meats.

- Clean hands and utensils thoroughly before starting.

- Use as little water as possible to wash the foods.

- Do not overcook because of the loss of heat-sensitive nutrients.

- Do not add salt; use sugar sparingly. Do not give honey to babies under 1 year of age because of the possibility of infant botulism.

- Use enough water to puree the food.

- Strain or puree the food.

- Pour puree into ice cube tray and freeze.

- Unfreeze and heat in serving container the amount of food needed for a single feeding. Heat in a microwave oven or a water bath.

throughout the world and is based on culture, iron-fortified cereals are often given first. The next food introduced is usually fruits or vegetables—it makes little difference which precedes the other. The sequence by which most foods are introduced to infants is presented in Table 12-7. Some advice on how to prepare infant foods at home is given in Table 12-8.

Some Bad Nutrition Habits of the First Year May Be Critical

Once it was thought, because of people's preoccupation with the dangers of obesity, that feeding a baby too much food during the first year of life was harmful, but now it does not seem to be so bad after all. Scientists are no longer so certain that an overfed baby becomes obese and that an obese baby will grow up to be an obese adult.[2] Research shows no relationship between excess fat in infancy and excess fat in adolescence (as your own family photo album may show).

Even so, a baby's body weight should still be kept within recommended levels during the first few years of life. Some suggestions here for the parents are:

- Balance the baby's food intake with activity.
- Don't use food and drink as a reward.
- Don't force the baby to empty its bowl, plate, or cup.

Another bad habit to avoid starting in infancy is cultivating a liking for salt and sweets. Infants can appreciate the natural flavors in fruits and vegetables just as they are; it is adults who feel food needs more sugar and salt (at least more than the baby needs) for it to "taste right." Since babies develop a liking for salt at about four months—when their kidneys can then cope with high sodium intakes—now is a time to go easy rather than heavy on salt in food. Not a lot is known about babies' taste buds, however, and the role of the sensory qualities of weaning and post-weaning diets has been largely overlooked.[30] We are learning that babies' food dislikes may be short-lived. Most complaints about adverse reactions to foods occur during the first year of life.[31] Most of these foods can be introduced into the diet without risk by the third year.

The time of weaning is also a time when adults can help their young head off tooth decay. Sometimes parents will check the temperature or taste of food by putting the baby's spoon in their own mouths. The trouble is that a baby's teeth, which are just erupting from its gums, are particularly sensitive to a bacterium called *Streptococcus mutans,* which causes dental caries.[32] Saliva from adults is the usual transmitter of the bacterium to the infant. Thus, if you wish to test the temperature of the baby's food, it's best to just touch it to your wrist so it will not come in contact with your saliva.

> Nutrition-related problems arise if the baby is born prematurely, is undernourished, or is weaned onto nutritionally poor food. Most of these problems arise in developing countries because of a lack of food, poor sanitation, or poor education about infant nutrition.

DECISIONS

1. Is a Crying Baby Complaining About His or Her Diet?

Of course, an infant may be crying for reasons unrelated to food, but feeding problems in infancy are among the most common seen in baby clinics. A mother may regard frequent crying to be the result of inadequate or unsuitable foods, which may lead her to try changing the baby's food several times—to the distress of both baby and mother. Unfortunately, there is no easy answer to give to the mother.

In the past, manufacturers of baby formula thought a high protein content was more satisfying to the infant. However, high protein makes no difference in the amount of crying or in the volume consumed when compared with formulas that are lower in protein and sodium.[33]

2. Is Exercise Harmful to Mother or Fetus During Pregnancy?

Weight-reducing diets should never be tried during pregnancy, but if a mother-to-be wishes to control her weight, physical exercise is a good way to do it—provided the following rules are observed:

- No physical contact sports—horseback riding, wrestling, and the like are out.
- Avoid excessive increases in body heat. Heat stress has been found in experimental animals to cause fetal growth retardation and central nervous system defects, although no such detailed information is available on humans.

Acute exercise normally is not a harmful stress for the fetus, so it seems that a little exercise during pregnancy will probably do no harm. As for the other extreme—the sedentary lifestyle commonly adopted in late pregnancy in most Western societies—this seems to be only a cultural rather than a physiological phenomenon.[34]

3. Should a Pregnant Woman Avoid Alcohol?

Yes. Although it has been suspected for centuries that alcohol intake during pregnancy could cause severe damage to the fetus, it was only in 1973 that the fetal alcohol syndrome was first described. Since then, FAS has been found in every racial group and in many countries.

The harmful physical effects of FAS were described in Figure 12-4. Some children with FAS have behavioral problems. These include low attention spans and hyperactivity. This may produce learning disabilities. Many have problems with gross and fine motor coordination. Children with FAS have a high incidence of infections. FAS is the third most common form of mental retardation.

How does alcohol get involved? Alcohol is a drug that crosses the placenta with ease, but there are differences of opinion as to *how much* alcohol causes the negative effects. Thus, the best (most cautious) advice is to abstain from alcohol before and during pregnancy. The amount of alcohol intake during the first few weeks of pregancy determines if FAS will occur in the infant. Here is what certain amounts are said to do:

- One ounce (30 ml) of pure alcohol per day causes low birth weight in the infant. (One ounce of *pure* alcohol is equivalent to 2 to 3 ounces, or two servings of hard liquor such as whiskey or vodka.)
- One ounce of pure alcohol per week increases the risk of spontaneous abortions.

You should be aware that over-the-counter medications have a surprisingly high alcohol content.[35] Nighttime cough syrups have up to 25% alcohol; the daytime versions have 5%-10%. Mouth washes range from 6% to 27% alcohol. These medications can be a problem if intake is abused.

4. Does Honey Cause Infant Botulism?

Infant botulism was reported first in 1976. Now cases are confirmed throughout the world.[36] Children between the ages of 2 weeks and 6 months with infant botulism may develop a mild paralysis with failure to thrive, a moderate paralysis requiring admission to hospital, or a rapid paralysis with sudden death resembling sudden infant death syndrome (SIDS). Infant botulism is characterized by constipation, followed by lethargy, weak sucking and crying, drooping eye-lids, paralysis of the eye muscles, facial weakness, and in some cases, difficulty in breathing.

Infant botulism occurs with both breast-fed and bottle-fed infants. There seems to be a relation between onset of the problem and the recent introduction of formula. How the microorganism *C. botulinum* gets into the child's system is unknown, but honey has been suggested as a possible source.

Less than one third of all patients with infant botulism were found to have been fed honey. Still, perhaps parents should play it safe and spare their infants the honey—at least until more is known about a problem that is no longer simply a medical curiosity.

5. Can "Bottle Caries" Be Eliminated By Being Careful About How Long the Baby Sucks the Bottle?

Bottle caries—also called "nursing bottle mouth," "nursing caries," and "night bottle syndrome"—is caused by infant formula or other substances that may cause dental caries if they remain in contact with the baby's teeth for a long period. It occurs when babies fall asleep with the bottle in their mouths for long periods or when parents give them pacifiers often dipped in sweeteners. One Canadian study showed that about 3% of children under 4 years of age have the disease.

Early signs of bottle caries consists of dull white or chalky areas on the teeth resulting from decalcification. As the problem gets worse, the color goes from yellow to brown to black, and the area increases in size. Bottle caries can be prevented by regular dental visits and good oral hygiene. If parents delay taking their children to the dentist until they are three years of age or older, the disease may be well advanced.[37]

Summary

PREGNANCY

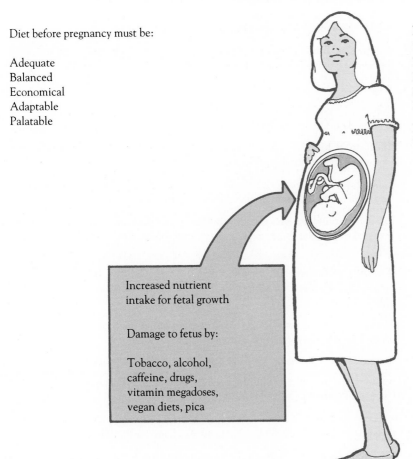

Diet before pregnancy must be:

Adequate
Balanced
Economical
Adaptable
Palatable

Nutrition risks at start of pregnancy
Under 15 years of age
Number of pregnancies
Low income
Smoking
Drugs
Alcohol
Disease

Optimal weight gain in
pregnancy is 24-28 pounds

Increased nutrient
intake for fetal growth

Damage to fetus by:

Tobacco, alcohol,
caffeine, drugs,
vitamin megadoses,
vegan diets, pica

LACTATION

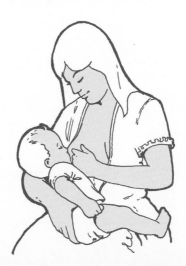

Decisions:

Breast-feed
Cow's milk
Formula

Decisions during first
year of life:

When to feed solid or
semisolid foods

Development of food
patterns in infant

Breast-feeding
benefits to mother:

Loss of fat
Birth control
Emotional satisfaction
Convenience
Economical

REFERENCES

1. Rosenfield, A., and Maine, D.: Maternal mortality: a neglected tragedy, Lancet **ii:**83, 1985.

2. Widdowson, E.M.: Food and health from conception to extreme old age. In G.G. Birch and K.J. Porter, editors: Food and health: science and technology, London, Applied Sciences Publishers, Ltd., 1981.

3. Anonymous: Influence of nutritional status on pharmacokinetics of contraceptive progestogens, Nutrition Reviews **42:**182, 1984.

4. Wegman, M.E.: Annual summary of vital statistics, 1985. Pediatrics **78:**983, 1986.

5. Duhring, J.L.: Nutrition in pregnancy, In Present knowledge in nutrition, 5th edition, Washington, D.C., The Nutrition Foundation, Inc., 1984.

6. Kliegman, R.M., and Gross, T.: Perinatal problems of the obese mother and her infant, Obstetrics and Gynecology **66:**299, 1985.

7. Taffel, S.M., and Keppel, K.G.: Advice about weight gain during pregnancy and actual weight gain, Amercian Journal of Public Health **76:**1396, 1986.

8. Committee on Nutrition of the Mother and Preschool Child: Alternative dietary practices and nutritional abuses in pregnancy, Washington, D.C., National Academy Press, 1982.

9. Worthington-Roberts, B.S., Vermeersch, J., and Williams, S.R.: Nutrition in pregnancy and lactation, 3rd edition, St. Louis, Times Mirror/Mosby College Publishing, 1985.

10. Malhotra, A., and Sawers, R.S.: Dietary supplementation in pregnancy, British Medical Journal **293:**465, 1986.

11. Truswell, A.S.: Nutrition for pregnancy, British Medical Journal **291:**263, 1985.

12. Schuster, K., and others: Morning sickness and vitamin B_6 status of pregnant women, Human Nutrition: Clinical Nutrition **39C:**75, 1985.

13. National Research Council: Alternative Dietary Practices and Nutritional Abuses in Pregnancy, Washington, D.C., National Academy Press, 1982.

14. Martin, T.R., and Bracken, M.B.: Association of low birth weight with passive smoke exposure in pregnancy, American Journal of Epidemiology **124:**633, 1986.

15. Streissguth, A.P., and others: Natural history of the fetal alcohol syndrome: a 10-year follow-up of eleven patients, Lancet **ii:**85, 1985.

16. Joffe, A., and Radius, S.M.: Breast versus bottle: correlates of adolescent mothers; infant-feeding practices, Pediatrics **79:**689, 1987.

17. Baranowski, T., and others: Social support, social influence, ethnicity and the breast-feeding decision, Social Science and Medicine **17:**1599, 1983.

18. Anonymous: Adequacy of lactation in well-nourished mothers, Nutrition Reviews **42:**8, 1984.

19. Anderson, G.H.: Human milk feeding, Pediatric Clinics of North America **32:**335, 1985.

20. Butte, N.F., and others: Longitudinal changes in milk composition of mothers delivering preterm and term infants, Early Human Development **9:**153, 1984.

21. Zmora, E., and others: Multiple nutritional deficiencies in infants from a strict vegetarian community, American Journal of Diseases of Children **133**:141, 1979.

22. Pratt, H.F.: Breastfeeding and eczema, Early Human Development **9**:283, 1984.

23. Committee on Nutrition, American Academy of Pediatrics, The use of whole cow's milk in infancy, Pediatrics **72**:253, 1983.

24. Anonymous: Advice about milk for infants and young children, Lancet **i**:843, 1987.

25. Agras, W.S., and others: Does a vigorous feeding style influence early development of adiposity? Journal of Pediatrics **110**:799, 1987.

26. Ashworth, A.: International differences in infant mortality and the impact of malnutrition: a review, Human Nutrition: Clinical Nutrition **36C**:7, 1982.

27. Gayle, H.D., and others: Malnutrition in the first two years of life: The contribution of low birth weight to population estimates in the United States, American Journal of Diseases of Children, **141**:531, 1987.

28. Haffejee, I.E., and Moosa, A.: Honey in the treatment of infantile gastroenteritis, British Medical Journal **290**:1866, 1985.

29. Beaton, G.H.: Nutritional needs during the first year of life, Pediatric Clinics of North America **32**:275, 1985.

30. Kare, M.R., and Beauchamp, G.K.: The role of taste in the infant diet, American Journal of Clinical Nutrition **41**:418, 1985.

31. Bock, S.A.: Prospective appraisal of complaints of adverse reaction to foods in children during the first 3 years of life, Pediatrics **79**:683, 1987.

32. Loesche, W.J.: Nutrition and dental decay in infants, American Journal of Clinical Nutrition **41**:423, 1985.

33. Brooke, O.G., and Wood, C.: Investigation of the 'satisfying' quality of infant formula milks, Archives of Disease in Childhood **60**:577, 1985.

34. Lotgering, F.K., and others: Maternal and fetal responses to exercise during pregnancy, Physiological Reviews **65**:1, 1985.

35. Hecht, A.: What's that alcohol doing in my medicine, FDA Consumer, page 16, November 1984.

36. Anonymous: Infant botulism, Lancet **ii**:1256, 1986.

37. Lane, B.J., and Sellen, V.: Bottle caries: a nursing responsibility, Canadian Journal of Public Health **77**:128, 1986.

13

Nutrition from Infancy to Adolescence
Years of Physical and Mental Growth

CONNECTIONS

We cover two extremes in this chapter: the child almost totally dependent on adults for food and the teenager making independent food choices. If the child received good nutrition during gestation and infancy, as described in the last chapter, a good foundation has been laid for the rapid growth to follow.

In developing countries, nutrition problems in young children arise from lack of food and from poor sanitation. In industrialized countries, the nutrient deficiencies that occur are usually mild. As we discussed in Chapter 11, people in industrialized countries are concerned about whether processed foods contain additives and sugar that will cause hyperactivity, but there is no cause for alarm.

At the end of the growing years, adolescents may have nutrition problems that are primarily self-inflicted—the results of smoking and alcohol and drug abuse, for instance. Other such problems are anorexia nervosa, bulimia, those associated with pregnancy, and even problems related to athletic performance, which were described in earlier chapters.

Because these activities may complicate otherwise normal diets, effective nutrition education is needed—suggesting how, for instance, to make good nutrition choices in fast foods and snacks. Perhaps one way to motivate nutrition interest in teenagers is to show the interrelationships between food and the body.

The period of growth from a child's first birthday, or the time he or she is weaned, to the end of adolescence is a time of high parental expectations. "We want you to grow big and strong," they say, "to be tops in learning, sports, and social activities—to be the best."

Part of being "the best" is eating right. But what if children don't *want* to eat the same thing as everyone else in the family? What if food is used to exert independence—if alcohol and drug use thwart parental hopes for school and athletics or anorexia, bulimia, and obesity are used to respond to social pressures? Obviously, during this period food becomes something else besides just food—a means of expressing protest, a device for meeting sensory satisfactions, a factor to be weighed in one's attractiveness. Yet all this pulling and hauling goes on at a time when nutrient requirements are quite high.

North Americans in particular are quite concerned about "normal growth" and "maximum growth" during this period from toddler to teen. But, as Dr. John Durnin points out, the idea of normal growth is only part science; it is also part emotion and prejudice. Certainly the idea that children should attain "maximum growth" is somewhat mythical. "To presume that maximum growth is always best," he writes, "and that the biggest people in the world, North Americans, should set the reference for the rest of the world's population, appears to me highly presumptuous." Let us begin to examine this presumptuousness.

TODDLER TO TEEN: GREAT NUTRITION CONTRASTS

What, in fact, *is* normal growth and what kind of nutrition is required to attain it? Some major nutrition highlights during this period are presented in this section.

Because the Cost of Feeding Children is High, It Should be Done Right

What would you guess it cost to feed *you* from birth to age 17? The U.S. Department of Agriculture took a look at what a child living in an urban area in the northeastern part of the United States, eating at only a moderately expensive level, would cost during these years, and came up with these figures:[1]

Economics

- Cost for food eaten at home: $20,514
- Cost for food eaten away from home: $2354

Do these numbers seem excessive? They may be slightly so, because costs were found to be a little less in other parts of the country. Even so, they do *not* include extra costs brought about by nutrition problems, such as medical costs during infancy due to treatment for diarrhea and infections or low protein intakes. Nor do they include the costs that will *result later* from faulty nutrition, such as reduced earning power brought about by slow brain development caused by malnutrition. And they do not include economic costs of teenage alcohol and drug abuse; anorexia nervosa and bulimia; the birth of a child to an unmarried, unemployed mother; money wasted on worthless weight-loss programs; and treatment in later life of diet-influenced "killer diseases" such as hypertension, coronary heart disease, and cancer.

The Quality and Quantity of Food Consumed Varies from Tot to Teen

Many factors influence the nutritional status of a child, as Figure 13-1 shows. Here are some of them:

Family economic and educational level

Family income is a major factor in determining the quantity and quality of food for each family member. Lower quantities of food are more likely if there are many

Economics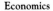

FIGURE 13-1
Many factors influence the dietary status of children.

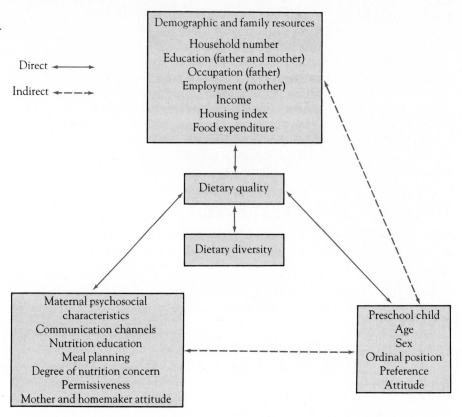

mouths to feed or if the wage earner or earners have low-paying jobs or are out of work. Higher incomes—quite often the result of higher education—also affect the nutritional quality of food, and educated parents are apt to live in places allowing better food storage conditions and to be able to have more knowledge about nutrition in general.

The parents' role

The parents' level of nutrition education, their ability to prepare nutritious meals that are interesting to the child, and their positive interaction with the child at all levels of home life are important. Ideally, the parents should be able to influence the child's food choices in a nonintimidating way, unhampered by fears, phobias, and tensions. Parents should also understand that the pattern of food intake changes as the child develops (Figure 13-2).

Birth order of the preschool child

Where the child stands in the birth order within the family (older or younger in relation to siblings) and whether he or she attends a day-care center may also affect dietary status. There may not be much food left for the youngest child of a large family.

Age and gender

The range of ages covered in this chapter—first birthday to end of adolescence—covers quite a range of nutrition possibilities: young children who may still be breast-feeding, children fed in schools and day care centers, and teenagers with money enough of their own to make independent decisions about what to eat. Whatever their age, not all American children are receiving the RDA for some nutrients; which nutrients are likely to be in short supply depends on age and gender.

Early Nutrition May Affect Later Quality of Life

What will your old age be like? A lot of the status of your health then depends on the quantity and quality of the diet you received during your early growing period and even your diet now, if you are still in adolescence. Obesity, hypertension, diabetes, coronary heart disease, and other health problems are thought to develop in early life. Indeed, the diet in early years may be a very important factor in determining how long we live. Experiments with animals show that they live longer if a nutritionally balanced diet is fed in amounts slightly lower than the amount normally eaten by the animal. If this is true for human beings, perhaps if we were to go through life always a little hungry we might live a bit longer. This generalization cannot hold for everyone, however; some people simply cannot tolerate hunger early in life.

Children Should be Taught that Food is Not Just a Toy

Although some adults seem to eat as though food were just simple fuel—like wood to a stove—many of us find a great deal of pleasure in eating. Young children find food objects of play; they use it to explore their developing senses and, at times, to express their growing independence from their elders. However, food is not *just* a toy, and parents should try to make their children understand this.

Mealtimes can be pleasurable or tense. That is, eating can be a focal point for happy family discussions; indeed, research shows that pleasant conversation with children during a meal increases the amount of food they eat. However, some parents also use food in ways to try to control their children—giving it out as reward or bribe or token of affection, withholding it as punishment. Nagging and fighting during mealtimes may well alter a child's view of food.

Adolescents take food beyond the realm of play or toys. Being able to make many of their food choices independently, they may pick foods that have some meaning in relation to body image, attractiveness, social impact, athletic performance—even pregnancy. Nutritionists working with teenagers must be sensitive to the mix of personal preferences and social pressures.

> The quantity and quality of foods eaten between the first birthday (weaning) and the end of the teenage years may have health effects throughout life. These decisions are influenced by economic, social, psychological, and sensory factors.

THE PRESCHOOL YEARS

The preschool years, ages 1 to 6, are the years when children are switched over from breast-feeding, cow's milk, or formula and put on a steady diet of semi-solid foods. The transition period is known as weaning.

Decisions Made at Weaning Affect the Child Later

⮐ "No simple, straightforward recommendations for weaning can be drawn," concluded a 1985 workshop on current issues in feeding normal infants.[2] Weaning practices, then, are as different as the human race. However it is done, weaning consists of a major switch in the make-up of the nutrients consumed by a body that is rapidly growing—and it is all influenced by various social and economic pressures as to what weaning should be and when it should occur. ⮐

Education 🔑

This does not mean there are no wrong ways of weaning a child. Indeed, some decisions can have profound consequences. For example, some mothers in developing countries wean their babies to a protein-poor, carbohydrate-rich milk substitute that can cause *kwashiorkor*—severe malnutrition characterized by swollen stomach, anemia, and loss of hair. As a result, these children usually do not catch up to the growth in children weaned to better nutrients.

Such mistakes are rare in developed countries because of the variety of commercial weaning foods available, but mistakes do happen. Kwashiorkor was once reported in infants in California, for example.[3] Because the babies were sensitive to milk protein, they were given a milk substitute of high-fat, low-protein nondairy creamer. Within 1½ to 6 months, the infants were hospitalized with all of the clinical signs of kwashiorkor.

Children with severe growth retardation during the early years of life usually survive.[2] The health implications over a lifetime caused by nutrient restrictions in these early years are not fully understood.

For Preschoolers, Food is Adventure

Food is fun during the preschool age, although there are dislikes as well as likes:

- *Flavors:* mild flavors are liked, strong or tart flavors are disliked
- *Colors:* green, orange, yellow, and pink are liked
- *Texture:* dry foods are difficult to eat. It is best to serve a variety of textures at each meal: one soft food, one crisp, one chewy
- *Familiarity:* children like familiar foods. New foods should be introduced in small amounts.

Nutritious snacks may be useful breaks from tensions at the family dinner table.

TABLE 13-1 Responses to the Question, "Is There Anything About Your Child's Current Eating Behavior That Bothers You?"

Problem	% of Responses
Child consumes a restricted range of foods[1]	37
Child's eating habits[2]	17
Child eats insufficient quantity of food	12
Child is not interested in eating[3]	10
Child likes "junk foods"	8
Child dislikes new foods	3
Other	13

[1]Includes refusals of a particular class of foods—for example, vegetables, meats.
[2]Includes dawdling, messiness, difficulty in chewing.
[3]Includes disinterest in eating particular meals—for example, breakfast.

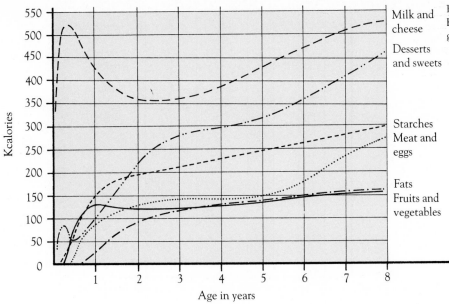

FIGURE 13-2
Food intake changes as the child grows.

At this age, children should be allowed to play with their food. The author recalls having fun using "boulders" of meat and "concrete" of mashed potatoes to hold back a "gravy lake"; peas plugged any leaks in the dam. While this spectacle might have annoyed the author's parents, eventually everything got eaten—and that is the point of allowing play with nutritious foods at this time in life. This is also a time when children use food to gain attention.

Parents should not be alarmed, however, if appetite and interest in food vary during this period, resulting in irregular weight gains. There are a number of normal changes taking place, including major adjustments in the frequency and type of food eaten (Figure 13-2). Children also are likely to discover the pleasures of snacking. In any case, many children are not ready biologically or psychologically to be regulated into an adult pattern of three meals per day.

Should Parents Worry About What Preschoolers Eat?

Some parents worry about what their preschoolers eat, but whether such concern is justified is not clear. Feeding problems in preschoolers have not been researched in detail. Still, one study of 80 mothers in a California suburb sheds some light on the problem.[4] Both mothers and fathers were upper-middle class and well educated, and their children ranged from 2 to 7 years. The mothers' responses to the question, "Is there anything about your child's current eating behavior that bothers you?" are shown in Table 13-1.

The results of the survey showed that:

- Children with problems in eating behavior had less exposure to novel foods
- They were more likely to be prodded and rewarded to eat and punished for not eating

FIGURE 13-3
Children get a third of their dietary
energy and fat from snacks. Breakfast
contributes only 10% to 15% of daily
energy and macronutrient intake.

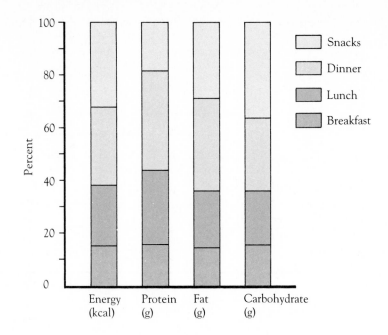

- They had greater problems resulting from aggressive behavior, toileting difficulties, and fearfulness
- The problem eaters were more likely to have developed a conditioned taste aversion

The researchers caution against too sweeping interpretations of the results. The study was based on the response of the mothers only. We still wait for a study involving direct observation of the children and their parents. This will be important because Dr. Frances Davidson of Georgetown University says "Mommies don't know what their children eat." Parents believed that their children consumed 500 kcalories less than what the children actually ate. Usually the extra kcalories were consumed in soft drinks and snack foods.[5]

Do Most North American Preschoolers Have an Adequate Diet?

The 1977-1978 Nationwide Food Consumption Survey by the U.S. Department of Agriculture found that for one- to two-year-olds the only nutrient for which intake was below the recommended level was iron. However, by ages 3-5, recommended intakes of iron, calcium, magnesium, and vitamin B_6 were below recommended intake. The reason iron is low is that it is difficult for the child to meet the RDA for iron by eating the family food. Notice that the RDA for toddlers is 15 mg of iron. It needs a high intake of iron-rich foods such as meat to attain this level of iron intake. The low level of calcium intake is due to reduced milk consumption.

The children in this age group have a high requirement for nutrients in order to maintain their rapid growth of tissues and increased physical activity, although such activity can vary widely. The need for most nutrients steadily increases as children grow from ages one to six.

Recommended intakes differ for some nutrients in Canada (see the chart on the inside back cover). In children ages 4-6, the Canadian values are lower for all nutrients listed, except for energy and vitamin A. Notice these are recommended values; the required amounts for nutrients are the same for all nationalities.

Preschoolers Need Balanced and Varied Diets

Preschoolers can fulfill their nutrient requirements by following the same advice every healthy person should follow: eat a balanced varied diet. This means:

- *Eat from the four food groups:* portions from the four basic food groups should be eaten every day. Table 13-2 shows the food pattern for preschool children.
- *Use variety:* there should be variety within each food group.
- *Restrict intake of unhealthy foods:* sweets, fats, and oils should be kept to a minimum.
- *Be careful about fiber:* fiber intake has to be handled carefully. Fiber intake in North American children of all ages is low because of low intakes of fruit and vegetables. However, the intake of high-fiber, low-kcalorie foods, to the exclusion of all other foods, should not be encouraged. Fiber-rich foods are bulky and filling, which causes problems because of the child's small stomach size. Fiber may also interfere with the absorption of much needed calcium, iron, magnesium, zinc, copper, and phosphorus.

For Normal Preschoolers, Dietary Supplements Are Unnecessary, Except for Iron

The Nutrition Canada survey in the early 1970s showed that 30% of children up to four years of age had a high probability of being iron-deficient. In the United States, there is iron deficiency among preschoolers from low-income families, but their iron status can be improved via the Special Supplemental Food Program for *Women, Infants and Children (WIC)*. The effects of deficiency of iron in the 1-6 year age group on later educational achievement are unknown; however, the deficiency affects educational achievement and the efficiency of problem solving in older children.[6]

Except for iron, dietary supplements are unnecessary for preschoolers if their growth is normal. However, children in low-income families may well need supplementation of other nutrients. In Denver, for instance, preschoolers of low-income families had zinc intakes that were only 52% of the RDA, which had the effect of decreasing their appetite and, hence, their intake of other nutrients as well. After they were given zinc supplements, they increased their intake of all nutrients.[7] Similarly, children of low-income families in Memphis were found to have low intakes of nutrients, which were corrected through federal supplementary food programs.[8]

Infants and preschoolers on vegan diets have been found to have dietary intakes deficient in energy, protein, calcium, iron, zinc, riboflavin, and vitamins D and B_{12}. There are four reasons for these deficiencies:

1. The stomachs of infants and preschoolers cannot carry a large volume of food. (This applies to all children, not just vegans.)
2. Most vegan diets consist mostly of foods with low kcaloric density.
3. Vegan diets offer limited food choices (remember the importance of variety in the well-balanced diet.)

Women's, Infant's, and Children's Program (WIC)
Nutritional and medical support from federal funds for low-income women with high risk pregnancies.

Economics

TABLE 13-2 Food Pattern for Preschool Children*

Food	Portion Size	Number of Portions Advised	
		Ages 2 to 4 Years	Ages 4 to 6 Years
Milk and Dairy Products			
Milk†	4 oz	3 to 6	3 to 4
Cheese	½ to ¾ oz	May be substituted for one portion of liquid milk	
Yogurt	¼ to ½ cup	May be substituted for one portion of liquid milk	
Powdered skim milk	2 tbsp	May be substituted for one portion of liquid milk	
Meat and Meat Equivalents			
Meat‡, fish§, poultry	1 to 2 oz	2	2
Egg	1	1	1
Peanut butter	1 to 2 tbsp		
Legumes—dried peas and beans	¼ to ⅓ cup cooked		
Vegetables and Fruits			
Vegetables		4 to 5 to include 1 green leafy or yellow‖	4 to 5 to include 1 green leafy or yellow
Cooked	2 to 4 tbsp		
Raw	Few pieces		
Fruit		1 citrus fruit or other vegetable or fruit rich in vitamin C	1 citrus fruit or other vegetable or fruit rich in vitamin C
Canned	4 to 8 tbsp		
Raw	½ to 1 small		
Fruit juice	3 to 4 oz		
Bread and Cereal Grains			
Whole grain or enriched white bread	½ to 1 slice	3	3
Cooked cereal	¼ to ½ cup	May be substituted for one serving of bread	
Ready-to-serve dry cereals	½ to 1 cup		
Spaghetti, macaroni, noodles, rice	¼ to ½ cup		
Crackers	2 to 3		
Fat			
Bacon	1 slice	Not to be substituted for meat	
Butter or vitamin A–fortified margarine	1 tsp	3	3 to 4
Desserts	¼ to ½ cup	As demanded by calorie needs	
Sugars	½ to 1 tsp	2	2

* Diets should be monitored for adequacy of iron and vitamin D intake.
† Approximately ⅔ cup can easily be incorporated in a child's food during cooking.
‡ Liver once a week can be used as liver sausage or cooked liver.
§ Should be served once or twice per week to substitute for meat.
‖ If child's preferences are limited, used double portions of preferred vegetables until appetite for other vegetables develop.

4. Vegan children usually eat fewer meals and snacks than nonvegan children. Diet counseling may improve intake, but this is difficult because of the food beliefs of the parents.[9]

Improper weaning procedures can lead to kwashiorkor and other nutrition problems. The preschool years are ones of food exploration. Parents tend to worry about food intake, but most preschoolers in the United States and Canada are eating an adequate diet. Iron is the only nutrient that might need supplementation.

THE MIDDLE YEARS OF GROWTH: AGES 6 TO 11

Compared to infancy and adolescence, the years 6-11 are peaceful both biologically and psychologically. Appetite and growth show no wide fluctuations. Children gradually widen their selection of foods. Energy is principally expended in physical activity such as sports. Children are not as preoccupied with body size as they will be in adolescence.

Of course, physical and psychological development varies; the range of 6-11 represents the average, and was rather arbitrarily chosen to fit the age brackets used in the RDA tables. Many boys and girls may show the first signs of puberty before the age of eleven.

Eating Habits Having Been Established, Nutrient Intakes Are Adequate for Most Children This Age

The recommended intake of most nutrients is higher than for the under-six age group. Surveys show that magnesium and vitamin B_6 are the only nutrients whose intake is low. Intakes of vitamins A and C and calcium are low in some children, but there is no evidence of clinical signs of deficiency. A recent study of elementary students in Kansas showed diet to be adequate. Almost all students ate grain products, high-protein foods, vegetables, and milk products.[10]

The reason nutrient intakes are adequate in this age group is that food preferences have become established for a wide variety of foods. Plate waste is much less in school lunch programs now than when children get older. Still, there is some waste—girls seem to do more of it than boys—and some food is refused. The lowest refusal rates are for milk, fruit, and desserts, the highest for vegetables and mixed casseroles.[11]

Despite the assertion that, in general, children ages 6-11 receive an adequate diet, there are many who are unfortunate casualties of economic recession. Even in the United States in the 1980s, poor, hungry children exist. The Citizens' Commission on Hunger in New England estimated in 1980 that there were 296,000 children between 5 and 17 years of age who lived below the poverty level.

Economics 🔑

This Age Group Greatly Benefits from School Breakfast and Lunch Programs

Begun in 1946, the National School Lunch Program was started after American military officials saw the numbers of young men suffering from malnutrition who had been drafted for World War II. Today the program provides subsidized lunches (either free or reduced in price) for needy school children and provides full-price lunches for nonneedy children. The School Breakfast program was started in 1966 for low-income children, and by 1972 was available to all children in school districts having the program.

School districts are required to provide a means for parents and students to become involved in the school lunch program. If you are a parent yourself, you may wish to become involved in menu planning, making improvements in eating locations, and educating children about better eating habits.

The minimum quantity of the four food groups required in school lunch programs is given in Table 13-3. The composition of the food groups may change with time. For example, the U.S. Department of Agriculture proposed a number of alternatives to meat in all Child Nutrition Programs—for example, it was proposed that nuts and seeds and nut and seed butters be allowed for half the meat/meat alternative requirement. The American Dietetic Association has agreed with this proposal and has suggested including yogurt and tofu in the category of meat/meat alternates.[12]

TABLE 13-3 School Lunch Pattern—Approximate per Lunch Minimums

| Food Group | Components | Minimum Quantities | | | | Recommended Quantities for Children 12 Years and Older; 7-12† |
		Age 1-2; Preschool	Age 3-4; Preschool	Age 5-8; K-3	Age 9 and Older; 4-12	
Milk	Unflavored, fluid lowfat, skim or buttermilk must be offered*	¾ cup (6 fl oz)	¾ cup (6 fl oz)	½ pint (8 fl oz)	½ pint (8 fl oz)	½ pint (8 fl oz)
Meat or meat alternate (quantity of the edible portion as served)	Lean meat, poultry, or fish	1 oz	1½ oz	1½ oz	2 oz	3 oz
	Cheese	1 oz	1½ oz	1½ oz	2 oz	3 oz
	Large egg	½	¾	¾	1	1½
	Cooked dry beans or peas	¼ cup	⅜ cup	⅜ cup	½ cup	¾ cup
	Peanut butter or an equivalent quantity of any combination of any of above	2 tbsp	3 tbsp	3 tbsp	4 tbsp	6 tbsp
Vegetable or fruit	2 or more servings of vegetable or fruit or both	½ cup	½ cup	½ cup	¾ cup	¾ cup
Bread or bread alternate (servings per week)	Must be enriched or whole-grain—at least ½ serving‡ for group I or one serving‡ for groups II-V must be served daily	5	8	8	8	10

* If a school serves another form of milk (whole or flavored), it must offer its children unflavored fluid lowfat milk, skim milk, or buttermilk as a beverage choice.

† The *minimum* portion sizes for these children are the portion sizes for group IV.

‡ Serving 1 slice of bread; or ½ cup of cooked rice, macaroni, noodles, other pasta products, other cereal product such as bulgur and corn grits; or as stated in the *Food Buying Guide* for biscuits, rolls, muffins, and similar products.

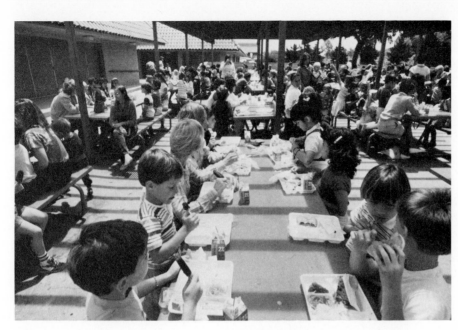

School lunches can be nutritious, inexpensive, and tasty.

The provision of nutritious snacks in the school environment is especially important. Snacking is common in this age group. In fact, 10-year-olds get a third of their energy and fat from snacks (Figure 13-3). Breakfast contributes only 10%-15% of daily energy and macronutrient intake.[13]

Nutritionists Are Showing Increasing Interest in Preteens (Ages 10 to 13)

In the last decade, there has been increasing recognition among scientists that nutrition problems of adults begin in childhood, and that a great many patterns are established in the preteen years—that is, ages 10-13. Some of the key findings are described below.

Less salt: easier than you think?

High dietary sodium intake may be linked to hypertension. Two reassuring experiments find that most elementary and high school students hardly notice that certain menu items are made with less salt than usual. In fact, it was discovered that students who *did* notice generally preferred the reduced-sodium foods.[14] This is encouraging news, because children ages 10-13 get almost one third of their daily sodium from school lunches.

Trying to control cholesterol through diet

It has been found that infants fed human milk or cow's milk during their first three months of life developed higher serum cholesterol levels at ages 7-12 than did children fed a commercial formula at infancy.[15] A diet high in cholesterol at the beginning of life may be the start of problems with high serum cholesterol levels during middle age.

➥ Actually, little information is available on the effect of early diet on blood cholesterol. To lower serum cholesterol, nutritionists recommend decreasing the intake of red meat, eggs, and dairy products. This solution may be acceptable for adults, but for preteens and teens it also will considerably lower the intake of iron and calcium in their diet—which is already low in these nutrients. A British study strongly recommended against any intervention in young childrens' diets, especially those under five years of age, as a way to reduce the risk of heart disease in later life.[16]

In addition, there are other reasons why pediatricians have not stressed these means of preventing coronary heart disease:[17]

- It is time consuming to explain all of the dietary and nondietary factors in the disease.
- Both the pediatrician and parents are more interested in immediate health problems rather than a problem that may develop 30-50 years later.
- There is no clear proof the problem is controlled by diet modification.
- Altering diet, especially in infants and young children, might adversely affect the growth and general health of the child.
- Hyperlipidemia is rare in children, and so testing serum cholesterol levels (at $10 to $15 a test) is a waste of time and money.
- Putting such emphasis on risk factors may cause needless anxiety in parents and child.

In short, diets that avoid extremes are probably safe for children for whom there is no special risk of developing coronary heart disease. The American Academy of Pediatrics recommends that the kcalories coming from fat be limited to 30%-40% of total kcalories.[18] ➥

Obesity is Rising Among Preteens

Despite years of medical advice against overfeeding infants and youngsters, more American children than ever before are obese. During the past two decades, obesity increased by 54% among children aged 6-11 and by 39% among those aged 12-17.[19] Among preadolescent black children, the prevalence of obesity increased almost twice as much as among preadolescent whites.

Forty percent of children who are obese at age 7 become obese adults. Seventy percent of obese adolescents become obese adults. What can be done about the problem?

➥ Unfortunately, not much, according to several top researchers in obesity; they saw no way to prevent obesity in children, nor could they determine who should be treated and at what age.[19] ➥

It is quite easy for children to become obese; only 50 kcalories extra a day will put on 5 lb in a year. There is no evidence that obese kids overeat by great amounts. They seem to be less active than children in the early 1900s, although it's difficult to know whether this is a consequence or a cause of obesity. North American children become less active as they get older. This problem could be alleviated if health and physical fitness were made a family affair.[20] Still, the amount of television watching seems to have a high correlation with obesity.[19] Not only are children inactive during the hours they are watching, but they also eat more while

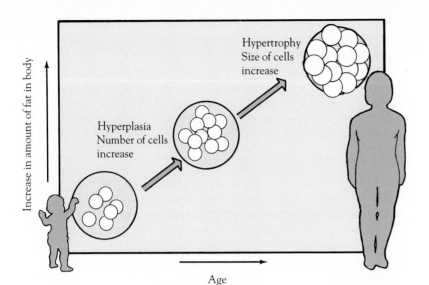

FIGURE 13-4
Why fat babies may become fat adults. The greater the number of fat cells (hyperplasia) the greater the possibility they will increase in size (hypertrophy) to cause obesity in teenagers and adults.

viewing television, and in fact they eat more of the foods that are *advertised* on TV.

No one knows when the cellular foundation is established for adult obesity. The first few years of life is a period of increases in the number of cells (hyperplasia), the size of cells (hypertrophy), or a combination of hyperplasia and hypertrophy. This is the way all tissues, including adipose tissue, increase in size. The greater the number of fat cells, then, the greater the possibility of obesity (Figure 13-4). Previously it was suggested that diet should be controlled to prevent an excessive increase in the number of fat cells. We are not so sure now if this is good advice.

Should there be a program to screen school children for obesity.[21] The author's feeling is "yes," because obesity is such a serious health problem in adults. Unfortunately, it is difficult to set up a screening process because there is no distinctive eating behavior associated with obesity.[22] However, there may be differences in the way obese, average, and slim children relate to the same foods.[23] Researchers have found boys from these three groups give different answers to questions about particular foods ("It's fattening"; "it makes you grow"; "it gives you energy" etc.) For example, unlike average or slim boys, obese boys linked cakes, sugar, and candy (which they identified as "high-energy" foods) to positive effects such as growth. Nutritionists need, then, to learn more about the processes in the body and the attractiveness of food before they can understand obesity in childhood. We must also invent ways to increase the involvement of a greater number of the nation's children in enjoyable physical activity.

Diet Has Little, If Any, Effect on Behavior Problems, Including Hyperactivity

Hyperactivity—also called *hyperkinesis, minimal brain dysfunction,* and *learning disability*—has many symptoms. Although the symptoms are ill-defined, they include overactivity, short attention span, distractedness, and impulsive behavior. However, the child's behavior patterns may appear different for parents than for teachers, and they may not appear consistent to observers.

It is even difficult to determine the prevalence of hyperactivity, the estimates running from 3%-20% of all American children of school age. Hyperactive children are of normal or above-average intelligence, despite their handicaps. The disorder is treated with educational techniques, psychotherapy, behavior modification therapy, and medication.

Do salicylates or food additives play a role?

Salicylates
Organic compounds occurring naturally in many foods of plant origin.

In the middle 1970s, Dr. Ben Feingold, an allergist, claimed that hyperactivity was caused by foods high in *salicylates* and foods containing additives. Since his ideas were popularized at a time of concern about environmental pollution, safety of food, and overuse of medications, they were favorably received by many parents of hyperactive children.

A wide variety of foods are high in salicylates: fruits (apples, oranges, and berries), vegetables (almonds and cucumbers), herbs and spices, tea, licorice and peppermint candies, and some honeys.[24] Salicylates also are found in oil of wintergreen (a food flavoring), aspirin, lotions, and liniments. In other words, they appear just about everywhere—which is why Feingold later changed his opinion about eliminating salicylates: it became clear that eliminating so many foods would cause nutrition problems. Interest in the role of salicylates in hyperactivity has now waned, although investigators are now focusing on the role of salicylates in some cases of asthma and itchy skin rashes.

Artificial colors and flavors, the second source of hyperactivity according to Feingold, were later found in some well-controlled studies of his "defined diets" to have no relationship at all. As a conference sponsored by the National Institutes of Health in 1982 stated: "Defined diets should not be universally used in the treatment of childhood hyperactivity at this time."[25] Medical opinion in the later 1980s has not changed on hyperactivity.

Does reducing sugar and aspartame intake or increasing vitamin intake help?

Wouldn't it be nice if parents could cure hyperactivity by simply reducing their children's sugar intake or giving them a megavitamin pill? However, most studies show no relationship between high sugar intake and hyperactivity—whether children are diagnosed normal[26] or hyperactive.[27] Many people feel that sugar is so harmful that they will find its exoneration here hard to believe. As one contributor to a pediatrics journal writes:

Beware of sugar under different, unfamiliar names.

> Despite the lack of data, the notion that sucrose is harmful is so widespread that patients bring this up frequently with their physicians. Health food stores promote fructose and honey as "natural" sweeteners, even though honey usually contains some sucrose. With parents of hyperkinetic children, the belief that sucrose is harmful . . . is quite common.[28]

Autism
A self-centered mental state from which reality tends to be excluded.

As for megavitamins, hyperactivity and attention disorders in children cannot be prevented or cured by megadoses of niacin, ascorbic acid, pyridoxine, and pantothenic acid.[29] Indeed, these high doses could cause liver damage and gastrointestinal upsets. However, vitamins may be helpful in treating something that is the *opposite* of hyperactivity—the neurological disorder known as *autism*. Although confirming research is needed, some recent evidence suggests that supplements of both vitamin B_6 and magnesium may be effective in autistic children.[30] Parents with autistic children should not experiment with nutrients as a means of treatment. Recent evidence suggests that autism may involve neurotransmitter imbalance.

Television Influences What Children Eat

In the United States, children of ages 2-12 watch about 25 hours of television per week. This means that the average child watches more than 20,000 commercials each year!

About two thirds of the TV commercials children watch are about food, most frequently high-sugar foods.[31] Food advertisements appeal to children's sense of fun, and 60% are in animated form. Children who watch more commercial televison have more requests for candy and sugared cereals when they are out food shopping with their parents. TV viewing is positively correlated to the intake of high-kcalorie snacks and to the prevalence of obesity.

In the noncommercial area, a great deal of eating and drinking occurs on many TV shows, yet obese actors are not common. Television shows also convey unrealistic messages about alcohol, tobacco, and other drugs and indirectly encourage their use.[32] All in all, it is clear that television has a great impact on nutrition, but the impact has not been quantified. The impact may not be good.

The Sense of Social Responsibility About Better Nutrition for Children Needs To Be Increased

The greatest effect of the world's economic recession of the 1980s is falling on the world's 1.8 billion citizens who are under age 15. One hundred million children go hungry—every day. Ten million infants and children die every year who could be saved with adequate nutrition and health care.[33]

In the latest literature on child nutrition, there are many writings about the responsibilities of nations for the health of their children. As you might expect, however, the major problem is money. The principal government program to assist poor children in the United States, Aid to Families with Dependent Children (AFDC), costs only one cent an hour for each of its 1.1 million recipients, but it is subject to budget cuts. Many pediatricians are concerned that cutbacks in child-related programs, not just in the United States but in all countries, will worsen the already austere conditions faced by many children.[34] In 1985, the U.S. Congress was urged by the American Dietetic Association to consider the negative consequences of budget cuts in school lunch and food stamp programs.

Economics

Nutrient deficiencies are rare in the 6-11 age group. Potential health problems in adult life can be influenced during this period by the development of eating patterns. Many adult health problems can be prevented by reducing the intake of sodium, cholesterol, and fat and reducing the incidence of hypertension and obesity. Hyperactivity is not strongly related to the intake of food additives, sugar, or salicylates. Television viewing can have negative effects on nutrient intakes in this group.

ADOLESCENCE: BEING UNCONVENTIONAL IS CONVENTIONAL

What do adolescents want? What makes teenagers so temperamental and inexplicable to adults? And why do they *eat* in such strange ways? These questions are important, because, according to Dr. Myron Winick of Columbia University, adolescence is the most crucial dietary period in a person's life. Diet is so important during adolescence because of the adolescent growth spurt, because eating habits formed during these years continue throughout adult life, and because eating disorders, if they do develop, are most likely to do so during this period.[5]

There Are Ten Reasons for Concern About Teenagers' Eating Habits

A useful way to begin is to run through the list of ten aspects of eating behavior in adolescents outlined by Dr. A.S. Truswell, as follows.[35]

Skipping meals

Teenagers often skip meals, especially breakfast. Yet their classroom performance is usually not affected because snacks are taken during the morning.

Eating snacks

Sixty to seventy percent of American children and teenagers eat snacks at least once a day. Snacks contribute 12% to 17% of the RDA for energy and nutrients for teenagers. Boys and girls have the same favorite snacks but in different order of preference:

- Girls like soft drinks, bakery products, milk desserts, salty snacks, fruit, milk, candy, bread, and meat.
- Boys like soft drinks, milk, bakery products, bread, milk desserts, salty snacks, meats, and fruit.

Many snacks will supply kcalories from fat and sugar (and sometimes alcohol). A snack of fruit will increase the intake of vitamin C and milk will increase calcium intake. Intake of calcium is particularly important to teenage girls (Table 13-3).

Nutritionally poor food is eaten sometimes because of peer pressure. Other reasons include convenience and taste.

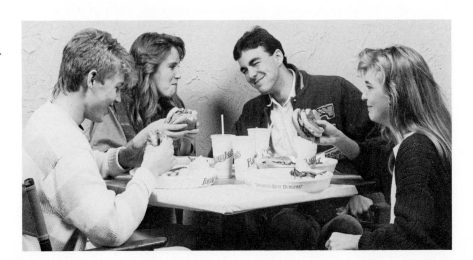

Fast foods

Fast foods, which include carry-out foods, are favorites of adolescents, and can actually provide adequate nutrients if selected wisely. (See Appendix O.) However, many selections are high in fat, kcalories, and sodium, and low in calcium and fiber. Health problems due to poor nutrition are most likely to occur if fast foods are the major portion of the diet.

Unconventional meals

Other family members may find an adolescent's sudden switch to, say, a vegetarian diet an annoyance or even a threat, but unconventional meals need not be short on nutrients.

Alcohol

Of all the new "foods" being investigated by adolescents, this is the most dangerous. Alcohol is a major contributor to premature deaths of teenagers.

Soft drinks

Obviously, soft drinks are a better alternative than alcohol, despite the fact that they provide kcalories and almost no other nutrients. A drawback is that they may replace milk in the diet, and so reduce the intake of calcium that is particularly important to teenage girls. Very large intakes of soft drinks may cause obesity and nutrient deficiencies, especially if coupled with other poor dietary habits.

Different tastes

Teenagers may develop different likes and dislikes, which may vary between boys and girls, between cultures, and between teenagers who suddenly have a major interest in, say, athletics or special diets.

Higher energy intakes

When girls reach approximately age 12 and boys reach age 14, they may suddenly need high energy intakes, reaching as much as 4000 kcalories per day.

Lower levels of nutrients

Teenagers are in danger of taking in lower levels of nutrients—calcium, iron, and vitamin B_6 in particular. Vitamin B_6 inadequacy seems to be prevalent in some black and white adolescent girls.[36] Low intakes of folacin and iron are common among teenage girls because of low intakes of leafy green vegetables, meat, and iron enriched foods, respectively. Ironically, this reduction occurs at a time when, because of rapid growth, authorities recommend that intakes of nutrients should be high. However, this is also a time of experimentation with eating styles, a period when food is used to express personal or social messages.

Adolescent dieting

For a discussion of the importance of this subject see Chapter 10.

Teenagers Have Different Nutrition Demands Today Than Adolescents Had a Century Ago

Considering the erratic eating behavior of teenagers today, it is remarkable that symptoms of severe nutrient deficiencies are rare in industrialized countries. In general, the major dietary deficiency seen today seems to be in iron.

How, then, does the nutrition status of teenagers today compare with their counterparts 100 years ago, when the term "junk food" had not yet entered the language and other aspects of life were considerably different? Let us consider the differences.

Beginning of puberty

Puberty begins at an earlier age now than it did in the 1880s. Menarche (the first menstruation) occurs at 12 or 13 today compared with about age 17 then. This means increased iron requirements at an earlier age to replace lost iron.

Size

Teenagers today are taller and weigh more at any given age compared to teenagers a century ago.

Weight-loss diets

This is an interesting area because it shows the tyranny of fashion. One hundred years ago, there was less emphasis among teenage girls on weight-loss diets, the principal reason being that the human body was covered with more clothes. Today, with advertising and fashion constantly setting standards for attractiveness and ideal bodies, an adolescent girl is often concerned about ideal body image and the best ways to achieve weight loss.[37]

Sugar

In the good old days (if that's what they were), high-sugar snack foods were not as available as they are now.

Surviving infancy

Fewer infants survived infectious diseases and diarrhea to become teenagers in the 1880s. In addition, infant malnutrition in North America then resembled that in many developing countries today.

Vitamin supplements

In the 1880s, people were still a quarter-century away from the discovery of the first vitamin. Vitamin deficiencies were common—too little niacin among the poor in the southern United States, for example, and too little vitamin D among the people in Britain.

Food additives

In the good old days, there were fewer food additives, which means the shelf life of foods was considerably less. On the other hand, sugar and salt were probably used less then than they are now.

Food advertising

In the 1880s there was no pressure from advertisers to buy nutritionally inferior foods.

Hyperactivity, anorexia nervosa, and bulimia

Did these modern disorders exist in the 1880s? Scientists don't know. Medical records give no indication, so we might guess they were not so troublesome then.

Alcohol, drugs, and cigarettes

Alcohol and drug abuse is certainly more common among teenagers now than it was a century ago. Nowadays about 70% of American twelfth graders have smoked cigarettes at least twice, and smoking is also a problem in other countries. For teenagers, smoking not only puts them more at risk to heart disease later in life, but also, at the time of adolescence, may cause decreased food intake, causing lower body weights and deficient nutrient intakes. For teenage girls who smoke, the risks are even greater if they take oral contraceptives, because doing so significantly increases their chances of having a stroke. Increased requirements for vitamin C in smokers result in lower tissue levels of vitamin C. This may be a problem for some teenagers because their diet may be low in vitamin C.

Pregnancy

The incidence of teenage pregnancies has been increasing recently, but why should it be any higher today than 100 years ago? Besides societal factors, one reason may be the earlier age of menarche today. In any event, the United States has a higher rate of teenage pregnancies than any other industrialized country. From a nutrition standpoint, a marginal diet in the teenage mother may pose problems for the child later. Moreover, teenagers are more likely to have low birth weight babies.

Oral contraceptives

There were no oral contraceptive agents (OCAs) in the 1880s, so there were no nutrition problems resulting from OCAs. Recently we learned that low blood levels of vitamin B_6 are not a major problem for adult women taking OCAs. However, intake of vitamin B_6 tends to be low for teenage girls and for women of all ages.[38]

Athletics and nutrition

Today there are probably more athletic events than there were in the 1880s that oblige athletes to control body weight, gymnastics being one example.[39] Twentieth-century athletes may think they benefit from the availability of nutrition supplements, like vitamin pills, but supplements are not needed if the diet is adequate—and a balanced diet was possible a century ago.

Family structure and work

There are more working mothers and teenagers today. Working teenagers are more likely to eat sandwich-type food, and to skip the evening meal. They have lower intakes of calcium and riboflavin than nonworking adolescents.

Nutrition and illness

As you might guess, modern medicine makes nutritional support available during illness in ways that could not have been imagined in 1880. If people cannot take in food through their mouths, they may receive nutrients through their veins, a process known as *total parenteral nutrition.* Moreover, there are ways in which handicapped children can eat their food more easily than was the case a century ago.[40] Availability of a number of mechanical devices now gives the child independence in eating and drinking.

Total parenteral nutrition
Infusion of all nutrients through a vein.

Acne

Teenagers' problems with *acne* must certainly go back further than 1880. Even today acne is a problem for 85% of teenagers at some point. Although there are

Acne
Inflammation of the skin causing pimples, cysts, and scars.

TABLE 13-4 Acceptable, Nutritious Foods for Teenagers

Servings	Foods
3-4	Milk and dairy products (people with lactose intolerance must take low lactose dairy products)
2	Meat, poultry, fish, legumes
4	Whole grain or enriched or fortified bread or cereal
2	Fruits, including citrus
2	Vegetables, including green leafy and yellow

nondietary reasons for acne, fatty foods, chocolate, soft drinks, and alcohol (especially beer) are popularly thought to contribute to it. However, since teenagers consume many of these foods anyway, it is difficult to isolate dietary causes. Reducing fatty foods, confectionary, and alcohol may improve the acne condition,[35] and this is good advice anyway for a still-growing teenager.

Today's adolescent has an advantage over his or her counterpart of the last century, however, in that a synthetic form of vitamin A, marketed as Accutane, is available on prescription to help clear up acne. Before you use Accutane, however, you need to have a medical examination, including blood and urine analysis, and you will not be allowed to take the drug if you are pregnant. You should also be aware of a host of side effects from Accutane: increased triglycerides and cholesterol in the blood, decrease in high-density lipoproteins, and decrease in body secretions—which in turn cause chapped lips, dry and itchy skin, mild nosebleeds, eye irritation, joint and muscle pain, rashes, and increased sensitivity to sunburn. If *all* of these were to happen to you, it would certainly be a heavy price to pay for clearing up your skin.

Control of metabolic diseases

One hundred years ago, metabolic diseases, including phenylketonuria (PKU), could not be controlled by diet. The control of PKU has eliminated this cause of mental retardation. But confusion on whether the child "outgrew" the need for restricted diet caused distress among parents and lower IQ scores in the children. Only recently was it suggested that phenylalanine restriction should continue after the age of eight years in children with PKU.[41]

Modern children and teens seem to "have it better" nutritionally than their ancestors of the same age.

Adolescents Should Be Encouraged to Eat Food that Is Not Only Palatable but Nutritious

With all the competition from fast-food restaurants, vending machines, convenience stores, and the like, it can be a real struggle to encourage teenagers to eat a healthy diet. The point, however, is that it does not matter *where* the teenager eats so long as the total intake provides the right kinds of foods and in the right amounts, as shown in Table 13-4.

Because adolescence is a time of rebellion against the authority of older people, experts suggest that the best way to convey good nutrition advice to teenagers is through suitable role models—especially since advertising makes junk-food alternatives so attractive. Some experts believe that teenagers are prone to accept nonsense about food because they don't know how to evaluate the claims made.[41]

Perhaps what is important is that whatever food is offered—as in school lunches—it should be not only nutritious but *palatable*. Otherwise, teenagers will tend to think that nutritious food isn't very interesting and doesn't taste very good.

Adolescence is a period of missed meals, snacking, and fast foods and can be the start of experiments with cigarettes, alcohol, and drugs. Psychological factors may be involved in obesity, anorexia nervosa, and bulimia. Teenage pregnancy places a premium on nutrient reserves in a body that is still growing.

Because this period of physical and mental development is so important, this chapter ends with a review of some important nutritional and environmental factors in child development (Table 13-5).

TABLE 13-5 **Summary of Nutritional and Environmental Factors in Child Development**

Stage of Development	Environmental Effects and Nutrition Consequences
1-year-old	Correct decisions on type and amount of food are important because this is a period of rapid growth Child begins to have fun with food Diarrhea and infections are problems if there is poor sanitation, hygiene, and diet
6- to 11-year-olds	Appetite and growth rates are more regular than in infants No major deficiencies; intake of vitamin B_6 and magnesium may be low Benefit from school lunch program and other supplemental feeding programs Hyperactivity can be a problem; there is no strong evidence that intake of sugar or additives is the reason Obese children have higher probability of becoming obese adults Television may communicate harmful messages about nutrition
Teenagers	Missed meals, snacking, fast foods, soft drinks are common dietary patterns; however, signs of clinical deficiencies are rare (exception is iron deficiencies in girls) Weight reduction diets undertaken because of obesity or for certain athletic events can cause problems Anorexia and bulimia can lead to death Cigarette smoking, alcohol, and drugs may upset nutrient intake Teenage pregnancy places stress on the girl's body because it adds to the body's own high nutrient requirements for growth

DECISIONS

1. Should Teenagers Diet?

Obesity is hazardous to health. Hypertension, increased serum cholesterol, and other blood factors related to a higher risk of coronary heart disease are undesirable even during the teen years.[43] Moreover, many fat children become fat adults. Is the solution, therefore, for a teenager to go on a weight-reducing diet?

There are two problems with teenage dieting:

- A teenager is growing rapidly. Enough kcalories and protein must be provided in the diet to allow lean tissue (including muscles) to grow. No one diet can be planned that will restrict kcalories and protein from fat cells, while providing the necessary nutrients to the other tissues.
- Some experts think that weight reduction after ages 4 to 6 years is too late.[19] Obese adolescents who struggle to become thin may have to continue that struggle throughout life. If this involves repeatedly losing and regaining weight—so-called yo-yo dieting—it becomes increasingly more difficult to lose the weight as the yo-yo pattern continues. It is as if after a few attempts the body is no longer fooled into losing weight. This pattern of repeated weight loss and gain is practiced by college wrestlers, and one expert predicts that such people will have difficulty throughout life in maintaining normal weight.[19]

For these reasons, prevention of obesity in childhood is important. If weight reduction is necessary, it should be done under medical supervision. The cooperation of family and school is important also, so that the teenager does not develop a body image that may lead to patterns of bulimia or anorexia nervosa.

2. Should Children Take Multivitamin Preparations?

If prescribed by a doctor, yes.

The problem is that many people believe the information about multivitamin-mineral preparations they see in television commercials and decide to take the supplements without medical advice.

Making decisions based on TV commercials is not the surest bet. One study of rural poor in Mississippi found the most often used vitamin was a sweetened multivitamin shaped like cartoon characters.[44] The same amount of nutrients could have been obtained from another product costing 60% less. In addition, a Canadian study found the same cartoon-shaped vitamin tablets were found to be the culprits for most of the severe overdosage in children.[45] Indeed, because of the high intake of iron, medical treatment was usually necessary, although no deaths occurred.

Actually, these vitamin-mineral supplements often *were* prescribed by doctors—but in response to pressure from parents. The parents felt vitamin pills would help because they felt their children were picky eaters, ate an unbalanced diet, suffered frequent infections, or were exposed to winter stress. In actuality, detailed studies in Canada found no widespread evidence of nutritional deficiency.

In summary, let the dietitian or doctor—not the television and not the parents—do any prescribing of vitamin supplements.

SUMMARY

1-6 YEAR OLD

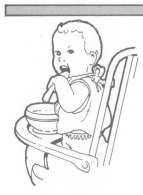

Explores food
Most preschoolers in North
  America have an
  adequate diet
Supplements unnecessary
  (except iron)

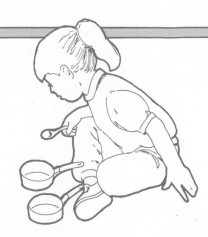

Growth slowed by
severe diarrhea

6-11 YEAR OLD

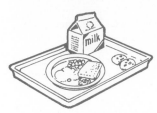

Peaceful time biologically
  and psychologically
Nutrient intake OK because
  eating habits are
  established
School feeding

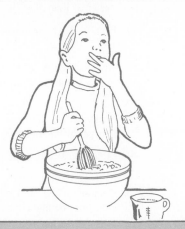

TV watching influences
  food intake
Hyperactivity poorly related
  to foods
Increased interest by
  scientists in this age group
  in studying heart disease,
  obesity, etc.

ADOLESCENT

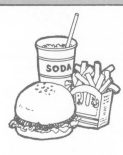

Nutrition concerns because
  of:
Missing meals, eating
  snacks, fast foods,
  unconventional meals,
  alcohol/smoking/drugs,
  soft drinks, distinct likes
  and dislikes, high energy
  intake, low nutrient
  intake, dieting, teen
  pregnancy

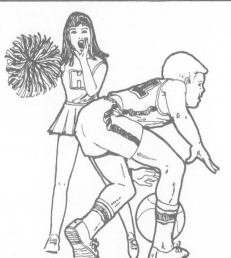

Emphasis on body weight
  Anorexia nervosa/bulimia
Pressure
  Athletic performance
  Appearance

REFERENCES

1. Anonymous: Updated estimates of the cost of raising a child, Family Economics Review, No. 2, page 32, 1985.

2. Finberg, L.: The weaning process, Pediatrics **75**(Suppl.):214, 1985.

3. Anonymous: Iatrogenic kwashiorkor in California, Nutrition Reviews **39**:397, 1981.

4. Pelchat, M.L. and Pliner, P.: Antecedents and correlates of feeding problems in young children, Journal of Nutrition Education **18**:23, 1986.

5. Hale, E.: Good nutrition for your growing child, FDA Consumer, page 21, April, 1987.

6. Pollitt, E., and others: Cognitive effects of iron-deficiency anaemia, Lancet **i**:158, 1985.

7. Krebs, N.F., and others: Increased food intake of young children receiving a zinc supplement, American Journal of Diseases of Children **138**:270, 1984.

8. Zee, P., and others: Nutritional improvement of poor urban preschool children: a 1983-1977 comparison, Journal of the American Medical Association **253**:3269, 1985.

9. Truesdell, D.D., and Acosta, P.B.: Feeding the vegan infant and child, Journal of the American Dietetic Association **85**:837, 1985.

10. Newell, G.K., and others: Food consumption and quality of diets of Kansas elementary students, Journal of the American Dietetic Association **85**:939, 1985.

11. Beal, V.A.: Nutrition in the life span, New York, John Wiley & Sons, Inc., p. 313, 1980.

12. American Dietetic Association: Comments on proposed rule for meat alternates used in child nutrition programs, Journal of the American Dietetic Association **86**:530, 1986.

13. Farris, R.P., and others: Macronutrient intakes of 10-year-old children, 1973 to 1982, Journal of the American Dietetic Association **86**:765, 1986.

14. Miller, R.W.: Low-sodium menus pass school tests, FDA Consumer, page 28, April, 1985.

15. Hodgson, P.A., and others: Comparison of serum cholesterol in children fed high, moderate, or low cholesterol milk diets during neonatal period, Metabolism **25**:739, 1976.

16. Taitz, L.S.: Diet of young children and cardiovascular disease, British Medical Journal **294**:920, 1987.

17. McNamara, D.G.: Can (should) the pediatrician wage preventive medicine war against coronary heart disease? American Journal of Diseases of Children **140**:985, 1986.

18. American Academy of Pediatrics, Committee on Nutrition: Prudent life-style for children: dietary fat and cholesterol, Pediatrics **78**:521, 1986.

19. Kolata, G.: Obese children: a growing problem, Science, **232**:20, 1986.

20. Strong, W.B.: Physical fitness in children, American Journal of Diseases of Children, **141**:488, 1987.

21. Peckham, C., and others: Obesity in school children: is there a case for screening? Public Health **99**:3, 1985.

22. Israel, A.C., and others: Eating behaviors, eating style, and children's weight status: failure to find an obese eating style, International Journal of Eating Disorders **4**:113, 1985.

23. Worsley, A., and others: Australian 10-year-olds' perceptions of food. III. The influence of obesity status, International Journal of Obesity **8**:327, 1984.

24. Swain, A.R., and others: Salicylates in foods, Journal of the American Dietetic Association **85**:950, 1985.

25. National Institutes of Health: Defined diets and childhood hyperactivity, National Institutes of Health Consensus Development Conference Summary, Volume 4, No. 3, 1982.

26. Fergusun, H.B., and others: Double-blind challenge studies of behavioral and cognitive effects of sucrose-aspartame ingestion in normal children, Nutrition Reviews **44**(Suppl.):144, May, 1986.

27. Wolraich, M., and others: Effects of sucrose ingestion on the behavior of hyperactive boys, Journal of Pediatrics **106**:675, 1985.

28. Gross, M.D.: Effects of sucrose on hyperkinetic children, Pediatrics **74**:876, 1984.

29. Anonymous: Megavitamins and the hyperactive child, Nutrition Reviews **43**:105, 1985.

30. Martineau, J., and others: Vitamin B_6, magnesium, and combined B_6-Mg: therapeutic effects in childhood autism, Biological Psychiatry, **20**:467, 1985.

31. Zuckerman, D.M., and Zuckerman, B.S.: Television's impact on children, Pediatrics **75**:233, 1985.

32. Holroyd, H.J.: Children, adolescents, and television, American Journal of Diseases of Children **139**:549, 1985.

33. Schmidt, B.J.: Current outlook for children around the world, Pediatrics **74**:294, 1984.

34. Strauss, A.: The arms race and children in fiscal 1985, Pediatrics **75**:1149, 1985.

35. Truswell, A.S.: ABC of nutrition: children and adolescents, British Medical Journal **291**:397, 1985.

36. Driskell, J.A., and others: Longitudinal assessment of vitamin B_6 status in Southern adolescent girls, Journal of the American Dietetic Association **87**:307, 1987.

37. Storz, N.S., and Greene, W.H.: Body weight, body image, and perception of fad diets in adolescent girls, Journal of Nutrition Education **15**:15, 1983.

38. Miller, L.T.: Do oral contraceptive agents affect nutrient requirements—vitamin B_6? Journal of Nutrition **116**:1344, 1986.

39. Perron, M., and Endres, J.: Knowledge, attitudes, and dietary practices of female athletes, Journal of the American Dietetic Association **85**:573, 1985.

40. Luiselli, J.K., and others: Contingency management of food selectivity and oppositional eating in a multiply handicapped child, Journal of Clinical Child Psychology **14**:153, 1985.

41. Holtzman, N.A., and others: Effect of age at loss of dietary control on intellectual performance and behavior of children with phenylketonuria, New England Journal of Medicine **314**:593, 1986.

42. Herbert, V.: Rebellion against parental authority: fad diets, "badditives," and food supplements. In E.W. Haller and G.E. Cotton, editors: Nutrition in the young and the elderly, Lexington, Mass., The Collamore Press, p. 135, 1983.

43. Freedman, D.S., and others: Relationship of changes in obesity to serum lipid and lipoprotein changes in childhood and adolescence, Journal of the American Medical Association **254:**515, 1985.

44. Sharpe, T.R., and Smith, M.C.: Use of vitamin-mineral supplements by AFDC children, Public Health Reports **100:**321, 1985.

45. Issenman, R.M., and others: Children's multiple vitamins: overuse leads to overdose, Canadian Medical Association Journal **132:**781, 1985.

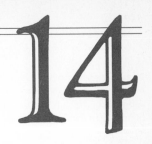

Nutrition For Adults
Young, Middle-Aged, and Elderly

CONNECTIONS

In adulthood the high nutrient demands required during growth are replaced by lower demands of maintenance. Higher intakes of nutrients then become required only during exceptional circumstances: during pregnancy and lactation, and after traumas like burns or surgery.

In industrialized countries, overnutrition is the principal nutrition problem of young and middle-aged adults; it leads to obesity. Diet may also have some relationship to cancer, hypertension, coronary heart disease, diabetes, and stroke.

Among the elderly, the principal nutrition problems may involve difficulties in getting and preparing food, difficulty in eating because of poor teeth, and problems with foods that cause constipation and indigestion.

Humanity has always searched for a "fountain of youth." Can changing the diet slow the aging process? Though scientists are not yet able to slow down the aging process, there are many entrepreneurs who claim their products or methods can.

"The desire to live as long as possible, and preferably as a young person, has stimulated a continuing search for an 'elixir of life,' " writes Dr. Alfred Harper. Even today, he says, "the assumption is still prevalent that it should be possible to delay the effects of aging and prolong life span through diet modification, the use of a nutritional supplement or treatment with some secret formula."

Are there any secret formulas? Here is an answer from Dr. Elsie Widdowson, an internationally respected nutritionist who has devoted over 50 years of her life to research on a number of nutrition problems:

From my personal experience, my recipe for food and health in extreme old age is small portions of ordinary meals, milk to drink with all of them, and anything the individual fancies, whether it be fish, fruit, cake or chocolate. Activity within the person's capacity is very important, especially in the sunshine out of doors. Tender loving care is as important in extreme old age as it is in infancy in promoting well-being and health.

Wise eating habits, physical activity, and positive interactions with others may be the best recipe for a healthy and happy old age. Plenty of rich food early in life leads to nutrition problems later in life. The aging clock cannot be turned back.

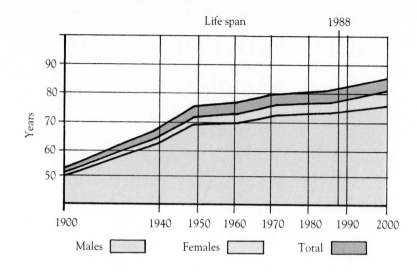

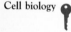

Some people think our modern diet is
bad, but there are fewer deficiencies
than at any other time in human
history.

NUTRITIONAL CHANGES OVER A LIFETIME

How long is it possible to live? You need to be skeptical about some claims for
exceptionally long lives (such as those for 120 years or more). Some societies have
no rigorous records of births and deaths and they may revere old age in a way that
induces individuals to exaggerate their age.

The maximum *documented* life span is 113 years.[1] Is it possible you could live
this long? Certainly you have a better chance than your grandparents of reaching
advanced old age. As Figure 14-1 shows, life expectancy at birth has increased in
the United States since the beginning of this century: a child born in 1900 was
expected to live only to age 50, whereas a child born in 1990 should live to age
75.

Of course, whether you live to old age is determined in part by your nutrition
habits during middle age. As Dr. Hamish Munro, then at the U.S. Department
of Agriculture's Human Nutrition Research Center on Aging, has written:

> Middle age is a time to establish health-related habits (including nutritional) in prep-
> aration for old age. Although emphasis tends to be placed on the age-associated diseases of
> adults (atherosclerosis, cancer, etc.), the progressive erosion of tissue function, though less
> dramatic, is commonly responsible for the eventual disabling of the individual.[2]

Cell biology 🔑

Cells age and die in all tissues in your body throughout your life. In most tissues
the dead cells are replaced. This cycle is at various stages in different cells within
your body at this moment. Each tissue is coordinated so that at any given time
some cells are "young" and some are "old." For example, the cells in the gastrointestinal tract are replaced every 3 to 4 days. Red blood cells are replaced every
120 days, so that (regardless of how old you are) some of your red blood cells right
now may be at days 1, 39, 109, or any other age up to approximately 120 days.

This cycle of aging and renewal is part of the normal functioning of the body.
In some tissues, such as muscle and brain, in older people the aged cells are not
replaced. This leads to decreased function in the tissue. Mechanisms causing these

losses are still a mystery. One text on the biology of aging has ten different theories of aging listed in the index. (Some have rather interesting names—"error catastrophe hypothesis," for example, or "programmed aging.")

Table 14-1 summarizes the various functional changes and tissue losses during certain periods of life and their nutritional implications. Some of these changes can influence decisions on the amount and type of foods to eat. This in turn will influence nutrient intake. Also, the ability to absorb and utilize some nutrients, and to excrete the end products of metabolism, may be affected.

Certain diseases occur in higher frequencies in middle age or old age, as Table 14-2 shows. Nutrient imbalances are at least partly responsible for arthritis, hypertension, heart conditions, atherosclerosis, deformities or orthopedic impair-

TABLE 14-1 Nutritional Implications of Loss of Tissue Function During Aging

Tissue	Functional Change	Nutritional Implications
Lean body mass	Loss of muscle and other soft tissue	Decreased energy requirements because of decreased basal requirements
Heart	Decreased output	Decreased oxygen for tissue metabolism
Lungs	Decreased maximum breathing capacity	Decreased oxygen for tissue metabolism
Muscles	Decreased strength and endurance	Difficulty in cutting some foods
Nerves	Decreased conduction velocity	Decreased muscle coordination—difficulty in cutting some foods
Kidneys	Decreased filtration rates	Possible difficulty in eliminating some end products of metabolism, e.g., nitrogen, from protein metabolism; water and electrolyte balance more difficult to control
Bones	Increased incidence of broken bones	Immobility to buy or prepare food
Mouth	Decreased saliva flow; loss of taste discrimination	Loss of ability to chew and taste food; may lead to different food choices
Teeth	Loss	Inability to chew certain foods; dentures may cause the same problem plus infections under the dentures due to lack of lubrication because of decreased saliva
Digestive system	Decreased digestive juices; decreased muscle activity	Difficulty in digesting some food; constipation because of loss of muscles in digestive system; decreased efficiency in absorbing some nutrients—fat, iron, vitamin B_{12}, and some medication
Eyes	Deterioration	Decreased ability to shop, prepare and appreciate food
Hearing	Deterioration	May prevent people from using food as a means of social interaction

TABLE 14-2 Selected Chronic Conditions Associated with Aging

Chronic Condition	Frequency of Persons Reporting Conditions (%)	Rate of Occurence per 1,000 Persons		
		Total	45-64 Years	65 + Years
Arthritis	44	121	247	465
Hypertension	39	113	244	379
Hearing impairments	28	83	143	284
Heart conditions	27	76	123	277
Visual impairments	12	40	55	137
Arteriosclerosis	12	—	—	—
Deformities or orthopedic impairments	—	82	118	128
Diabetes	8	24	57	83
Diseases of urinary system	—	25	32	56
Asthma	—	32	34	29

ments, and diabetes. Notice how the prevalence of these diseases increases between the 45-64 and the 65-plus age groups. Add to this list some cancers, osteoporosis, and periodontal disease. The list is extensive. However, many of these problems are only *in part* due to faulty diets. Other factors influencing the rate of aging are the amount and type of exercise, the physical environment, and the person's genetic makeup (Figure 14-2).

Some common causes of nutritional problems in old age include inadequate dietary intake, altered absorption and metabolism of nutrients, and degenerative diseases caused by dietary and nondietary factors.

FIGURE 14-2
Factors influencing aging. Many factors, dietary and nondietary, influence the aging process. Notice that only some of them are under our control.

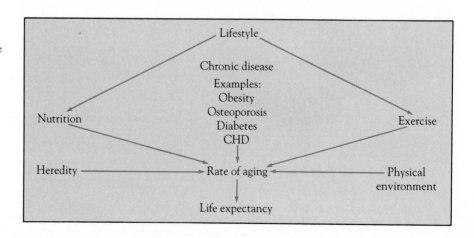

NUTRITION IN YOUNG AND MIDDLE-AGED ADULTS

Young adults are those in the 21 to 40 year age range; middle-aged adults are in the 40 to 60 year age range. We will discuss these two groups together; the elderly (over 60) will be discussed separately.

What is satisfactory nutrition for adults? Basically, the key words are "varied" and "appropriate amounts": one should eat appropriate amounts of a variety of foods. The American Dietetic Association has issued the following recommendations for food selections for women (the recommendations made for men are almost identical):

1. Eat a daily variety of foods from all major food groups.

   3-4 low-fat servings of dairy foods.

   2 low-fat servings of meat/meat alternatives.

   4 servings of vegetables/fruits.

   4 servings of whole-grain breads/cereals.

2. Maintain healthy body weight.

   For adults to lose weight safely and effectively: do not go below 10 kcal per pound of present weight, do not skip meals, and increase physical activity (exercise).

   To gain weight, increase caloric intake and exercise in moderation.

3. Exercise regularly.

   3 days per week.

4. Limit total fat to no more than one-third of daily calories.

   Select variety of fat sources: saturated, polyunsaturated, monounsaturated.

   Limit nonfat group foods, such as margarine, butter, cooking oils, salad dressing, cookies, cakes, and cream.

   Choose low-fat selections of meat and milk food groups.

5. Eat at least one half of daily calories from carbohydrates.

   Select complex carbohydrates, such as beans, peas, pasta, vegetables, nuts, and seeds.

6. Eat a variey of fiber-rich foods.

   Make daily selections from fresh fruit with skin, vegetables, legumes (navy, pinto, and kidney beans), whole grains (brown rice, oatmeal, oat and wheat bran).

   Increase intake of fiber gradually.

   Avoid excess fiber intake, especially from one source.

7. Include 3 to 4 daily servings of calcium-rich foods.

   Consume low-fat milk, yogurt, cheese.

   Increase milk in cooking.

   Eat broccoli, sardines with bones, canned salmon with bones, collard greens.

8. Include plenty of iron-rich foods.

   Make daily selections from lean meat, liver, prunes, pinto and kidney beans, spinach, leafy green vegetables, enriched and whole-grain breads/cereals.

9. Limit intake of salt and sodium-containing foods.

   Limit intake of salt added to food preparation.

   Limit use of salt.

   Watch food labels for monosodium glutamate, sodium bicarbonate, sodium citrate, and other sodium sources.

10. Rely on foods for necessary nutrients, using vitamin and mineral supplements only under specific circumstances.

FIGURE 14-3
Adult women tend to have lower intakes of some nutrients when compared to the intakes for men. Data are based on the USDA Nationwide Food Consumption Survey, 1977–1978.

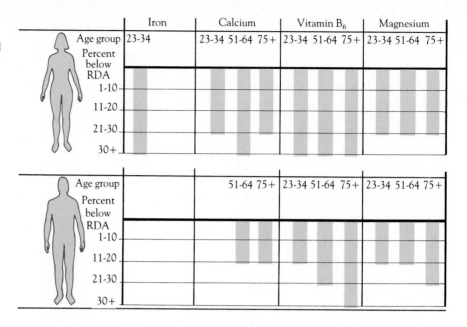

	Iron	Calcium	Vitamin B$_6$	Magnesium
Age group	23-34	23-34 51-64 75+	23-34 51-64 75+	23-34 51-64 75+

		51-64 75+	23-34 51-64 75+	23-34 51-64 75+

11. If you drink alcohol, limit intake to 1-2 drinks daily.
12. Avoid smoking.
13. Adjust diet, exercise, and other health promotional behaviors to correspond with an individual's own identified risk factors.
    Diet is only one risk factor; others include heredity, lifestyle, and environment
    Consult a physician with risk factor questions
14. If you have questions about the adequacy of your diet, consult a dietitian.

It is rare that people in middle age die from undernutrition, even in developing countries (provided they are not experiencing famine). Contrast this with the high death rates from undernutrition among infants and children described in Chapter 13. One reason is a lower requirement for nutrients in adults because nutrients are needed for maintenance rather than for growth. Another reason is the higher resistance to infection in adults.

Death from undernutrition is rare in developed countries.

Still, even in the United States, some adults experience low intake of certain nutrients, as Figure 14-3 illustrates. Women have lower intakes than men of the same age for vitamin B$_6$, magnesium, calcium, and iron (in the premenopausal group). Zinc and folacin intakes are also below recommended intakes.[3] The most visible signs of low iron intake are a lack of energy and a pale appearance; low calcium intake may result in severe osteoporosis.[4] Nutrient intakes are lowest among the poor, Canadian Eskimos, and Native Americans.

There are some encouraging signs of dietary improvements among American women and men. Data for women were quantified recently.[3] In the years 1977-1985, there was a 20% increase in carbohydrate intake and a 5% reduction in fat intake. There were increased intakes of low-fat and skim milk; mixtures with meat, poultry, or fish; grain products, especially pastas and mixtures with grains; and nonalcoholic (but also alcoholic) beverages. Decreased intakes were reported for whole milk, beef, pork, and eggs. Where this food is eaten is changing also. In 1985, women took in over a quarter of their dietary intake away from home.[3]

Not all young and middle-aged adults have specific nutritional problems. Let us discuss the nutrition problems faced by college students, women, men, and adults in general.

College Students Have Certain Specific Nutrition Problems

If you are a college student yourself, think of the kind of life you lead. The varying nutritive value of dining hall food, the busy study schedules, the kind of food permissible with a limited budget, the inducements of junk food or fast food advertising, the lack of nutrition knowledge, the pressure to alter one's diet for athletic reasons or to lose weight or to adhere to a particular religious or cultural creed—any and all of these can produce nutritional abuse to a college student's body.

Typical nutrition-related problems include dental caries, obesity, anemia (especially in women), acne, alcoholism, and drug abuse. Despite their extra years of education, eating disorders seem to be as prevalent among female graduate students as in other students and nonstudents.[5] Students who view themselves as being more maladjusted than their peers may run a higher risk of bulimia. All in all, concluded one study, college students simply don't eat right: they don't eat the right type or amount of food and they don't take the right amount of time to consume food.[6]

Now that you are nearing the end of this book, perhaps you are in a position to look at your own eating behavior and judge how it compares with the general student behavior described above.

Women Experience Some Nutrition Problems More Often than Men Do

The food choices that women make are influenced by weight-control problems, money, and time pressure, and by nutrition-related concerns.[7] Apart from nutrition matters related to pregnancy and lactation (Chapter 12), the greatest nutrition-related problems of women have to do with obesity, cancer, osteoporosis, various anemias, side effects from taking oral contraceptives, *premenstrual syndrome*, and goiter.

Premenstrual Syndrome
Several unpleasant symptoms occurring before and thought to be related to menstruation.

Obesity

We examined the causes and treatments of obesity in Chapter 10. Obesity is related closely to hypertension, hypercholesterolemia, type II (maturity onset) diabetes, certain cancers, and to a number of other problems (Figure 14-4), as well as to a decrease in life span.[8]

During pregnancy, many obese women also suffer from hypertension, diabetes, gallstones, blood clots, and aches in the back, legs, and joints. Obese pregnant women are also apt to have toxemia (characterized by excesssive vomiting and convulsions) and difficulties during childbirth.[9]

About one in every four adult American women is more than 20% above ideal

FIGURE 14-4
Many parts of the body are affected by obesity.

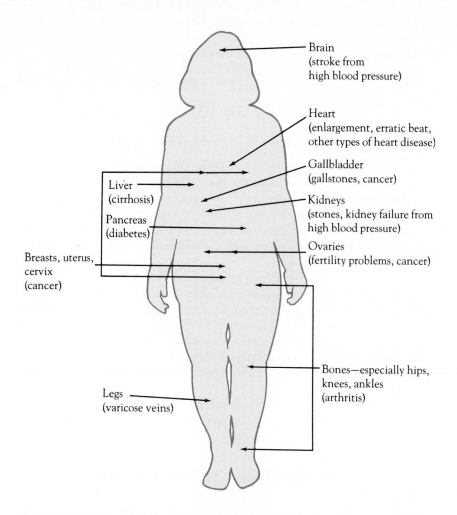

Brain
(stroke from
high blood pressure)

Heart
(enlargement, erratic beat,
other types of heart disease)

Gallbladder
(gallstones, cancer)

Liver
(cirrhosis)

Kidneys
(stones, kidney failure from
high blood pressure)

Pancreas
(diabetes)

Ovaries
(fertility problems, cancer)

Breasts, uterus,
cervix
(cancer)

Bones—especially hips,
knees, ankles
(arthritis)

Legs
(varicose veins)

body weight. As Figure 14-5 shows, Americans ages 20 to 64 (whether women or men) are more apt to be obese than their counterparts in Canada and Great Britain, perhaps because of differences in the relative level of affluence among the three countries. The reason obesity seems to increase with age is that kcaloric intake is not balanced by energy expenditure.

Why is there a higher incidence of obesity in poor adult women—particularly blacks and Native Americans—but not poor adult men or in poor children of both sexes? Evidently, the switch from being thin to being fat begins to take place when a girl is about 15, and by age 50 a low-income woman averages 17 lb more than her higher-income counterpart—even though the poorer woman is generally shorter in height.[10] In Chapter 10, we described some of the theories of obesity— that people gain weight because they like food and it tastes good (the sensory hypothesis), that each person has a set weight he or she will attain in life (the set-point theory), that the number of fat cells of fat babies leads to fat adults (adipocyte size and number theory), and some other genetic and physiological explanations. However, Dr. S.M. Garn of the University of Michigan examined these theories in relation to obesity in poor women and found that none seemed to apply.[10] Could it be that poor adult men are engaged in hard manual labor with high energy expenditure? ⇦

Some cancers

The National Cancer Institute estimates that diet and tobacco are major causes of many types of cancers. Here let us consider lung and mouth cancer and breast cancer.

As cigarette smoking becomes more popular among young women, health officials have expressed concern about increased incidences of lung cancer in women. Diet seems to have no bearing on this form of cancer, but it does in cancer of the mouth and larynx (part of the throat). When increased alcohol consumption is added to cigarette smoking, the rate of mouth and larynx cancer increases.

More North American women die from breast cancer than from any other form of cancer. Indeed, it is the highest cause of death among women aged 40-44. Some of the factors involved in breast cancer are:[11]

- *Race.* Breast cancer is more common among Jewish women in the United States than among women of Asian or African descent.
- *Geography.* Breast cancer is more common in developed nations such as the United States. It is rare in Japan and in developing countries; perhaps, it is speculated, because fat intake there is low. This means that total kcaloric intake is usually low also.
- *Time of menarche and menopause.* Women who experience early menarche or late menopause have a higher risk of breast cancer.
- *Family history.* Cancer tends to occur more in some families than in others, suggesting a genetic component to the disease.

FIGURE 14-5
Prevalence of overweight and obesity in the United States, Canada, and Great Britain.

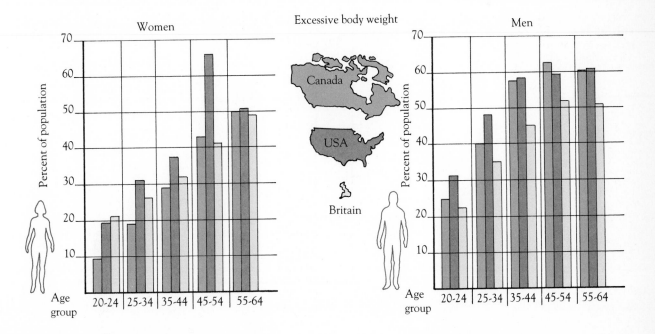

Is there a relationship between dietary fat and breast cancer? This theory is now called into question.[12] Because the average American woman has a rather high dietary fat intake—40% of total kcalories—it was thought to be connected to the high incidence of breast cancer among American women. However, a recent study found that over a 4-year period there was no increased incidence in breast cancer for women whose dietary fat intake ranged from 32% to 44% of kcalories. This observation needs to be confirmed.

What is the evidence linking high dietary fat and breast cancer? Women in Japan and in most of Africa and Asia have a low intake of fat. They also have a low incidence of breast cancer. Is there a direct relationship between dietary fat and breast cancer in women? Maybe, but the diets differ in other ways, for instance in the degree of saturation of the dietary fat and in the intake of minerals and vitamins. Other differences in diet that may affect the incidence of breast cancer in women include different intakes of alcohol, fish oils, vegetables, and kcalories. Some clues may come from the health records of Seventh Day Adventists. Members of this sect are vegetarian and do not drink alcohol. Their dietary fat intake is low, partly because they do not eat meat. Yet their total kcalorie intake is fairly high. Seventh Day Adventists in the United States have an incidence of breast cancer almost identical to the total American population.

At present, a number of women are maintaining dietary fat at 20% of the kcalories in their diet (Figure 14-6), in an 8½-year study of the National Cancer Institute to test the relationship of this low-fat diet to breast cancer. However, such a diet is difficult to maintain, and the women are having to prepare most of their own food and stay clear of restaurant and holiday meals.[12] Even in vegetarian diets the intake of fat is around 30% of total kcalories. A nonvegetarian low-fat diet means that one must eat small portions of meat well-trimmed of fat, low-fat salad dressings, and low-fat cheeses.

FIGURE 14-6
Diets low in energy from fat are difficult to achieve.

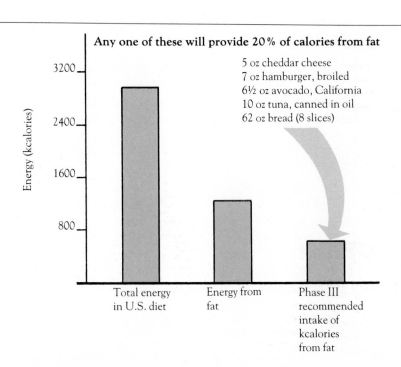

Any one of these will provide 20% of calories from fat

5 oz cheddar cheese
7 oz hamburger, broiled
6½ oz avocado, California
10 oz tuna, canned in oil
62 oz bread (8 slices)

Energy (kcalories)

3200

2400

1600

800

Total energy
in U.S. diet

Energy from
fat

Phase III
recommended
intake of
kcalories
from fat

Osteoporosis

Loss of calcium from the bones, which was decribed in Chapter 7, occurs during various stages of aging. Osteoporosis is an expensive disease for the United States, costing about $1 billion a year. The reason is that by age 80, osteoporosis accounts for 15% of the spine fractures in women, 24% of the wrist fractures, and 33% of the hip fractures. By age 85, about 93% of women will have broken at least one bone, whereas only 20% will have had cardiovascular disease, 15% diabetes, 15% hypertension, 10% central nervous system disorders, including Alzheimer's disease, and 5% rheumatoid arthritis.[13]

 Economics

Osteoporosis gets progressively worse as women go from middle to old age. It is calculated that the yearly rate of bone loss ranges from 2% (arms) to 8% (chest).[14] But even women in their late twenties report that after pregnancy they show such symptoms of osteoporosis as bone loss, low back pain, and hip pain.[15] However, osteoporosis associated with pregnancy usually improves after delivery, which means its cause is probably nondietary.

Among the recommendations for preventing osteoporosis are the following:

- *Calcium.* Consume adequate (1500 mg per day) calcium, beginning early in life. Starting to take calcium later, for instance 1000-2000 mg per day in the early menopause, is not effective in preventing bone loss.[16] Still, high calcium intake does not necessarily mean less chance of broken hips, as data developed by Dr. Mark Hegsted for various countries show (Figure 14-7). Hegsted remarks: "It will be embarrassing enough if the current calcium hype is simply useless; it will be immeasurably worse if the recommendations are actually detrimental to health."[4] Thus, much remains to be done to determine the exact role of added calcium in osteoporosis.
- *Fluoridation.* Fluoridation of drinking water also may be helpful in preventing bone fractures in the elderly.[17]
- *Smoking.* Smoking should be avoided.
- *Coffee, soft drinks, and alcohol.* Excessive use of caffeine should be avoided. Soft drinks substituted for milk will interfere with the availability of calcium. Alcohol abuse increases bone fragility even in adult men.[18]
- *High protein.* High intakes of protein should be avoided. High protein intakes, irrespective of dietary source, causes a loss of calcium through the urine.
- *Estrogen.* Anorexia nervosa and excessive exercise causes amenorrhea. Sufficient estrogen is not secreted in these situations. Estrogen is effective in preventing osteoporosis.[14]
- *Milk.* People, such as elderly blacks and Mexican-Americans, with lactase deficiency can consume some dairy products, including lactose-reduced milk.

Be cautious of some advertised claims for calcium supplements. There may be more effective ways to prevent osteoporosis.

The importance of exercise in preventing bone loss must be emphasized here. Additional advantages of exercise are the control of body weight and the social aspect of many exercise programs. For example, many cities in Canada and in other countries offer such activities as elderobics for 60-plus people.

Anemias

Blood loss such as that brought about by menstruation, bleeding ulcers, or childbirth can cause anemia.

Women who are pregnant or who are postmenopausal do not lose iron through menstruation. Some forms of anemia may be caused by dietary deficiencies of iron,

FIGURE 14-7
Calcium and hip fractures. The amount of calcium available in the food supply compared with the incidence of hip fractures in women in many countries. Such data serve as a warning against enthusiastic use of high calcium intakes to prevent osteoporosis. Notice that the intake of calcium by women in the United Kingdom and the United States are similar, yet American women suffer from a much higher rate of hip fractures.

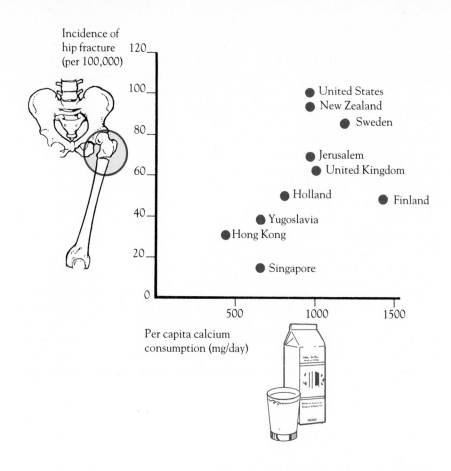

folacin, vitamin B_{12}, or vitamin B_6, or when diets have low iron bioavailability. Symptoms of severe folacin deficiency are probably uncommon.[19]

Economics

As many as 40% of women of ages 20 to 50 may suffer from the symptoms of iron deficiency. Black women whose incomes are below the poverty level have the lowest iron intake. Ferrous sulfate is the form in which iron is most frequently prescribed, and it may be obtained in a "slow release" form. One study showed that prices for ferrous sulfate varied even for the same preparation.[20] Prices per gram of iron varied from $0.32 to $20.28—a $19.96 difference! As you might guess, generic pills were cheaper than brand-name pills. However, there were no savings to be had by shopping at chain pharmacies, which charged as much or more for the pills as individually owned pharmacies.

Oral contraceptives

Oral contraceptive agents (abbreviated OCAs) have varying effects on adult women's health, depending on the type of OCA and the length of time the woman has been taking it. OCAs may slightly decrease the level of vitamin B_6 and folacin in the blood, especially if the woman has a borderline deficiency of these nutrients. Women taking OCAs who eat a balanced diet have no special need for nutrient supplements.

A British study reports that women taking OCAs have higher incidences of inflammation of the intestines, which can interfere with normal digestion and absorption of nutrients.[21] A recent study showed that among women aged 20-44 OCA users had lower body fat content but a higher total kcaloric intake. This apparent contradiction is explained by differences in lifestyles and in behavior.[22]

Premenstrual syndrome

Many unpleasant symptoms, including breast tenderness, pelvic pain, headache, abdominal bloating, an impression of weight gain, irritability, constipation, anxiety, aggressiveness, depression, fatigue, insomnia, and a craving for sweet or salty foods are attributed to premenstrual syndrome (PMS).

Scientists have been aware of PMS for over fifty years, yet they still do not precisely understand the effects of the complicated series of hormonal changes involved in the menstrual cycle. What is known is that the incidence of PMS increases the older a woman is, the more children she has had, and the less she exercises.[23] Advances in reproductive physiology allow investigators to follow the hormonal changes that occur before and during menstruation.

Unfortunately, the roles of specific nutrients in treating PMS are ill defined, owing partly to poorly designed studies. Although megadoses of vitamin B_6 are popularly recommended to treat PMS, this treatment has not been confirmed as being truly helpful. Indeed, high intakes of vitamin B_6 can produce toxic effects; although some so-called authorities recommend up to 2000 mg per day of the vitamin, the vitamin B_6 RDA for adult women is 2 mg.

Other treatments are also promoted to fight PMS—sodium restriction; high complex-carbohydrate diets; and supplements of vitamin E, magnesium, and primrose oil (which contains vitamin E, unsaturated fatty acids, and other components)—but there is no evidence that they are effective. More good experimental work must be done before reliable dietary recommendations about PMS can be made.

Menstrual cycle and food cravings

A recent study of young college women found that menstruation caused an increase in craving for chocolate but no craving for high-sugar or low-carbohydrate foods. There was no evidence that chocolate was craved for its pharmacologic effect (stimulant) or its nutritive value. Much remains to be learned about food cravings just before and during menstruation.[24]

Goiter

This disorder, which is mostly a problem in developing countries, where iodine is not added to salt, is more common in girls and in young women than it is in young men.

The most prevalent nutrition-related problems for women in developed countries are obesity, certain cancers, and anemia.

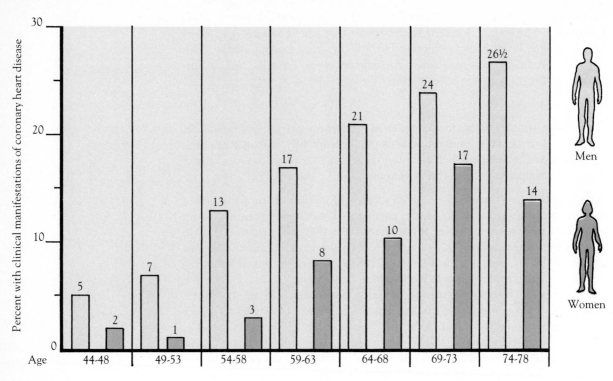

FIGURE 14-8
Coronary heart disease. Data show the incidence of coronary heart disease in American men and women. The increase in incidence for women occurs after the menopause.

Men Experience Some Nutrition-Related Problems More Often Than Women Do

Things are not equal between the sexes: men may live shorter lives, but while they are living them they do not seem to have as much of a problem obtaining enough nutrients as women do (Figure 14-3). However, men seem to suffer more from problems brought on by excesses in their diet. Most deaths of adult males in industrialized countries are caused by coronary heart disease and cancer.

Coronary heart disease

Symptoms of coronary heart disease are present in over 5½ million Americans. Many others are believed to have undiagnosed coronary heart disease. Over 550,000 lives are lost to this disease each year in the United States. As Figure 14-8 shows, coronary heart disease is more common among middle-aged men than among middle-aged women. One reason is that men have lower levels of the protective high-density lipoprotein than women do.

Characterized by a British magazine as "The Western way to die" (Figure 14-9), coronary heart disease is much more common in North America and Europe than it is in Japan and in developing countries. Japanese emigrants to the United States eventually have increased rates of coronary heart disease, which suggest that the different incidences in the two countries don't result from genetic differences. Still, the Japanese in Japan have a higher death rate from strokes (see Figure 14-9), which is brought on by hypertension, which in turn is related to the diet. The Japanese diet is low in saturated fat and cholesterol but high in sodium.

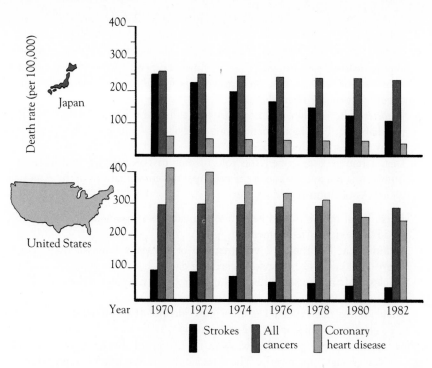

FIGURE 14-9
"The Western way to die." Death rates from coronary heart disease, cancers, and strokes differ widely in the United States and Japan.

In a study of nutrition, it should frequently be noted that there are many *nondietary* risk factors in diseases, particularly heart disease. This means you should be careful about making comparisons between countries because matters other than food and drink may influence the incidence of disease.

Some factors that may contribute to heart disease can be controlled; others cannot.

You *cannot control* the following:

- *Gender.* The incidence of coronary heart disease is higher in men than in women.
- *Age.* As Figure 14-8 shows, coronary heart disease increases in incidence in males after ages 35 to 39 and in females after ages 40 to 44.
- *Genetics.* People who have a history of heart disease in their families and forebears have a higher probability of developing it themselves.

You *can control* the following:

- *Smoking.* One of the greatest causes of heart disease, cigarette smoking reduces HDL cholesterol—the "good" cholesterol. However, this can be changed; the trend is reversed when people quit smoking.[25] In 1986, the Chicago Heart Association found cigarette smoking and cholesterol were the least frequently recognized risk factors in coronary heart disease.
- *Coffee.* The apparent effect of coffee drinking may be due to smoking, since many smokers are also heavy consumers of coffee. Nevertheless, there is a two- to threefold increase in the risk of coronary heart disease in heavy coffee drinkers.[26]
- *Obesity.* Weight loss causes a reduction in serum cholesterol.
- *Hypertension.* In 1986, the Chicago Heart Association found hypertension to

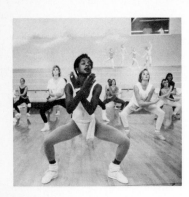

Much of the prevention of coronary heart disease is within our control.

be the most frequently recognized and understood risk factor among the general public.

- *Exercise.* Although beneficial, exercise provides no absolute guarantee of escaping heart disease in middle age.[27] However, people who exercise are more conscious of body weight, diet, and smoking—the other important matters affecting coronary heart disease.
- *Diabetes.* The incidence of coronary heart disease is higher in diabetics than nondiabetics. Diet recommendations for diabetes include a reduction in total fat intake, especially saturated fat.
- *Diet.* Chapter 4 described the role of diet in coronary heart disease. The following summarizes some of the principal recommendations of the American Heart Association regarding diet:

Fats: Total intake should be 30% of all calories consumed, down from 30% to 35% previously recommended.
Sodium: Eat less than a level teaspoon of salt daily (equivalent to 1 g for every 1,000 calories), not to exceed 3 g daily.
Cholesterol: Intake should be 100 mg per 1,000 calories consumed each day (one egg).
Alcohol: Do not exceed 1½ oz of pure alcohol (two mixed drinks, or two 4-oz glasses of wine, or two 12-oz beers).

Public Health 🔑

How much does the public know about these controllable factors in this killer disease? Not enough, apparently. The Chicago Heart Association found that few people could identify all three of the major risk factors—cigarette smoking, hypertension, and cholesterol. Moreover, men are less likely than women to believe that dietary and lifestyle factors contribute to the incidence of heart disease.[28] As the authors of this finding write: "Taking food and nutrition out of the realm of women's responsibility, and teaching the importance and interrelationships of nutrition, fitness, and health for all individuals should be a public health priority."

Some cancers

Lung cancer is the most common form of cancer in men, for two main reasons: cigarette smoking and occupation.

Aside from giving up smoking and staying clear of occupations involving, say, the installation of asbestos, is there anything you can do to decrease your risk of developing lung cancer? Actually, you might try increasing your intake of beta-carotene and vitamin E, although these will not give you a magic shield against lung cancer.

Beta-carotene, the vitamin A precursor, may protect against the common type of lung cancer known as squamous cell carcinoma. Researchers at Johns Hopkins University now claim that vitamin E may help reduce the risk of any type of lung cancer.[29] Why beta-carotene and vitamin E have this protective effect is not known, but you might try eating more beta-carotene–rich foods like carrots, sweet potatoes, squash, and pumpkins, and other vegetables and fruits with a deep orange or yellow color. For vitamin E, you may eat whole grains, nuts, egg yolk, and plant oils like wheatgerm oil. All of these foods are excellent additions to the diet anyway. Intake of egg yolks should be limited by persons controlling their cholesterol intake.

Two important statements must be made about this exciting research.

- A high intake of beta-carotene and vitamin E *does not* make cigarette smoking risk-free.[29] Even if beta-carotene decreased lung-cancer deaths by half, lifelong smokers would still have a 10 to 15 times greater risk than nonsmokers (the risk is 20 to 30 times greater now).
- Beta-carotene and vitamin E may not be what's doing the trick anyway. The positive effects on lung cancer could be due to some other undiscovered component in foods rich in beta-carotene and vitamin E. This suggests that supplements may not be worthwhile; you should eat the foods rich in beta-carotene and vitamin E instead of taking vitamin supplements.

> The most prevalent diet-related diseases in men are coronary heart disease and certain types of cancer.

Certain Nutrition-Related Problems Are Common to Both Men and Women

Getting older means getting *better* in a number of ways, but in some ways it does not. Let us consider some of the principal nutrition-related problems of young and middle-age adults: hypertension, dental disorders, diabetes, arthritis, and a few others.

Hypertension

Also called high blood pressure, hypertension is associated with a high incidence of stroke and is one of many factors in coronary heart disease. In the United States, its highest incidence is among blacks of all ages. Places where hypertension is low or nonexistent are a few isolated communities in Africa, Brazil, and some Pacific Islands.

Knowing your own blood pressure is useful, and many medical paraprofessionals are equipped to measure it for you. There are even coin-operated machines in some drugstores that allow you to test your own blood pressure. Blood pressure is expressed as two numbers. The upper number indicates *systolic pressure*, which is the pressure against the arterial walls when the heart pumps blood. The lower number is *diastolic pressure*, the pressure between heartbeats. Normal values for healthy young people are 100/60 mm to 120/80 mm.

The following factors are correlated with hypertension:[30]

- *Genetics.* High blood pressure is a disease that runs in families.
- *Age.* Blood pressure increases as people get older.
- *Emotional state.* Tension from anxiety can raise blood pressure.
- *Diet.* Increased hypertension has been linked to overweight and obesity, high sodium intake in some people, and high alcohol intake.

A few years ago calcium deficiency was considered a major factor in hypertension, and increased calcium intake was urged as a double-barreled solution for

Systolic Pressure
Blood presure measured when the heart is contracting.

Diastolic Pressure
Blood pressure measured when the heart is relaxed.

treating hypertension while preventing osteoporosis. However, much of the original enthusiasm for calcium has waned.[31] Because evidence of the beneficial effects of calcium on hypertension is inconclusive, calcium supplements should be used with caution.

To decrease hypertension, it is recommended that one increase the intake of potassium, which is found in high amounts in vegetables, and increase the intake of polyunsaturated fatty acids, which is found in high amounts in foods of plant origin.[30] Under no circumstances should non-dietary supplements of either potassium or polyunsaturated fatty acids be self-medicated.

Nutritional intervention alone, without the use of antihypertensive drugs, seems to be effective in lowering high blood pressure.[32] This was achieved by reducing overweight and excessive salt and alcohol intakes. The researchers are enthusiastic because this form of treatment lessens the necessity for treatment with drugs that can have unwanted side effects.

Dental and gum disorders

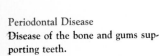

Dentistry

Over 98% of Americans have dental caries—cavities—and repair of damaged teeth costs over $4 billion a year. Loss of teeth before age 35 is due mainly to dental caries. After age 35 the primary reason for the loss is periodontal disease.

Three factors contribute to dental caries:

- Saliva. Some people have more trouble with cavities despite observing all precautions. One reason may be differing rates of production of saliva. Saliva washes bacteria from surfaces in the mouth. These bacteria are then swallowed and killed by the strong acid in the stomach. The more saliva produced, the more bacteria killed.
- Plaque. This contains decay-causing bacteria. *Streptococcus mutans* is the most important. These micro-organisms convert sugar into an acid that erodes the enamel.
- Sugar. The stickier the source of the sugar, the more decay-causing acid is produced by these bacteria.

Fluoride from the diet, drinking water, and toothpaste is beneficial in preventing caries.

Periodontal disease

Periodontal Disease
Disease of the bone and gums supporting teeth.

The major cause of tooth loss in adults over 35, *periodontal disease* affects the gums and causes loss of bones surrounding the teeth. Diets low in calcium, protein, vitamin C, and zinc are thought to increase the incidence of periodontal disease. These are nutrients needed for the production of collagen and dentin, both important in the structure of teeth.

Dietary deficiency of protein or vitamin C is not a problem for most Americans. Plaque activity is involved in periodontal disease, so reduced sugar consumption might help prevent tooth loss. There is some speculation that food high in fiber, and coarse, chewy foods are beneficial in this disease, but much remains to be learned.

Diabetes

There are two kinds of diabetes, type I and type II.

Type I, insulin-dependent diabetes, requires life-long diet modification. The diet should provide enough energy for growth and maintenance, but not for weight gain. Timing of meals is important. Smaller and more frequent meals, and eating carbohydrate-rich foods about every three hours is recommended. Restriction of carbohydrate intake is not as severe as was once recommended. A bedtime snack prevents hypoglycemia (low blood glucose level) from developing during the night.

Diabetes is a risk factor for coronary heart disease; therefore, dietary factors in coronary heart disease should be considered. These include reductions in kcalories and the amount of fat, especially saturated fat, in the diet, a moderate use of alcohol, and perhaps a high-fiber intake. The diet must fit in with the person's lifestyle, socioeconomic and ethnic factors, food preferences, and personality.

Type II or noninsulin-dependent diabetes occurs in many obese adults. It accounts for more than 90% of all diabetes in the United States. It is a major cause of death as well as blindness, kidney failure, and limb amputations.[33] Losing weight usually reduces the presence of this kind of diabetes. Because it occurs mainly in overweight, sedentary adults the type of lifestyle may be a major cause of type II diabetes. The best way to reduce the problem is to lose weight, exercise regularly (*not* occasionally), and avoid fad diets.

However restrictive some diets seem to diabetics, at least they should be glad they were arrived at by some scientific routes. If you had been a diabetic soldier in the Royal Artillery of the British Army in 1797, for instance, John Rollo, the surgeon-general, would have prescribed the following diet.

History

Breakfast	1½ pints milk and ½ pint lime water, mixed together; Bread and butter
Noon	Plain blood pudding, blood and suet only
Dinner	Game or old meats; Fat and rancid old meats "as fat as the stomach may bear"
Supper	Same as breakfast

Thinking diabetes was a disease of the stomach, he eliminated all fruits and vegetables from the diet. Today there is more emphasis on limiting fat intake, consuming no more than the RDA for protein, and attending to sodium intake. Still, the refinement of knowledge about diabetes and diet continues.[34]

Arthritis

Slight relief from arthritis may be obtained with high intakes of polyunsaturated fat. A supplement of the fatty acid called eicosapentaenoic acid (better known as omega-3 fatty acid—found mainly in fish oils) also helps and will reduce morning stiffness and tenderness in the joints, but the disease is not eliminated. When this diet is allowed to lapse, the original arthritic condition will return. What remains to be worked out is the optimal dose and duration of fish oil supplementation.

Multiple sclerosis

Multiple sclerosis (MS) is a progressive disease of the nervous system. Diet, especially dairy products, may contribute to the condition, but no conclusive evidence is available. Minor relief can be obtained from supplements of the essential fatty acid called linoleic acid.

Multiple Sclerosis
A chronic, slowly progressive disease of the central nervous system.

Migraine

Although migraine is not considered a disease, the pain of migraine headache can be worse than the pain of many diseases. Migraine may run in families, but there are also some dietary contributors. The migraine may be produced by an allergic reaction to certain foods, through chemical triggers in the food that act on the vascular system, or by hypoglycemia. ⬅

Crohn's disease

Crohn's Disease
Chronic inflammation of the intestine.

⬅ An inflammation of the gastrointestinal tract, *Crohn's disease* may be associated with high sugar intake. For serious conditions, patients are treated by giving them all nutrients in their simplest, elemental form. Thus, protein is given as amino acids, carbohydrates are given as glucose, and fats are given as fatty acid. ⬅

Dysgeusia

Dysgeusia
Impairment or perversion of the normal sense of taste.

Dysgeusia is the technical name for taste distortion, which may result in low intakes in energy, calcium, and vitamins A and C. It can occur in people deficient in zinc and vitamin A or people suffering from infections, cancer, and disorders of kidneys, nerves, and hormonal secretions.

Heartburn

⬅ Heartburn may not be high on the list of sufferings, but it is certainly unpleasant. Smoking a cigarette after a meal may cause heartburn, but so may a whole host of foods: fatty foods, spicy foods, fried foods, peppers, tomatoes, radishes, salad dressings, orange juice, tomato juice, coffee (even decaffeinated), alcohol, food seasonings, flavorings (including oils of spearmint, peppermint, garlic, and onion). ⬅

Severe burns

Burns, of course, are not the exclusive province of adults, but they cause increased nutritional requirements for adults. There are dietary ways of helping patients recover from burns. Burn patients should receive adequate dietary energy and protein and also vitamin and mineral supplements—particularly vitamin C and zinc.

Childhood diseases in adulthood

Cystic Fibrosis
Hereditary disease that affects most glands, causing abnormal secretions.

Down's Syndrome
Preferred name for mongolism; a form of mental retardation.

There are a great many diseases and disorders present at birth that seriously affect the person's adult life. Let us discuss three of the most serious: *cystic fibrosis, Down's syndrome,* and mental retardation.

Cystic fibrosis This genetic disorder consists of alterations in gland secretions that obstruct pancreatic and bile ducts, intestines, and bronchi. Obstructions of the intestines interfere with digestion, causing malabsorption of fat, protein, and fat-soluble vitamins, as well as poor absorption of calcium, phosphorus, and sodium. An adult who has had cystic fibrosis will show the effects of reduced growth rate and possibly undernutrition. The good news, however, is that the number of people with cystic fibrosis now living to adulthood is much greater than in years past.

Down's syndrome This is the preferred name for mongolism, a form of mental retardation. Children with Down's syndrome show multiple deficiencies of vitamins and minerals, but treatment with amino acids, vitamins, minerals, and/or hormones has no affect on the disorder. Still, with improved medical treatment, more people with Down's syndrome are living to adulthood.

For mental retardation in general, it has been shown that vitamin and mineral supplements have no affect on IQ or behavior in institutionalized mentally retarded, whether children or adults.

> The major causes of death in adults in industrialized countries are coronary heart disease, cancer, and stroke. Diet is only one of many factors causing these diseases. Some nutrition-related diseases are more common in women—obesity, osteoporosis, breast cancer, nutritional anemias, goiter, premenstrual stress. Men have a higher incidence of coronary heart disease and lung cancer. Dietary changes may be beneficial in arthritis and in multiple sclerosis, but worthless in other adult disorders.

NUTRITION IN THE ELDERLY

We have defined the elderly as those age 60 or over—a somewhat arbitrary range. It is important to know about the nutrition requirements in those over 60 because, as Figure 14-9 indicates, so many more people are surviving into this stage of life.

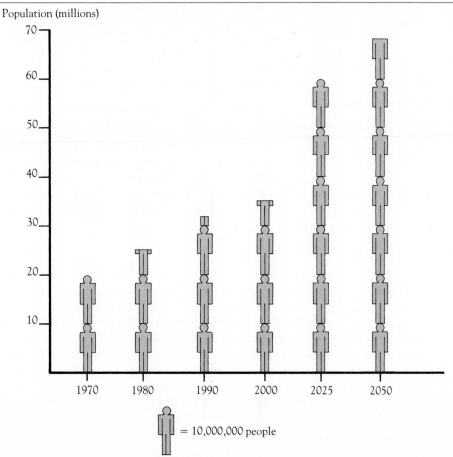

Population (millions)

= 10,000,000 people

FIGURE 14-10
U.S. population distribution. Clearly, the American population is aging rapidly.

No doubt about it, people are living longer—25-30 years longer than they were at the beginning of this century. Today life expectancy at birth in the United States is 78 for white females and 71 for white males; for nonwhite females it is 73, and for nonwhite males it is 64. There are more elderly people now than at any time in history, and that proportion will continue to increase (Figure 14-10).

Let us begin to describe the nutrition needs of the elderly by pointing out that three significant changes have taken place since youth:

- Changes in body composition and physiological functioning of the tissues that occurred gradually during aging may have an effect in old age (Table 14-1). These may cause difficulties in obtaining food and utilizing the nutrients. Some changes during aging may make a person less prepared for some of life's stresses such as a death in the family or extensive surgery.
- Chronic diseases and disabilities are more common at this age. These include most of the diseases discussed above.
- Total food intake is reduced as you grow older. This may lead to problems in the choice of a nutritious diet.

Let us examine the nutritional consequences of each of these.

Changes in Body Composition and Physiological Functioning of Tissues Affect Nutritional Status

Physiology

Significant changes in body composition and decreases in physiological functions usually begin around age 30, although the rates of change vary for different tissues. Let us look at the changes in the entire body, changes in how the elderly perceive and handle food, and changes in how the tissues transport, use, and store nutrients. We must bear in mind that the following changes in the body do not occur to the same extent in all people.

Decrease in lean body mass

The reduction in lean body mass, most of it due to loss of skeletal muscle, also means a reduction in basal metabolic rate. As a result, fewer total kcalories are required in the diet to meet one's energy requirements. However, the nutrients required are still high (see the RDA table), which means the elderly must choose food with a high nutrient density to meet these requirements. Excess alcohol and foods high in sugar and fat should be avoided.

Decrease in sensory function

As Table 14-1 shows, as one ages, one is less able to see, hear, and even smell and taste. Indeed, as Figure 14-11 indicates, the elderly are not as good as young people at detecting bitter and spicy tastes and smooth and crunchy textures in foods.

The decline in the sensory functions affects the kind of nutrition elderly people receive. Declining vision affects a person's ability to get to the store and to read labels and menus. Poor hearing may make people less inclined to eat with friends. Decline in ability to smell means food odors are not detected as well and the sense of taste diminishes. All of these may make older people less interested in food.

Some studies report that zinc deficiency is a problem among the elderly; a lack of zinc has an adverse effect on the sense of taste. However, a recent study of hospitalized elderly people in Canada showed their zinc status to be satisfactory.

Persons preparing food for either very young or very old people should consider age-related differences in sensory reactions to food.

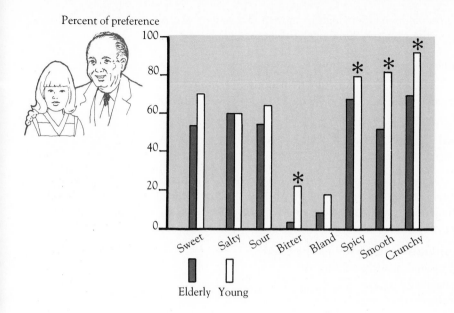

FIGURE 14-11
Different tastes. The chart shows the differences in taste and smell in the elderly and the young.

Decrease in nerve-muscle coordination

If you are young, it may not even cross your mind that cutting and eating food depends very much on nerve-muscle coordination. In preparing food for the elderly, it is necessary to be aware that this decline makes eating difficult.

Decrease in chewing and swallowing ability

Half of all Americans have lost all their teeth by age 65. Think how this restricts one's ability to eat. Dentures help, of course, but they do not take away the risk of certain nutrition problems.[35] For instance, the elderly eat fewer fruits and raw vegetables. This means they also get less fiber—which is why the elderly suffer from constipation and why Americans spend so much money ($390 million a year) on laxatives.

Dentistry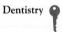

Decrease in digestion and absorption

Another reason elderly people have problems with constipation is loss of activity in the smooth muscles of the intestine. (Intestinal cancer may also be a problem.)

Older people also suffer from intestinal gas, which some seek to alleviate by avoiding such gas-inducing foods as cabbage and legumes. However, much of the problem is actually due to swallowing air along with food.

Information on digestion and absorption of nutrients by the elderly is limited.[36] Absorption of fat, calcium, vitamin C, and vitamin B_{12} may be reduced. Elderly people secrete less hydrochloric acid in the stomach. This may reduce the amount of iron absorbed into the blood.

Decrease in kidney function

The elderly are less able to produce urine (either concentrated or diluted), which makes it more difficult for them to maintain water and electrolyte balance. Older people should avoid diets high in protein and sodium because they put an added strain on the excretory functions of their aging kidneys.

Decrease in heart and respiratory functions

As the heart and respiratory functions decline, they reduce the flow of oxygen to the tissues.

Chronic Diseases and Disabilities Are More Common Among the Elderly

We mentioned that coronary heart disease, cancer, hypertension, obesity, diabetes, and osteoporosis affect adults earlier in life. Because some of these diseases have a high mortality rate in middle age rather than old age, the most common problems among people over 60 are the following:[37]

- Arthritis—affects 38% of the elderly
- Impaired hearing—29%
- Impaired vision—20%
- Hypertension—20%
- Heart conditions—20%

Total Food Intake Is Reduced as People Get Older

Many factors account for the reduced food intake among the elderly—physiological, psychological, and social.

Physiological factors

The loss of sensory abilities and of teeth can translate into a loss of appetite. Limitations in physical abilities (including ability to exercise) can affect one's ability to obtain food. Chronic diseases may require special diets.

Psychological factors

Ignorance or lack of nutrition knowledge, aversion to certain kinds of foods, fad diets, and concerns about the symbolism of food can affect food choices and nutrition. Factors contributing to the symbolism of food include inputs from a person's social, racial, cultural, or religious background.

Retirement frequently means isolation, loss of self-esteem, bitterness, and depression.[38] Loss of a spouse, children, or lifelong friends and eating companions leads to loneliness and increased isolation. This may mean a lack of interest in food, with a resulting reduction in nutrient intake.[39]

Social factors

Some elderly people are isolated from family and friends. Some cannot get to food stores, and others lack the facilities to store and cook food. Others abuse alcohol and drugs. A number of studies show that many old people regard social contact with other people during meals as important as the nutritive value of the food.

Low income from pensions and retirement funds may determine nutrient intake. Many elderly live in old neighborhoods in the inner city. This makes the purchase of food difficult. They frequently cannot take advantage of reduced-price specials

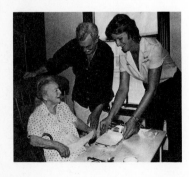

Meals on Wheels provide attractive, nutritious food to many house-bound older Americans.

offered in the larger supermarkets. Shopping may also add to the fears of criminal assault.

Malnutrition in the elderly can be brought about by one or more of the causes shown in Table 14-3.

TABLE 14-3 Causes of Malnutrition in the Elderly

Primary Causes	Secondary Causes
Food not available due to:	**Nutrients not available due to:**
Ignorance	Impaired appetite
Social isolation	Inability to chew food
Physical disability	Malabsorption of nutrients
Mental disturbance	Alcoholism
Certain diseases	Drugs
Poverty	Increased requirements

Most Older People Get Sufficient Nutrients, but Some Risk Factors Exist

Despite all of these hindrances, the elderly in industrialized countries seem to receive adequate amounts of most nutrients. Low intakes of calcium, vitamin C, vitamin B_6, magnesium, and possibly zinc have been observed in a number of surveys. However, osteoporosis (due to insufficient calcium) is the only common clinical manifestation of a serious deficiency. We saw that many of the young and women of childbearing years had problems with iron deficiency. This is not the case with the elderly—one study showed that men and women over 84 years of age had normal hemoglobin levels.[40]

Still, there are some potential nutritional risk factors among older people, as follows[38]:
1. Sometimes less than one meal per day
2. Small amount of milk—less than a half pint (0.28 liter) per day
3. Low intake of vitamin C because of low intake of fruit and vegetables
4. Wasting of food—even that supplied by "meals-on-wheels" services
5. Long periods in the day without food or drink
6. Depression or loneliness
7. Unexpected weight change—a significant gain or loss
8. Shopping difficulties
9. Low income
10. Physical and mental disabilities
11. Alcoholism

Society Can Offer Ways to Help the Elderly Obtain Sufficient Nutrients

In 1972, Title VII of the Older Americans Act established nutrition programs for people 60 years and older. Reorganization of this program in 1978 created Title

Economics

III-C. This dealt with home-delivered meals, congregate dining, nutrition services, and nutrition education for the elderly. Although this federally funded program has had its funding changed over the years, it has been significant in reducing nutritional problems among the elderly.

Services of home-delivered meals for the elderly, which may be paid for by federal or community funds,[37] usually offer a hot meal delivered five days per week. Sometimes a cold meal is added that may be eaten later. However, now there is a problem because more women have entered the work force and are unavailable as volunteer "meals-on-wheels" drivers. Delivery delays can result in micro-organisms creating food-safety problems.

> Decreased lean body mass means less dietary energy is required by the elderly. Loss of sensory discrimination and teeth limit food choices. Loss of tissue function decreases the availability of some nutrients. Mealtime is an important social occasion for many lonely old people.

EXTENDING YOUR LIFE: ARE THERE NUTRITIONAL SECRETS?

Perhaps the answer to this question was given away earlier in the chapter. Nevertheless, it is worth examining it in detail because the mass media continually bring us stories about nutrients and substances—vitamins, amino acids, skin creams, and so on—that are supposed to extend life. Antiaging nostrums are now a $10 billion form of quackery.

Yet, seriously: *are* there dietary ways to extend human life? The answer is not a firm "no" but rather "yes and no":

- *Yes*—proper diets early in life can avoid infant and child mortality and perhaps minimize the risk of killer diseases like heart disease, stroke, and cancer.
- *No*—there is no magic pill to prevent aging.

Common sense and good nutrition rather than so-called magic pills may slow the aging process.

Let us examine some attempts to achieve a slow-down in aging.[41]

Restricting Kcalories Has Helped Laboratory Animals Live Longer

In the late 1930s, Dr. Clive McCoy at Cornell University showed that if young rats were given a reduced intake of a nutritionally balanced diet they lived longer than rats fed the same diet in unlimited amounts. Chronic diseases, including cancers, were less common in animals fed the reduced food intake.

But what human parents are going to restrict significantly the food intake of their young children in hope that the child will live longer? This type of research is, however, useful in forming a better understanding of the complex mechanisms of aging.

Lower body weight results when kcaloric intake is restricted. The question remains as to whether lower body weight alone causes the increase in longevity. Dr. John Beasley of the University of Wisconsin also notes that the extent of physical activity and social status are important factors in longevity.[42] Evidence for this conclusion comes from the higher mortality rate in people with lower social status. These people also tend to have higher body weights. All of the foregoing leads us to conclude that the relationship between body weight and longevity is complex.

Exercise May Make You Healthier but Might Not Extend Your Life

Cultural attitudes toward exercise have undergone many changes. Consider that a century ago exercise was believed to cause damage to the body and to inhibit longevity. It would be difficult to find anyone who believes that today.

Still, the claim that exercise will lead to longevity is not supported by scientific evidence. Indeed, it might require a lifetime of physical activity to effectively prolong life. Of course, that doesn't means that a jog, or even a walk, around the neighborhood is not beneficial. The benefit of exercise is that it will increase kcalorie expenditure in relation to body weight, slow down the loss of bone mineral, and improve the cardiovascular and muscular systems.[43] These benefits will give you a healthier life but not necessarily a longer one.

Antioxidants Should Be Treated with Caution

Many antioxidants have been tested for antiaging properties. They include vitamins A, E, and C, the amino acid cysteine, and the mineral selenium. Also included is the food additive butylated hydroxytoluene (BHT), which is added to food to prevent spoilage. All these compounds make free radicals harmless. Free radicals are produced in certain metabolic reactions in the body. Antioxidants make free radicals harmless. If this does not happen the free radicals cause aging in a tissue by damaging the membranes of cells in the tissue. This may cause individual cells to die, and therefore lead to the aging of the tissue.

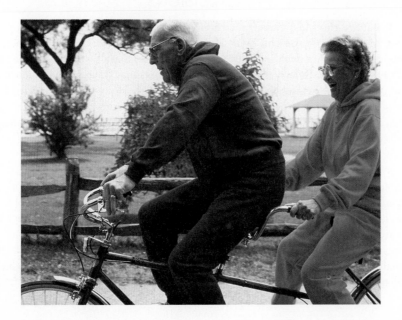

Proper nutrition and adequate exercise are important in ensuring a healthy and enjoyable old age.

Experiments with antioxidants on laboratory animals produced some increase in life expectancy, but the animals also lost body weight. If you choose to take some of the substances mentioned here, be sure to be cautious about limiting your intakes. Large intakes of these vitamins and selenium may cause toxicity.

Some Other Chemicals Have Slowed Aging in Animals

The following chemicals have somewhat slowed the aging process in experimental animals, but there is no evidence that they would do so in humans[41]:

- *Centrophenoxine.* This chemical is thought to prevent the deposition of the age pigment, lipofuscin, in tissues.
- *Levodopa.* High doses of this chemical reduce the symptoms of Parkinson's disease, an age-related disorder of the nervous system.
- *Gerovital-H3.* This supposed antiaging drug, which was first used over 30 years ago in Romania, is worthless.
- *Dehydroepiandrosterone (DHEA).* This is a weak male sex hormone that should not be taken by humans.

Immunologic Interventions Might Provide Insights into Aging

Decay of the immune system may be an important cause of aging. Transplantation of cells and tissues from young into old animals has provided researchers with useful information about the mechanisms of aging, but this is hardly a process that could be done with humans. More promising is the use of chemicals to prevent the aging of the immune system, but work in this area is only beginning.

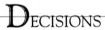

DECISIONS

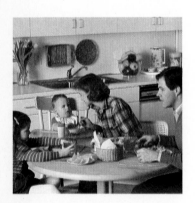

The influence of family is just one of the factors associated with our food choices.

1. What are the Most Important Influences on Food Decisions?
Cost of food, body weight, and concerns about personal health are the most important factors in deciding which foods to buy, no matter what the phase of the family's life cycle. Relatives, friends, and neighbors may have some influence, but family members themselves are the most influential. However, this influence decreases when members live in different parts of the country. Information gleaned from advertisements, food articles, television/radio, and government pamphlets is only moderately important.[44]

2. Will Nutrition Improve the Quality of Aging Skin or Make Nails Stronger?
Older people may be tempted to try collagen-based cosmetics, but they offer no benefits beyond softening and moisturizing of the skin. A significant problem is the large number of medications taken by the elderly, some which interact with nutrients that affect skin quality. For example, penicillamine makes zinc (and copper) unavailable and causes a zinc-deficient dermatitis. Isoniazid, an antibacterial agent used against tuberculosis, interferes with vitamin B_6 and produces a pellagra-like skin rash.[1]

Gelatin is promoted as a means of toughening fingernails, but there is poor clinical evidence for this.[45] Although it is in fact a protein from the bones and hides of cattle, gelatin is a poor-quality protein. Moreover, there is no reason why one should expect it to be absorbed intact and taken straight to the nails; when taken orally, gelatin is broken down like any other protein (just as insulin is) (see Chapter 5).

3. With all the Debate about Diet in Relation to Coronary Heart Disease, What Type of Diet Should I Be Eating?

Nutritionists and medical researchers speak of the "prudent diet," meaning a diet that is low in saturated fat and cholesterol. However, this diet comes in for criticism. "I cannot accept the recommendation that the prudent diet be adopted by everyone over the age of 2 years," says Dr. E.H. Ahrens, Jr. of Rockefeller University. There is, he says, a "paucity of data available to us with regard to risk/benefit ratios of the prudent diet. . . . "[46] Ahrens sees support for this view in the good success rates when diet modification involves the entire family, not just the individual at risk.

Other experts say there are no good ways to screen the population for risks of heart disease.[47] For instance, eggs have been criticized as a source of cholesterol (250 mg of cholesterol in one egg yolk, the amount of cholesterol recommended per day in the "prudent diet"), yet it has been found that eating as many as 3-6 eggs a day increases plasma low-density lipoprotein in only 50% of the population.[48] In addition, studies show that the type of fatty acids found in fish oil are beneficial against coronary heart disease,[49] yet researchers also point out that fish consumption is "also correlated, perhaps unfavorably, with mortality from cancer and other diseases."

One recent large study that looked at evidence over a 20 year period concludes that "the results tend to support the hypothesis that diet is related, albeit weakly, to the development of coronary heart disease."[50] With that the case must rest.

4. If I Decide To Take Calcium Supplements To Prevent Osteoporosis, Do I Risk Getting Kidney Stones?

There is a dilemma here because we have seen some evidence for, and some against, the ability of calcium supplementation to prevent osteoporosis. Some assistance in reaching a decision on the danger of getting kidney stones comes from an endocrinologist (a physician whose specialty is hormones) and a kidney specialist.[51]

Kidney stones are composed of calcium. However, a low intake of calcium may actually be harmful even for someone with kidney stones. People with kidney stones continue to lose a lot of calcium through their urine. Therefore, low calcium intake would only increase calcium loss from bone. The experts recommend treatment with a drug called thiazide rather than reducing dietary calcium intake as the appropriate method of treatment for kidney stones. They suggest also that the cause of the problem should be determined first.

The experts stress that an adequate dietary intake of calcium should provide no problems for people with no kidney stones. Problems with extra calcium supplements should not arise because estrogen treatment rather than additional calcium is the preferred treatment for osteoporosis.

SUMMARY

FOOD INTAKE

Influenced by:
Social isolation
Physiological changes
Psychological reasons

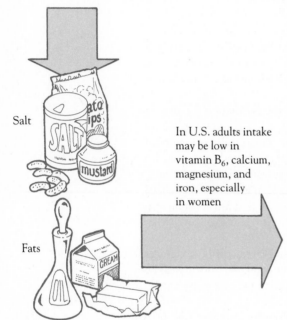

Salt

Fats

Sugar

In U.S. adults intake
may be low in
vitamin B_6, calcium,
magnesium, and
iron, especially
in women

Diet may play a role in:

Coronary heart disease	Osteoporosis
Cancer (breast, lung)	Anemia
Hypertension	Oral health
Diabetes	Other medical
Obesity	problems

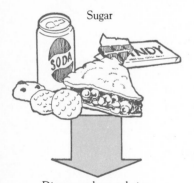

Nutrition implications
in reduced intake:

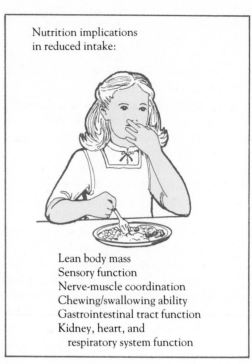

Lean body mass
Sensory function
Nerve-muscle coordination
Chewing/swallowing ability
Gastrointestinal tract function
Kidney, heart, and
   respiratory system function

Factors that may
slow aging:

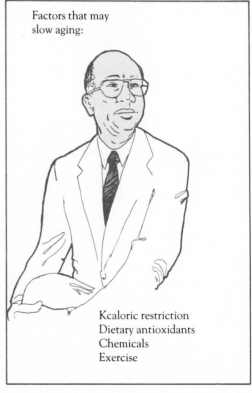

Kcaloric restriction
Dietary antioxidants
Chemicals
Exercise

REFERENCES

1. Morrison, S.D.: Nutrition and longevity. In Present knowledge in nutrition, 5th ed. The Nutrition Foundation, Washington, D.C., p. 646, 1984.

2. Munro, H.N.: Nutrition-related problems of middle age, Proceedings of the Nutrition Society **43**:281, 1984.

3. Peterkin, B.B.: Women's diets: 1977 and 1985, Journal of Nutrition Education **18**:251, 1986.

4. Hegsted, D.M.: Calcium and osteoporosis, Journal of Nutrition **116**:2316, 1986.

5. Herzog, D.B., and others: Frequency of bulimic behaviors and associated social maladjustment in female graduate students, Journal of Psychiatric Research **20**:355, 1986.

6. Marrale, J.C., and others: What some college students eat, Nutrition Today, page 16, January/February, 1986.

7. Herrmann, R.O., and others: Patterns of nutrition concerns and dietary constraints among adult women, Journal of the American Dietetic Association **84**:1478, 1984.

8. Burton, B.T., and Foster, W.R.: Health implications of obesity: an NIH Consensus Development Conference, Journal of the American Dietetic Association **85**:1117, 1985.

9. Weck, E.: The dangerous burden of obesity, FDA Consumer, page 16, November, 1986.

10. Garn, S.M.: Family-line and socioeconomic factors in fatness and obesity, Nutrition Reviews **44**:381, 1986.

11. Wynder, E.L.: Nutrition and cancer, Federation Proceedings **35**:1309, 1976.

12. Kolata, G.: Dietary fat: breast cancer link questioned, Science **235**:436, 1987.

13. Barber, H.R.K.: Osteoporosis: the challenge of protection, Geriatrics **40**:19, April 1985.

14. Gotfredsen, A., and others: Bone changes occurring spontaneously and caused by oestrogen in early postmenopausal women: a local or generalised phenomenon? British Medical Journal **292**:1098, 1986.

15. Sone, M.W., and Smith, R.: Osteoporosis and pregnancy, Journal of the American Medical Association **255**:2495, 1986.

16. Nilas, L., and others: Calcium supplementation and postmenopausal bone loss, British Medical Journal **290**:156, 1985.

17. Simonen, O., and Laitinen, O.: Does fluoridation of drinking-water prevent bone fragility and osteoporosis? Lancet **ii**:432, 1985.

18. Bikle, D.D., and others: Bone disease in alcohol abuse, Annals of Internal Medicine **103**:42, 1985.

19. Beaton, G.H.: Nutritional conditions in Canada, In Nutrition in the 1980s: constraints on our knowledge, N. Selvey, and P.L. White, editors, Alan R. Liss, Inc., New York, p. 221, 1981.

20. Boggs, D.R.: Fate of a ferrous sulfate prescription, American Journal of Medicine **82**:124, 1987.

21. Vessey, M., and others: Chronic inflammatory bowel disease, cigarette smoking, and the use of oral contraceptives: findings in a large cohort study of women of childbearing age, British Medical Journal **292**:1101, 1986.

22. Wallace, R.B., and others: Contrasting diet and body mass among users and nonusers of oral contraceptives and exogenous estrogens: The Lipid Research Clinics Program Prevalence Study, American Journal of Epidemiology, **125**:854, 1987.

23. Anonymous: Nutrition and women's health concerns, Dairy Council Digest **57**:(1) January/February, 1986.

24. Tomelleri, R., and Grunewald, K.K.: Menstrual cycle and food craving in young college women, Journal of the American Medical Association **87**:311, 1987.

25. Fortmann, S.P., and others: Changes in plasma high density lipoprotein cholesterol after changes in cigarette use, American Journal of Epidemiology **124**:706, 1986.

26. LaCroix, A.Z., and others: Coffee consumption and the incidence of coronary heart disease, New England Journal of Medicine **315**:977, 1986.

27. Leon, A.S.: Physical activity levels and coronary heart disease, Medical Clinics of North America **69**:3, 1985.

28. Kline, R.L., and Terry, R.D.: Differences in beliefs about heart disease risk factors between men and women, Journal of the American Dietetic Association **86**:786, 1986.

29. Anonymous: Foods may reduce the risk of lung cancer, Tufts University Diet & Nurition Letter **4**(12), February, 1987.

30. Truswell, A.S.: Diet and hypertension, British Medical Journal **291**:125, 1985.

31. Kaplan, N.M., and Meese, R.B.: The calcium deficiency hypothesis of hypertension: a critique, Annals of Internal Medicine **105**:947, 1986.

32. Stamler, R., and others: Nutritional therapy for high blood pressure, Journal of the American Medical Association **257**:1484, 1987.

33. Kolata, G.: Diabetics should lose weight, and avoid diet fads, Science **235**:163, 1987.

34. Crapo, P., and Vinik, A.I.: Nutrition controversies in diabetes management, Journal of the American Dietetic Association **87**:25, 1987.

35. Wayler, A.H., and others: Masticatory performance and food acceptability in persons with removable partial dentures, full dentures, and intact natural dentition, Journal of Gerontology **39**:284, 1984.

36. Bowman, B.B., and Rosenberg, I.H.: Digestive function and aging, Human Nutrition: Clinical Nutrition **37C**:75, 1983.

37. Schlenker, E.D.: Nutrition and aging, Times Mirror/Mosby College Publishing, St. Louis, p. 11, 1984.

38. Davies, L.: Nutrition and the elderly: identifying those at risk, Proceedings of the Nutrition Society **43**:295, 1984.

39. Institute of Food Technologists' Expert Panel on Food Safety & Nutrition: Nutrition and the elderly, Food Technology, **40**:81, September 1986.

40. Zauber, N.P., and Zauber, A.G.: Hematologic data of healthy very old people, Journal of the American Medical Association **257**:2181, 1987.

41. Schneider, E.L. and Reed, J.D.: Life extensions, New England Journal of Medicine **312**:1159, 1985.

42. Beasley, J.W.: Body weight and longevity, Journal of the American Medical Association **257:**1895, 1987.

43. Lane, N.S., and others: Aging, long-distance running and the development of musculoskeletal disability, American Journal of Medicine **82:**772, 1987.

44. Schafer, R.B., and Keith, P.M.: Influences on food decisions across the family life cycle, Journal of the American Dietetic Association **78:**145, 1981.

45. Worthington-Roberts, B., and Breskin, M.: Fads or facts: a pharmacist's guide to controversial 'nutrition' products, American Pharmacy **NS23:**30, August 1983.

46. Ahrens, E.H., Jr.: The diet-heart question in 1985: has it really been settled? Lancet **i:**1085, 1985.

47. Oliver, M.F.: Strategies for preventing coronary heart disease, Nutrition Reviews **43:**257, 1985.

48. Anonymous: Influence of eggs on plasma lipoproteins, Nutrition Reviews **43:**263, 1985.

49. Glomset, J.A.: Fish, fatty acids, and human health, New England Journal of Medicine **312:**1253, 1985.

50. Kushi, L.H., and others: Diet and 20-year mortality from coronary heart disease: the Ireland-Boston diet-heart study, New England Journal of Medicine **312:**811, 1985.

51. Favus, M.J.: The calcium stone former with osteoporosis, Journal of the American Medical Association **257:**2215, 1987.

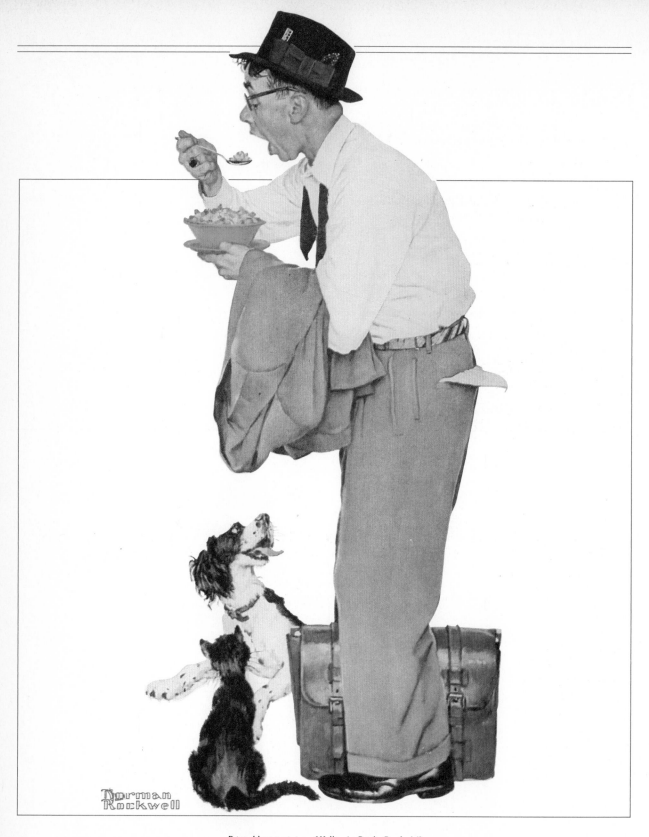

PART IV

Applications and Implications

Is nutrition important in helping your body's response to psychological stress, such as that associated with taking an exam, maintaining a tight schedule, driving in heavy traffic, or dealing with problems with the boss? Probably not, but it is important in the response to physical stress, such as recovery from illness, burns, surgery, and infections. The use of alcohol, tobacco, and other drugs also has a role in our nutritional status. In addition to stress, our lives are affected by changing family structures. In Chapter 15 we will examine the effects on nutrient intake of single parent families, flextime and shift working, eating out, day-care facilities, and homes for the elderly.

We will also explore exciting recent developments, such as the growth in popularity of exotic foods (kiwi fruit, for example) and ethnic foods, and investigate nutritional "rip-offs" such as food faddism and nutritional quackery.

Does government have a role as a provider of food? The importance of various food assistance programs will be examined.

To predict the future we must understand the past. Chapter 16 includes a brief review of the history of nutrition as a science, an examination of the credentials of the people who provide nutrition information, and a look at how they obtain that information.

The future of nutrition is exciting—eating in outer space, nutritional support for artificial heart patients, dietary control of heart disease and some cancers, and the availability of more and better food as a result of genetic engineering, biotechnology, food technology and improved food labeling.

Some nutrition-related issues remain in question: Is it legally and morally justified to remove nutrient support for terminally ill patients? Can certain nutrients control mood and behavior? Can nutrients reverse some effects of environmental contamination? Can we provide enough food to feed a rapidly expanding world population? We will consider these important questions that will need to be answered in the near future.

15

Nutrition and Current Lifestyles

CONNECTIONS

Many people have hectic lifestyles. Is there a way that nutrition can lessen the stress on their nerves? The proper functioning of nerves requires certain vitamins and minerals, but unfortunately it does not follow that these same nutrients will make one feel less stressed.

Other kinds of stress certainly affect the kind of nutrients needed. Physical stress that requires tissue rebuilding, such as the stress suffered from injury, burns, infection, malnutrition, and surgery, involves all nutrients. Drugs and medications, both legal and illegal, affect the absorption and use of nutrients and dietary intake. What, then, can we say about nutrients and nervous stress?

Chapters 12 to 14 described nutrient requirements during the various stages of the life cycle. Chapters 9 and 10 described how the body uses energy. Now let us see how energy use relates to lifestyles, the organization of the modern family, and the pressures to "eat on the run." We will also look at the emotionally charged topic of food faddism.

People's lifestyles are often a series of contradictions. They may worry about stress in their lives, but they may use unproven nutrition remedies to try to counter that stress. They may say they want more nutritious foods, yet junk foods and fast foods are available everywhere. They say they want foods free of chemicals, yet they themselves may take chemicals such as street and over-the-counter drugs. They may want to lose weight, but rush to fad diets despite the fact that there is plenty of free, reliable information on weight loss.

Of course, there is much that is good about nutrition in today's society, and it's not as though one has no choice as to what one should eat. Still, it is important to examine the pressures you may experience and what they mean for nutrition.

Nutritional values of D-Lites food products.

	CALORIES	PROTEIN (g)	PROTEIN*	CARBOHYDRATES (g)	FAT (g)	VITAMIN A*	THIAMINE*	RIBOFLAVIN*	NIACIN*	CALCIUM*	IRON*
D'Lites Sandwiches on Lite Multi-Grain Bun											
Chicken Filet Sandwich (On Multi-Grain Bun)	311	26	40	27	11	•	7	4	29	4	44
1/4 lb[1] Fish Filet Sandwich (On Multi-Grain Bun)	377	23	35	38	14	•	3	2	28	4	76
Hot Ham 'N Cheese Sandwich (On Multi-Grain Bun)	307	29	45	26	9	•	23	7	19	19	38
Little D-Lite (On Multi-Grain Bun)	231	15	23	23	9	•	3	6	17	4	18
1/4 lb[1] D'Lite Burger (On Multi-Grain Bun)	331	25	38	23	16	•	3	11	27	4	25
Double D-Lite (On Multi-Grain Bun)	558	44	67	23	31	•	3	20	47	4	38
D'Lites Nutritious and Lite Products											
Fresh, Domestic Ground Beef (4 oz,[1] 80% lean)	218	19	29	0	15	•	•	9	20	•	13
Litely Breaded Chicken Filet (Average 80g as served)	158	20	31	5	6	•	3	2	21	•	31
Litely Breaded Natural Fish Filet (Average 100g as served)	205	17	26	14	8	•	•	•	21	•	64
Extra-Lean, Specially-Trimmed Ham/3 oz (85g)	133	19	29	1	5	•	20	•	12	•	26
Lite White Sesame-Seed Bun (50g)	122	6	9	23	1	•	3	2	7	4	12
Lite Multi-Grain Bun (50g)	113	6	9	21	1	•	8	3	11	4	13
Lite Cheese (3/4 oz serving)	52	4	11	2	3	4	•	5	•	15	•
Lite Mayonnaise (1 T serving)	40	0	•	1	4	•	•	•	•	•	•
Lite Tartar Sauce (1 T serving)	50	0	•	1	5	•	•	•	•	•	•
Other Delicious D'Lites											
Vegetarian D'Lite (174g)	230	14	21	24	13	5	14	5	10	2	42
Soup D'Lite (265g)	127	12	18	16	3	11	5	6	7	12	85
Baked Potato (Plain, average 10 oz)	264	10	16	69	1	•	19	5	23	3	11
Baked Potato with Cheese & Broccoli (412g)	404	15	23	71	11	•	24	7	35	2	69
Baked Potato with Beef & Mushrooms (454g)	458	14	20	73	13	•	24	11	36	4	71
French Fries (3.25 oz serving)	283	5	7	36	14	•	5	2	5	•	46
French Fries (4 oz serving)	348	6	9	45	17	•	6	2	6	•	57
Potato Skins (Serving of 1 skin average 37g)	89	2	3	10	4	•	•	•	•	3	16
Salad Bar[2] (292g serving)	91	9	14	8	5	23	13	47	7	9	25
Chocolate D'Lite (5.5 oz serving)	204	5	11	41	4	2	•	10	•	19	•

CONDIMENTS, approximate calories per serving:
Ketchup-19, Mustard-5, Pickles-3, Onions-2, Tomatoes-9, Lettuce-2.

TOPPINGS, calories: Sour Cream (2 oz)-112, Cheddar Cheese (1 oz)-108, Bacon Bits (1 oz)-74, Sliced Almonds (½ oz)-35, Granola (1 oz)-128, Coconut (1 oz)-83, *Nutritional data based on tests conducted November 1983 by Law & Company Laboratories, an independent laboratory in Atlanta, Georgia. Nutritional values may vary depending on suppliers and preparation procedures.*

• Contains less than 2% of R.D.A.
* Percent of U.S. R.D.A. (Recommended Daily Allowance)
[1] Approximate Pre-cooked Weight
[2] Add approximately 40 calories per tablespoon of reduced calorie dressing. Salad includes 4 ounces of Iceberg lettuce and ½ ounce each of carrots, tomatoes, cucumbers, cheese, alfalfa sprouts, broccoli, bell pepper, eggs, mushrooms, onions, spinach, Romaine lettuce, and red cabbage. Other items available.

An adequate diet should make nutrient supplements unnecessary even during periods of stress.

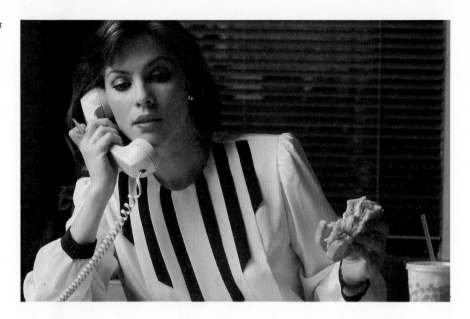

LIFE STRESSES: NOT ALL CURABLE WITH STRESS PILLS

In articles about contemporary lifestyles, the word "stress" invariably appears. TV commercials say the solution to stress is to run out and buy some pills, often pills containing vitamins and minerals.

Is it true that most North Americans lead stressful lives, and will vitamin and mineral supplements help? Let us examine both of these questions.

Stress Means Different Things to Different People

What, exactly, *is* stress? One definition is that stress is "the nonspecific response of the body to any demand." Translated, this means the response of the body to psychological and physical stresses. Psychological stresses include emotional tension and anxiety. Physical stresses include responses to injury, burns, infections, trauma, surgery, and temperature extremes.

If we concentrate on psychological stresses, we see that different people respond in different ways to the same kind of stress. You, for instance, may not be bothered driving 10 miles to work or school every day, even under conditions of heavy traffic, whereas someone else might be very tense at the end of the commute. The same is true of jobs: some people thrive on stressful jobs, but other people can't handle them. In sum, people have different personalities and different ways of coping with stress.

Long-term psychological stresses may be a cause of some diseases such as coronary heart disease, hypertension, and stomach ulcers. It is hypothesized, for instance, that there is a relationship between the so-called type A personality— people who are impatient, highly competitive, and obsessive with deadlines—and coronary heart disease. However, this association can be argued either way: does stress cause the behavior or does the behavior cause the stress? Moreover, people who have type A personalities are also often heavy smokers and coffee drinkers, two factors that may be involved in coronary heart disease.

Nutrient Supplements Do Not Cure Psychological Stress

Vitamin-pill manufacturers have found out that stress is good business for them—that, in fact, what they call the "stress segment" of drugstore vitamin sales is an estimated $75 million a year business. Actually, however, only about a third of all vitamins are sold through drugstores, so you can see what big business stress control has become.[1]

Although vitamin pills seem to sell fastest during times of stress and worry, do they in fact ease tensions? Scientists have much to learn about how the body copes with stress, but it is currently believed that the body's reserves of nutrients are probably sufficient to meet the stresses and strains of daily living.[2] You are also helped by hormonal and metabolic responses that enable you to cope with these regular stresses. Although some psychological disturbances *may* be associated with some nutrient deficiencies—for example, a deficiency of folacin has been linked to certain psychiatric disorders, including depression[3]—there is no evidence that nutrient supplements will correct minor stresses. It is far better to cope with such stresses by eating a healthy diet (Figure 15-1), finding time for relaxation, avoiding caffeine (which can make one nervous), and avoiding salt because of its relationship to hypertension.

People who persist in trying to cure the many stressful irritations in their lives with "stress tablets" should be aware that not all brands are alike in nutrient content (Table 15-1). Moreover, they should be aware that the manufacturers of such pills may try to say that the tablets really are not intended to relieve psychological stress

TABLE 15-1 Contents of Leading Stress Tablets (Percent of USRDA)

	Stresstabs (Lederle)	Stressgard (Miles)	Megastress (Schiff)	Superstress (Thompson)	Ultrastress (Nature's Plus)
Vitamin C	1000%	1000%	1666%	1000%	833%
Vitamin B_1	1000	1000	5000	3333	8333
Vitamin B_2	882	588	4167	2941	7532
Niacin	500	500	500	1250	625
Vitamin B_6	250	250	2500	2500	6250
Vitamin B_{12}	200	200	833	833	8333
Folic Acid	100	100	100	100	100
Pantothenic Acid	200	200	500	2500	2000
Biotin	15	10	—	83	41
Vitamin E	100	100	—	—	—
Vitamin A	—	100	—	100	—
Vitamin D	—	100	—	—	—
Zinc	—	100	—	66	—
Iron	—	100	—	—	111
Copper	—	100	—	—	—

* Data in this column are daily recommended vitamin allowances for persons suffering from severe physical trauma, as given in the National Academy of Sciences publication *Therapeutic Nutrition* (1952).

FIGURE 15-1
Proper eating habits can take care of
some of the stresses in life.

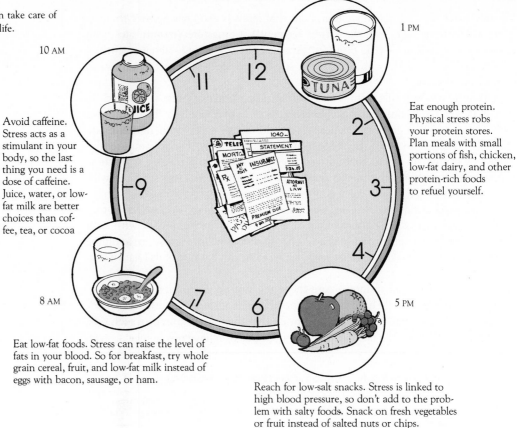

Avoid caffeine.
Stress acts as a
stimulant in your
body, so the last
thing you need is a
dose of caffeine.
Juice, water, or low-
fat milk are better
choices than cof-
fee, tea, or cocoa

Eat enough protein.
Physical stress robs
your protein stores.
Plan meals with small
portions of fish, chicken,
low-fat dairy, and other
protein-rich foods
to refuel yourself.

Eat low-fat foods. Stress can raise the level of
fats in your blood. So for breakfast, try whole
grain cereal, fruit, and low-fat milk instead of
eggs with bacon, sausage, or ham.

Reach for low-salt snacks. Stress is linked to
high blood pressure, so don't add to the problem with salty foods. Snack on fresh vegetables
or fruit instead of salted nuts or chips.

all the while their advertising suggests that they are in fact intended for such use.
For instance, a spokesman for the manufacturer of Stresstabs, one of the best-
selling tablets in the stress-control market, says they don't recommend the product
"for psychological stress. . . . We make it clear in the ads we're talking about
physiological stress, such as alcohol consumption, smoking, pregnancy, drug ther-
apies, and severe malnutrition from hospital stays and surgery." Still, an ad that
talks about "if you're burning the candle at both ends" would seem to be promoting
pills that *are* for the relief of psychological stress.[1] Notice how the word "stress"
is emphasized in the names of all these vitamin supplements.

Physical Stress Is of Greater Concern to Nutritionists

A more legitimate concern is for nutrient intake during physiological stress. Infections, burns, accidents, injuries, and operations may all cause major metabolic
changes involving a breakdown of some body tissues. Infections and burns also
cause increases in body temperature, which cause greater energy loss from the body.
A further complication is a loss of appetite during many kinds of physical stress.

Nutritionists know that the requirement for kcalories, protein, and many vitamins and minerals increases after physical stress (Table 15-2). However, the
amount of the increase in the basal requirements for vitamins and minerals has
not yet been determined.

TABLE 15-2 Effects of Physical Stress on the Basal Requirements for Selected Nutrients

Nutrient	Effect of Stress on Requirement*
Kcalories	Up to 200% increase
Protein	60%-500% increase
Calcium	Increase
Phosphorus	Increase
Zinc	Increase
Vitamin A	Increase
Vitamin C	Increase
Thiamin	Increase
Riboflavin	Increase
Niacin	Increase

*Requirement is defined as the intake below which deficiency symptoms occur.

Psychological stresses, especially those of short-term duration, have little nutritional significance. Physical stresses caused by illness and injury require nutrient replacement for losses during the stress.

DRUG USE AND NUTRIENT UTILIZATION

About 75 million Americans are regular users of over-the-counter and prescription drugs. Drugs, legal and illegal, are everywhere, or so it would seem from the number of ads, articles, and television documentaries that have appeared. People take drugs or pills for the slightest discomfort. Athletes take drugs to improve performance. Street drugs seem to be ever-increasing. Let us take a look at these areas of concern.

Prescription and Nonprescription Drugs Affect Nutrition

Many prescription and over-the-counter drugs may affect the intake of food and the absorption, utilization, and excretion of nutrients.[4] As Table 15-3 indicates, the nutrients most affected by such drugs are certain vitamins and minerals.

Some of the drugs listed in Table 15-3 may be taken for long periods of time. Thus, if any nutrient deficiencies are experienced during the course of drug therapy, a physician should be notified.

Although it's unlikely this would happen to you, you should be aware that some unscrupulous doctors have prescribed illegal drugs and chemicals. One Texas physician was ordered to stop prescribing 2,4-dinitrophenol for weight-loss treatments, a chemical that is a "severe explosion hazard when dry"[5] and that is used not only in explosives but also in photographic developers and weed killers.

Some Athletes Take Drugs To Improve Performance

Some college football players may see nothing wrong (either from a health or ethical point of view) with taking anabolic steroids, but such drugs can produce harmful effects.[6] Athletes taking the steroid Deca-Durabolin, for instance, are generally not aware that certain foods should be avoided when the steroid is taken. These include anchovies, dill pickles, sardines, green olives, canned soups and vegetables, TV dinners, soy sauce, processed cheeses, and salty snack foods such as potato chips and cold cuts—quite a range of foods![4] The side effects of abuse of steroids include edema and irregular heartbeat.

Street Drugs Affect Nutrition

Street drugs, or illegal drugs, have several effects on the user's nutritional status. For one thing, because of their high price, the drugs often drain off funds that might otherwise be spent on nutritious foods. In addition, drugs may decrease one's appetite, change the taste of food, or otherwise affect a person's interest in food. Marijuana, for instance, causes changes in the sense of taste and sense of smell, and marijuana users find themselves craving sweet foods.

TABLE 15-3 **Potential Drug-Nutrient Interactions for Some Commonly Used Drugs**

Drug	Use	Nutrient	Potential Side Effect
Alcohol		Thiamin	Deficiency
		Vitamin B$_6$	Deficiency
		Folate	Deficiency
		Zinc	Deficiency
		Calcium	Deficiency
		Magnesium	Deficiency
Aluminum hydroxide	Antacid	Phosphorus	Binding
		Calcium	Deficiency
Antacids	Antacid	Thiamin	Decreased absorption due to altered gastrointestinal pH
		Calcium	
		Iron	
Anticoagulants	Prevention of blood clots	Vitamin K	Deficiency
Antihistamines	Treatment of allergies and nausea; as local anesthetic		Weight gain
Amphetamines	Appetite suppressant	Low nutrient intake	Appetite suppression Weight loss
Aspirin	Anti-inflammatory	Iron	Anemia
Cathartics	To induce bowel movements	Calcium	Impaired gastrointestinal motility
		Potassium	Impaired gastrointestinal motility

TABLE 15-3 Potential Drug-Nutrient Interactions for Some Commonly Used Drugs—cont'd

Drug	Use	Nutrient	Potential Side Effect
Cholestyramine	Reducing cholesterol	Vitamins A, D, E, K	Deficiencies
Cimetidine	Treatment of ulcers	Vitamin B_{12}	Deficiency
Clofibrate	Reducing cholesterol	Carbohydrate Vitamin B_{12} Carotene Iron	Enzyme inactivation Decreased absorption
Colchicine	Treatment of gout	Vitamin B_{12} Carotene Magnesium	Decreased absorption due to damaged intestinal mucosa
Corticosteroids	Anti-inflammatory	Zinc Calcium Potassium	Damage to intestinal mucosa Gastrointestinal loss
Ethacrynic acid	Diuretic	Sodium	Depletion
Furosemide	Diuretic	Calcium Potassium Sodium	Diuretic effect Depletion
Gentamicin	Antibiotic	Potassium Sodium	Depletion
Levodopa	Treatment of Parkinson's disease	Protein	Competition for absorption
Neomycin	Antibiotic	Fat Protein Sodium Potassium Calcium Iron Vitamin B_{12}	Decreases pancreatic lipase and binds bile salts and interferes with absorption
Penicillamine	Antibiotic	Zinc Vitamin B_6 Sodium	Altered nutrient excretion
Phenobarbital	Sedative; treatment of epilepsy	Vitamin D Folate	Impaired metabolism and utilization
Phenytoin	Treatment of epilepsy	Vitamin D Folate	Impaired metabolism and utilization
Tetracycline	Antibiotic	Protein Iron	Impaired uptake and utilization General malabsorption
Tricyclic antidepressants	Antidepressant		Weight gain due to appetite stimulation

Drug abusers are often alcohol abusers as well, and people who drink a lot of alcohol take in kcalories, but they don't take in nutrients (see Chapter 8). Indeed, many drug users suffer from a variety of illnesses that affect their nutritional status— AIDS, the most recent to be added to a long list, is spread by the use of unsterile hypodermic needles—that affect their nutritional status.

> Whether legal over-the-counter or prescription drugs, steroids used to try to enhance athletic performance, or illegal street drugs, any drugs may interfere with the intake of food and the absorption and utilization of nutrients.

DRINKING AND SMOKING: NUTRITIONAL IMPLICATIONS

Although the health effects of alcohol were described in Chapter 8 and the effects of tobacco have been alluded to here and there, let us next describe the influence on lifestyle on the use of these two drugs.

The Notion that Moderate Drinking Is Healthful Has Not Been Proven

Alcohol abuse costs the United States about $120 billion a year—more than the cost of *any other health problem*. Still, the alcoholic beverage industry has mounted a vigorous campaign to convince us all that moderate drinking is beneficial to health.[7]

What is "moderate drinking?" Some say it means only one or two drinks a day, and it has been suggested that people drinking this amount actually run less risk of coronary heart disease than people who do not drink at all. However, this notion relies on inconclusive evidence concerning alcohol and heart disease. At present, 83% of all men and 95% of all women in the United States drink less than two drinks a day.

Since the 1940s, drinking has become more socially acceptable for women, but alcohol problems have also increased. This is a cause for concern to physicians, according to Dr. Sheila Blume and colleagues.[8]

Cigarette Smoking Is a Global Problem

Tobacco is a profitable crop. In many developing countries, in fact, forests are cleared and food crops neglected in order to plant tobacco plants.[9] This kind of agriculture diverts money not only from food crops but also from improvements in sanitation and housing, all of which affect health.

Smoking, of course, has no health benefits whatsoever. From a nutrition standpoint, for instance, it has an adverse effect on osteoporosis (bone loss) in women after menopause, and physicians are advised to consider a woman's smoking habits when evaluating how much estrogen should be given to prevent osteoporosis.[10] (Along this line, a physician must now ask not how many packs a day a person smokes, but the number of cigarettes per day, since the tobacco industry has recently begun upping the number of cigarettes in a pack from 20 to 25 or 30). Vitamin E is an important protective agent against lung damage in all smokers.[11]

Unfortunately, smoking harms not only smokers but also the nonsmokers who must spend a lot of time with them. For instance, it has been reported that such "passive smoking" may produce low birth weight in babies and early menopause in women, although these results need to be confirmed with further studies.

> Advertising and other marketing techniques make alcohol and cigarette consumption appear attractive. However, the diversion of money and the harmful health effects of these drugs have important nutritional consequences.

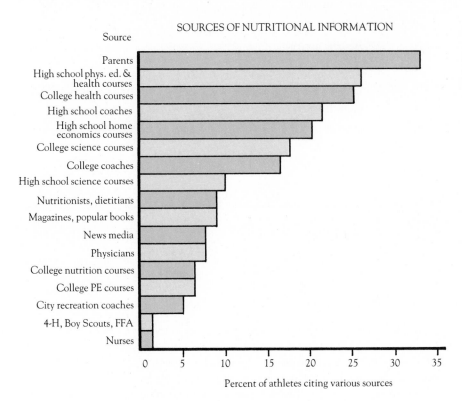

SOURCES OF NUTRITIONAL INFORMATION

FIGURE 15-2
Sources of nutrition information most frequently identified by male college athletes. Sources used most frequently may not always be the best.

Percent of athletes citing various sources

EXERCISE, NUTRITION, AND LIFESTYLES

How knowledgeable are Americans about fitness and nutrition? The answer would seem to be: not very. Most people, for instance, don't know the frequency, duration, and intensity of exercise that is recommended in order to strengthen heart and lungs.[12] Even college athletes often get nutrition information from sources (including parents and coaches) whose reliability is questionable (Figure 15-2).

TABLE 15-4 National Sporting Goods Association 1985 Sports Participation Survey Top 20

Rank	Sport	Number of People (millions)*
1	Swimming	73.3
2	Bicycle riding	50.7
3	Camping (vacation/overnight)	46.4
4	Fishing (fresh water)	43.4
5	Exercise walking	41.5
6	Bowling (tenpin)	35.7
7	Exercising with equipment	32.1
8	Boating (motor)	26.6
9	Running/jogging	26.3
10	Calisthenics	26.1
11	Aerobic exercising	23.9
12	Billiards/pool	23
13	Hunting/shooting	22
14	Softball	21.6
15	Hiking	21.1
16	Volleyball	20.1
17	Basketball	19.5
18	Tennis	19
19	Golf	18.5
20	Roller skating	18.1

*Number of people, aged 7 and older, who participated more than once during the year. For swimming, bicycling, exercise walking, exercising with equipment, running/jogging, calisthenics, and aerobics, participation is defined as engaging in the activity six times or more within the year.

Still Americans are active participants in sports activities (Table 15-4). Moreover, many Americans—women in particular—are doing more walking instead of driving, climbing stairs instead of taking elevators, and parking far away and deliberately walking to their destinations (Figure 15-3). Even children are apparently exercising more: "In living rooms, in church basements, in high-profile franchise outlets with trampolines and balance beams," says one report, "toddlers across America are stretching, climbing, rolling, and running to the music."[13] Is such exercise valuable? Perhaps the answer is, as one physician states, that "children do not need structured exercise as much as they need the stimulus to turn off the television and do the things that kids have always done—play."[13]

The modern obsession with exercise and body weight has produced some unconventional eating patterns. For example, whether a vegetarian diet actually improves athletic performance is unknown, although a study in Israel shows no difference in aerobic or anaerobic capacities of vegetarian men and women compared to nonvegetarians.[14] An unfortunate result of the preoccupation with body weight, as you have seen, is anorexia nervosa. As Table 15-5 shows, many female athletes are now showing characteristics similar to those seen in anorexics, including anemia, slow heart rates (bradycardia), and low blood pressure (hypotension).

Americans do not seem to have much knowledge of exercise and diet, despite participation in many sports. Exercise programs for toddlers are of questionable value. Vegetarianism does not seem to affect athletic performance. Some female athletes show symptoms similar to those of anorexia nervosa.

HOW TODAY'S FAMILY LIFESTYLES AFFECT NUTRIENT INTAKE

Your family's lifestyle is probably quite a bit different from that your parents grew up with. Not only is the family structure itself changing, but more people are eating out and the entire environment of food and eating is different. Let us consider some of these changes.

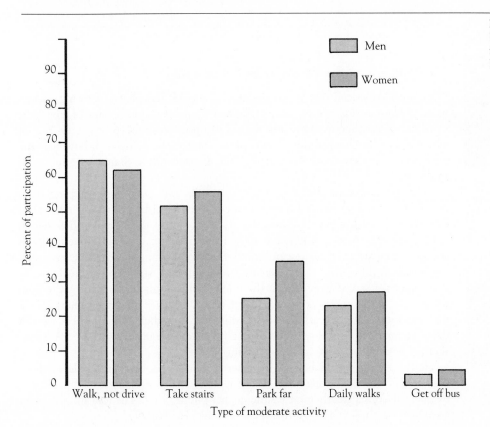

FIGURE 15-3
Increased participation in different forms of physical activity leads to healthier lives.

TABLE 15-5 The Anorectic Versus the Athletic Female

Shared Features

- Dietary faddism
- Controlled calorie consumption
- Specific carbohydrate avoidance
- Low bodyweight

- Slow heart rate and low blood pressure
- Increased physical activity
- No or few menstrual periods
- Anemia (may or may not be present)

Distinguishing Features

Athletic:

- Purposeful training
- Increased exercise tolerance
- Good muscular development
- Accurate body image
- Body fat level within defined normal range
- Increased plasma volume
- Increased O_2 extraction from blood
- Efficient energy metabolism
- Increased HDL_2 (high-density lipoprotein)

Anorectic:

- Aimless physical activity
- Poor or decreasing exercise performance
- Poor muscular development
- Flawed body image (believes herself to be overweight)
- Body fat level below normal range
- Electrolyte abnormalities if abusing laxatives and/or diuretics
- Cold intolerance
- Dry skin
- Irregular heartbeat
- Downy hair covering the body
- White blood cell dysfunction

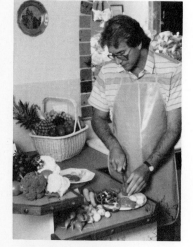

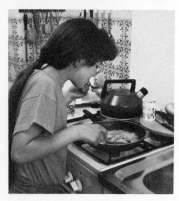

Current lifestyles can cause significant changes in who prepares the food in many households.

The Structure of the Family is Different Today

The North American family has undergone a good deal of restructuring—more working mothers, more single parents, more financial pressures because of job losses, more use of flextime in the work place—so nutritionists have begun to look at whether this has changed nutrition patterns. More data are needed; however, the available evidence to date suggests that the effect is not as dramatic as might be supposed.

Single-person households and larger households still spend the same proportion of the home food dollar on different types of food, according to recent research.[15] For instance, both groups allocate slightly over half of the home food dollar to nonconvenience foods, which contribute more nutrients than convenience foods do. In a comparison of adolescent children of nonworking mothers, it was found there was no difference in the percentage of children who skipped breakfast, in the number of snacks eaten, or in the number of evening meals eaten away from home.[16] In addition, there were few differences between the two groups in the nutrient intake at the various meals. Moreover, whether their mothers worked days, evenings, or nights seemed to have no effect on nutrient intake.[17] All this, then, should be welcome news to working mothers.

However, busy work schedules often mean people miss breakfast. Indeed, about a quarter of the adult population in the United States regularly skips breakfast.[18] Regular breakfasts greatly increase the quality of one's diet. The four most popular breakfasts for those who take this meal on a regular basis are:

- Eggs, bread, and coffee
- Ready-to-eat cereal with milk
- Coffee and bread
- Eggs, bread, and milk

More People are Eating Out

Busy people also seem to eat out more, but this does not mean they are not concerned about nutrition. According to the National Restaurant Association, 77% of consumers say they are more interested in nutrition than they were a year previously.[19]

The primary concerns about food of people eating in restaurants have been categorized as follows:

- 32%—nutrition and fitness
- 22%—conventional tastes
- 22%—convenience
- 20%—dieting

Let us examine those in the first category: what is the buying behavior of the consumer interested in nutrition? These seem to fall into five categories:

- Restrictive dieters
- Those requiring diet modifications because of health concerns
- Those interested in fitness and long-term health benefits
- The elderly
- Vegetarians

The restaurant industry is trying to meet the demands of the consumer for "healthy" food by making menu changes that feature fresher, lighter foods, by changing food preparation methods, by providing nutrition information, and by making use of special promotions regarding health, diet, and fitness.[19]

Eating out is also done in increasing numbers by people visiting foreign countries as tourists. Studies show that the majority of tourists continue to eat foreign dishes upon their return home.

Of course, your work or studies don't necessarily *require* you to eat lunch in a restaurant. Many people bring their own lunch to work, and the advantages are that you can not only eat nutritiously but also eat whatever *you* feel like eating. If you are able to "brown-bag" it, you might want to consider some of the food and drink items shown in Table 15-6 when you pack your lunch.

When packing lunches, keep the following rules in mind:

- Keep work areas clean
- Use foods that are thoroughly cooked and unlikely to spoil if they are unrefrigerated for a time
- Make a balanced meal with nutritious foods that provide more kcalories
- Keep them cool as long as possible

The foregoing advice was offered by Annabel Hecht of the public affairs staff of the Food and Drug Administration.[20]

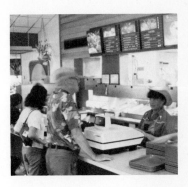

Fast-food outlets in the United States now number over 140,000; annual sales, over $34 billion.

Tourism usually expands our eating horizons.

Food likely to spoil should not be kept unrefrigerated for more than 2 to 3 hours at 60°-125° F. (Room temperature is 65°-75° F.)

Brown-bagging can be nutritious, convenient, economical, and palatable.

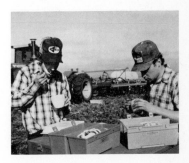

TABLE 15-6 Putting a Little Punch in Your Lunch

Almost anything goes when it comes to lunch, as long as one item is selected from each of the four basic food groups and no item is excessive in sugar, fat, or sodium. Here are a few sample menus; mix them up or add any of your family favorites and enjoy.

Chopped egg on whole-wheat bread	Apples stuffed with peanut butter
Celery and carrot sticks	Sesame crackers
Nuts and raisins	Green salad (lettuce, green pepper, cucumber)
Milk	Unsalted sunflower seeds
Peanut butter mixed with chopped dried fruit or walnuts on zucchini bread	Milk
Broccoli florets	Lettuce wrapped around sliced turkey
Yogurt with fruit	Sliced, buttered Boston brown bread
Vegetable juice	Banana and plain yogurt
Ham and cheese cubes	Fruit juice
Bran muffin	Chicken noodle soup
Fresh tomato slices	Swiss cheese sandwich on rye bread
Berries	Three-bean salad
Oatmeal cookies	Fruit bars
Milk	Milk

The Young and the Elderly Have Different Eating Requirements

Over 8 million women with children under 6 years of age are in the work force in the United States. More than half of these children are cared for outside the home. Indeed, most mothers who work full time place their children in full-time day-care programs.

Concerned about the nutritional adequacy and quality of food provided in day-care programs, the American Dietetic Association has recommended the following specific standards[21]:

- *Food-service and meal plans:* Meals and snacks should be nutritious and day-care personnel should consider the child's cultural food patterns. A child in a part-day program (4 to 8 hours) should receive a quantity of food that fulfills at least one third of daily nutrition needs. A child in a full-day program (8 hours or more) should receive food that fulfills at least one half to two thirds of the day's nutritional needs. Programs that serve three meals a day should meet 100% of the RDA.
- *Emotional climate:* The staff should maintain a positive emotional climate at mealtimes, so that children may accept and enjoy their food.
- *Physical environment:* Chairs, tables, and eating utensils should be appropriate for the age, size, and developmental level of the children being served, with special provisions made to meet the needs of the handicapped.
- *Nutrition education:* Day-care providers should develop and implement a nutrition-education plan that will help children, parents, families, and people caring for the children make informed decisions about issues affecting their health.
- *Nutrition consultation and guidance:* A registered dietitian or qualified nutritionist should regularly consult with the day-care provider. Guidance is es-

pecially needed in nutrition assessment, including growth and development of each child, as early as possible after the child is placed in the day-care program.

- *Compliance with state and local regulations:* Day-care centers must comply with local and state regulations related to sanitation matters and to the preparation, safety, and wholesomeness of food.

Considering the large number of children now in day-care programs, these are important guidelines. Disturbing reports regularly appear in medical journals about the occurrence of diarrheal diseases in such centers, often because the staff members who change the infants' diapers are the same people who prepare food.[22]

At the other end of the life cycle is the equally important task of feeding the elderly. Group meals in a community setting are an effective way of dealing with the health and nutrition problems of noninstitutionalized older Americans, especially the elderly poor. Unfortunately, however, the people managing such programs sometimes don't have the same ideas about quality that their participants expect.[23]

Of course it goes without saying that institutionalized elderly should have the best nutrition possible. However, a recent study showed that over half of the people in a nursing home suffered from protein-calorie malnutrition.[24] This is totally unacceptable.

> Changes in the structure of the family and the fact that more mothers work outside the home seem to have had minimal effects on children's patterns of nutrient intake. Many people, children and adults, miss breakfast. Restaurants are changing their menus to respond to changing food preferences. Food-service providers in children's day-care programs and in programs for the elderly need to follow nutrition guidelines if health problems are to be avoided.

EATING THE "MODERN WAY"

Food expenditures as a percentage of disposable income have steadily declined since the 1960s (Figure 15-4). This means that people have more money available to buy nutritious foods, to experiment with new and exotic foods, and, unfortunately, to pursue food fads. Let us examine some of the new patterns of eating.

It Is Possible to Eat Nutritiously Even if You Live a Fast-Paced Life

You may be one of those who eats in restaurants a lot—many people do. If so, you should be aware of the following (Figure 15-5):

- Chinese food is high in sodium.
- Mexican food and French food are high in fat.
- Look for fresh ingredients, cooked lightly, with little sauce; this will maximize your nutrient intake while minimizing your energy intake.
- Consider eating fish instead of meat. Meat has had adverse publicity in relation to coronary heart disease, whereas omega-3 fatty acids found in fish have had favorable effects in relation to coronary heart disease.

FIGURE 15-4
Food expenditure as a percentage of disposable personal income. Notice that more disposable income is available than in 1956.

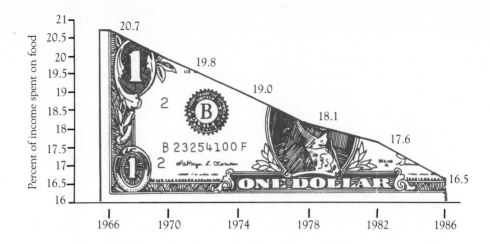

Not all fast foods are hazardous. Many restaurant chains have introduced salad bars (watch it, though, on those high-kcalorie salad dressings) and have tried to scale back the amount of sodium and fat in their offerings. Nutritive values for fast food are given in Appendix O.

Even if you live life on the run, however, it is not necessary to eat in restaurants. Here are some tips:

- *Inexpensive food:* If you are on a budget, you should know that the most nutritious foods are the least expensive. Whole grains, fresh fruits, and vegetables usually come without fancy packaging and with no processing, two factors that make food expensive.
- *Shop near the walls:* In the supermarket, avoid the center aisles, where the canned, processed, and frozen foods are usually kept. Shop the aisles along the walls, where the fresh foods are usually displayed.
- *Freeze casserole portions:* If you are single, it's worthwhile cooking a casserole, then freezing individual servings for later meals.
- *Avoid airline food:* If you travel a lot, take fresh fruit or vegetables and a home-made sandwich with you. Airline food is usually high in fat, sugar, and sodium.
- *Slow down:* Eating is one of life's greatest pleasures. If you're too busy to eat, slow down and take time for a banana or other fresh fruit or a piece of toast (easy on the butter or margarine). If you don't, skipping meals will slow you down anyway.

People are Choosing More Exotic, Natural, and Ethnic Foods

In most supermarkets, the range of foods has increased in recent years. Depending on where you live, you may now be able to buy fresh kiwi fruit, okra, Chinese mustard cabbage, snow peas, and other contributors to what you might call "the fruit and vegetable revolution." Once yogurt was considered pretty unusual, but now there are all kinds of exotic yogurts and cultured milks.[25]

Of course the food industry is well aware of the nation's changing palate and has noticed that the sales volume of certain products is impressive when sodium and sugar are reduced (Table 15-7). You may expect to see many more foods using natural ingredients, more vitamin fortification, fewer preservatives and kcalories, and lower saturated fat, sodium and cholesterol contents.

Regional ethnic differences still exist, as Figure 15-6 shows. On the Pacific coast, Hispanic and Asian foods are popular. In the mid-Atlantic states, veal and pasta dishes are popular, reflecting the Italian influence in that area.

Are You Really Using Your Refrigerator?

Nutritionists at Oregon State University found the average household threw away $150 worth of food every year.[26] Of course, some people threw away nothing, but others discarded as much as $1689 worth of food in a year!

The major reasons people threw out food were:

- Poor quality of fruits and vegetables—which means they may not have stored them at the right temperature or stored them over too long a time.
- Meat, fish, and poultry were stored too long—which means they may not have known how to get the most out of their refrigerators.
- Leftovers were not used for combination dishes—probably because people didn't take time to do so or didn't exercise their imagination.
- Plate waste for cereals and dairy products was not used—which may mean the parent wasn't saying, "Clean your plate or else!"

FIGURE 15-5
Eating properly is possible with any lifestyle.

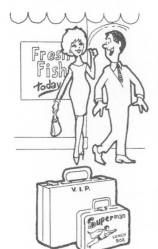

If you eat out often, choose your restaurants wisely. Most French and Mexican food is high-fat; Chinese is high-salt. Look for fresh ingredients, cooked lightly, with little sauce.

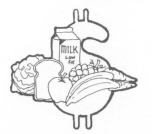

If you travel frequently, take along a home-made sandwich and fresh fruit whenever you can. Airline food is highly processed and loaded with fat, sugar, and salt.

If you're on a budget, good news. The foods that are most nutritious—whole grains, fresh vegetables—are least expensive. It's the processed foods that boost your bill.

If you're single, take the time to cook a fresh casserole and freeze individual servings. You'll waste less time in fast-food lines and be eating less fat and salt, and more fiber.

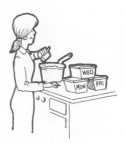

If you're a homemaker, shop the perimeter of the supermarket first, where fresh foods are on display. Avoid the center aisles, where canned, frozen, and processed foods are shelved.

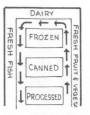

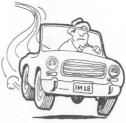

If you're too busy to eat...Wait a minute, no one's too busy to eat. Try "quick foods" like toast, a bean taco, or a fruit frappe. Skipping meals drains your energy and concentration.

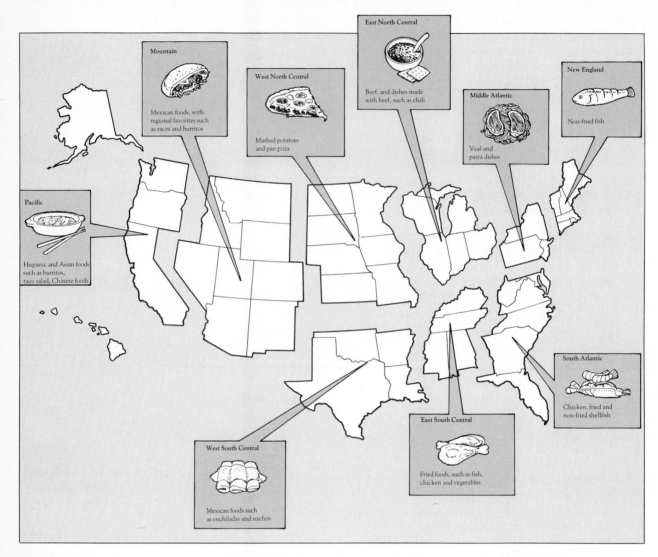

FIGURE 15-6
Regional food preferences, United States.

Some food is thrown away for the wrong reasons.

Nearly one third of the food thrown away was considered by the householder to be unsafe to eat. Young people threw away food mainly because it did not look good. More than half of the older people studied said they discarded food because of food storage reasons. The bottom line seems to be that, even with today's refrigerators and freezers, people are unable to evaluate how safe their stored food is.

With your knowledge of food and nutrition, you can pick your way successfully through the many choices in grocery shopping and restaurants. The popularity of exotic, natural, and ethnic foods will increase. People throw away a lot of food at home because of ignorance about food safety.

FOOD FADDISM: FED BY FOOD FEARS

Food faddism—also known as *food quackery* and *nutrition cultism*—usually refers to unsubstantiated ideas and practices about nutrition.[27] Modern food faddism arose from the movement in the 19th century toward health reform. In this movement, diet was considered essential to a disease-free life and was felt to determine one's mental health, behavior, intelligence, sexual passion, spirituality, and other important aspects of living. In the form it takes today, food faddism usually overestimates the beneficial effects of organic foods, health foods, and raw foods and underestimates the nutritive value of white flour and sugar.

How do you recognize a food faddist or quack? There are several guidelines:

- *Spurious degrees:* Nutrition quacks may have simply bought their college diplomas from "diploma mills." The scrutiny with which such institutions pass on their applicants is so rigorous that in one instance a poodle from New York and a basset hound from California received degrees as "nutrition counselors"—simply because their owners each sent the degree mill $50.[28] A doctorate in nutrition can be obtained from such establishments for $4000.
- *Composition of advisory board:* Sellers of nutritional supplements have often listed some impressive names on their advisory boards. In the 1980s, a number of reputable scientists resigned from such boards when they discovered the nature of the enterprise they were advising.[29]
- *Use of invalid tests:* Nutrition quacks use invalid tests to try to convince people of their special nutrition needs—for example, hair analysis (discussed earlier), cytotoxic testing for food allergies, computerized analyses that are impressive but misleading, and analysis of crystal patterns formed by a person's saliva.
- *Questionable prescriptions:* Quacks often claim they are using food as medicine, and therefore prescribe megadoses of vitamins and minerals, herbs, enzymes,

TABLE 15-7 New Products Analysis—Manufacturers' Sales of Selected Reduced Sodium and Sugar Foods (in millions of dollars)

	1982	1986[E]	1995[P]
Soft drinks	$1,871	$3,486	$11,378
Cereal	535	898	2,426
Candy and gum	278	625	1,638
Sugar substitutes	101	307	683
Canned fruit	124	251	610
Canned vegetables	56	151	478
Hot cocoa mixes	12	93	193
Sauces and dressings	42	83	232
Spreads and syrups	59	80	108
Meats and seafoods	27	58	265
Salt substitutes	36	30	50

E, estimate; P, projection.

or extracts from the brain and from glands such as the pancreas and adrenals. All of these treatments are useless or dangerous.

- *Something to sell:* Nutrition quacks always have something to sell. Often the product is sold by direct sales to the public or through magazine advertisements, rather than through a physician or pharmacy. The cost of the product is often high—not just in the consumer's wasted dollars but also in a depressing list of other things: malnutrition, toxic overdoses, nutritional imbalances, delay or neglect in getting proper medical care, unnecessary anxiety about false diagnoses, and conversion of the person to deviant views about health and medical care.[28]

Food faddism and nutritional quackery can be medically harmful and economically wasteful. Nutrition quacks frequently have bogus qualifications.

GOVERNMENT AND FEEDING THE NEEDY

Economics

Does the U.S. government have the obligation to feed the hungry in this country? That is a matter of debate between people of different political beliefs, and that debate won't be settled here. It has been discovered, however, that people attending church-sponsored soup kitchens—people who were forced to this choice because of finding themselves unemployed in an economic recession—are usually deficient in several nutrients.[30] That is, the soup-kitchen meals were not adequate to meet all their nutrient requirements.

But such privately sponsored operations are not the only ways of feeding the needy. Food-assistance programs administered by the U.S. Department of Agriculture amount to about $20 billion a year. Nearly 20 million people are on food stamps. About 3.3 million people participate in the Food Program for Women, Infants and Children (WIC).

The WIC Program Shows How Government Food-Assistance Programs Work

A description of the WIC program shows how government food-assistance programs are administered. The WIC program was introduced in 1972 because Congress realized the importance of proper nutrition and health care during pregnancy and during the child's early development. WIC is available to pregnant and lactating women and to infants and children whose health may be at risk because of nutritional needs and low income. WIC provides nutritional education and supplemental foods and encourages regular health care.

Eligibility requirements are as follows:

- *Who is eligible:* Pregnant women, breast-feeding women up to 12 months postpartum, and infants or children up to age 5.
- *Nutritional need:* Candidates must undergo a nutritional evaluation that includes measurements of height and weight, hemoglobin/hematocrit analysis, and diet and medical history.
- *Income:* Less than 185% of current poverty guidelines.

Other Government Programs Are Available for Children and the Elderly

Other food programs administered by the Department of Agriculture are the School Lunch and Breakfast programs and the Child Care Food Program. This is for children in both day-care centers and day-care homes.

The elderly also have specific nutrition needs requiring government assistance. For many older Americans, income, transportation, storage and preparation of food, health and dental matters, and family problems are all nutrition-related problems. For example, increased mobility has scattered many families throughout the country so that some elderly people suffer social isolation and loneliness. Elderly people have difficulty meeting RDA values for certain nutrients, especially calcium, magnesium, and vitamin B_6.

One form of governmental assistance designed to address some of these problems is the Nutrition Program for Older Americans (Title III). This program provides lunches for a small fee (and often the fee is optional) in a congregate-dining setting. Hot meals are served to the elderly in community halls, churches, schools, and other centers. The assistance not only gives old people nutritious meals that meet one third of their RDAs but also provides them with social opportunities to meet other people.

> About 20 million Americans are on food stamps. Nutrition-support programs for the young include the Food Program for Women, Infants and Children, the School Lunch and Breakfast programs, and the Child Care Food Program. The Nutrition Program for Older Americans (Title III) is designed to assist the elderly.

Decisions

1. Does AIDS Have a Nutrition Connection?

Some initial research hinted that there might be a nutrition connection with acquired immune deficiency syndrome (AIDS). African AIDS patients showed chronic diarrhea, fever, and weight loss, and the disorder was initially called "slim disease." However, it is now believed that nutrition has no connection as a cause of AIDS but nutrition problems can be consequences of the disease.

Because of the chronic diarrhea, nutrient malabsorption is common in AIDS patients.[31] In particular, zinc is one nutrient that such patients do not absorb well—an especially unfortunate occurrence because zinc plays a major role in various immune functions. Clearly, the zinc deficiency puts the already impaired immune system in even worse shape.

2. How Can I Decide What Food Is Best to Eat at Work?

According to one study, people said they chose the food they ate at work according to the following criteria and in the following ranking: sensory appeal, health value, expediency, and the influence of others.[32] Much of the food served around work places is very seductive, but it is sweet and salty and contains plenty of hidden fat. Thus, if the main reason people make their food choices is sensory appeal, you might do well to take a nutritious brown-bag lunch that you make yourself (and you can make it early in the morning when perhaps your senses aren't fully awake yet).

Changing food habits means modifying one's taste. Men seem to be more consistent than women in deciding what they want to eat.

3. Are There Any Precautions I Should Take Before Buying Imported Ethnic Foods?

The increased popularity of ethnic food has added wonderful possibilities for diversity to the North American diet. However, until recently, ethnic food stores usually were not given much attention by local health inspectors,[33] and there is evidence that product defects were unacceptably high, posing possible hazards to consumers.

When shopping for ethnic foods (or any foods), watch for the following defects:

- Swollen, leaky, rusty, or otherwise damaged containers
- Moldy and decomposed foods
- Dry foods in plastic bags contaminated by insects and vermin
- Use of undeclared food additives
- Products short of the stated weight
- Products labeled only in the language of the country from which they were shipped

Foods sold in ethnic food stores may have been prepared under conditions not acceptable in North America. Moreover, they may be outdated because of slow sales turnover. One survey of ethnic food stores found that most unsafe food was in cans and glass jars and that some containers had discolored, moldy, or partly decomposed food.[33]

With all this, we don't mean to scare you off of ethnic foods. Using your knowledge of food safety learned from this book, feel free to try any ethnic and exotic foods that capture your fancy. And *bon appetite!*

SUMMARY

IMPACT OF CURRENT LIFESTYLES ON NUTRITION

Family structure:
Single parent, flex time
Limited evidence
suggests little impact

Eating away from home:
Increased "brown bagging"
Day care, and nursing homes—
nutrition problems sometimes
"Eating on the run"—
better nutrition choices
now ethnic, natural,
exotic foods
popular

Stress: are supplements needed?
Physical, maybe
Psychological, no

Government feeding programs:
Food stamps,
school lunch
and breakfasts,
nutrition
programs for elderly

Drugs:
Interfere with
nutrient use
Money spent on
drugs instead of
foods

Alcohol, cigarettes:
Messages from industry
Increased intakes by
women cause nutrition
problems

Food faddism:
Misleading
nutrition
information

Exercise:
Increased interest,
but nation not fully fit yet

REFERENCES

1. Liebman, B.: Stress pills: burning the consumer at both ends. Nutrition Action **12:**1, April 1985.

2. Berdanier, C.D.: The many faces of stress. Nutrition Today, p. 12, March-April 1987.

3. Abou-Saleh, M.T., and Coppen, A.: The biology of folate in depression: implications for nutritional hypotheses of the psychoses. Journal of Psychiatric Research **20:**91, 1986.

4. Morgan, B.L.G.: The food and drug interaction guide. Simon & Schuster, Inc., New York, p. 13, 1986.

5. Hecht, A.: Diet drug danger déjà vu. FDA Consumer, p. 22, February 1987.

6. Cowart, V.: Steroids in sports: after four decades, time to return these genies to the bottle? Journal of the American Medical Association **257:**421, 1987.

7. Blume, S., and others: The risks of moderate drinking. Journal of the American Medical Association **256:**3213, 1986.

8. Blume, S.B.: Women and alcohol. Journal of the American Medical Association **256:**1467, 1986.

9. The cost of smoking. Lancet **i:**514, 1986.

10. Jensen, J., and others: Cigarette smoking, serum estrogens, and bone loss during hormone-replacement therapy early after menopause. New England Journal of Medicine **313:**973, 1985.

11. Pacht, E.R., and others: Deficiency of vitamin E in the alveolar fluid of cigarette smokers. Journal of Clinical Investigation **77:**789, 1986.

12. Cinque, C.: Are Americans fit? Survey data conflict. Physician and Sportsmedicine **14:**24, November 1986.

13. Ward, A.: Born to jog: exercise programs for preschoolers. Physician and Sportsmedicine **14:**163, December 1986.

14. Hanne, N., and others: Physical fitness, anthropometric and metabolic parameters in vegetarian athletes. Journal of Sports Medicine **26:**180, 1986.

15. Richardson, S., and others: Convenience and nonconvenience food use in single-person and multi-person households. Home Economics Research Journal **14:**11, 1985.

16. Skinner, J.D., and others: Relationship between mother's employment and nutritional quality of adolescents' diets. Home Economics Research Journal **13:**218, 1985.

17. Pearson, J.M., and others: Food use in households in three work-shift categories. Home Economic Research Journal **13:**400, 1985.

18. Morgan, K.J., and others: The role of breakfast in diet adequacy of the U.S. adult population. Journal of the American College of Nutrition **5:**551, 1986.

19. Carlson, B.L., and Tabacchi, M.H.: Meeting consumer nutrition information needs in restaurants. Journal of Nutrition Education **18:**211, 1986.

20. Hecht, A.: Healthy lunches for the brown bag set. FDA Consumer, p. 8, September 1986.

21. Position of the American Dietetic Association: nutrition standards in day-care programs for children. Journal of the American Dietetic Association **87:**503, 1987.

22. Sullivan, P., and others: Longitudinal study of occurrence of diarrheal disease in day care centers. American Journal of Public Health **74:**987, 1984.

23. Harris, L.J., and others: Comparing participants' and managers' perception of service in a congregate meals program. Journal of the American Dietetic Association **87:**190, 1987.

24. Pinchcofsky-Devin, G.D., and Kaminski, M.V.: Incidence of protein calorie malnutrition in the nursing home population. Journal of the American College of Nutrition **6:**109, 1987.

25. Zamula, E.: Beyond yogurt: milking the public's taste for exotic health foods. FDA Consumer, p. 12, November 1986.

26. Van Garde, S.J., and Woodburn, M.J.: Food discard practices of householders. Journal of the American Dietetic Association **87:**322, 1987.

27. Jarvis, W.T.: Food faddism, cultism, and quackery. Annual Review of Nutrition **3:**35, 1983.

28. Jarvis, W.T.: Recognizing today's nutrition quacks. Nutrition and the M.D. **11:**1, December 1985.

29. Stare, F.J.: Marketing a nutritional "revolutionary breakthrough": trading on names. New England Journal of Medicine **315:**971, 1986.

30. Laven, G.T., and Brown, K.C.: Nutritional status of men attending a soup kitchen: a pilot study. American Journal of Public Health **75:**875, 1985.

31. Malabsorption in AIDS. Nutrition and the M.D. **12:**1, February 1986.

32. Dalton, S.S., and others: Worksite food choices: an investigation of intended and actual selections. Journal of Nutrition Education **18:**182, 1986.

33. Lecos, C.W.: Imported ethnic foods: exotic fare but buyer beware. FDA Consumer, p. 24, December 1986/January 1987.

16   Nutrition and the Future

CONNECTIONS

The previous chapters described 46 essential nutrients, hundreds of chemicals in every meal, different nutrient requirements during one's life, different methods of preserving and preparing food, and different social and cultural attitudes toward food. With this background, perhaps you can understand why some questions about nutrition are difficult to answer.

One reason is the explosive growth of nutrition knowledge in this century, knowledge constantly refined by new discoveries. Another reason is the different attitudes people have toward food. Yet another reason is the commercial manipulation of information of nutrition terms—for instance, in advertising nutrition supplements that may not be beneficial and may even be harmful.

This final chapter will consider some of the exciting challenges that lie ahead: nutrition requirements for space exploration and for artificial heart recipients, the ethics of withholding nutrient support for terminally ill patients, the use of biotechnology and genetic engineering to provide more nutritious food.

Let us state an obvious but often overlooked point—or rather, let's have Reay Tannahill state it: "Food is not only inseparable from the history of mankind but essential to it. Without food there would be no history, no mankind."

With something as important as food, then, somehow you would expect that we would know more about it. But, as Harold Orlans points out, "Knowledge of the nation's health and nutritional status is dated, uncertain, incomplete, and complex, whereas politicians demand simplicity, and administrators, practicability; and everyone wants more and better information."

So where do we go from here? The answer, in Elizabeth Whelan's words: "Serve up scientific facts, not placebos." Ultimately, if nutritionists are to please the politicians, administrators, and everyone else, they must deal with truths, not wishful thinking.

THE LESSONS OF NUTRITION HISTORY

Meals have been eaten on the moon,[1] yet hunger remains common on earth. Nutrient deficiencies once were the preponderant concern, and still are to a great extent, but now people in industrialized nations need to worry that the diets that eliminate deficiencies in turn lead to "killer diseases": hypertension, coronary heart disease, diabetes, and cancer.

Clearly, a lot has been learned, but not enough. Table 16-1 summarizes some of the landmark nutrition discoveries made during the past 60 years:

- In the 1930s and 1940s, there was new knowledge about vitamins and minerals
- In the 1950s, studies examining complex diseases such as coronary heart disease were started
- In the 1960s, the importance of nonnutrient components in the diet, such as fiber, was suggested
- In the 1960s and 1970s, national surveys of the nutritional status of the population of Canada and the United States were begun
- In the 1980s, nutrient support systems for people who are ill were improved; much was learned about the effect of malnutrition on body cells and their components

TABLE 16-1   Some Major Discoveries in Nutrition from the 1920s to the 1970s

1929	Essential fatty acid deficiency described
1931	Magnesium and manganese essential nutrients (demonstrated in rats)
1932	Vitamin C extracted from lemon juice; crystalline (pure) vitamin D prepared
1933	Riboflavin and pantothenic acid shown to be B vitamins
1934	Vitamin K discovered; zinc determined to be essential in rats
1935	First coenzyme shown to be related to niacin
1936	Thiamin synthesized
1938	Riboflavin deficiency identified in humans
1941	First RDAs published in the United States
1947	Vitamin B_{12} discovered
1949	Major study to identify the risk factors in heart disease started in Framingham, Massachusetts
1957	Selenium determined to be essential for farm animals
1963	Effects of zinc deficiency in humans described
1964	Pyridoxin deficiency described in adults
1966-74	Role of fiber in the diet described
1968	Total life support of a young child by total parenteral nutrition; Ten-State Nutrition Survey started
1970	Nutrition Canada National Survey started
1971	Active hormonal form of vitamin D3 identified

Note from the table how knowledge has been developed and refined over time: in 1934 zinc was found to be essential in rats, but it was not until 1963 that it was similarly found to be important in humans. Note also the historical pattern: discoveries of the vitamins and minerals led to recommendations for intakes of nutrients, descriptions of their metabolic functions and then their role in cancer, heart disease, and other complex diseases, then determinations of nutrient intakes at the national level, and finally incorporation of all nutrients in such a way that they may be provided to some ill people through veins rather than orally.

There are lessons to be learned from this kind of development. You can see this in studying the development of infant feeding practices over time.

The Development of Infant Feeding Practices

Every increase in nutrition knowledge usually brings modifications in eating behavior. Consider infant feeding practices during the last 100 years.

History

First there was concern about the possible harmful effects of feeding babies too much. Then there was concern over the effects of feeding them too little. Finally there was the phase of how it should best be done—when to wean, when to start solid foods. Today nutritionists are in the phase of "the search for perfection"—fine-tuning the study of infant nutrition.[1]

Let's look back at this. Why were people originally concerned about feeding babies too much? At one time, babies were said to suffer from the "summer complaint"—digestive problems caused by cow's milk. As chemical analysis became more sophisticated and it was found that cow's milk has high amounts of protein, fat, and carbohydrate, each of these constituents in turn was blamed for the infant distress. It took years, however, before it was discovered that it was not the nutrients in the milk but the filth in it and in the infant's bottle—the result of lack of hygiene and refrigeration.[1] Years later, in the 1970s, the concern about feeding babies too much resurfaced in another form—namely, that overfeeding infants might lead to adult obesity. This concern is debated still.

What about the issue of feeding babies too little or, more specifically, too little of the wrong nutrients? In the first quarter of this century, rickets was a problem in up to three-quarters of infants in the urban slums of the northern United States. When it was first proposed that cod liver oil be given to cure the bone problems caused by rickets, the suggestion was greeted with amusement—a "faddist idea," it would be called now. But it worked, and rickets has been nearly eliminated today. The success with cod liver oil led to the present practice of adding vitamin D to milk.

By now, the study of infant nutrition has advanced so that nutritionists have a pretty good understanding of the requirements of premature babies and of starving infants. The benefits of such understanding are demonstrated in the correct way to treat a starving baby: despite humanitarian instincts, one should not simply cram it with food, for this only increases the risk of death. Instead, during the first 2 to 3 days the baby should be given only enough food to sustain it and allow the damaged digestive system to recover its ability to metabolize larger intakes of nutrients. This information was discovered only within the last ten years, but its application has saved numerous starving babies.

Other Areas of Nutrition Knowledge Are Constantly Being Refined

How far have nutritionists come in specific knowledge? Consider a few examples:

- *Fiber:* Nutritionists no longer believe that it irritates the gastrointestinal system, but some still question its role in preventing colon cancer.[2]
- *Sugar:* Though it is not healthy for the teeth, nutritionists don't believe that high sugar intake causes diabetes. Consumption of a modest amount of sucrose is acceptable for diabetics, according to the American Diabetes Association, provided the diabetic continues to maintain metabolic control.
- *Molds in food:* These were once thought to cause certain nerve disorders. It is now believed that these disorders are caused by a deficiency of some of the B-complex vitamins.

The RDA values first outlined in 1941 are now in the 9th edition, but scientific evidence has dictated changes. For example, recommended intakes of protein are greatly reduced from the original values—although even today many lay people erroneously believe that protein supplements are necessary even if they already have a high protein intake. The publication of the 10th edition of the RDAs was delayed because of disagreements on the amounts of some nutrients to be recommended—for instance, in lowering the values for vitamins A and C.[3]

The lesson of all this is that nutrition information comes in fits and starts and often amid much debate. Small wonder that the lay person is often bewildered and is dazzled by promises held out by various food-related fads. Yet the chances for getting truthful, safe information are certainly higher than they have been in earlier times.

> Nutrition is a science in a constant state of transition. Research emphasis has moved from the discovery of new nutrients to the role these nutrients play in health and in disease. Nutrient intake is monitored now at the national level in many countries.

NUTRITION MISINFORMATION: THE MISUSE AND MANIPULATION OF LANGUAGE

Nutrition knowledge has grown, but so has the manipulation of language to support supposed nutrition claims. Some misuse of language is hair-splitting, but some is fraudulent. Examples:

- *Organic, health,* and *junk* are terms without formally agreed-upon definitions.
- *Malnutrition* may be understood by the general public to mean "undernutrition" or even "starvation," but the *mal* in malnourished means "bad," which applies to those who are overfed as well as underfed.
- *Fluoride* has been used as a scare word, as when, in 1985, voters in San Francisco were asked on their ballots "Shall fluorides, pesticides, or other toxic substances for water purification be added to the San Francisco drinking water supply?" Fluoride added to public water supplies (as it has been to San Francisco's for 30 years, with no ill effects) has actually been a good thing; it has reduced the incidence of dental caries, but some people still mistakenly

believe it causes cancer.[4] Certainly pesticides and other toxic substances are never intentionally added to drinking water. But the fluoride issue has been a powerful one in many places, leading to violence in Australia, for instance, when pro- and antifluoridation supporters came to blows during a parade.[5]

Some Food Labels Misrepresent the Amount of Water and Other Substances

Some words used in discussing food and nutrients have emotional impact.

There is nothing illegal about using unfamiliar terms on food labels to describe certain chemicals in foods—provided they are used correctly and scientifically. But, of course, most people don't know what those terms mean, even though the food industry estimates that 60% of Americans read labels. For instance, the word *sucrose* is used to obscure the word *sugar,* as we have seen, because the public associates sugar with obesity, empty calories, and dental caries. Indeed, the idea of sugar in *any* amount is bad to most consumers, even though problems only arise when the intake is high.

Food processors have discovered that it helps to hide a long (and presumably intimidating) chemical name, such as butylated hydroxytoluene or butylated hydroxyanisole, behind an abbreviation, such as BHT and BHA. Both are widely used food additives that act as preservatives and antioxidants and are on the approved GRAS (generally recognized as safe) list published by the Food and Drug Administration. There is no evidence they cause cancer.[4] Yet most people evidently would rather eat the abbreviation than the full chemical name.

Marketing 🔑

Now let us move on to a more serious matter of misrepresentation—soy *drinks* versus soy *milk.* Children are not supposed to be given soy drinks, at least not as the sole source of their nourishment.[6] If these are the exclusive source of nutrients, soy drinks (which usually contain water, soybeans, vegetable oil, kelp, pearl barley, barley malt, and salt) can lead to severe deficiencies in protein, kcalories, minerals, and vitamins. However, soy drinks are sometimes marketed as *soy milk.* The marketers hope to mislead by the word "milk," but these products should *not* be confused with the perfectly acceptable soy-based infant formulas available, which are designed to meet all infant nutritional needs.

Consumer Science 🔑

Sometimes the most useful information is in the fine print in advertisements and nutrition labels. Consider so-called grapefruit pills, advertised as aids to losing weight.[7] Not stated in the ads but stated on the label, however, is that, in order for the pills to work, you must reduce your food intake and increase your exercise. So what do you think is the *real* cause of your losing weight? There are many such examples of advertisements that cheat consumers in this way.[8]

Advertising is a significant means of making nutrition claims, and so, as the *Wall Street Journal* has headlined, the "Rise in Health Claims in Food Ads Can Help—and Mislead—Shoppers." In considering advertising, one must not only consider the manipulation of words and the interest of consumers but also the power of law and of regulatory agencies.[9,10]

Because People and Diets Differ, Generalizations Are Hard to Make

Advertising is always directed to each of us as individuals. Ads try to speak to "you." Of course, there are many different "yous" in the population and, with regard to nutrition wants and needs, even different "yous" within one's own lifetime.

People

Everyone is influenced by a number of variables that determine food intake and nutrient requirements: genetics, age, sex, race, culture, socioeconomic status, occupation, religion, and health status. Because everyone is unique, a nutrition experiment on one individual, or even a handful of individuals, is usually worthless. Thus, for nutrition experiments on people to be valid, they must be conducted on large numbers—often difficult to do, for reasons of economics, logistics, and ethics. Still, many advertising claims are based on the results performed on just a few people.

As examples of individual differences, consider the following:

- Nutrient intake differs between healthy young men and women, even between husband and wife.[11] One study found that husbands consumed slightly less vitamin C than did their wives but more kcalories, protein, fat, carbohydrate, cholesterol, and vitamin A; thus, the food intake data for one spouse could not be substituted for the other.
- Even babies vary in their food intake. It is simply not true that all infants during the first 18 months consume the same amount of food energy.[12] The amount of food eaten varied the least in fully breast-fed infants and increased as solids were introduced, but by 18 months the variations approached those of adults.

Statistics

How many people constitute an adequate representation for a nutrition experiment? This is the decision statisticians have to make. For example, statisticians for the National Health and Nutrition Examination Survey (HANES) felt they needed over 28,000 people in their sample if the results were to be representative for the entire population of the United States. HANES is an ongoing surveillance program to provide constant monitoring of the nutritional status of Americans.

In sum, you may think you are just "regular folks" like everyone else, but everyone has all kinds of variations in levels, for example, of hemoglobin, insulin, and growth hormone—even in just one day. Serum cholesterol levels can vary widely in a short period of time. Even nutrient intake varies from day to day. With so many variables to control, nutrition research on human subjects is difficult, expensive, and often requires many years. Thus, you should be cautious in accepting any statements or generalizations about nutrition because the number of people surveyed may not be sufficient.

Food

Those people living in industrialized countries may well have over 10,000 different foods available to them. Clearly, analyzing the nutrient content of this many foods every year would be an expensive process. To get around this, the Food and Drug Administration has devised a system whereby it obtains a certain combination of foods that is representative of American diets. For instance, it has determined that 50 particular foods represent 58% of the weight of the average American's total diet, 3500 particular foods represent 99.09% of the weight. The numbers of foods by which the FDA makes its analyses are shown in Table 16-2.

It is interesting that you may have 10,000 foods available to you, but 3500 of them will cover 99.09% (by weight) of those that are eaten. Clearly, not much is gained by the FDA's trying to include in its sample those 6500 other foods that are consumed so infrequently.

TABLE 16-2 Number of Different Foods the Food and Drug Administration Considers Representative of the Total Diet (by Weight) of the Average American

Number of Different Foods	Weight (%) of Total Diet Accounted For
50	58
100	68
250	82
500	90
1000	96
2000	98.4
3500	99.1

Knowledge about nutrition has grown considerably in the last 60 years, and it continues to grow. But we must guard against the spread of misinformation about nutrition.

SCIENTIFIC METHODS USED IN NUTRITION RESEARCH: HOW ACCURATE?

Chapter 1 provided an overview of the methods used in obtaining nutrition information, and responsible scientists use the best of these. But reliable information comes not only from accurate methods but also from representative samples.

Consider obesity. Although the usual measurement of obesity in a population sample is by skin-fold measurements, this method is not as accurate as some other methods (as described in Chapter 10). For one thing, many people object, for reasons of modesty, to having skin-fold measurements made on certain parts of their bodies. Incomplete measurement affects the outcome of the studies. More accurate kinds of obesity measurements require equipment found only in laboratories, which means people must suffer the inconvenience of journeying to the laboratory—another factor that may affect the outcome of any studies. Are measurements of obesity in the population done with the most accurate methods available? Clearly not—but they are the best methods that can be applied to the study of large groups. Once the faults intrinsic to such methods are understood, however, nutritionists are in a better position to interpret research data.

Despite the drawbacks, methods used in nutrition research have improved in recent years. Two of the most exciting new methods can be used to study coronary heart disease and anemia:

- *Coronary heart disease:* A number of years ago, only total serum cholesterol and triglyceride levels were measured. Today measurements of high density lipoprotein (HDL) and low density lipoprotein (LDL) concentrations give more information about the disease process.
- *Anemia:* Although anemia is widespread, little was known about how iron

enters the body from different foods until recently. Researchers discovered that if plants were grown in a water solution containing all needed nutrients plus mildly radioactive iron—which became incorporated into the plant and thus entered the body when the plant was eaten—then researchers could trace the passage of the isotope of iron through the body.

Although research methods have become more sophisticated, at times the greatest barrier to progress is that food is not uniform. For example, there is little variation in the measurements of nutrients in boiled potatoes, but much more variance when the potatoes are mashed and mixed with butter—especially in fat content, because of the lack of uniformity in the amount of butter mixed into the potatoes. Another example: How can you cut slices of roast beef so that each slice has the same content of fat and other nutrients?

> Nutrition information is usually more reliable if large numbers of people or of foods are examined. This reduces variance due to individual variation among people and lack of uniformity among certain foods. Because of this variation, one can never expect to have a very high degree of accuracy in the measurement of population characteristics or in the measurement of nutrient content of foods consumed by people.

INFORMATION FROM EXPERIMENTAL ANIMALS: CAUTION IS THE WATCHWORD

Which experimental animals provide the most valuable information in human nutrition research? Human beings.

But there are not only sampling problems but also ethical problems in working with human subjects—especially with the important matters in nutrition. Who among the readers of this book, for example, would allow their heart or liver to be taken out and dissected in the name of nutrition research? This is not to say that human beings have not provided valuable information under health-threatening circumstances—for example, studies on human starvation were performed by Ancel Keys of the University of Minnesota, mostly on World War II conscientious objectors.

Because of these limitations, experimental animals have provided the evidence for the discovery of many of the vitamins and minerals.[13] The most frequently used animals are rats, mice, chickens, hamsters, and guinea pigs and, less frequently, monkeys and pigs. The advantages of working with animals are that:

- Whole tissues can be removed for examination and the animal killed
- Their small size makes sampling easy
- Their short life-span allows nutritionists to more readily study the aging process
- Diet, environmental temperature, and genetic influences can be controlled

In applying the results of animal experiments to humans, however, special precautions must be taken. One of them is in generalizing from the particular animal species. Oftentimes, the choice of species is dictated by cost and convenience (rather than sound biological principles), which is why rats are so often used. However, rats are poor models for the study of some important areas of nutrition. For example, pregnancy and lactation cause greater metabolic strain in rats than they do in human females. Moreover, rats have multiple births—over 10 in a litter usually. In addition, the chemical composition of the rat's body at birth is different from that of a human infant, and there is great difference in the chemical composition of rat milk compared to human milk.

Many of the present concerns in human nutrition cannot be addressed adequately in animal experiments.[13] For example:

- Which animal, if any, would you suggest for studying the interaction between nutrition and brain development?
- Protein-energy malnutrition in human children is important, but animal models do not represent all the same clinical signs.
- The dietary ratio of phosphorus and calcium is handled differently by animals than by humans.
- Atherosclerosis is hard to induce in rats, partly because these animals have high levels of high density lipoproteins.
- Different animal models have varied responses to dietary cholesterol and so have only limited use in providing answers about heart disease in humans.
- Vitamin E deficiency is almost unknown in humans, yet it is easily induced in some animals.
- Rats are useless in the study of niacin metabolism because they do not develop pellagra.
- Protein requirements are greater in the growing rat than in growing humans.
- Alcoholism is a great cause of nutrient deficiencies in industrialized countries, yet rats refuse to consume alcohol in the amounts that will cause liver damage of the sort that affects human alcoholics.

This list is long and could be made longer, but the point has been made: experimental animals can help researchers find answers to some human nutritional problems but not to some of the most serious ones.

Some people object to the use of animals in nutritional experiments and in other areas of medical research. There is obvious conflict between the pain inflicted and the need for the information that can help humans; however, standards are rigid to minimize suffering and maximize the information gained.

> Experimental animals provided much useful information in the discovery of some vitamins and minerals. Despite some differences in growth rate and metabolic functions, they continue to produce valuable information applicable to human nutrition. They are of less value in studying complex diseases such as heart disease and cancer.

CHECKING CREDENTIALS: WHO GIVES NUTRITION INFORMATION?

Anyone who has training in nutrition from a recognized university should be able to analyze nutrition information. The following background is considered qualified training in the science of nutrition:

- Registered dietitians—graduate training in nutrition, leading to M.S. or Ph.D. degrees. Registered dietitians receive a wide range of courses in nutrition and food preparation, attend an internship (or the equivalent) for one year, and pass examinations in a number of areas of competency set by the American or Canadian Dietetic Association.
- Medical doctors—usually receive some training in nutrition, although this was not always true in the past. Nutrition is now becoming established in most medical schools; however, one nutrition test showed significant variation in nutrition knowledge among medical students,[14] and many medical students expressed dissatisfaction with the quantity and quality of their nutrition education.
- Graduates in biochemistry, biology, or food science—usually have the basis for further training in nutrition. As for that further training, you should be aware that many nonaccredited institutions and "universities" exist that will sell you a degree in nutrition.[15] This is possible because *anybody can call himself or herself a "nutritionist."*

The qualifications of many "pop" nutritionists make alarming reading.[16] One such person had a background in communications and education, another had experience as a tax auditor and later co-owned an electrical equipment business. Neither had *any* training in nutrition, yet they have written books, contributed to magazines, and appeared on television as "experts" on the subject.

How do unqualified people like these get away with this? There are six reasons.

Beware: Unfortunately, anybody can use the title of "nutritionist."

Nutrition Scientists Often Are Not Dramatic Communicators

Indeed, many scientists in general are poor communicators because they are isolated from the public's daily concerns and because they communicate with other scientists in a technical language.

The public, however, is not interested in listening to technical language and does not want to hear a long pro-and-con evaluation of the latest nutrition discovery. The most important question to lay people is: "Will it work?"—and they hope for an answer that is short and simple.

Unqualified people posing as "nutritionists" seem always to manage to keep their answers short and simple, which makes them very attractive in a medium such as television. However, if used correctly, television has possibilities for conveying truly useful and truthful nutrition information.[17]

Nutrition Research Must Pass a Rigid Review Process

All research papers published in reputable scientific journals, including nutrition journals, must go through a review process. Two or three experts in the area of research evaluate each paper. If they consider it scientifically correct, based on existing knowledge, the paper is published; otherwise, it is not.

This process tends to make nutrition scientists cautious, and rightly so. But that does not help them communicate with the public. Nutrition quacks, by contrast, are popular and successful because they have quick, easy answers.

Malnutrition Is Not Always Visible

In developing countries, one can often see the signs of malnutrition—the evidence of low-quantity, low-quality diets is there to see among the people on the streets. In advanced nations, by contrast, the diseases of malnutrition—which are mostly the diseases of affluence, such as coronary heart disease, hypertension, and some trace mineral deficiencies—are not so visible and do not usually appear until later in life.

In developed countries, therefore, quacks may be able to convince people that they might be nutritionally in danger, but they attract susceptible individuals by simply allowing them to continue with their old eating habits, eating their favorite foods, but sell them some magical supplement purported to correct their nutrition problems.

People Can't Relate Personally to Nutrition Information

Not everyone will die of heart disease, hypertension, and cancer, although these nutrition-related problems have been found in a large percentage of the population. Because most people have difficulty considering themselves part of a "statistical set,"[18] many are likely to figure "it won't happen to me—let other people worry about that." In general, then, people are more apt to eat food for satisfaction than for reasons of nutrition or prevention of disease.

There Are Few Real Restrictions on Diet

Essentially you have the freedom to eat almost anything you want, so long as you can afford it. This is a freedom that goes unappreciated until one is forced for medical reasons to go on a restricted diet. Because the freedom until then is so nearly absolute, many tend to be resentful of recommendations by government or nutrition or medical experts as to what they should eat; they often view such advice as attempts to control their freedom.

Nutrition Information in the Mass Media Is Sometimes Suspect

How accurate is nutrition information in the popular press? In Table 1-2 we saw that some popular magazines provided sound nutrition information and others did not. There is an encouraging trend in the improvement of nutrition information in the mass media. Many qualified nutritionists have regular newspaper features on nutrition. Sources of nutrition information in scientific journals appear in Appendix E.

It is necessary to ask many questions before accepting nutrition information.

EXCITING FUTURE TRENDS

How well can the future be predicted? In predicting future trends in nutrition, keep in mind that in 1946 Oxford University in England refused to accept a large donation for nutrition research because it was thought that all of the major discoveries in nutrition had already been made! As you have seen, however, there is still a lot that has to be learned.

Here are some areas in which research will continue:

- Nutritional improvement in foods
- The effects of food additives (although some of the concern about them is irrational)
- Low-cost foods that provide fresh flavor, aroma, and color
- Improved convenience foods
- Foods free from infestations and filth
- Better control of food quality by regulatory agencies
- Improved nutrition information (see Figure 16-1)

If the preceding areas seem a bit uninteresting, consider the following, where changes are apt to be more dramatic.

Space exploration

The short history of feeding people in space has been an interesting search on how to package food for and eat food in a weightless environment. Now the challenge moves to the more complicated process of providing attractive and nutritious foods for long voyages in space.[19]

FIGURE 16-1
What we will eat in the year 2000. Experts predict many changes in the food and how it will be prepared.

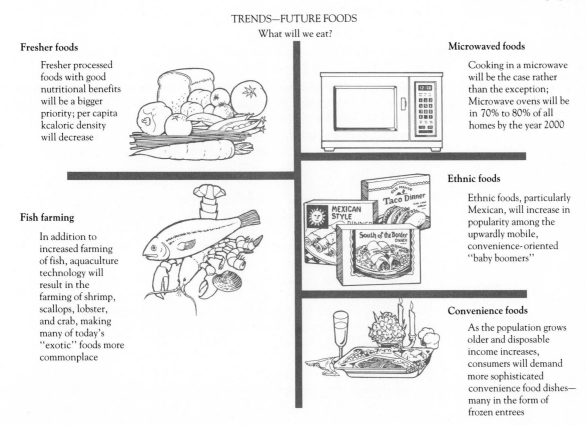

TRENDS—FUTURE FOODS
What will we eat?

Fresher foods

Fresher processed foods with good nutritional benefits will be a bigger priority; per capita kcaloric density will decrease

Microwaved foods

Cooking in a microwave will be the case rather than the exception; Microwave ovens will be in 70% to 80% of all homes by the year 2000

Fish farming

In addition to increased farming of fish, aquaculture technology will result in the farming of shrimp, scallops, lobster, and crab, making many of today's "exotic" foods more commonplace

Ethnic foods

Ethnic foods, particularly Mexican, will increase in popularity among the upwardly mobile, convenience-oriented "baby boomers"

Convenience foods

As the population grows older and disposable income increases, consumers will demand more sophisticated convenience food dishes—many in the form of frozen entrees

Astronauts tell us that eating in a
weightless environment causes none of
the expected problems.

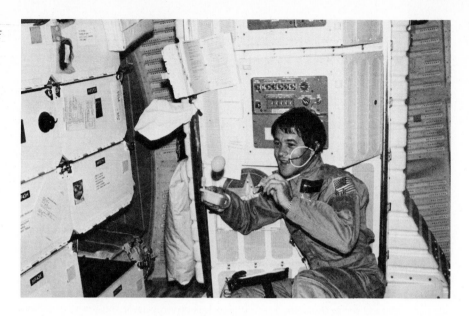

Diets for artificial heart patients

Medicine

Observations of the first artificial heart implant patient, Barney Clark, revealed
that he had special nutrition requirements. Surgical teams for this kind of operation
now include a nutritionist to monitor nutrition needs.[20]

Withholding nutrition for terminal patients

Law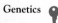

Is failure to provide sufficient food and water for a terminally ill patient any different
from withdrawing medical treatment? There is no difference, according to a New
Jersey Supreme Court ruling. Emotional and ethical problems must be resolved,
but guidelines have been developed in this area.[21] What about the opposite: Is it
ethical to force-feed a person who is voluntarily fasting to death?[22] These are topics
you will hear more about in the future.

Genetic engineering

Genetics

This area of research offers exciting possibilities in nutrition. For example, there
is discussion about genetic therapy for phenylketonuria (PKU), a disease that
requires dietary modification.[23] Gene expression—the process by which genetic
information is transferred in the cell—may perhaps be controlled by food components and essential nutrients.[24]

   Genetic engineering has also been used to increase the protein content of
potatoes and to produce genetically engineered insulin to control blood glucose
levels. Both developments address a supply problem—the first the shortage of
protein in the diets of people of many countries, the second the dependence on
the pancreases of cattle for a source of insulin.

Food technology

New breakthroughs will certainly be seen in this area.[25] Whatever developments
occur, however, will be determined by the cost and availability of resources, de-

mographics, government policies and regulations, sponsorship of agricultural re-search, corporate management policies and practices, and consumer desires and opinions.

Food microbiology

Researchers in this area will probably be in for a busy time in the future. Any time illness or death occurs as a result of food-related business, it seems to catch the public's attention. For instance, a recent outbreak of food-borne disease known as listeriosis, caused by the micro-organism *Listeria monocytogenes,* caused meningitis, inflammation of the membranes of the brain or spinal cord. It has also caused miscarriages, generally in the last half of pregnancy, and even death. The con-taminated foods included cheese, unpasteurized milk, poached eggs, and cole slaw.

To prevent food-borne diseases, food-service workers and homemakers need to be educated in proper food handling. According to the Centers for Disease Control, about 75% of these disease outbreaks occur in food-service establishments, 20% in homes, and 3% in food-processing plants. To get an idea of the sheer numbers involved, consider that 70% of $300 billion that Americans spend on food each year is for processing, transporting, and marketing.[26] This food moves through about 25,000 food manufacturers, 35,000 wholesalers, 250,000 food stores, and 270,000 eating establishments. That doesn't even include the number of homes in the country. Thus, it is not surprising that bacteria can enter somewhere along this long chain.

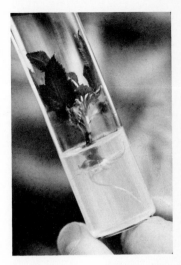

New methods of food production must be developed if the world population is to be adequately nourished. One prom-ising method is hydroponics—growing plants in a water medium containing all required nutrients.

Biotechnology

Most food processing companies are interested in using biotechnology to lower costs by increasing processing efficiencies. Some are interested in opening up new markets with better tasting foods.[27] One European company is trying to grow micro-organisms having the texture, flavor, and protein composition of hamburger, which would have the advantage of offering a product low in saturated fat. By the year 2000, it is estimated, biotechnology will be responsible for producing over $11 billion worth of microbically derived foods and food ingredients.

Food Technology

Behavior and mood

Nutrition researchers have been giving increasing attention to the role of behavior and mood in eating. Consider the following areas:

Psychology

- *Tryptophan and sleep:* In a symposium on diet and behavior,[28] it was pointed out that high intakes of tryptophan induce sleep, but the effects of levels of this amino acid in a typical meal on human sleep patterns are unknown. In any case, the relationship between tryptophan and sleep may be the basis for the bit of folklore that drinking a glass of warm milk at bedtime will induce sleep. (Some people claim it works better if nutmeg is added to the milk.)
- *Carbohydrates and concentration:* High carbohydrate intake tends to make peo-ple (women in particular) less alert. For instance, it is reported that when older adults eat a high-carbohydrate lunch, their concentration decreases in the afternoon. Performance and mental capacity is improved with small bal-anced meals.
- *Sugar and behavior:* Contrary to popular belief, sugar does not aggravate hy-peractivity or contribute to behavior or learning problems in children.

■ *Diet and criminality:* Does diet cause criminal behavior and can diet control it? There is no evidence for this. The American Dietetic Association has pointed out that the belief that diet can control criminality has a number of problems: Not only does it waste public funds and detract from other, more effective kinds of treatment, it also may lead to nutritional deficiencies and to the mistaken notion that individuals have no control over their own behavior.

The topic of food in relation to mood and behavior is covered here at length because it has become such a popular issue in the mass media (see Figure 16-2). In reporting on this area, *Newsweek* (October 14, 1985) correctly pointed out that there are large gaps in our knowledge about how food influences behavior. Despite this, there will probably always be someone to try to sell you a food or diet that will "put you in a good mood."

Nutrition and harmful chemical environments

Technology

Researchers in the Soviet Union are investigating how certain foods and vitamins may be used to control the harmful effects of toxic chemical occupational environments.[29] Whether nutrition can really be used in the detoxification and elim-

FIGURE 16-2
Does diet affect mood? Maybe, according to some research.

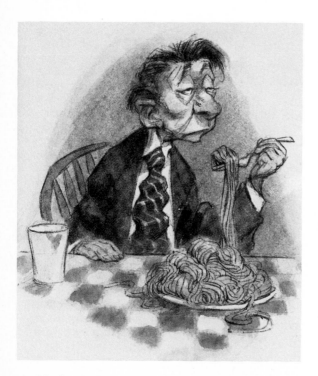

Mind and matter: Nodding off with carbohydrates?

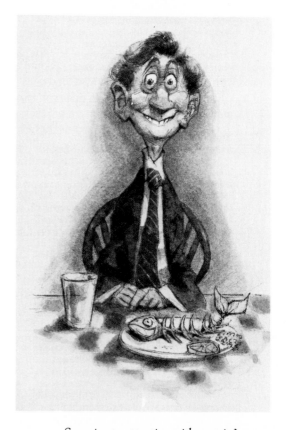

Snapping to attention with protein?

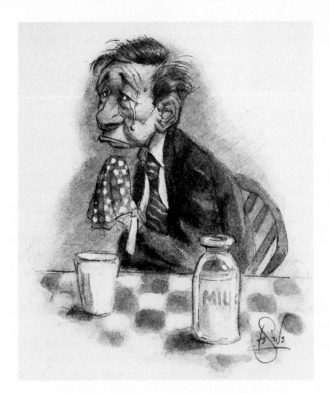

Down in the dumps with a glass of milk?

ination of environmental chemicals remains to be seen, but it is known that many of the constituents of food influence the metabolism of drugs and toxicants.[30] This is an area of active research.

Food pill for killer diseases

You will probably see foods packaged in pill form that will supposedly counteract the risk of killer diseases. Many of these products will be produced by opportunists, such as the company that manufactured pills made from a combination of cabbage, Brussels sprouts, carrots, cauliflower, spinach, and broccoli. Closed down for making false medical claims and false advertising, the company promoted its products on the basis of reports by the National Academy of Sciences that a regular diet of these vegetables is associated with a reduction in certain types of cancers.[31] Although the association may be valid, the components of these foods responsible for the beneficial effects have not been isolated. The belief in magical medical properties in some foods, however, will continue.

Medicine

Better food labeling

We may see increased amount of nutrition information on food labels in the future. Although such labels currently give you useful information on the amount of sodium, fiber, and cholesterol and the amount and type of fat and other nutrients, there are still concerns about the *type* of nutrition information given. Consider sugar, for example. One Canadian nutritionist lists the following concerns about the public's demand for more labeling information about sugar[32]:

- Is there legislative authority to require sugar labeling of foods? This will vary between countries.
- What is the exact nature of the health concern? Sugar causes dental caries, for instance. When eaten in excess, it may cause obesity.
- Are all sugar-containing foods equally cariogenic—that is, are they all equally likely to cause dental caries? The answer is no, which presents a problem if a person's main health concern is avoiding dental caries.
- Is the risk to health posed by sugar sufficient to justify the cost of such labeling? This point is debatable.
- How should sugar be legally defined? Chapter 3 listed a variety of terms used to describe "sugar." The problem becomes obvious.
- What labeling format is best understood? Much work remains to be done on educating the public as to the correct use of information from labels.

Epidemiology

Medicine

More research in epidemiology will try to explain the relationship between diet and disease in different parts of the world.[33] For example, why is it that executives of American companies are more likely to die of heart disease than executives of Japanese companies?[34] Part of the answer is that the Americans have higher body weights, eat more kcalories from animal fat, and have higher levels of serum cholesterol. On the other hand, why are the same Japanese executives more likely to suffer a stroke compared to their American counterparts? Part of the answer here is that the Japanese have a higher rate of cigarette smoking, a higher sodium intake, and a greater increase in blood pressure with age.

Another example of how epidemiology influences guidance about food: It was thought that there was a close relationship between low levels of fiber in the diet and some diseases such as cancer of the colon. However, researcher Ian MacDonald points out that in the two centuries between 1770 and 1970 the intake of fiber *decreased* dramatically yet life expectancy *increased* dramatically—the opposite of what we might expect.[35] Sugar consumption also increased during that time, a development we might have considered would not enhance longevity. Clearly, factors other than fiber and sugar must be involved in increasing life expectancy.

Nutrition and infection

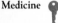
Medicine

In the future, there will probably be more research on nutrition and its relationship to people's resistance to infections.[36] Undernourished people are more prone to getting infections and many infectious diseases cause death. However, nutrition is not the only factor, of course. As Figure 16-3 shows, there are many others: the environment, illness, child care, medical care, and food availability. The relative importance of each of these factors remains to be determined.

Nutrition and the cell

Cell Biology

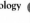

Future investigators will probably direct major attention to the cellular aspects of nutrition, such as how nutrients cross the blood-brain barrier. The results of this research should provide more information about how the brain uses certain nutrients and how drug metabolism in the brain is influenced by nutrition.

There may also be some breakthroughs in the understanding of the cellular basis

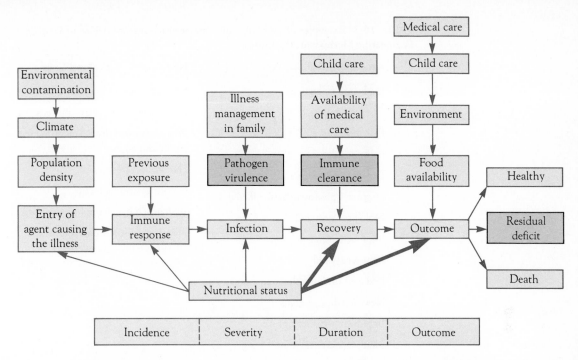

FIGURE 16-3
Infant mortality from infectious disease
is a problem in many countries. Contributing factors include environment,
other illness, child care, medical care,
and food availability.

of obesity. For instance, Rudolph Leibel of Rockefeller University is studying the
influence of small molecules on the surface of fat cells.[37] All fat cells have alpha
receptors that stimulate the uptake of fat into the cell and beta receptors that
stimulate fat breakdown. This may explain why fat accumulates more in some areas
than in others. A better understanding of how this works may enable people to
"spot reduce"—for instance, take fat off hips or thighs but not elsewhere—if ways
can be found to increase the activity of beta receptors and decrease the activity of
alpha receptors.

Statistics, interpretations, and nutrition

Does calcium lower hypertension? Nutritionists used to think so, but now we are
not so sure.[38] The reason is that there have been conflicting interpretations of data
because different statistical techniques were used. Thus, in the future you may
expect to see more accurate use of statistics in advancing the science of nutrition.

Disputes over interpretations can have serious consequences.[39] For instance, the
10th edition of the Recommended Dietary Allowances (RDAs) was supposed to
have been published in the fall of 1985, but some nutritionists disputed the recommendation that the RDAs be lowered for vitamins A and C, thinking that this
change might be seen as approval for reduced consumption of fruits and vegetables,
major sources of these two vitamins. In addition, reduced intake would be the
opposite of the recommendations made in the National Academy of Science's 1982
report *Diet, Nutrition, and Cancer.*

This RDA dispute has economic and political consequences because RDA values   Economics
are used in many federal, state, and private nutrition programs. Thus, reduced
RDA values could lead to reduced funding for school lunches, food stamps, and
institutions for the chronically ill. Moreover, lower RDAs might be cited as evidence that fewer Americans are hungry and used to redefine definitions of poverty
level and eligibility for welfare programs.

TABLE 16-3 Examples of Agriculturally Important Targets for Use of Genetic Engineering Methods in the Future

Agricultural Characteristics	New Uses for Agricultural Crops
Herbicide tolerance	Specialty oils and waxes
Disease resistance	Pharmaceutically active proteins
Pest resistance	Pharmaceutical drugs (plant secondary products)
Salinity tolerance	
Drought tolerance	Flavors and fragrances
Improved photosynthetic efficiency	Colorings and pigments
Biological pesticides	Biomass (e.g., alcohol production)
Improved storage characteristics	New horticultural characteristics (flavor, color, size, etc.)
Improved yield	
Reduced undesirable characteristics	
New breeding systems	
Improved fertilizer uptake	
Metal toxicity tolerance	
Cold tolerance	
Frost resistance	
Heat tolerance	
Improved nitrogen fixation	

Agriculture, governments, and the food supply

Political Science

The amount of food available to the world's people will no doubt be increased. In part this will be achieved through the use of genetic engineering methods, as Table 16-3 indicates. However, the prospects for improved agricultural practices are not good in those parts of the world where they are needed most: the poor countries. Although methods for predicting and preventing famines have been greatly improved,[40] the real difficulty, unfortunately, lies in persuading officials in agencies and governments to view food crises as *socioeconomic and political events* rather than simply climatic and agricultural catastrophes.

Politics and economics are powerful influences on nutrition, but many nutritionists do not seem to be concerned about this. Famed nutritionist Jean Meyer, now president of Tufts University, scolds members of his profession for not recognizing their social responsibilities.[41] He urges them to get more involved in the political process in order to improve funding for basic nutrition research and for the alleviation of world hunger. Because governmental influence on food policies is often controversial,[42] nutritionists should get involved more in questioning government subsidies of foods of doubtful nutritive value, such as sugar, butter, and wine.

TABLE 16-4 Nutrition-Related Objectives Selected for Achievement by the Year 1990

Nutrition-Related Objective	Level of Success (1980-1986)
Areas Selected for Reduction or Elimination	
Reduction of mean serum cholesterol in the adult population to 200 mg/dl (5.17 mmol/L) or less	On track for 1990
Reduction of average daily sodium consumption to at least the 3- to 6-g range, and reduction of sodium levels in processed food by 20%	Not achieved, or insufficient data
Reduction of iron deficiency anemia in pregnant women to 3.5%	Not achieved, or insufficient data
Elimination of growth retardation caused by inadequate diets in infants and children	Not achieved
Reduction of significant overweight to 10% of men and 17% of women	Not achieved
Areas Targeted for Increases or Improvement	
Knowledge by 70% of adults of the major foods low in fat, low in sodium, high in kcalories, high in sugars, and good sources of fiber	On track for 1990
Knowledge by more than 75% of the population of the principal dietary factors known or strongly suspected to be related to heart disease, high blood pressure, dental caries, and cancer	On track for 1990
Increase in breast-feeding to 75% at hospital discharge and 35% at 6 months of age	On track for 1990
Understanding by 90% of adults that weight loss requires fewer kcalories or increased physical activity or both	On track for 1990
A comprehensive national nutrition monitoring system, including the capability to monitor nutrition problems in special population groups	On track for 1990
Awareness and promotion of the *Dietary Guidelines for Americans* by greater than 50% of school and employee cafeteria managers	Not achieved, or insufficient data
Kcalorie and other nutrient labeling of all packaged foods	Not achieved
Adoption of weight-loss regimens, combining diet and exercise, by 50% of the overweight population	Not achieved
Some nutrition education as part of required school health education at elementary and secondary levels in all states	Not achieved
Some nutrition education and counseling included in virtually all routine health contacts	Not achieved

Forward march

There is no lack of avenues of investigation for nutritionists. What is the relationship between nutrition and drugs, of nutrition and exercise, of food extracts such as omega-3 fatty acids and heart disease? What is the interaction between nutrients? How can nutritionists better determine a person's true nutritional status? What is the influence of chronobiology on the use of nutrients?

How well are we doing in meeting some present objectives? The results are mixed according to a recent report.[43] In 1979 the Surgeon General's report, *Healthy People*, identified specific goals for improving the health of the American public by the year 1990. The mid-term report card is in on the nutrition-related aspects of this report (Table 16-4). As a nation we seem to be doing a good job in reducing serum cholesterol, in increasing our knowledge about diet and disease, and in increasing the number of people who breast-feed; we are also on track for establishing a comprehensive national nutrition monitoring system.

We await more information on how well we are doing on reducing sodium, on reducing the incidence of iron deficiency anemia, and on increasing awareness of the *Dietary Guidelines for Americans*.

It is unfortunate that some important goals have not been achieved by 1987. The possibility of success by 1990 looks remote for the following: The elimination of growth retardation caused by inadequate diets in infants and children, the reduction of the incidence of overweight in both men and women, requiring kcalorie and other nutrient labeling on packaged foods, getting many of the people who are overweight to adopt a combination of diet and exercise to achieve weight loss, having nutrition education required in school health education in elementary and secondary levels in all states, and having some nutrition education and counseling included in almost all routine health contacts.

These are important goals for people in the United States and in other industrialized countries. But there is one question of utmost significance to every person in the world. What is the maximum number of people in the world that *can* be fed? If future generations of people are to survive, a satisfactory answer to this question must be found. In a 1985 article, Kenneth Blaxter, using realistic estimates of land area that can be used for agriculture and its potential food yield, estimated that the world has the capacity to feed 7 to 8 billion people.[44] Unfortunately, there are already 5 billion people on earth right now, and there will probably be 6 billion people by the end of the century—very few years away. From this standpoint, time seems to be running out. Still, that master of gloom and doom, Thomas Malthus, prophesied that the world would become too populated to support itself by the 1870s. Thus, although there is, no doubt, an upper limit to how many people the world can feed, that limit is a matter of debate among experts.

It would be a shame to end this book without a word of encouragement. Clearly, a lot has been learned about the nutrient needs of the human body in recent years, and that learning process will continue. Thus, the information on all the preceding pages is not static; although some of it may remain unchanged in the future, much of it will be modified. As nutrition knowledge becomes more sophisticated, nutritionists will be better able to make recommendations that will enhance the quality and healthfulness of the food you eat.

Future expansion in nutrition information will come from space exploration and surgery. There will be significant changes in the legal aspects of life termination, and in food production, processing, and labeling. In addition, we will learn more about nutrition and the control of mood and behavior, the effects of environmental pollutants, the control of killer diseases, and how to cope with over-population.

DECISIONS

1. Should I Consider Nutrition as a Career?

If it seems to suit you, the author can heartily recommend it. As you have just seen, there is no shortage of nutrition problems to be solved. People have enjoyable, profitable careers in nutrition even though their training may at first seem far removed from the field.

Nutrition relates to many aspects of the natural and social sciences. It is a subject built on strong foundations of natural sciences because it involves transfer of chemicals from foods to the human body. However, decisions about which foods to eat is determined by the social animal within everyone, the subject of study of the social sciences. Thus, whichever you specialize in, natural or social sciences, you can develop a nutrition career using these skills. The natural sciences are put to use in the careers of registered dietitian, public health nutritionist, physician, dentist, nurse, physical therapist, food-service worker, health educator, physical educator, and nutritional researcher, whether for agriculture, the food industry, or the government. The social sciences are put to use in careers in nutritional anthropology, developmental psychology, and social, economic, and political aspects of food production and distribution.

Even if you do not choose a nutrition-related career, however, a knowledge of nutrition will clearly lead to better health habits and thus, it is to be hoped, a happier and more productive life.

2. Will Nutritional Requirements be Different for Space Travelers?

It is entirely possible that space flight will become a reality not just for astronauts but for ordinary people, and as a result, nutritionists will need to learn about changes in nutrient requirements and metabolism. The following new experiences all have a nutrition component: extravehicular activity, physiological responses to microgravity that influence metabolism and energy needs, in-flight nutritional experience, space menus, food packaging, in-flight food-service methodology, water supply, and disposal of food wastes.[45]

However, before you get on board a spacecraft, consider what nutritionists don't know. The following are gaps in nutrition knowledge:

- Lack of RDA values for some micronutrients considered essential in long-term space missions
- An understanding of space-associated changes in body compositions
- Whether calcium supplements prior to departure will counteract space-related bone loss
- Problems in providing food for long (greater than 3 to 4 hours) extravehicular activity
- Any benefits of supplementation with individual amino acids (as found by Soviet researchers, but not confirmed elsewhere)
- The advantages of athletic levels of fitness in resisting space deconditioning
- The nutritional significance, if any, of digestive disturbances experienced by people early in space flights
- Whether preflight supplementation with minerals, vitamins, proteins, or amino acids will prevent muscle loss
- Factors influencing the bioavailability of essential micronutrients
- In-flight eating behavior—essential information for food-service planning
- What food will taste like in space in flights longer than 90 days
- Technology for providing a microbe-free on-board water supply
- A safe range of dietary vitamin D for long-term missions
- Whether bone calcium is released during spaceflight and deposited in soft tissue
- Possible harmful effects of spaceflight on glucose metabolism

Should these and other questions be resolved during your lifetime, have a good flight!

SUMMARY

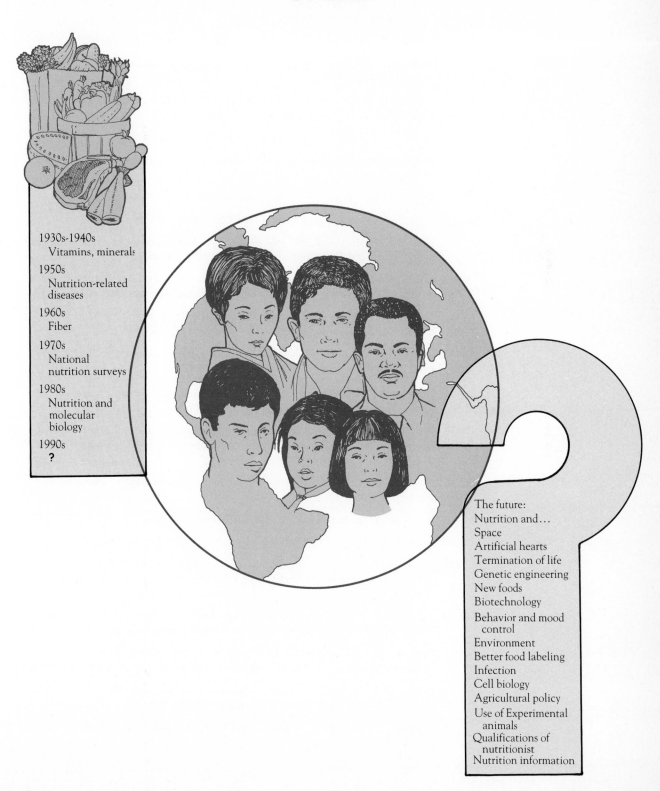

1930s-1940s
Vitamins, minerals

1950s
Nutrition-related
diseases

1960s
Fiber

1970s
National
nutrition surveys

1980s
Nutrition and
molecular
biology

1990s
?

The future:
Nutrition and…
Space
Artificial hearts
Termination of life
Genetic engineering
New foods
Biotechnology
Behavior and mood
control
Environment
Better food labeling
Infection
Cell biology
Agricultural policy
Use of Experimental
animals
Qualifications of
nutritionist
Nutrition information

REFERENCES

1. Pratt, E.L.: Historical perspectives: food, feeding, and fancies. Journal of the American College of Nutrition **3:**115, 1984.

2. Jacobs, L.R.: Dietary fiber and cancer, Journal of Nutrition **117:**319, 1987.

3. Olson, J.A.: Vitamins A and C: proposed allowances. Nutrition Today, p. 26, September-October, 1986.

4. National Academy of Sciences: Diet, nutrition, and cancer. Washington, D.C., National Academy Press, 1982, p. 162.

5. Smith, G.: Tapping into the fluoride debate. New Scientist, p. 50, August 1, 1985.

6. Nightingale, S.: Soy drink warning. Journal of the American Medical Association **254:**1428, 1985.

7. The fine print with grapefruit pills. FDA Consumer, p. 5, June 1985.

8. Miller, R.W.: Critiquing quack ads. FDA Consumer, p. 11, March 1985.

9. Howell, R.T., Jr.: Legal and policy issues of health claims for foods: an unhealthy prescription. Food Drug Cosmetic Law Journal **40:**22, 1985.

10. Cooper, R.M.: Health claims on foods: reflections on the food-drug distinction and on the law of misbranding. American Journal of Clinical Nutrition **44:**560, 1986.

11. Lee, J., and Kolonel, L.N.: Nutrient intakes of husbands and wives: implications for epidemiological research. Journal of Epidemiology **115:**515, 1982.

12. Black, A.E., and others: Daily variation in food intake of infants from 2 to 18 months. Human Nutrition: Applied Nutrition **37A:**448, 1983.

13. Hegarty, P.V.: Use of experimental animals in human nutrition research: some justification and precautions. Contemporary Nutrition **6:**(no. 3), March 1981.

14. Weinsier, R.L., and others: Nutrition knowledge of senior medical students: a collaborative study of southeastern medical schools. American Journal of Clinical Nutrition **43:**959, 1986.

15. Aronson, V.: You can't tell a nutritionist by the diploma. FDA Consumer, p. 28, August 1983.

16. Rynearson, E.H.: Americans love hogwash. Nutrition Reviews **32**(suppl no. 1):1, 1974.

17. Cross, A.T.: Television's role in nutrition education. Nutrition Update **2:**251, 1985.

18. Yarbrough, P.: Ineffective communication. In Nutrition in the 1980's: constraints on our knowledge, Salvey, N., and White, P.L., editors, New York, Alan R. Liss, Inc., 1981, p. 539.

19. Sauer, R.L., editor: Food service and nutrition for the space station. NASA Conference Publication 2370, National Aeronautics and Space Administration, 1985.

20. Raymond, J., and others: Nutrition for the first total artificial heart patient: implications for future patients. Journal of the American Dietetic Association **84:**532, 1984.

21. Curran, W.J.: Defining appropriate medical care: providing nutrients and hydration for the dying. New England Journal of Medicine **313:**940, 1985.

22. Frommel, D., and others: Voluntary total fasting: challenge for the medical community. Lancet **i:**1451, 1984.

23. Cederbaum, S.D., and others: Symposium on genetic engineering and phenylketonuria. Pediatrics **74:**406, 1984.

24. Rucker, R. and Tinker, D.: The role of nutrition in gene expression: a fertile field for the application of molecular biology. Journal of Nutrition **116:**177, 1986.

25. Kirk, J.R.: Unlimited horizons in new food technology. Food Drug Cosmetic Law Journal **39:**109, 1984.

26. Liska, B.J.: New bacteria in the news. Food Technology **40:**16, August 1986.

27. Taylor, D.L.: Biotechnology comes of age in the food industry. Food Engineering, p. 28, September 1985.

28. Summary, diet and behavior symposium proceedings, Nutrition Reviews **44** (Supplement):252, May 1986.

29. Sutphen, E.I.: Soviet prophylactic nutrition for workers in toxic chemical occupational environments. American Journal of Clinical Nutrition **42:**746, 1985.

30. Omaye, S.T.: Effects of diet on toxicity testing. Federation Proceedings **45:**133, 1986.

31. Ballentine, C.: On cabbages and cancer. FDA Consumer, p. 29, 1984.

32. Cheney, M.C.: Food regulations as obstacles to success in nutrition intervention programs. In Selvey, N., and White, P.L., editors: Nutrition in the 1980s: constraints on our knowledge. New York, Alan R. Liss, Inc., 1981, p. 549.

33. Woteki, C.E., and others: Nutritional epidemiology and national surveys, Journal of Nutrition **117:**401, 1987.

34. Comstock, G.W., and others: Cardiovascular risk factors in American and Japanese executives. Journal of the Royal Society of Medicine **78:**536, 1985.

35. MacDonald, I.: Nonsense and nonscience in nutrition. Proceedings of the Nutrition Society **42:**513, 1983.

36. Symposium: nutrition and resistance to infection. Proceedings of the Nutrition Society **45:**289, 1986.

37. Kolata, G.: Weight regulation may start in our cells, not psyches. Smithsonian, p. 90, January 1986.

38. Larkin, T.: Evidence vs. nonsense: a guide to the scientific method. FDA Consumer, p. 27, June 1985.

39. Marshall, E.: The academy kills a nutrition report. Science **230:**420, 1985.

40. Mellor, J.W.: Prediction and prevention of famine. Federation Proceedings **45:**2427, 1986.

41. Mayer, J.: Social responsibilities of nutritionists. Journal of Nutrition **116:**714, 1986.

42. Acheson, E.D.: Food policy, nutrition and government. Proceedings of the Nutrition Society **45:**131, 1986.

43. Sorenson, A.W., and others: Health objectives for the nation, Journal of the American Dietetic Association **87:**920, 1987.

44. Blaxter, K.: Food and people. Nutrition Today, p. 15, September-October 1985.

45. Altman, P.L. and Talbot, J.M.: Nutrition and metabolism in space flight. Journal of Nutrition **117:**421, 1987.

Nutrition and the Human Body

The human body must have mechanisms to obtain, use, and control the nutrients from food. An order or system is necessary to maximize the use of nutrients. In this appendix we compare this system with the normal workings of a modern city. This approach gives you a sort of "road map" to the human body. If you have studied these systems in biology or physiology courses, a glance at this "map" is all that is needed. If this is unfamiliar territory, more details than are provided here can be found in any introductory physiology text.

Let us look at the whole map first, before focusing on certain areas. Cities have distribution centers where products made outside the city are repackaged, or put into other forms suitable for distribution throughout local neighborhoods. In the same way the digestive system takes the nutrients from food, processes many of the nutrients into a form that can be sent into the transportation system—the blood—for distribution to different neighborhoods—the tissues.

A signal system is needed for this elaborate flow of nutrients. There are about 46 different nutrients, all important to the body, that must be delivered on time to the correct destination. Watch early morning television traffic reports and see the disruption when traffic signals malfunction in a city. The body has a number of signal systems to tell us when we need food, when we have enough food, and what to do with the nutrients from the food. Wrong signals, or no signals, are as disastrous to the human body as they are to the functioning of a city. For example, one theory of obesity is that the signals from the brain to control the amount of food eaten are sent incorrectly, or not sent at all. Another example is the signal for the removal of glucose from the blood by the action of insulin. Glucose is the preferred source of energy for tissues, especially the brain and the central nervous system. Loss of glucose in the urine in insulin-dependent (type I) diabetes is serious. In summary, the control system for most signals in the human body is the brain. These signals are carried by the nervous system, and hormones have an important role in implementing these signals.

The transportation system must take nutrients to all parts of the body—it would be too bad for us if nothing went beyond the liver, for instance. The circulatory system distributes throughout the body the nutrients from the digestive tract and the oxygen in the air. In addition, waste is produced, so that must be dumped. If it accumulates in our body it may produce toxic symptoms. Energy must be used efficiently in the transport of nutrients, the maintenance of tissues, and the regulation of body temperature.

Aren't the topics discussed so far familiar areas of debate for voters, city councils, and city workers? Quality of life for a city is determined by all parts of the city working properly—good distribution, clean environment, and adequate utilization of resources. Likewise, good nutrition is the adequate supply and utilization of *all* nutrients to *all* cells in the body. This enables the tissues made up by these cells to function properly. Good health means all tissues are working optimally. To ensure the proper utilization of nutrients by cells, the following systems play important roles.

DIGESTIVE SYSTEM

The digestive system is the first of a series of systems in the transfer of nutrients from food into nutrients in the human body. The digestive system releases nutrients from the diet (see Chapter 2, Metabolism Notes). This is achieved by a series of specialized enzymes. These and other digestive juices are provided by cells lining the digestive tract, by the liver (especially bile), and by the pancreas. Other secretions protect the cells lining the digestive tract. This secretion, called mucus, forms the mucous membrane coating the cells of the intestines.

Nutrients are absorbed at specific sites along the digestive tract. Not many nutrients are absorbed in the stomach or in the lower part of the large intestine. The upper portion of the small intestine is the site of greatest absorption. People who have this portion of small intestine surgically removed must have many nutrients provided directly into their veins.

The lower part of the intestinal system, the colon, is a storage area for the waste products of digestion. Here the feces remain until excretion.

A nervous system connection between the brain and the digestive system triggers contractions in the stomach. These are the familiar hunger pangs that we experience from time to time. After you have eaten a certain amount of food, another signal from the brain decreases the desire to eat.

CIRCULATORY SYSTEM

Nutrients from digestion (and oxygen from the air inhaled through the lungs) are distributed to the cells by the circulatory system. After digestion nutrients in the blood pass through the liver. This is a marvelous biochemical processing machine. Some nutrients are stored in the liver—glucose is converted into fat; fatty acids and glycerol are converted into fat; fat-soluble vitamin A is stored; and alcohol is detoxified.

The blood next passes through the kidneys. Body wastes carried by the blood are removed for excretion. Excess intakes of water-soluble nutrients and other substances are excreted also. For example, much of the vitamin C from a large volume of vitamin C–enriched fruit drink or a tablet of vitamin C will be filtered out of the blood by the kidney if the body has enough vitamin C. The water-soluble substances are then excreted in the urine.

Blood also delivers oxygen to the cells and removes the carbon dioxide produced by metabolism. Blood also helps regulate body temperature. Heat is produced by metabolism—the breakdown of carbohydrate, fat, and protein for energy. Some of this heat must be removed from the body, and the blood supply plays a major role in heat loss from the body. Blood also is important in regulating the effect of environmental temperature. In a cold environment the blood flow to the limbs is reduced (that is why your fingers and toes look white). Excess heat is removed from the body by increasing blood flow to the skin, and to the limbs.

Dehydration has severe consequences on blood volume. Human beings are the only animals that will voluntarily restrict fluid intake. When this happens, lost fluids are not replaced adequately. Athletes should be encouraged to drink more fluids to avoid dehydration. This is especially important in prolonged activity. Otherwise performance is lowered because dehydration causes a decrease in blood volume from loss of water from perspiration. Fatigue is one of many symptoms of dehydration.

EXCRETORY SYSTEM

Body waste is removed from the body through the digestive tract, kidneys, skin, and lungs.

Undigested food and some secretions into the digestive system (bile, for example) are excreted in the feces. The kidneys produce urine after purification of the blood. Urine is stored in the urinary bladder before excretion. Some hormones influence the working of the kidney. One example is aldosterone, which regulates the elimination of sodium.

The main function of the skin in excretion is the elimination of excess body heat. The lungs eliminate carbon dioxide produced when carbohydrates, fats, and proteins are broken down for energy.

STORAGE SYSTEMS

It is important that the human body has reserves of nutrients. Otherwise we would need to eat continuously. The amount of storage capacity varies depending on the nutrient (see Chapter 2). The way the nutrient is stored differs also. Storage may be at a particular site designed specifically for storage. Adipose tissue, for example, is used for long-term storage of fat. Other tissues store nutrients as well as performing other important functions. Short-term stores of carbohydrate are in muscle and liver glycogen, while blood has a small reserve of amino acids.

Some nutrients must be obtained in a period of deficiency by the destruction of a tissue containing high concentrations of the nutrient. Examples include calcium in bone and protein in muscle. Both of these nutrients are important in the proper functioning of bones and muscles, respectively. However, in emergencies caused by inadequate intake, calcium is released from bone and amino acids are released from muscle proteins. This is not storage in a strict sense of the word because loss of these nutrients harms the tissues involved in the loss.

CONTROL SYSTEMS

The hormones and the nervous system are two control mechanisms in the body having significant influences on nutrients.

Nutrition and Hormones

The importance of one hormone, insulin, is shown early in the book. Insulin is secreted by the pancreas. It enables the transfer of glucose from blood to cells where it is converted into glycogen or fat. Glucagon is a hormone causing the opposite effect of insulin—the breakdown of glucose and the conversion of some amino acids into glucose. Since glucose is such an important nutrient for the proper functioning of all cells in the body, it is important that there is this check-and-balance control system on glucose use.

Some important hormonal systems and their relation to nutrition are:

Anterior pituitary gland

This gland is located at the base of the brain and secretes the following hormones.

Growth hormone (GH)—affects all tissues, growth, fat breakdown, and antibody formation.

Thyroid-stimulating hormone (TSH)—manufactures and releases thyroid hormone; requires iodine to function; regulates energy metabolism.

Prolactin—secreted by women after the birth of a baby; involved in milk production.

Adrenocorticotropin (ACTH)—stimulates the adrenal cortex to release its hormones (see below).

Hypothalamus

A part of the brain, the hypothalamus controls the release of hormones by the pituitary gland. For example, it produces hormones that enhance the release of ACTH and TSH and hormones that inhibit the release of GH and prolactin.

Posterior pituitary gland

Among the hormones produced by the posterior pituitary gland is the antidiuretic hormone (vasopressin), which prevents water loss through kidneys and regulates sodium levels.

Gastrointestinal tract

Hormones produced by the gastrointestinal tract include the following.

Gastrin—stimulates secretion of digestive juices and the hydrochloric acid in stomach in response to food.

Cholecystokinin—stimulates emptying of gallbladder and pancreas secretions for digestion in the small intestine.

Secretin—produced by the pancreas to neutralize the acid contents of digestion as they arrive in the duodenum (upper small intestine) from the acid environment of the stomach.

Energy regulation

Hormones involved in energy regulation include the following.

Insulin and glucagon—produced by pancreas; functions are described at the introduction to the hormones previously.

Thyroxin—produced by the thyroid gland; increases metabolic rate by increasing energy metabolism.

Growth hormone (GH)—see description previously in anterior pituitary gland section.

Glucocorticoids—secreted by the adrenal cortex; protect against stress; involved in carbohydrate and protein metabolism.

Epinephrine (adrenaline) and norepinephrine (noradrenaline)—produced in the adrenal medulla; main function is to react to flight or fright by increasing blood flow especially to muscles, increasing the breakdown of glycogen, glucose, and fat.

Other hormones

Other hormones with important interactions with nutrition include the following.

Prostaglandins—fatty acid–related compounds present in many tissues; require vitamin E for proper functioning; affect cardiac and smooth muscle; and stimulate the uterus to contract.

Aldosterone—causes kidneys to secrete less sodium and less water; raises blood pressure.

Calcitonin (CT), parathyroid hormone (PTH), vitamin D—involved in bone formation; CT removes excess calcium in blood and deposits it in bones; PTH has the reverse effect of CT on bones; vitamin D and PTH are essential for calcium absorption from the gastrointestinal tract.

Nutrition and the Nervous System

Muscles and organs within the body are under either direct or indirect control by the nervous system. All voluntary movements of muscle are under a nervous reflex—pulling your hand away from an excessive source of heat is triggered by nerve impulses from the brain. Of course the energy to pull the hand away must come from the energy nutrients.

Involuntary muscle function (we do not knowingly cause the muscles to function) is important during digestion. Shivering in the cold is an involuntary movement of muscles to generate body heat. That heat comes from the energy nutrients involved in the movement of the muscles during the shivering.

Some nutrients are important in nerve functioning. Among them are the type of fat—especially cholesterol—in membranes around nerve cells, and some of the B-complex vitamins in nerve functioning—especially thiamin and niacin. Glucose is the only source of energy for nerves.

There are exciting developments in research on the effects of nutrients on behavior and moods. We await further developments in this important area.

Calculating Your Nutrient Intake

We hope that you will use this Appendix as you read through the book. Some of the questions you can answer by accurate measurement of nutrient intakes include: Is your nutrient intake adequate? Does your nutrient intake vary greatly between the weekend and the rest of the week? Do you eat poorly "on the run"? Is your elderly neighbor, your pregnant friend, or your toddler cousin getting the required amount of nutrients?

These are important questions, so attention to detail is needed if they are to be answered accurately. You need to do the following:

Decide how long a period of dietary intake you will study

A period of three days or more is best—a 24-hour period may or may not be typical of your regular dietary intake (see Chapter 2 for more details).

Keep a *complete* record of *all* foods *and* beverages consumed

Longer time periods should give you a more representative analysis of your dietary intake. Methods available include the following:

Twenty-four-hour recall. All foods and beverages taken in the past 24 hours. This may be more difficult than you think—how good is your memory? Many of us regard yesterday's food as history; did you drink that big glass of orange juice yesterday or the day before?

Food records. Record all of the food you eat. This avoids your dependence on memory. Be careful not to bias your answer by eating what you should eat rather than what you usually do eat.

Daily food summary. This is a listing of how much and how often you eat certain foods. How many times per day or per week do you consume the following foods and drinks?

Milk or cheese
Nuts and seeds
Fruits
Meat, poultry, fish
Legumes (beans, peas)
Fats (butter, margarines, oils)
Eggs
Vegetables
Starchy foods (cereals, bread, potatoes, rice)

Fried snacks (corn and potato chips, etc.)
Desserts and sweet baked goods
Sugar and salt added to food
Coffee, tea, carbonated drinks (not diet)
Fruit drinks
Alcoholic beverages

Describe the food as completely as possible

The form of the food. Meat trimmed of fat; skim or whole milk; sweetened or unsweetened fruit juices; butter added to bread, vegetables, potatoes; cake with or without icing. These examples influence the amount of fat or sugar and the number of kcalories in each serving.

Method of preparation. Was the food raw, fried, baked, broiled (see Chapter 11 for more details)?

Condiments. Mayonnaise and salad dressings; cream and sugar used in coffee and tea; syrups and jellies; catsup and mustard.

Estimate the serving size

This is important, and it may require some practice. See the inside front cover for further details on conversion factors for weights and measures.

Volume—cups, tablespoons, teaspoons
Weight—pounds, ounces
Units—one orange, one frankfurter, one cookie

Calculate your nutrient intake from the data in Appendixes G, H, I, J, K, O, and P

Use of all of these tables gives you an indication of your nutrient intake. No nutrition texts give nutrient content of *all* foods available to us. However, if you do require information on a food not listed here, consult *Composition of Foods,* Agriculture Handbook Nos. 8-1 through 8-16, United States Department of Agriculture, Washington, D.C. This handbook provides the nutrient profile for over 4000 foods.

Calculations

Nutrient content

The nutrient composition of foods is measured in either serving size (Appendixes G, K, O, and P) or per 100 g of food (Appendixes, H, I, and J). Serving size is useful in defining typical amounts of food eaten. Nutrient content per 100 g of food is useful in comparing nutrient concentration in different foods. The two sets of values are interconvertible. The following examples are for the calcium content of cheddar cheese. The same calculation applies for all foods and nutrients.

Converting nutrients per serving to nutrient content per 100 g of food. In Appendix P we saw that 1 oz of cheddar cheese had 204 mg of calcium. One ounce is equivalent to 28 g. Therefore, if 28 g of cheddar cheese contains 204 mg calcium then 100 g of cheddar cheese contains

$$\frac{204 \times 100}{28} = 729 \text{ mg calcium}$$

B

Converting nutrients per 100 g of food into nutrients per serving. Let's continue with cheddar cheese as the example. There is 105 mg cholesterol in 100 g of cheddar cheese (Appendix H). To convert this to the amount of cholesterol in one ounce or 28 g (Appendix P): if 100 g of cheddar cheese contains 105 mg cholesterol then 28 g of cheddar cheese contains

$$\frac{105 \times 28}{100} = 29.4 \text{ mg cholesterol}$$

Calculating the polyunsaturated fatty acid to saturated fatty acid ratio (P/S ratio). In Chapters 4 and 14 the importance of different types of fat in the possible cause or prevention of coronary heart disease is discussed. Briefly, saturated fat increases and polyunsaturated fat decreases serum cholesterol. Coronary heart disease is correlated with high serum cholesterol levels. To determine the amount of saturated and polyunsaturated fat in a food the P/S ratio is calculated (monounsaturated fat has a neutral role in heart disease so it is not included in the calculations). Experts believe the ideal ratio is 1:1.

Still with cheddar cheese as the example, we see in Appendix P that one ounce has 0.3 g of polyunsaturated fatty acids and 6.0 g saturated fatty acids, which yields a P/S ratio of 0.3/6.0 or 0.05:1. Usually the ratio is expressed when S = 1. We see that cheddar cheese has a high proportion of saturated fat.

Now let's look at the P/S ratio in safflower oil. This is a rich source of polyunsaturated fatty acids. This oil is used in some margarines. One cup of safflower oil has 162.4 g of polyunsaturated fat and 19.8 g of saturated fatty acids. Therefore, the P/S ratio is 10.4/1.3 or 8:1.

Interconverting nutritive values in different weights of food. Supposing you ate 1¼ oz of cheddar cheese. Appendix P gives the nutrient content in 1 oz cheddar cheese. You want to know how much protein was in that 1¼ oz:

1 oz of cheddar cheese contains 7 g of protein

$$1\tfrac{1}{4} \text{ oz contains } \frac{7 \times 1\tfrac{1}{4}}{1} = \frac{7 \times 5}{1 \times 4} = \frac{35}{4} = 8.75 \text{ g protein}$$

Other conversion factors used by nutritionists are listed inside the front cover.

Profile of Nutrient Supplement Users

Have you used vitamin supplements in the past? Do your friends use them now? Are vitamin and mineral supplements necessary for health and beauty? Results from a recent large survey are summarized in this Appendix and should help you in answering these questions.

Information in this Appendix relates especially to information in Chapter 6 on the vitamins, Chapter 7 on the minerals, and Chapter 15 on current lifestyles.

Many supplement users visit health food stores with little or no information about the products or their health status. About three out of four people use nutrient supplements without the involvement of their doctor. What seems surprising is that over one third of people surveyed saw no benefits from taking these supplements. Frequently people made up their own minds to take these supplements without any influence from their physician, family and friends, or from books and magazines. Clearly, there is much to learn about why well-nourished people are attracted to self-prescribed vitamin and mineral supplements.

Profile of Nutrient Supplement Users

	Vitamin and Mineral Supplement Usage Groups	
	Light	Heavy
Health Food Store Visits		
None	63.0	43.7
Less than once a month	26.3	37.6
One to three times a month	7.3	12.7
Once or more a week	3.3	6.1
Total	100.0	100.0
Source of Purchase Information		
None	82.9	71.5
Popular media	9.4	4.1
Health magazines/books	5.7	20.6
Others	2.1	3.8
Total	100.0	100.0

Source: Adapted from Levy, A.S. and Schucker, R.E., Patterns of nutrient intake among dietary supplement users: Attitudinal and behavioral correlates. *Journal of the American Dietetic Association*, **87**:754, 1987. *Continued.*

C

Profile of Nutrient Supplement Users—cont'd

	Vitamin and Mineral Supplement Usage Groups	
	Light	Heavy
Source of Health Information		
None	52.9	44.0
Popular media	30.3	24.4
Health magazines/books	8.6	23.4
Others	8.2	8.2
Total	100.0	100.0
Physician Involvement		
Physician prescribed product	13.7	11.6
Physician recommended product	16.7	10.3
No physician involvement	69.6	78.1
Total	100.0	100.0
Perceived Product Benefits		
None	39.7	34.8
General health	44.1	32.8
Specific health	16.2	32.4
Total	100.0	100.0
Source of Influence on Purchase		
Myself	40.1	29.0
Physician	25.6	18.8
Family/friend	30.7	41.1
Books/magazines	7.1	19.4
Total	103.5	108.3
Place of Purchase		
Grocery store	14.2	9.6
Drugstore/pharmacy	53.3	35.2
Health food store	9.4	24.2
Mail order	2.9	15.7
Direct sales	8.8	7.6
Other	8.8	7.6
Total	97.4	99.9
Daily Exercise		
Yes	51.8	54.7
No	48.2	45.3
Total	100.0	100.0

Biochemical Indicators of Good Nutrition Status

Tests discussed in this appendix indicate if there is an adequate level of certain nutrients in the body. This information relates to the discussion on assessment of nutritional status in Chapter 2. Most nutrients measured are vitamins and minerals, and these are examined in detail in Chapters 6 and 7. Background information on why blood and urine are important in nutritional status studies is given in Appendix B.

Notice the importance of whole blood, plasma and serum (the liquid remaining when the cells are removed from blood), and erythrocytes (red blood cells) in determining the nutritional status of a person.

The concentration of a nutrient in blood is determined in a number of ways. One is by measuring the concentration of a particular chemical in the blood. The best example is the measurement of iron status by hemoglobin measurement. This is the biochemical indicator most familiar to people. The heme part of hemoglobin contains iron. Therefore, a person deficient in iron cannot make sufficient iron-requiring heme. In turn, the hemoglobin level drops. Another way is to measure the amount of the nutrient circulating in the blood. Examples include the level of sodium and potassium. For some nutrients the most accurate measure comes from measuring an enzyme requiring a particular nutrient for its activity. For example, one enzyme requires riboflavin as a coenzyme. If a person's diet is low in riboflavin, the activity of this enzyme is reduced.

Urine samples are used to determine the status of some of the water-soluble vitamins. The reason is that intakes in excess of the requirements of the body are excreted in the urine.

Some of the tests listed here are performed before surgery and other clinical procedures. Ask for these results—they should be made available to you. These values may be useful for future reference.

Biochemical Indicators of Good Nutrition Status

Nutrient or Measurement	Test	Normal or Acceptable Levels	
		Men	Women
Iron	Hemoglobin (g/100 mL)	≥14.0[1]	≥12.0
	Infants (under 2 years)	≥10.0	≥10.0
	Children (6-12 years)	≥11.5	≥11.5
	Pregnancy (2nd trimester)		≥11.0
	(3rd trimester)		≥10.5
Protein	Serum albumin (g/100 mL)	≥3.5	≥3.5
Normal lipid metabolism	Serum cholesterol (mg/100 mL)	<240	<240
	Serum triglyceride (mg/100 mL)	40-160	35-135
Normal carbohydrate metabolism	Serum glucose (mg/100 mL)	75-110	75-110
Sodium	Serum sodium (mEq/L)	130-150	130-155
Potassium	Serum potassium (mEq/L)	3.5-5.3	3.5-5.3
Vitamin A	Plasma vitamin A (μg/100 mL)	>20	>20
Vitamin C	Serum vitamin C (mg/100 mL)	≥0.3	≥0.3
Riboflavin	Erythrocyte glutathione peroxidase (% stimulation of activity by added riboflavin cofactor)	<20	<20
Vitamin B_6	Tryptophan load test—increase in excretion of xanthurenic acid (mg/day)	<25	<25
Folacin	Serum folacin (nanogram/mL)	>6.0	>6.0
Thiamin	Urinary thiamin (μg/g creatinine)	>65	>65
Zinc	Plasma zinc (μg/100 mL)	80-115	80-115

Source: Some information obtained from: Roe, D.A.: *Drug-induced nutritional deficiences*, AVI Press, Westport, Conn., 1976, and Sauberlich, H.E., Skala, H.H., and Dowdy, R.P.: *Laboratory tests for the assessment of nutritional status*, CRC Press, Inc., Cleveland, 1974.

Sources of Nutrition Information

The reference section at the end of each chapter of *Decisions in Nutrition* gives some idea of the amazing number of sources of nutrition information. We have emphasized throughout that only sources of reliable nutrition information should be consulted. The following is a list of some of the most frequently used sources of information. For your convenience it is divided into the following groups: dictionaries and encyclopedias, professional journals, newsletters, professional resources.

DICTIONARIES AND ENCYCLOPEDIAS OF NUTRITION

Detailed descriptions of most of the terms used in nutrition are given in the following two books:

Ensminger, A.H., Ensminger, M.E., Konlande, J.E., and Robson, J.R.K.: *Food for Health—A Nutrition Encyclopedia*, Pegus Press, Clovis, California, 1986.

Yudkin, J.: *The Penguin Encyclopaedia of Nutrition*, Viking Penguin Inc., New York, 1985.

Descriptions and definitions of foods, and nutrient changes due to the production, preparation, and processing of foods are given in:

Bender, A.E.: *Dictionary of Nutrition and Food Technology*, 5th edition, Butterworth Publishers, Boston, 1982.

Concepts in biochemistry as it relates to nutrition are given in:

Hamilton, E.M.N., and Gropper, S.A.S.: *The Biochemistry of Human Nutrition—A Desk Reference*, West Publishing Company, St. Paul, 1987.

PROFESSIONAL JOURNALS DEALING WITH NUTRITION
General

The following journals deal with many different topics in nutrition:

Annual Review of Nutrition
FDA Consumer
Journal of the American College of Nutrition
Journal of the American Dietetic Association
Journal of the Canadian Dietetic Association
Journal of Nutrition
Journal of Nutrition Education

Nutrition Reviews
Nutrition Today
Proceedings of the Nutrition Society (British)

Clinical Nutrition

The following journals deal mainly with clinical nutrition issues. Examples are the role of diet in diseases such as coronary heart disease, cancer, hypertension, diabetes, and obesity.
American Journal of Clinical Nutrition
American Journal of Medicine
British Medical Journal
Canadian Medical Association
Human Nutrition: Clinical Nutrition (British)
Journal of the American Medical Association
Lancet (British)
New England Journal of Medicine

Food—Nutritive Value

How food processing and preparation affect nutritive value is covered in the following journals:
Food Chemical Toxicology
Food Engineering
Food Technology
Journal of Food Science
National Food Review

Nutrition and Behavior

Major issues in this area are eating disorders and obesity. The following journals frequently have articles of interest to nutritionists:
American Journal of Psychology
Appetite
International Journal of Obesity
Journal of Clinical Psychology
Physiology and Behavior

Family and Public Health Nutrition

Articles here deal with the effects of family structure, sanitation, and education on the nutritional status of the population. Included also are comparisons of nutrition and nonnutrition factors in nutrition-related diseases (coronary heart disease, cancer, etc.) in different countries.
American Journal of Epidemiology
American Journal of Public Health
Canadian Journal of Public Health
Home Economics Research Journal
Journal of Epidemiology

Nutrition and the Young

Archives of Disease in Childhood
Journal of Pediatrics
Pediatrics

Nutrition and the Elderly

Geriatrics
Gerontology
Journal of Gerontology

Nutrition and the Athlete

International Journal of Sport Medicine
Journal of Sports Medicine
Journal of Applied Physiology
Medicine and Science in Sports and Exercise
The Physician and Sportsmedicine

Major Journals that Frequently Have Articles in Nutrition

American Journal of Physiology
Federation Proceedings
New Scientist (British)
Nature (British)
Science

NEWSLETTERS DEALING WITH NUTRITION

Nutrition information written for an audience without a strong background in the
sciences. Those indicated with an (*) are free to nutrition professionals.

Newsletters dealing with one topic in nutrition in each issue, and written by
an expert on the topic:

Contemporary Nutrition*
   General Mills, Inc.
   Production Manager
   P.O. Box 1112, Dept. 65
   Minneapolis, Minnesota 55440

Dietetic Currents*
   Ross Laboratories
   Director of Professional Services
   625 Cleveland Avenue
   Columbus, Ohio 43216

Dairy Council Digest
   National Dairy Council
   6300 North River Road
   Rosemont, Illinois 60018

Food and Nutrition News*
   National Livestock and Meat Board
   444 North Michigan Avenue
   Chicago, Illinois 60610

The following newsletters deal with a number of nutrition topics in each issue:

Nutrition & the M.D.
P.O. Box 2160
Van Nuys, California 91404

Tufts University Diet & Nutrition Letter
P.O. Box 10948
Des Moines, Iowa 50940

PROFESSIONAL RESOURCES IN NUTRITION

Organizations publishing information include:

American Cancer Society
777 Third Avenue
New York, New York 10017

American Dental Association
211 East Chicago Avenue
Chicago, Illinois 60611

American Geriatrics Society
10 Columbus Circle
New York, New York 10010

American Heart Association
7320 Greenville Avenue
Dallas, Texas 75231

American Home Economics Association
5010 Massachusetts Avenue, N.W.
Washington, DC 20036

Consumer Information Center
U.S. General Services Administration
Pueblo, Colorado 81009

Food and Nutrition Information and Education Resources Center
National Library of Congress
Beltsville, Maryland 20705

Food and Nutrition Board
National Research Council, National Academy of Sciences
2101 Constitution Avenue N.W.
Washington, DC 20418

Institute of Food Technologists
221 N. LaSalle Street
Chicago, Illinois 60601

Office of Cancer Communications
National Cancer Institute
Building 31, Room 10A18
9000 Rockville Pike
Bethesda, Maryland 20205

INDIVIDUALS ABLE TO PROVIDE RELIABLE NUTRITION INFORMATION

Dietitians—in private practice, hospitals, and nursing homes

Extension agents—in county extension offices

Home economists—in various food-related businesses

Nutritionists—in universities (mainly in food science and nutrition); in city, county, and state public health departments

E

Vitamin and Mineral Intake

Estimated Safe and Adequate Daily Dietary Intakes of Selected Vitamins and Minerals

	Age (Years)	Vitamins		
		Vitamin K (μg)	Biotin (μg)	Pantothenic Acid (mg)
Infants	0-0.5	12	35	2
	0.5-1	10-20	50	3
Children and adolescents	1-3	15-30	65	3
	4-6	20-40	85	3-4
	7-10	30-60	120	4-5
	11+	50-100	100-200	4-7
Adults		70-140	100-200	4-7

	Age (Years)	Trace Elements					
		Copper (mg)	Manganese (mg)	Fluoride (mg)	Chromium (mg)	Selenium (mg)	Molybdenum (mg)
Infants	0-0.5	0.5-0.7	0.5-0.7	0.1-0.5	0.01-0.04	0.01-0.04	0.03-0.06
	0.5-1	0.7-1.0	0.7-1.0	0.2-1.0	0.02-0.06	0.02-0.06	0.04-0.08
Children and adolescents	1-3	1.0-1.5	1.0-1.5	0.5-1.5	0.02-0.08	0.02-0.08	0.05-0.1
	4-6	1.5-2.0	1.5-2.0	1.0-2.5	0.03-0.12	0.03-0.12	0.06-0.15
	7-10	2.0-2.5	2.0-3.0	1.5-2.5	0.05-0.2	0.05-0.2	0.10-0.3
	11+	2.0-3.0	2.5-5.0	1.5-2.5	0.05-0.2	0.05-0.2	0.15-0.5
Adults		2.0-3.0	2.5-5.0	1.5-4.0	0.05-0.2	0.05-0.2	0.15-0.5

Source: *Recommended Dietary Allowances,* 9th edition, National Academy Press, Washington, D.C., 1980.

Estimated Safe and Adequate Daily Dietary Intakes of Selected Vitamins and Minerals—cont'd

	Age (Years)	Electrolytes		
		Sodium (mg)	Potassium (mg)	Chloride (mg)
Infants	0-0.5	115-350	350-925	275-700
	0.5-1	250-750	425-1275	400-1200
Children and adolescents	1-3	325-975	550-1650	500-1500
	4-6	450-1350	775-2325	700-2100
	7-10	600-1800	1000-3000	925-2775
	11+	900-2700	1525-4575	1400-4200
Adults		1100-3300	1875-5625	1700-5100

Dietary Fiber in Foods

Information in this appendix relates to the detailed discussion on fiber in Chapter 3, the discussion on the production and processing of foods in Chapter 11, and the discussion of fiber as a protective factor in a number of diseases is discussed in Chapter 14.

These are the most up-to-date figures on the fiber content of foods. The table was compiled by experts at the National Cancer Institute, National Institutes of Health, from a critical evaluation of the scientific literature on fiber. To get the full benefit of the information presented here it is important to observe the following cautions from the experts:[1]

- There are many technical problems in getting accurate measures on the amount of fiber in different foods.
- Usually only a few samples of each food were used (and sometimes only one sample).
- Sometimes food samples are not described properly—for instance, genetic information, the stage of maturity, and whether the fiber-rich skin was peeled from the plant. These factors can influence fiber content.
- Changes in the fiber content of foods during food processing have not been well documented.

This information should not intimidate you from using this appendix to examine the fiber content of your own diet. Rather, the information is given to show that there is much to be learned in the future about an important component in our diet.

[1]Lanza, E. and Butrum, R.R.: A critical review of food fiber analysis and data, *Journal of the American Dietetic Association* **86**:732, 1986.

Dietary Fiber in Foods

Food	Serving Size	Fiber (g)/ Serving	Food	Serving Size	Fiber (g)/ Serving
Breakfast Cereals			Dates	3	1.9
All-Bran	⅓ c (1 oz)	8.5	Grapefruit	½	1.6
Bran Buds	⅓ c (1 oz)	7.9	Grapes	20	0.6
Bran Chex	⅔ c (1 oz)	4.6	Orange	1	2.6
Cheerios-type	1¼ c (1 oz)	1.1	Peach (w/skin)	1	1.9
Corn Bran	⅔ c (1 oz)	5.4	Peach (w/o skin)	1	1.2
Cracklin' Bran	⅓ c (1 oz)	4.3	Pear (w/skin)	½ large	3.1
Crispy Wheats n' Raisins	¾ c (1 oz)	1.3	Pear (w/o skin)	½ large	2.5
40% Bran-type	¾ c (1 oz)	4.0	Pineapple	½ c	1.1
Frosted-Mini Wheats	4 biscuits (1 oz)	2.1	Plums, damsons	5	0.9
Graham Crackos	¾ c (1 oz)	1.7	Prunes	3	3.0
Grape-Nuts	¼ c (1 oz)	1.4	Raisins	¼ c	3.1
Heartland Natural Cereal, plain	¼ c (1 oz)	1.3	Raspberries	½ c	3.1
			Strawberries	1 c	3.0
Honey Bran	⅞ c (1 oz)	3.1	Watermelon	1 c	0.4
Most	⅔ c (1 oz)	3.5	*Juices*		
Nutri-Grain, barley	¾ c (1 oz)	1.7	Apple	½ c (4 oz)	0.4
Nutri-Grain, corn	¾ c (1 oz)	1.8	Grapefruit	½ c (4 oz)	0.5
Nutri-Grain, rye	¾ c (1 oz)	1.8	Grape	½ c (4 oz)	0.6
Nutri-Grain, wheat	¾ c (1 oz)	1.8	Orange	½ c (4 oz)	0.5
100% Bran	½ c (1 oz)	8.4	Papaya	½ c (4 oz)	0.8
100% Natural Cereal, plain	¼ c (1 oz)	1.0			
			Vegetables		
Raisin Bran-type	¾ c (1 oz)	4.0	*Cooked*		
Shredded Wheat	⅔ c (1 oz)	2.6	Asparagus, cut	½ c	1.0
Tasteeos	1¼ c (1 oz)	1.0	Beans, string, green	½ c	1.6
Total	1 c (1 oz)	2.0	Broccoli	½ c	2.2
Wheat n' Raisin Chex	¾ c (1⅓ oz)	2.5	Brussels sprouts	½ c	2.3
Wheat Chex	⅔ c (1⅓ oz)	2.1	Cabbage, red	½ c	1.4
Wheaties	1 c (1 oz)	2.0	Cabbage, white	½ c	1.4
Oatmeal, regular, quick, and instant, cooked	¾ c (1 oz)	1.6	Carrots	½ c	2.3
			Cauliflower	½ c	1.1
Wheat germ	¼ c (2 oz)	3.4	Corn, canned	½ c	2.9
Cornflakes	1¼ c (1 oz)	0.3	Kale leaves	½ c	1.4
Rice Krispies	1 c (1 oz)	0.1	Parsnip	½ c	2.7
Special K	1⅓ c (1 oz)	0.2	Peas	½ c	3.6
Sugar Smacks	¾ c (1 oz)	0.4	Potato (w/o skin)	1 med.	1.4
			Potato (w/skin)	1 med.	2.5
Fruits			Spinach	½ c	2.1
Apple (w/o skin)	1 med.	2.7	Squash, summer	½ c	1.4
Apple (w/skin)	1 med.	3.5	Sweet potatoes	½ med.	1.7
Apricot (fresh)	3 med.	1.8	Turnip	½ c	1.6
Apricot, dried	5 halves	1.4	Zucchini	½ c	1.8
Banana	1 med.	2.4	*Raw*		
Blueberries	½ c	2.0	Bean sprout, soy	½ c	1.5
Cantaloupe	¼ melon	1.0	Celery, diced	½ c	1.1
Cherries, sweet	10	1.2	Cucumber	½ c	0.4

Source: Lanza, E. and Butrum, R.R., A critical review of food fiber analysis and data, *Journal of the American Dietetic Association*, **86**:732, 1986. Reprinted with permission.

Continued.

Dietary Fiber in Foods—cont'd

Food	Serving Size	Fiber (g)/ Serving	Food	Serving Size	Fiber (g)/ Serving
Lettuce, sliced	1 c	0.9	Crisp bread, wheat	2 crackers	1.8
Mushrooms, sliced	½ c	0.9	French bread	1 sl	0.7
Onions, sliced	½ c	0.8	Italian bread	1 sl	0.3
Pepper, green, sliced	½ c	0.5	Mixed grain	1 sl	0.9
Tomato	1 med.	1.5	Oatmeal	1 sl	0.5
Spinach		1.2	Pita bread (5″)	1 piece	0.4
			Pumpernickel bread	1 sl	1.0
Legumes			Raisin bread	1 sl	0.6
Baked beans, tomato sauce	½ c	8.8	White bread	1 sl	0.4
			Whole wheat bread	1 sl	1.4
Dried peas, cooked	½ c	4.7	*Pasta and rice (cooked)*		
Kidney beans, cooked	½ c	7.3	Macaroni	1 c	1.0
Lima beans, cooked/ canned	½ c	4.5	Rice, brown	½ c	1.0
			Rice, polished	½ c	0.2
Lentils, cooked	½ c	3.7	Spaghetti (regular)	1 c	1.1
Navy beans, cooked	½ c	6.0	Spaghetti (whole wheat)	1 c	3.9
Breads, Pastas, and Flours			**Nuts**		
Bagels	1 bagel	0.6	Almonds	10 nuts	1.1
Bran muffins	1 muffin	2.5	Peanuts	10 nuts	1.4
Cracked wheat	1 sl	1.0	Filberts	10 nuts	0.8
Crisp bread, rye	2 crackers	2.0			

G

Cholesterol in Foods

The importance of the chemistry of cholesterol is discussed in Chapter 4, and its relationship in coronary heart disease is discussed in Chapter 14.

You can make a direct comparison between the various foods listed in this appendix because all values are expressed as milligrams of cholesterol per 100 g of food. High sources of cholesterol are liver, egg yolk, butter, fish oils, shellfish, and some processed meats. If you wish to convert values in this appendix into serving sizes or into other unit weights, use the calculations in Appendix B.

Look for some surprising sources of cholesterol in the section headed "Other Foods." Cakes, cookies, and cupcakes will have cholesterol if eggs and butter are used in their preparation. Saltines have cholesterol because they are made with animal shortening. Contributing cholesterol to doughnuts are eggs; to French fries edible tallow (if used); to pizza cheese and meat (if a meat topping is used); to some salad dressings mainly cheese (in blue cheese dressing), and eggs (in the mayonnaise-type dressings). Not all salad dressings contain cholesterol—Italian, French, Thousand Island, and homemade vinegar and soybean oil dressings have no cholesterol.

Cholesterol in Foods

Food Item	Cholesterol (mg/100 g)	Food Item	Cholesterol (mg/100 g)
Meat, Poultry, Fish			
Beef, ground, raw	85	Chicken, dark meat, w/o skin, raw	80
Beef, round, raw	66	Chicken, skin only, raw	109
T-bone steak, lean and fat, raw	71	Turkey, with skin, roasted	82
Pork, cured, bacon, raw	67	Bologna (beef and pork)	57
Pork, cured salt pork, raw	86	Braunschweiger	157
Pork, fresh ham, raw	74	Frankfurters (beef)	47
Lamb	71	Salami, cooked (beef and pork)	64
Veal	71	Liver, beef, fried	438
Chicken, broiler fryers, flesh	90	Catfish	67

Sources: Adapted from Hepburn, F.N., Exler, J., and Weihrauch, J.L.: Provisional tables on the content of omega-3 fatty acids and other fat components of selected foods, *Journal of the American Dietetic Association* **86:**788, 1986; and Weihrauch, J.L.: Provisional table on the fatty acid and cholesterol content of selected foods, Data Research Branch, Consumer Nutrition Division, United States Department of Agriculture, Washington, D.C., 1984.

Continued.

Cholesterol in Foods—cont'd

Food Item	Cholesterol (mg/100 g)	Food Item	Cholesterol (mg/100 g)
Meat, Poultry, Fish—cont'd		**Dairy and Egg Products—cont'd**	
Cod	40	Yogurt, with added milk solids:	
Herring	55	with low-fat milk	5
Mackerel	55	with nonfat milk	2
Perch	85	with whole milk	13
Salmon	74	Egg yolk, chicken, raw	1,602
Trout	58	**Fats and Oils**	
Tuna	46	Butter	219
Crab	88	Butter oil	256
Clam	31	Chicken fat	85
Lobster	112	**Other Foods**	
Oyster	39	Cakes:	
Shrimp	130	pound	206
Fish oils:		yellow, 2 layer	52
cod liver oil	570	Cookies:	
herring oil	766	brownies, with chocolate icing	52
menhaden oil	521	chocolate chip	53
salmon oil	484	Crackers:	
Dairy and Egg Products		graham	0
Cheese, cheddar	105	saltines	27
Cheese, Roquefort	90	Cupcakes, with chocolate icing	42
Cream, heavy whipping	137	Doughnuts	40
Milk, whole	14	French fries (fried in edible tallow)	12
		Pizza with cheese	22
		Salad dressing:	
		blue cheese	17
		mayonnaise-type	26

H

Omega-3 Fatty Acids in Foods

Information in this appendix is particularly relevant to the discussions on the fatty acids in Chapter 4 and to the evaluation of dietary factors in coronary heart disease in Chapter 14.

Nutritionists are interested in omega-3 fatty acids because of recent evidence linking high intakes of these fatty acids with a lower incidence of coronary heart disease. Investigations are proceeding on the specifics of this relationship.

Some technical details will help you if you want to follow this active area of study during the next few years. The most common dietary sources of the omega-3 fatty acids are fish oils, which contain eicosapentaenoic acid (20:5ω3) and docosahexaenoic acid (22:6ω3), and soybean oil, which contains linolenic acid (18:3ω3). In compiling this appendix I have combined all three fatty acids under the general heading "omega-3 fatty acids."

Articles and advertisements in the popular press stress fish oils as important sources of omega-3 fatty acids. But notice that soybeans, soybean oil, and certain nuts are high in these fatty acids. Different margarines and salad oils have varying concentrations of omega-3 fatty acids because of different ingredients.

Omega-3 Fatty Acids in Foods

Food Item	Edible Portion, Raw (g/100 g)	Food Item	Edible Portion, Raw (g/100 g)
Fish Oils			
Cod liver oil	19.2	Dogfish, spiny	1.9
Herring oil	12.0	Herring, Atlantic	1.7
Menhaden oil	21.7	Herring, Pacific	1.8
Salmon oil	20.9	Mackerel, Atlantic	2.6
		Mackerel, king	2.2
Finned Fish			
Anchovy, European	1.4	Mullet, unspecified	1.1
Bluefish	1.2	Sablefish	1.5

Source: Hepburn, F.N., Exler, J., and Weihrauch, J.L.: Provisional tables on the content of omega-3 fatty acids and other fat components of selected foods, *Journal of the American Dietetic Association* **86**:788, 1986. *Continued.*

Food Item	Edible Portion, Raw (g/100 g)	Food Item	Edible Portion, Raw (g/100 g)
Finned Fish—cont'd		**Fats and Oils—cont'd**	
Salmon, Atlantic	1.4	Salad dressing, commercial, blue cheese, regular	3.7
Salmon, Chinook	1.5		
Scad, Muroaji	2.1	Salad dressing, commercial, Italian, regular	3.3
Sprat	1.3		
Sturgeon, Atlantic	1.5	Salad dressing, commercial, mayonnaise (imitation), soybean, without cholesterol	4.6
Trout, lake	2.0		
Tuna, albacore	1.5	Salad dressing, commercial, mayonnaise, safflower and soybean	3.0
Tuna, bluefin	1.6		
Whitefish, lake	1.3	Salad dressing, commercial, mayonnaise, soybean	4.2
Fats and Oils		Salad dressing, commercial, mayonnaise-type	2.0
Butter	1.2		
Butter oil	1.5	Salad dressing, commercial, Thousand Island, regular	2.5
Chicken fat	1.0		
Duck fat	1.0	Salad dressing, home recipe, French	1.9
Lard	1.0		
Linseed oil	53.3	Salad dressing, home recipe, vinegar and soybean oil	1.4
Margarine, hard, soybean	1.5		
Margarine, hard, soybean oil and hydrogenated soybean oil	1.9	Shortening, special purpose, for bread, soybean (hydrogenated) and cottonseed	4.0
Margarine, hard, hydrogenated soybean oil and palm oil	2.3	Shortening, special purpose, heavy-duty, frying, soybean (hydrogenated)	2.4
Margarine, hard, hydrogenated soybean oil and cottonseed oil	2.8		
Margarine, hard, hydrogenated soybean oil and hydrogenated palm oil	3.0	Soybean lecithin	5.1
		Soybean oil	6.8
		Walnut oil	10.4
Margarine, liquid, hydrogenated soybean oil, soybean oil and cottonseed oil	2.4	**Legumes**	
		Soybeans, dry	1.6
Margarine, soft, hydrogenated soybean oil and cottonseed oil	1.6	**Nuts and Seeds**	
		Beechnuts, dried	1.7
Margarine, soft, hydrogenated soybean oil and palm oil	1.9	Butternuts, dried	8.7
		Chia seeds, dried	3.9
Margarine, soft, soybean oil, hydrogenated soybean oil and hydrogenated cottonseed oil	2.8	Walnuts, black	3.3
		Walnuts, English/Persian	6.8
Rapeseed oil (canola)	11.1	**Vegetables**	
Rice bran oil	1.6	Soybeans, green, raw	3.2
		Soybeans, mature seeds, sprouted, cooked	2.1

Sodium, Potassium, Zinc, Selenium, and Iodine Content of Food

Information in this appendix relates especially to the information on the minerals in Chapter 7 and to the information on relationship between certain minerals and diseases during the life cycle, discussed in Chapters 12, 13, and 14.

Nutritive values are expressed as milligrams per 100 g of food. Use the calculations in Appendix B to convert values in this appendix into other units of measurement.

Sodium is included because some people have to control sodium intake because of hypertension and kidney failure. Some fast foods are high in sodium (Appendix O). Potassium is included because it contributes to a decrease in hypertension.

Zinc is a nutrient whose importance has been appreciated more in recent years as understanding of its functions in the body has increased. Some evidence suggests that its intake may be marginal for some people in the United States. Selenium is included because of its interdependence with vitamin E and an as yet unproven usefulness in preventing cancer. Notice how many foods have zero selenium. Iodine is included because deficiency was a problem for people living in the center of great land masses—for example, the central United States and central Canada. Now the concern is that we may be getting too much iodine—in part from the widespread use of iodized salt and from iodine in detergents used to clean some food processing machinery.

Sodium, Potassium, Zinc, Selenium, and Iodine Content of Food (mg/100 g)

Food Item	Sodium	Potassium	Zinc	Selenium	Iodine
Milk and Milk Products					
Whole milk, fluid	43	141	0.36	0	0.025
Low-fat milk, 2% fat, fluid	44	153	0.40	0	0.027
Chocolate milk, fluid, low-fat milk	72	157	0.40	0	0.033
Skim milk, fluid	45	153	0.36	0	0.026
Buttermilk, fluid	100	158	0.42	0	0.023

Source: Pennington, J.A.T., Young, B.E., Wilson, D.B., Johnson, R.D., and Vanderveen, J.E.: Mineral content of foods and total diets: The selected minerals in foods survey, 1982 to 1984, *Journal of the American Dietetic Association* **86**:876, 1986.   *Continued.*

Sodium, Potassium, Zinc, Selenium, and Iodine Content of Food (mg/100 g)—cont'd

Food Item	Sodium	Potassium	Zinc	Selenium	Iodine
Milk and Milk Products—cont'd					
Yogurt, plain, low-fat	66	221	0.62	0	0.032
Milkshake, chocolate, fast-food type	93	198	0.42	0	0.056
Evaporated milk, canned	100	309	0.84	0	0.032
Yogurt, sweetened, strawberry, pre-stirred	53	171	0.42	0.001	0.019
Cheese, American, processed	1,598	79	3.41	0.011	0.033
Cottage cheese, creamed, 4% milk-fat	351	88	0.41	0.004	0.024
Cheese, cheddar, (sharp/mild)	562	76	3.80	0.012	0.067
Meat, Poultry, Fish, and Eggs					
Beef, ground, regular hamburger, cooked in patty shape	76	310	5.82	0.016	0.019
Beef chuck roast, oven roasted	69	293	8.10	0.018	0.015
Beef, round steak, stewed in water	33	195	6.85	0.024	0.035
Beef, (loin/sirloin) steak, pan cooked with added fat	60	323	5.58	0.021	0.015
Pork, ham, cured, not canned, oven cooked	1,274	290	2.77	0.024	0.011
Pork chop, pan-cooked with added fat	73	371	3.04	0.027	0.007
Pork sausage, (link/bulk), oven cooked	916	260	3.08	0.015	0.019
Pork, bacon, oven-cooked	1,595	278	2.77	0.017	0.010
Pork roast, loin, oven-cooked	58	334	3.04	0.030	0.011
Lamb chop, pan-cooked, with added fat	89	324	5.39	0.017	0.014
Veal cutlet, breaded, pan cooked with added fat	120	321	3.12	0.012	0.016
Chicken, drumsticks and breasts, breaded and fried with added fat, homemade	81	293	1.68	0.021	0.032
Chicken, oven roasted	83	273	1.81	0.024	0.021
Turkey breast, oven roasted	122	317	1.59	0.026	0.019
Liver (beef/calf), pan fried with added fat	82	353	6.11	0.048	0.042
Frankfurters, (beef/beef and pork), boiled	714	121	2.90	0.009	0.013
Bologna	1,038	186	2.00	0.010	0.034

Sodium, Potassium, Zinc, Selenium, and Iodine Content of Food (mg/100 g)—cont'd

Food Item	Sodium	Potassium	Zinc	Selenium	Iodine
Meat, Poultry, Fish, and Eggs—cont'd					
Salami, lunch meat type, regular, not hard	1,241	233	2.53	0.013	0.028
Cod/haddock fillet, (fresh/frozen), oven cooked	176	375	0.54	0.034	0.175
Tuna, canned in oil, drained	353	211	0.90	0.078	0.028
Shrimp (fresh/frozen), breaded and fried with added fat, homemade	284	102	1.48	0.043	0.029
Fish sticks, commercial, frozen, oven cooked	565	236	0.54	0.016	0.055
Eggs, scrambled with added milk and fat	306	133	1.22	0.018	0.065
Eggs, fried with added fat	145	147	1.76	0.026	0.071
Eggs, soft boiled	122	129	1.42	0.024	0.040
Legumes					
Pinto beans, boiled from dried	0	413	1.04	0.006	0.055
Pork and beans, canned	372	272	1.56	0.001	0.005
Cowpeas (blackeyed peas), boiled from dried	2	303	1.38	0	0.092
Lima beans, mature, boiled from dried	0	508	0.91	0.001	0.032
Lima beans, immature, frozen, boiled	77	289	0.78	0	0.114
Navy beans, boiled from dried	0	404	1.03	0	0.086
Red beans, boiled from dried	0	432	1.00	0	0.069
Peas, green, canned	248	117	0.74	0.001	0.012
Peas, green, frozen, boiled	63	102	0.59	0	0.005
Nuts and Nut Products					
Peanut butter, creamy, commercial in jar	498	640	2.92	0.003	0.006
Peanuts, dry roasted in jar, salted	800	686	3.31	0.001	0.011
Pecans, packaged, unsalted	2	524	5.39	0.001	0.001
Grains and Grain Products					
Rice, white, enriched, cooked	259	34	0.68	0.009	0.046
Oatmeal, cooked	191	81	0.79	0.009	0.019
Farina, enriched, cooked	161	20	0.15	0.001	0.021
Corn grits (hominy grits), enriched, cooked	206	19	0.13	0.002	0.071

Continued.

Sodium, Potassium, Zinc, Selenium, and Iodine Content of Food (mg/100 g)—cont'd

Food Item	Sodium	Potassium	Zinc	Selenium	Iodine
Grains and Grain Products—cont'd					
Corn, (fresh/frozen), boiled	0	193	0.54	0	0.001
Corn, canned	190	154	0.42	0	0.007
Corn, cream style, canned	301	129	0.55	0.001	0.008
Popcorn, popped in oil	0	226	2.83	0.003	0.055
White bread, enriched	558	110	0.77	0.026	0.099
Rolls, white, soft, enriched	542	134	0.84	0.023	0.045
Corn bread, southern style, home-made	453	139	0.66	0.010	0.058
Biscuits, baking powder, enriched, refrigerated type, baked	1,137	251	0.47	0.017	0.047
Whole wheat bread	552	234	1.83	0.029	0.114
Tortilla, flour	376	142	0.72	0.018	0.057
Rye bread	710	166	1.21	0.035	0.063
Muffins (blueberry/plain)	478	123	0.46	0.012	0.114
Saltine crackers	1,248	137	0.76	0.007	0.077
Corn chips	518	147	1.57	0.003	0.043
Pancakes made from mix with addition of egg, milk, and oil	574	183	0.84	0.009	0.036
Noodles, egg, enriched, cooked	5	35	0.68	0.019	0.004
Macaroni, enriched, cooked	1	36	0.47	0.015	0.024
Corn flakes	1,001	95	0.16	0.001	0.060
Fruit-flavored, presweetened cereal	456	103	14.56	0.006	7.421
Shredded wheat cereal	2	374	3.12	0.001	0.054
Raisin bran cereal	566	533	7.97	0.005	0.019
Crisped rice cereal	1,035	91	1.32	0.015	0.160
Granola, with raisins	174	336	1.97	0.019	0.013
Oat ring, unsweetened cereal	1,076	350	3.09	0.038	0.095
Fruits					
Apple, red with peel, raw	0	98	0.02	0	0.001
Orange, raw, (navel/Valencia)	0	149	0.05	0	0.001
Banana, raw	0	352	0.17	0.001	0
Watermelon, raw	1	106	0.05	0	0
Peach, canned in heavy syrup	7	100	0.06	0	0.003
Peach, raw	0	160	0.14	0	0.003
Applesauce, canned, sweetened	5	78	0.01	0	0

Sodium, Potassium, Zinc, Selenium, and Iodine Content of Food (mg/100 g)—cont'd

Food Item	Sodium	Potassium	Zinc	Selenium	Iodine
Fruits—cont'd					
Pear, raw	0	108	0.08	0	0.001
Strawberries, raw	1	129	0.12	0	0.009
Fruit cocktail, canned in heavy syrup	5	97	0.05	0	0.039
Grapes (purple/green), raw	2	185	0.03	0	0
Cantaloupe, raw	16	289	0.15	0	0.004
Pear, canned in heavy syrup	6	64	0.06	0	0.003
Plums, purple, raw	0	145	0.09	0	0
Grapefruit, raw	1	107	0.04	0	0
Pineapple, canned in juice pack	2	105	0.06	0	0.001
Cherries, sweet, raw	0	200	0.07	0	0
Raisins, dried	9	769	0.21	0	0.005
Prunes, dried, uncooked	1	725	0.45	0	0.021
Avocado, raw	5	505	0.61	0	0.002
Fruit Juices and Drinks					
Orange juice, frozen, reconstituted	1	172	0.02	0	0.001
Apple juice, canned, unsweetened	2	94	0.04	0	0.004
Grapefruit juice, frozen, reconstituted	1	132	0.03	0	0.001
Grape juice, canned	2	75	0.06	0.001	0.001
Pineapple juice, canned	2	117	0.08	0	0
Prune juice, bottled	5	175	0.12	0	0.003
Orange drink with added vitamin C, canned	16	20	0.01	0	0.001
Lemonade, frozen, reconstituted	1	14	0.01	0	0
Vegetables and Vegetable Products					
Spinach, canned	196	224	0.44	0.002	0.003
Spinach, (fresh/frozen), boiled	25	144	0.45	0	0.002
Collards, (fresh/frozen), boiled	12	104	0.22	0	0
Lettuce, raw	9	121	0.17	0	0
Cabbage, boiled from raw	7	97	0.09	0	0
Coleslaw with dressing, homemade	460	167	0.17	0	0.001
Sauerkraut, canned	591	151	0.15	0	0.001
Broccoli, (fresh/frozen), boiled	16	132	0.20	0	0
Celery, raw	80	282	0.13	0	0.001

Continued.

Sodium, Potassium, Zinc, Selenium, and Iodine Content of Food (mg/100 g)—cont'd

Food Item	Sodium	Potassium	Zinc	Selenium	Iodine
Vegetables and Vegetable Products—cont'd					
Asparagus, (fresh/frozen), boiled	1	153	0.36	0.001	0
Cauliflower, (fresh/frozen), boiled	10	132	0.15	0	0
Tomato, raw	3	242	0.11	0	0
Tomato juice, canned	237	228	0.13	0	0
Tomato sauce, canned	526	334	0.17	0	0.001
Tomatoes, canned	152	203	0.13	0	0.003
Beans, snap green, (fresh/frozen), boiled	0	126	0.23	0	0.002
Beans, snap green, canned	266	87	0.25	0	0.003
Cucumber, raw, pared	2	148	0.13	0	0
Squash, summer, (fresh/frozen), boiled	0	144	0.20	0	0.001
Sweet pepper, green, raw	1	162	0.11	0	0.001
Squash winter, (hubbard/acorn), (raw/frozen), boiled	0	166	0.20	0	0
Carrots, raw	56	319	0.23	0	0
Onion, raw	3	160	0.20	0	0.002
Vegetables, mixed, canned	242	160	0.30	0	0.001
Mushrooms, canned	328	98	0.73	0.001	0.001
Beets, canned	136	160	0.27	0	0
Radish, raw	24	200	0.18	0	0.001
Onion rings, breaded and fried, frozen, commercial, heated	482	145	0.46	0.003	0.066
French fries, frozen, commercial, heated	22	427	0.39	0	0.026
Mashed potatoes prepared with margarine and milk, from instant	253	236	0.24	0	0.028
Boiled potato without peel	2	265	0.22	0	0.004
Baked potato with peel	3	480	0.36	0	0.029
Potato chips, commercial	497	1,319	1.08	0.003	0.013
Scalloped potatoes, homemade	232	300	0.37	0	0.028
Sweet potato, baked in skin	33	473	0.27	0	0
Sweet potato, candied, homemade	173	357	0.26	0	0.015
Mixed Dishes					
Spaghetti with meat sauce, homemade	181	185	0.73	0.009	0.018
Beef and vegetable stew, homemade	299	280	2.16	0.005	0.023

Sodium, Potassium, Zinc, Selenium, and Iodine Content of Food (mg/100 g)—cont'd

Food Item	Sodium	Potassium	Zinc	Selenium	Iodine
Mixed Dishes—cont'd					
Pizza, cheese, frozen, commercial, heated	579	190	1.51	0.017	0.020
Chili con carne, beef and beans, canned	413	300	1.27	0.001	0.003
Macaroni and cheese, prepared from box mix	370	116	0.52	0.014	0.041
Quarter-pound hamburger sandwich on white roll with garnish, fast-food type	390	211	2.64	0.015	0.017
Meat loaf, beef, homemade	391	308	4.02	0.012	0.123
Spaghetti in tomato sauce, canned	277	81	0.44	0.009	0.072
Chicken noodle casserole, homemade	303	114	0.89	0.012	0.008
Lasagna, homemade	447	264	1.64	0.012	0.032
Potpie, frozen, commercial, chicken, oven heated	478	98	0.53	0.005	0.028
Pork chow mein, homemade	316	183	0.82	0.006	0.026
Frozen dinner—fried chicken, mashed potatoes, corn bread and/or vegetable, heated	614	253	0.71	0.010	0.015
Soups					
Chicken noodle soup, canned, reconstituted with water	283	14	0.32	0	0.002
Tomato soup, canned, reconstituted with whole milk	309	159	0.27	0	0.007
Vegetable beef soup, canned, reconstituted with water	263	45	0.66	0	0.007
Beef bouillon, canned, reconstituted with water	348	31	0.33	0	0.004
Condiments, Fats, and Sweeteners					
Gravy, brown, from mix	538	41	0.05	0	0.005
White sauce, medium, homemade	301	128	0.40	0.001	0.019
Pickles, dill, bottled	854	79	0.09	0	0.005
Margarine made with partially hydrogenated vegetable oil, stick type	767	14	0.01	0	0.003
Salad dressing, Italian, bottled	223	3	0.01	0	0.002
Butter, stick type	539	16	0.04	0.005	0.005
Vegetable oil, corn	1	2	0.01	0	0.002

Continued.

Sodium, Potassium, Zinc, Selenium, and Iodine Content of Food (mg/100 g)—cont'd

Food Item	Sodium	Potassium	Zinc	Selenium	Iodine
Condiments, Fats, and Sweetners—cont'd					
Mayonnaise, bottled	376	5	0.08	0.001	0.005
Cream, half-and-half, fluid	46	111	0.33	0	0.024
Cream substitute, powdered	130	915	0.15	0	0.013
Sugar, white, granulated	0	2	0	0	0.001
Syrup, pancake, bottled	75	16	0.20	0	0.007
Jelly, grape, bottled	47	48	0.02	0	0.011
Honey, bottled	3	52	0.18	0	0.014
Catsup, bottled	1,032	427	0.20	0	0.006
Desserts					
Ice cream, chocolate	83	255	0.52	0	0.071
Pudding, chocolate, instant, made with whole milk	289	191	0.63	0	0.035
Ice cream sandwich	253	176	0.47	0.001	0.046
Ice milk, vanilla	92	224	0.46	0.001	0.034
Beverages					
Soft drink from powder, cherry flavor, presweetened	5	0	0	0	0.002
Carbonated soda, low calorie, cola, artificially sweetened, canned	15	1	0.01	0	0.001
Coffee beverage, from instant	1	39	0	0	0
Coffee beverage, from instant decaffeinated	1	37	0	0	0
Tea beverage, hot, made with tea bag	0	14	0.01	0	0
Beer, canned	4	24	0	0	0
Wine, table, 12.2% alcohol	10	80	0.07	0	0.002
Whiskey, 80-proof	1	1	0	0	0
Water	3	0	0.01	0	0
Infant Foods					
Milk-based infant formula with iron, canned, ready-to-serve	23	83	0.75	0	0.010
Milk-based infant formula without iron, canned, ready-to-serve	25	85	0.78	0	0.011
Infant mixed cereal, prepared from dry with whole milk	5	47	0.36	0.002	0.006
Beef, (st/jr)	47	226	3.29	0.005	0.021
Pork, (st/jr)	40	225	2.21	0.011	0.017
Chicken/turkey, (st/jr)	44	177	1.72	0.013	0.061

J

Sodium, Potassium, Zinc, Selenium, and Iodine Content of Food (mg/100 g)—cont'd

Food Item	Sodium	Potassium	Zinc	Selenium	Iodine
Infant Foods—cont'd					
High meat (chicken/turkey) and vegetables, (st/jr)	23	88	1.05	0.006	0.050
High meat (beef) and vegetables, (st/jr)	26	126	1.37	0.003	0.007
High meat ham and vegetables, (st/jr)	18	138	1.00	0.003	0.001
Vegetables with beef, (st/jr)	12	91	0.40	0	0
Vegetables with (turkey/chicken), (st/jr)	11	59	0.34	0	0.004
Vegetables with (bacon/ham), (st/jr)	30	91	0.26	0	0.001
Chicken and noodles, (st/jr)	12	68	0.40	0.002	0.009
Tomatoes, beef and macaroni, (st/jr)	11	78	0.35	0.002	0.003
Turkey and rice, (st/jr)	12	67	0.39	0	0.005
Oatmeal with applesauce and bananas, (st/jr)	1	69	0.30	0	0.001
Carrots, (st/jr)	40	214	0.17	0.001	0.001
Green beans, (st/jr)	1	149	0.21	0	0.001
Mixed vegetables/garden vegetables, (st/jr)	11	110	0.19	0	0.002
Sweet potatoes/yellow squash, (st/jr)	18	254	0.16	0	0
Corn, creamed, (st/jr)	9	92	0.29	0	0.003
Peas, (st/jr)	6	107	0.49	0	0.001
Spinach, creamed, (st/jr)	34	176	0.55	0	0.011
Applesauce/applesauce with other fruit, (st/jr)	1	84	0.01	0.001	0.001
Peaches, (st/jr)	4	167	0.09	0	0.001
Pear/pear and pineapple, (st/jr)	1	102	0.08	0	0.002
Bananas and pineapple with tapioca, (st/jr)	4	95	0.04	0	0
Prunes/plums with tapioca, (st/jr)	5	146	0.09	0	0
Apple/apple cherry/apple grape juice, strained	6	106	0.02	0	0.006
Orange/orange pineapple juice, strained	3	186	0.04	0	0.002
Pudding/custard, any flavor (st/jr)	20	71	0.24	0	0.012
Fruit dessert with tapioca, any fruit (st/jr)	5	103	0.05	0	0
Dutch apple/apple Betty (st/jr)	12	40	0.02	0	0.001

J

APPENDIX K

Vitamin B$_6$, Vitamin B$_{12}$, and Folacin Content of Foods

These nutrients were not included in the Table of Food Composition so that they could be discussed in detail here. Values are presented per serving size. To convert to concentration of the nutrient per 100 grams of food refer to Appendix B.

In Chapter 6 is a description of some recent developments in vitamin B$_6$ nutrition. These include evidence that some college students may have low intakes of this nutrient. The dangers of very high intakes of vitamin B$_6$ and the relationship between body levels of the vitamin and premenstrual stress syndrome (PMS) are other areas of interest. Note that foods in the meat group are the richest sources of vitamin B$_6$.

Vitamin B$_{12}$ occurs only in foods of animal origin and in fermented foods. The meat group is the richest source of this vitamin. Vegan and other diets containing foods of plant origin only must be monitored closely.

Low folacin intakes are a problem especially in teenagers and during pregnancy. The table clearly shows the reason—low vegetable intakes.

Vitamin B₆, Vitamin B₁₂, and Folacin Content of Foods

Food	Serving Size	Weight (g)	Vitamin B_6 (mg)	Vitamin B_{12} (µg)	Folacin (µg)
Dairy Products					
Milk, whole	1 cup	244	0.10	0.87	12
nonfat	1 cup	244	0.10	0.93	13
Cheese, cheddar	1 oz	28	0.02	0.23	5
cottage	4 oz	112	0.09	0.80	15
Swiss	1 oz	28	0.02	0.25	2
Ice cream	1 cup	133	0.06	0.63	3
Butter	1 pat	5	—	—	0.4
Meat, Poultry, Fish, Eggs					
Beef, ground	3 oz	84	0.36	1.68	3
Chicken	3.5 oz	98	0.47	0.33	6
Ham	3.5 oz	98	0.34	0.83	3
Frankfurter	1	45	0.08	0.74	2
Tuna Fish	3 oz	84	0.39	2.02	13
Eggs, boiled	1	50	0.06	0.68	24
Fruit					
Apple	1	138	0.07	—	4
Banana	1	114	0.66	—	22
Peach	1	87	0.03	—	3
Orange juice	4 oz	112	0.01	—	14
Vegetables					
Broccoli	½ cup	78	0.12	—	52
Peas	½ cup	80	0.17	—	51
Corn	½ cup	83	0.18	—	19
Potatoes, baked	1 (large)	202	0.18	—	6
Cereal Products					
Bread, whole wheat	1 slice	25	0.05	—	14
enriched	1 slice	25	0.01	—	8
Rice	1 cup	185	0.02	—	1

Source: Adapted from Guthrie, H.A.: Introductory nutrition, ed. 6, Times Mirror/Mosby College Publishing, St. Louis, 1986.

K

APPENDIX

L

Dietary Guidelines for Reducing Cancer Risk

The role of diet in cancer is discussed in Chapter 14.

People want to know what major changes must be made in their diet to protect them against the possibility of cancer while still eating a nutritionally sound diet. Researchers at the U.S. Department of Agriculture used the 1977–1978 Nationwide Food Consumption Survey as a reference point for what most Americans are eating.[1]

If you eat the typical American diet and you want to follow the guidelines for reducing cancer risk you must increase your intake of whole-grain cereals, fruits, vegetables, peas and beans. Large reductions must be made in the intake of bacon, sausage, luncheon meats, nuts, fats and oils, cheese, and ice cream.

Following the guidelines for reducing cancer risk while meeting all the RDAs means even greater changes in the amounts of certain foods eaten. Women usually have the bigger dietary adjustments to make.

Eating a healthy diet usually costs more—diets following the cancer guidelines or following the cancer guidelines while meeting the RDAs are more expensive than diets that follow the national dietary pattern of people in the United States. For example, womens' diets that both follow cancer guidelines and meet all RDAs cost 23% more than diets that follow the present consumption pattern. The reason for this extra cost is the increased amount of red meat, vegetables, fruits, poultry, and fish.

[1]Cleveland, L.E. and Pfeffer, A.B.: Planning diets to meet the National Research Council's guidelines for reducing cancer risk; *Journal of the American Dietetic Association* **87**: 162, 1987.

Percent Change from Quantities of Food Groups in Consumption Pattern To Meet Guidelines for Reducing Cancer Risk and the RDAs

Food Group*	Men 20 to 50 years old		Women 20 to 50 years old	
	Diet Meeting Guidelines	Diet Meeting Guidelines and RDAs	Diet Meeting Guidelines	Diet Meeting Guidelines and RDAs
Vegetables†	24	24	22	37
Fruits‡	31	31	30	28
Whole-grain products#	71	71	64	157
Non-whole-grain products#	77	77	68	44
Bakery products¶	20	20	12	−73
Milk, yogurt	10	10	9	26
Cheese, ice cream‖	−23	−23	−18	−80
Bacon, sausage, lunch meat	−63	−63	−45	−66
Red meats**	0	0	0	82
Poultry, fish††	17	17	11	62
Eggs	−5	−5	−5	−37
Dry beans and peas	86	86	75	232
Nuts	−64	−64	−82	−90
Commercial mixtures‡‡	17	17	16	21
Fats and oils	−51	−51	−51	−51
Sugar and sweets	−11	−11	−11	−24
Cost	4	4	5	23

*Excludes three food groups that were used in developing sample diets: coffee and tea; soft drinks, punches, and ades; and seasonings.
†Combines four food groups that were used in developing sample diets: potatoes; high-nutrient vegetables; other vegetables; and mixtures, mostly vegetables and condiments. High-nutrient vegetables were classified according to their nutritive value per 1,000 kcal and per serving for vitamin A, vitamin C, vitamin B-6, magnesium, and iron; they are asparagus, bean sprouts, broccoli, Brussels sprouts, cabbage, carrots, cauliflower, green peppers, leafy greens, okra, sauerkraut, squash, sweet potatoes, tomatoes, turnips, and tomato and vegetable juices.
‡Combines two food groups used in developing sample diets: vitamin C-rich fruits and other fruits.
#Combines three food groups that were used in developing sample diets: breakfast cereals; flour, meal, rice, and pasta; and breads. Whole-grain cereals were defined as those with a whole-grain or high-fiber ingredient listed first on the label ingredient list. Whole-grain breads were defined as those containing any whole-grain or high-fiber ingredient.
¶Includes cakes, pies, cookies, crackers, pastries, pretzels, and corn and wheat snacks.
‖Combines two food groups that were used in developing sample diets: cheese and mixtures that were mostly milk.
**Combines two food groups that were used in developing sample diets: lower-cost red meats and higher-cost red meats.
††Combines two food groups used in developing sample diets: poultry and fish, including shellfish.
‡‡Combines two food groups that were used in developing sample diets: grain mixtures and mixtures that were mostly meat, poultry, fish, egg, or legumes. Examples are pizza, macaroni salad, frozen plate dinners, and pot pies.

L

Food Exchange Lists (United States)

The U.S. exchange system was introduced in Chapter 2.

The amount of energy nutrients in the U.S. exchange system was modified in 1986. Details of the amounts are given below and in the table on page 44. A person required to follow the exchange lists for health reasons should consult *Exchange Lists for Meal Planning,* American Diabetes Association, Chicago, revised 1986.

Starch/Bread

Eighty kcalories, 15 grams carbohydrate, 3 grams protein, trace of fat.

Included in this group are cereals, breads, crackers, pasta, fried beans, snack foods with fat, starchy vegetables (corn, potatoes, rice).

Meat and Substitutes

Lean—55 kcalories, zero carbohydrate, 7 grams protein, 3 grams fat.
Medium-fat—75 kcalories, zero carbohydrate, 7 grams protein, 5 grams fat.
High-fat—100 kcalories, zero carbohydrate, 7 grams protein, 8 grams fat.

There is zero carbohydrate on this list because meat has no carbohydrate. Frankfurters (hot dogs) and peanut butter are on the high-fat meat exchange list.

Vegetables

Twenty-five kcalories, 5 grams carbohydrate, 2 grams protein, zero fat.

This includes all vegetables, including those used in ethnic cooking (Chinese, Mexican, etc). The serving size for all vegetables is ½ cup cooked vegetables or vegetable juice, or 1 cup raw vegetables.

Fruits

Sixty kcalories, 15 grams carbohydrate, zero protein and fat.

There is almost zero protein and fat in fruits. The list includes all fruits, dried fruits, and fruit juices.

Fats

Forty-five kcalories, 5 grams fat, zero protein and carbohydrate.

This includes butter, margarine, oils, nuts, bacon, cream, salad dressings, and salt pork.

Milk

All types of milk have 12 grams carbohydrate, 8 grams protein, and the following amounts of energy and fat:
Skim—90 kcalories, trace of fat
Low-fat—120 kcalories, 5 grams fat
Whole—150 kcalories, 8 grams fat

Free Foods

The exchange lists provides certain free foods. These can be consumed in unlimited amounts because they provide no energy (kcalories).

They include diet drinks, coffee, tea, bouillon without fat, unsweetened pickles and gelatin, salt and pepper, paprika, garlic, lemon, other seasonings, and certain raw vegetables including Chinese cabbage, endive, lettuce, parsley, radishes, and watercress.

Average Values per Serving of All Foods and Most Commonly Used Foods[*]
on the 1986 Exchange Lists

Food Group	Energy (kcal)	Carbo-hydrate (g)	Protein (g)	Fat (g)	Dietary Fiber (g)
Starch/Bread					
Cereals (no. = 13)	78	18.7	2.7	0.4	3.4
Other cereals (no. = 9)	74	16.0	1.8	0.3	1.1
Hot cereals (no. = 6)	68	13.3	2.4	0.6	1.4
Pasta, other grains (no. = 12)	81	16.2	2.6	0.5	1.2
Dried beans (no. = 7)	73	13.3	4.7	0.3	4.0
Starchy vegetables (no. = 23)	79	17.5	2.5	0.5	3.5
Breads (no. = 17)	76	14.7	2.6	0.8	1.5
Crackers (no. = 12)	82	15.7	2.1	1.0	—
All breads/starches (no. = 99)	78	16.2	2.6	0.6	2.3
Snack foods with fat (no. = 12)	123	16.9	2.9	4.9	—
Most commonly used (no. = 32)	78	15.9	2.6	0.8	2.4

[*]Most commonly used foods determined from total diet study (14). *Continued.*

Average Values per Serving of All Foods and Most Commonly Used Foods on the 1986 Exchange Lists—cont'd

Food Group	Energy (kcal)	Carbo-hydrate (g)	Protein (g)	Fat (g)	Dietary Fiber (g)
Meat and Substitutes					
All lean meats (no. = 51)	52	0.4	8.2	1.7	—
All medium-fat meats (no. = 44)	69	0.3	7.8	3.8	—
All high-fat meats (no. = 24)	96	0.8	5.4	7.9	—
Most commonly used lean meats (no. = 8)	54	—	8.3	1.9	—
Most commonly used medium-fat meats (no. = 9)	74	—	8.4	4.2	—
Most commonly used high-fat meats (no. = 6)	97	—	5.2	8.2	—
Vegetables					
All vegetables in data base (no. = 60)	25	5.1	1.6	0.2	2.0† 3.0‡
Most commonly used (no. = 19)	25	5.3	1.5	0.2	1.9† 3.0‡
Fruits					
Fruits (no. = 41)	60	15.1	0.8	0.3	2.3
Dried fruits (no. = 6)	60	15.9	0.6	0.1	3.6
Juices (no. = 9)	55	13.5	0.5	0.1	0.2
All foods on fruit exchange (no. = 56)	59	15.3	0.8	0.2	2.1
Most commonly used (no. = 23)	58	14.3	0.7	0.2	1.4#
Fats					
All unsaturated fats (no. = 41)	48	1.6	0.5	4.6	—
All saturated fats (no. = 12)	46	1.3	0.6	4.3	—
All fats (no. = 53)	48	1.6	0.5	4.5	—
Most commonly used (no. = 11)	45	1.1	0.6	4.4	—
Milk					
Skim and very-low-fat (no. = 7)	93	12.1	8.4	1.0	—
Low-fat (no. = 2)	132	13.8	10.0	4.1	—
Whole (no. = 3)	153	11.5	8.2	8.4	—

†Cooked.
‡Raw.
#Six fruit juices included.

The Canadian Food Guide

APPENDIX

N

This information relates to material in Chapter 2. While of specific interest to Canadian readers, it is useful for other nationalities to see how dietary guides are constructed in different countries.

Features of this system include:

- The six food groups based on the content of carbohydrates, proteins, and fats.
- Measured amounts given for most foods.
- Foods are interchangeable between groups.
- The number of kcalories provided by each group is given.
- The difference between complex and simple carbohydrates is distinguished.
- The protein group emphasizes protein-rich foods low in fat, while those high in fat are identified.

Further details are provided in *Good Health Eating Guide,* Canadian Diabetes Association, Toronto, Ontario, 1981.

The Canadian Food Guide

		Nutrient Values per Serving			
Food Group System	**Exchange System**	**Carbohydrate (grams)**	**Protein (grams)**	**Fat (grams)**	**Energy (kcal)**
1 protein foods choice[1]	1 meat exchange	0	7	3	55
1 starchy foods choice	1 bread exchange	15 (starch)	2	0	68
1 milk choice	1 milk exchange				
	skim	6	4	0	40
	2% fat	6	4	2	58
	whole	6	4	4	76
1 fruits and vegetables choice	1 vegetable exchange (group A)	10 (simple)	1	0	44
1 fats and oils choice	1 fat exchange	0	0	5	45
Extra vegetables[2]	1 vegetable exchange (group B)	3.5	0	0	14
Extras (unmeasured)[3]	Energy-free foods (list A)	0	0	0	0
Extras (small measures)[4]	Energy-poor foods (list B)	2.5	0	0	15

[1]Choice = exchange or portion in U.S. food exchange system.

[2]Includes: asparagus, bamboo shoots, beans, bean sprouts, broccoli, Brussels sprouts, cabbage, cauliflower, celery, cucumber, eggplant, greens (beets, mustard, turnip, etc.), leeks, lettuce, mushrooms, okra, onions, parsley, pepper (red or green), radish, rhubarb, spinach, tomato, vegetable marrow, watercress, zucchini.

[3]Includes: bouillon, coffee, tea, and other low-calorie beverages, condiments, herbs and spices, and artificial sweeteners.

[4]Includes: barbecue sauce, bran, brewers yeast, chili sauce, cocoa powder, cranberry sauce (unsweetened), ketchup, dietetic fruit spreads, nuts, non-dairy creamer, relish, sugar substitutes, whipped topping, yogurt, plain.

Fast Foods—Table of Food Composition

Information in this appendix is relevant throughout the book—in particular Chapter 11 (dealing with modern food production and preparation), and Chapter 15 (in which nutrition and current lifestyles are discussed).

The following numbers are given to impress on you the importance in understanding the nutritive value of fast foods—they are here to stay.

- Between 1970 and 1980 fast food sales in the United States[1] increased by more than 300 percent from $6.5 to $23 *billion per year*
- The number of fast food outlets increased from 30,000 to 140,000.

[1]Young, E.A., Sims, O., Bingham, C. and Brennan, E.H.: Fast foods 1986: nutrient analyses. *Dietetic Currents* **13**: No. 6, 1986.

Fast Foods—Table of Food Composition

	Weight (g)	Energy (kcal)	Protein (g)	Carbohydrate (g)	Fat (g)	Cholesterol (mg)
Arby's						
Roast Beef, reg	147	350	22	32	15.0	39.0
Roast Beef, jr	86	218	12	22	8.0	20.0
Roast Beef, super	234	501	25	50	22.0	40.0
Roast Beef, deluxe	247	486	26	43	23.0	59.0
Beef'n Cheddar®	190	490	24	51	21.0	51.0
Chicken Breast Sandwich	210	592	28	56	27.0	57.0
Potato Cakes (2)	85	201	2	22	14.0	1.3
French Fries	71	211	2	33	8.0	6.0

Source: Arby's Inc, Atlanta, Georgia. Nutritional analyses by Arby's Laboratory and other independent testing laboratories.
— = no data available; × = less than 2% US RDA; tr = trace

- By 1983 annual sales amounted to $34 billion per year. This figure is nearly 40 percent of the annual sales for *all* U.S. eating establishments. Two hundred customers order one or more hamburgers *every second,* which translates into 6.7 billion patties worth $10 billion supplied annually by fast food chains alone.

Answer the following questions if you want to measure the impact of fast foods on your nutrient intake:

- How often do you consume fast foods?
- What are your financial resources? (Remember you are buying convenience also—limited money may be better spent on other foods.)
- Which fast foods do you buy and why? How important are nutritive value, price, family preference, convenience, cleanliness, quality, and taste to you?
- What is the nutrient content of your fast food selections?

The answer to the last question is given in the appendix.

Be aware of the following important point—you usually cannot make direct comparisons for the nutritive value of the same food item in the various fast food chains. The reason is simple—hamburgers, French fries or any other food do not weigh the same amount between the different fast food chains. For example, this appendix shows you that a hamburger in McDonald's weighs 100 grams, in Wendy's 117 grams, and in Dairy Queen 148 grams. Another example is the variation in the weight of a regular serving of French fries—in McDonald's 68 grams, Wendy's 98 grams, and Whataburger 85 grams.

If you want to make direct comparisons in nutritive value between the chains just convert the nutritive value of all products you are interested in into the nutrient content per 100 grams. In that way you are comparing apples with apples (or hamburgers with hamburgers!). Details of how to do these calculations are given in Appendix B.

Vitamin A (IU)	Thiamin (mg)	Riboflavin (mg)	Niacin (mg)	Vitamin C (mg)	Calcium (mg)	Iron (mg)	Phosphorus (mg)	Sodium (mg)	Zinc (mg)
×	0.23	0.43	7.6	×	80	3.6	—	590	—
×	0.15	0.26	4.0	×	40	1.8	—	345	—
750	0.38	0.60	9.0	36.0	100	4.5	—	800	—
×	0.30	0.34	5.0	×	100	6.3	—	1288	—
×	0.12	0.34	5.0	×	80	5.4	—	1520	—
×	0.23	0.26	10.0	×	100	3.6	—	1340	—
×	0.09	×	1.6	3.6	×	1.1	—	425	—
×	0.09	×	2.0	6.0	×	1.1	—	30	—

Continued.

O

Fast Foods—Table of Food Composition—cont'd

	Weight (g)	Energy (kcal)	Protein (g)	Carbohydrate (g)	Fat (g)	Cholesterol (mg)
Arby's—cont'd						
King Roast Beef	192	467	27	44	19.0	49.0
Bac'n Cheddar Deluxe	225	561	28	36	34.0	78.0
Hot Ham 'n Cheese	161	353	26	33	13.0	50.0
Turkey Deluxe	197	375	24	32	17.0	39.0
Baked Potato, plain	312	290	8	66	0.5	0
Superstuffed Potato, deluxe	312	648	18	59	38.0	72.0
Broccoli and Cheddar	340	541	13	72	22.0	24.0
Mushroom and Cheese	300	506	16	61	22.0	21.0
Taco	425	619	23	73	27.0	145.0
Vanilla Shake	250	295	8	44	10.0	30.0
Chocolate Shake	300	384	9	62	11.0	32.0
Jamocha Shake	305	424	8	76	10.0	31.0
Roasted Chicken Breast	150	254	43	2	7.0	200.0
Roasted Chicken Leg	161	319	41	1	16.0	214.0
Chicken Salad Sandwich	156	386	18	33	20.0	30.0
Chicken Salad and Croissant	150	472	22	16	36.0	12.0
Chicken Salad w/Tomato & Lettuce	270	515	25	24	36.0	12.0
Chicken Club Sandwich	210	621	26	57	32.0	108.0
Rice Pilaf	120	123	3	23	2.0	—
Scandinavian Vegetables, sauce	120	56	2	9	2.0	—
Tossed Salad, plain	210	44	3	7	tr	0
Tossed Salad w/20 Calorie Italian Drsg	240	57	3	9	1.0	0
Burger King						
Whopper Sandwich®	265	640	27	42	41	94
Whopper® w/Cheese	289	723	31	43	48	117
Double Beef Whopper®	351	850	46	52	52	—
Double Beef Whopper® w/Cheese	374	950	51	54	60	—
Whopper Junior®	136	370	15	31	17	41
Whopper Junior® w/Cheese	158	420	17	32	20	52
Hamburger	109	275	15	29	12	37

O

Burger King Corp Inc. Nutritional analyses by Hazelton Laboratory of America (formerly Raltech Scientific Services Inc), Madison, Wisconsin, and Campbell Laboratories, Camden, New Jersey.

Vitamin A (IU)	Thiamin (mg)	Riboflavin (mg)	Niacin (mg)	Vitamin C (mg)	Calcium (mg)	Iron (mg)	Phosphorus (mg)	Sodium (mg)	Zinc (mg)
100	0.30	0.60	10.0	2.4	100	4.5	—	765	—
×	0.15	0.26	6.0	3.6	100	2.7	—	1385	—
200	0.98	0.51	6.0	24.0	200	1.8	—	1655	—
300	0.23	0.43	12.0	4.8	80	2.7	—	850	—
×	0.30	0.14	5.0	63.0	20	1.8	—	12	—
1000	0.23	0.43	6.0	63.0	300	2.7	—	475	—
500	0.30	0.34	6.0	63.0	150	2.7	—	475	—
750	0.23	0.43	7.0	63.0	300	2.7	—	635	—
3000	0.38	0.26	8.0	63.0	450	3.6	—	1065	—
400	0.12	0.60	×	2.4	300	0.7	—	245	—
400	0.12	0.60	0.4	2.4	300	1.1	—	300	—
300	0.09	0.51	3.0	×	300	1.1	—	280	—
—	—	—	—	—	—	—	—	930	—
—	—	—	—	—	—	—	—	995	—
—	—	—	—	—	—	—	—	630	—
—	—	—	—	—	—	—	—	725	—
—	—	—	—	—	—	—	—	745	—
—	—	—	—	—	—	—	—	1300	—
—	—	—	—	—	—	—	—	438	—
—	—	—	—	—	—	—	—	465	—
—	—	—	—	—	—	—	—	23	—
—	—	—	—	—	—	—	—	465	—
618	0.33	0.41	7.0	14	80	4.9	237	842	4.50
1001	0.34	0.48	7.0	14	210	4.9	360	1126	5.10
617	0.34	0.56	10.0	14	91	7.3	387	1080	8.50
1001	0.35	0.63	10.0	14	222	7.3	510	1535	9.10
296	0.23	0.25	4.0	6	40	2.8	127	486	2.30
488	0.23	0.29	4.0	6	105	2.8	189	628	2.60
150	0.23	0.25	4.0	3	37	2.7	124	509	2.40

Continued.

O

Fast Foods—Table of Food Composition—cont'd

	Weight (g)	Energy (kcal)	Protein (g)	Carbohydrate (g)	Fat (g)	Cholesterol (mg)
Burger King—cont'd						
Cheeseburger	120	317	17	30	15	48
Bacon Double Cheeseburger	159	510	33	27	31	104
French Fries, reg	74	227	3	24	13	14
Onion Rings, reg	79	274	4	28	16	0
Apple Pie	125	305	3	44	12	4
Chocolate Shake, med	273	320	8	46	12	—
Vanilla Shake, med	273	321	9	49	10	—
Vanilla Shake, added syrup	284	334	9	51	10	—
Chocolate Shake, added syrup	284	374	8	60	11	—
Whaler® Fish Sandwich	189	488	19	45	27	84
Whaler® w/Cheese	201	530	21	46	30	95
Ham and Cheese	230	471	24	44	23	70
Chicken Sandwich	230	688	26	56	40	82
Chicken Tenders®	95	204	20	10	10	47
B'kfast Croissanwich®						
Bacon, Egg, Cheese	119	355	15	20	24	249
Sausage, Egg, Cheese	163	538	19	20	41	293
Ham, Egg, Cheese	145	335	18	20	20	262
Scrambled Egg Platter	195	468	14	33	30	370
Scrambled Egg Platter						
w/Sausage	247	702	22	33	52	420
w/Bacon	206	536	18	33	36	378
French Toast Platter						
w/Bacon	117	469	11	41	30	73
w/Sausage	158	635	16	41	46	115
Salad, plain	148	28	2	5	0	0
w/House Dressing	176	159	3	8	13	11
w/Bleu Cheese	176	184	3	7	16	22
w/1000 Island	176	145	2	9	12	17
w/French	176	152	2	13	11	0
w/Golden Italian	176	162	2	7	14	0
w/Creamy Italian	176	—	—	—	—	—
w/Reduced-Calorie Italian	176	42	2	7	1	0
Cherry Pie	128	357	4	55	13	6
Pecan Pie	113	459	5	64	20	4

Vitamin A (IU)	Thiamin (mg)	Riboflavin (mg)	Niacin (mg)	Vitamin C (mg)	Calcium (mg)	Iron (mg)	Phosphorus (mg)	Sodium (mg)	Zinc (mg)
341	0.23	0.29	4.0	3	102	3.8	186	651	2.60
384	0.31	0.42	6.0	×	168	3.8	328	728	5.10
×	0.10	0.30	7.5	×	×	0.5	114	160	×
×	×	×	×	×	124	0.8	195	665	0.40
×	0.27	0.16	0.6	5	×	1.2	31	412	×
×	0.13	0.55	×	×	260	1.6	262	202	1.00
×	0.11	0.57	×	×	295	×	284	205	1.00
—	—	—	—	—	—	—	—	213	—
×	0.12	0.51	×	×	248	1.6	264	225	1.05
36	0.28	0.21	4.0	×	×	2.2	249	592	0.09
227	0.27	0.24	4.0	×	112	2.2	311	734	1.10
725	0.87	0.42	6.0	7	195	3.2	384	1534	2.40
126	0.45	0.31	10.0	×	79	3.3	274	1423	1.20
95	0.08	0.08	7.0	×	18	0.7	236	636	0.60
426	0.32	0.30	2.0	×	136	2.0	249	762	1.50
426	0.36	0.32	4.0	×	145	2.9	292	1042	2.40
426	0.49	0.32	3.0	×	136	2.2	317	987	1.90
375	0.31	0.35	3.0	3	102	2.7	271	808	1.50
375	0.42	0.40	5.0	3	112	3.7	335	1213	2.70
375	0.39	0.38	4.0	3	103	2.8	299	975	1.90
×	0.24	0.24	3.0	×	59	2.7	118	448	1.30
×	0.29	0.27	6.0	×	70	3.7	164	686	2.30
1583	0.06	0.12	1.0	42	37	1.2	57	23	0.42
1604	0.06	0.15	1.0	42	44	1.3	74	293	0.52
1638	0.06	0.15	1.0	42	66	1.3	83	333	0.59
1659	0.06	0.13	1.0	43	42	1.4	66	251	0.50
1689	0.06	0.12	1.0	43	40	1.4	60	330	0.45
1598	0.05	0.12	1.0	42	40	1.3	60	292	0.43
—	—	—	—	—	—	—	—	—	—
1591	0.05	0.12	1.0	42	40	1.4	59	430	0.42
370	0.24	0.16	0.5	8	×	1.1	37	204	×
×	0.28	0.18	0.6	×	24	1.1	84	374	×

Continued.

O

Fast Foods—Table of Food Composition—cont'd

	Weight (g)	Energy (kcal)	Protein (g)	Carbohydrate (g)	Fat (g)	Cholesterol (mg)
Church's						
Fried Chicken						
Breast	93	278	21	9	17	—
Wing-Breast Cut	97	303	22	9	20	—
Thigh	93	306	19	9	22	—
Leg	56	147	13	5	9	—
Crispy Nuggets®						
Regular	18	55	3	4	3	—
Spicy	18	52	3	3	3	—
Southern Fried Catfish®	21	67	4	4	4	—
Hush Puppies	23	78	1	12	3	—
Dinner Roll	30	83	2	15	2	—
French Fries	90	256	4	31	13	—
Corn on the Cob (buttered)	270	165	5	29	3	—
Jalapeno Pepper	—	4	1	1	1	—
Pecan Pie	90	367	4	44	20	—
Cole Slaw	90	83	1	6	7	—
Dairy Queen						
Cone, sm	85	140	3	22	4	10
Cone, reg	142	240	6	38	7	15
Cone, lg	213	340	9	57	10	25
Dipped Cone, sm	92	190	3	25	9	10
Dipped Cone, reg	156	340	6	42	16	20
Dipped Cone, lg	234	510	9	64	24	30
Sundae, sm	106	190	3	33	4	10
Sundae, reg	177	310	5	56	8	20
Sundae, lg	248	440	8	78	10	30
Shake, sm	291	490	10	82	13	35
Shake, reg	418	710	14	120	19	50
Shake, lg	588	990	19	168	26	70

Source: Church's Fried Chicken, San Antonio, Texas. Nutrient analyses of chicken and catfish by Texas Testing Laboratories Inc, San Antonio; of hush puppies, Pioneer Flour Mills Inc, San Antonio. Other products calculated from Pennington JA, Church HN (eds): *Food Values of Portions Commonly Used,* ed. 14, Harper & Row, 1985.

Source: International Dairy Queen Inc, Minneapolis, Minnesota. Nutrient analyses by Hazelton Laboratory of America (formerly Raltech Scientific Services Inc). Madison, Wisconsin.

— = no data available; × = less than 2% US RDA; tr = trace

Vitamin A (IU)	Thiamin (mg)	Riboflavin (mg)	Niacin (mg)	Vitamin C (mg)	Calcium (mg)	Iron (mg)	Phosphorus (mg)	Sodium (mg)	Zinc (mg)
—	—	—	—	—	—	—	—	560	—
—	—	—	—	—	—	—	—	583	—
—	—	—	—	—	—	—	—	448	—
—	—	—	—	—	—	—	—	286	—
—	—	—	—	—	—	—	—	125	—
—	—	—	—	—	—	—	—	91	—
—	—	—	—	—	—	—	—	151	—
—	—	—	—	—	—	—	—	55	—
—	—	—	—	—	—	—	—	—	—
—	—	—	—	—	—	—	—	—	—
—	—	—	—	—	—	—	—	—	—
—	—	—	—	—	—	—	—	—	—
—	—	—	—	—	—	—	—	—	—
—	—	—	—	—	—	—	—	—	—
100	0.03	0.17	×	×	100	0.4	100	45	—
200	0.06	0.34	×	×	150	0.7	200	80	—
400	0.12	0.51	×	×	250	1.4	300	115	—
100	0.03	0.17	×	×	100	0.4	100	55	—
200	0.06	0.34	×	×	150	0.7	200	100	—
400	0.12	0.51	×	×	250	1.4	300	145	—
100	0.03	0.17	×	×	100	0.4	150	75	—
200	0.06	0.34	×	×	200	1.1	200	120	—
400	0.12	0.43	×	×	250	1.4	300	165	—
500	0.15	0.60	×	×	350	1.8	400	180	—
750	0.23	0.77	0.4	×	450	2.7	500	260	—
1000	0.30	1.02	0.8	×	700	3.6	800	360	—

Continued.

O

Fast Foods—Table of Food Composition—cont'd

	Weight (g)	Energy (kcal)	Protein (g)	Carbohydrate (g)	Fat (g)	Cholesterol (mg)
Dairy Queen—cont'd						
Malt, sm	291	520	10	91	13	35
Malt, reg	418	760	14	134	18	50
Malt, lg	588	1060	20	187	25	70
Float	397	410	5	82	7	20
Banana Split	383	540	9	103	11	30
Parfait	283	430	8	76	8	30
Peanut Buster Parfait	305	740	16	94	34	30
Double Delight	255	490	9	69	20	25
Hot Fudge Brownie Delight	266	600	9	85	25	20
Strawberry Shortcake	312	540	10	100	11	25
Freeze	397	500	9	89	12	30
Mr. Misty®, sm	248	190	0	48	0	0
Mr. Misty®, reg	330	250	0	63	0	0
Mr. Misty®, lg	439	340	0	84	0	0
Mr. Misty® Kiss	89	70	0	17	0	0
Mr. Misty® Freeze	411	500	9	91	12	30
Mr. Misty® Float	411	390	5	74	7	20
Buster Bar	149	460	10	41	29	10
Dilly Bar	85	210	3	21	13	10
DQ Sandwich	60	140	3	24	4	5
Single Hamburger	148	360	21	33	16	45
Double Hamburger	210	530	36	33	28	85
Triple Hamburger	272	710	51	33	45	135
Single w/Cheese	162	410	24	33	20	50
Double w/Cheese	239	650	43	34	37	95
Triple w/Cheese	301	820	58	34	50	145
Hot Dog	100	280	11	21	16	45
Hot Dog w/Chili	128	320	13	23	20	55
Hot Dog w/Cheese	114	330	15	21	21	55
Super Hot Dog	175	520	17	44	27	80
Super Hot Dog w/Chili	218	570	21	47	32	100
Super Hot Dog w/Cheese	196	580	22	45	34	100

O

Vitamin A (IU)	Thiamin (mg)	Riboflavin (mg)	Niacin (mg)	Vitamin C (mg)	Calcium (mg)	Iron (mg)	Phosphorus (mg)	Sodium (mg)	Zinc (mg)
500	0.15	0.60	0.4	×	350	2.7	400	180	—
750	0.30	0.85	0.8	×	450	4.5	600	260	—
1000	0.38	1.19	1.2	×	700	5.4	800	360	—
200	0.06	0.26	×	×	200	1.1	200	85	—
750	0.15	0.51	0.4	15.0	250	1.8	350	150	—
400	0.09	0.43	×	3.6	250	1.4	300	140	—
300	0.15	0.43	2.0	×	250	1.8	450	250	—
300	0.15	0.34	0.4	×	200	1.4	300	150	—
300	0.12	0.34	×	×	200	1.8	300	225	—
400	0.23	0.51	×	12.0	250	1.8	300	215	—
400	0.15	0.51	×	×	300	1.8	350	180	—
×	×	×	×	×	×	×	×	10	—
×	×	×	×	×	×	×	×	10	—
×	×	×	×	×	×	×	×	10	—
×	×	×	×	×	×	×	×	10	—
400	0.12	0.51	×	×	300	1.4	200	140	—
200	0.06	0.26	×	×	200	0.7	200	95	—
100	0.12	0.17	2.0	×	100	1.1	250	175	—
100	0.03	0.17	×	×	100	0.4	100	50	—
×	0.03	0.07	0.4	×	60	×	60	40	—
100	0.30	0.17	5.0	×	100	3.6	150	630	—
100	0.45	0.34	9.0	×	100	6.3	300	660	—
200	0.60	0.51	14.0	×	100	9.0	450	690	—
200	0.30	0.17	5.0	×	200	3.6	250	790	—
400	0.45	0.43	9.0	×	350	6.3	500	980	—
400	0.60	0.60	14.0	×	350	9.0	700	1010	—
×	0.12	0.14	3.0	×	80	1.4	80	830	—
×	0.15	0.26	4.0	×	80	1.8	150	985	—
100	0.12	0.17	3.0	×	150	1.4	200	990	—
×	0.23	0.26	5.0	×	150	2.7	150	1365	—
×	0.23	0.43	6.0	×	150	2.7	250	1595	—
100	0.23	0.26	5.0	×	250	1.4	300	1605	—

Continued.

O

Fast Foods—Table of Food Composition—cont'd

	Weight (g)	Energy (kcal)	Protein (g)	Carbohydrate (g)	Fat (g)	Cholesterol (mg)
Dairy Queen—cont'd						
Fish Filet Sandwich	170	400	20	41	17	50
Fish Filet Sandwich w/Cheese	177	440	24	39	21	60
Chicken Sandwich	220	670	29	46	41	75
French Fries, sm	71	200	2	25	10	10
French Fries, lg	113	320	3	40	16	15
Onion Rings	85	280	4	31	16	15
Hardee's						
Hamburger	110	305	17	29	13	—
Cheeseburger	116	335	17	29	17	—
Big Deluxe®	248	546	29	48	26	77
¼-Pound Cheeseburger®	190	506	28	41	26	61
Roast Beef Sandwich	143	377	21	36	17	57
Big Roast Beef®	167	418	28	34	19	60
Hot Dog	120	346	11	26	22	42
Hot Ham & Cheese	148	376	23	37	15	59
Fisherman's Fillet Sandwich®	196	514	20	50	26	41
Chicken Fillet	192	510	27	42	26	57
Bacon Cheeseburger	224	686	35	42	42	295
Sausage Biscuit	1123	413	10	34	26	29
Sausage & Egg Biscuit	162	521	16	34	35	293
Steak Biscuit	134	419	14	41	23	34
Steak & Egg Biscuit	162	527	20	41	31	298
Ham Biscuit	108	349	12	37	17	29
Ham & Egg Biscuit	184	458	19	37	26	293
Bacon & Egg Biscuit	114	405	13	30	26	305
French Fries, sm	71	239	3	28	13	4
French Fries, lg	113	381	5	44	21	6
Apple Turnover	87	282	3	37	14	5
Milkshake	326	391	11	63	10	42

Source: Hardee's Food Systems Inc, Rocky Mount, North Carolina. Nutrient analyses by Webb Food Laboratory, Raleigh, North Carolina.

Vitamin A (IU)	Thiamin (mg)	Riboflavin (mg)	Niacin (mg)	Vitamin C (mg)	Calcium (mg)	Iron (mg)	Phosphorus (mg)	Sodium (mg)	Zinc (mg)
×	0.15	0.26	3.0	×	60	0.7	200	875	—
100	0.15	0.26	3.0	×	150	0.4	250	1035	—
×	0.06	×	0.8	9	×	0.4	60	870	—
×	0.06	×	0.8	9	×	0.34	60	115	—
×	0.09	0.03	1.2	15	×	1.08	100	185	—
×	0.09	×	0.4	2.4	20	0.72	60	140	—
57	0.55	0.58	6.4	2.0	23	3.6	—	682	—
749	0.51	0.32	5.5	2.0	48	2.7	—	789	—
398	0.50	0.73	10.6	42.0	98	6.7	—	1083	—
508	0.35	0.60	14.0	33.0	103	6.5	—	1950	—
542	0.93	0.19	3.7	3.0	55	6.3	—	1030	—
648	1.03	0.22	5.2	8.0	74	8.1	—	1770	—
tr	0.29	0.22	4.2	0	43	2.5	—	744	—
178	0.37	0.74	2.5	1.0	207	3.8	—	1067	—
1152	1.33	1.51	7.2	5.0	88	5.1	—	314	—
1098	0.52	0.63	9.5	12.0	83	4.8	—	360	—
832	0.04	0.40	6.4	3.0	152	6.3	—	1074	—
45	0.36	0.22	2.8	1.0	139	2.8	—	864	—
755	0.41	0.37	2.9	1.0	169	4.0	—	1033	—
62	0.34	0.43	3.3	1.0	121	4.6	—	804	—
772	0.39	0.58	3.4	1.0	151	5.8	—	973	—
127	0.60	0.42	1.8	1.0	181	3.2	—	1415	—
837	0.65	0.57	1.9	1.0	211	4.0	—	1584	—
145	0.10	0.17	1.8	2.1	144	3.0	—	823	—
tr	0.07	0.03	1.0	10.0	14	1.0	—	121	—
tr	0.11	0.05	0.6	16.0	22	1.0	—	192	—
tr	0.03	0.04	0.4	21.67	19	1.0	—	—	—
0	0.20	0	0.2	0	450	1.0	—	—	—

Continued.

O

Fast Foods—Table of Food Composition—cont'd

	Weight (g)	Energy (kcal)	Protein (g)	Carbohydrate (g)	Fat (g)	Cholesterol (mg)
Jack in the Box						
Hamburger	98.0	276	13.0	30.0	12	29.0
Cheeseburger	113.0	323	16.0	32.0	15	42.0
Jumbo Jack®	205.0	485	26.0	38.0	26	64.0
Jumbo Jack® w/Cheese	—	630	32.0	45.0	35	110.0
Bacon Cheeseburger Supreme	231.0	724	34.0	44.0	46	70.0
Swiss & Bacon Burger	—	643	33.0	31.0	43	99.0
Ham & Swiss Burger	—	638	36.0	37.0	39	117.0
Mushroom Burger	178.7	477	28.0	30.0	27	87.0
Moby Jack®	137.0	444	16.0	39.0	25	47.0
Regular Taco	81.0	191	8.0	16.0	11	21.0
Super Taco	135.0	288	12.0	21.0	17	37.0
Club Pita	177.0	284	22.0	30.0	8	43.0
Chicken Supreme	228.0	601	31.0	39.0	36	60.0
Supreme Crescent	146.0	547	20.0	27.0	40	178.0
Sausage Crescent	156.0	584	22.0	28.0	43	187.0
Pancakes Breakfast	630.0	626	16.0	79.0	27	85.0
Scrambled Eggs Breakfast	720.0	719	26.0	55.0	44	260.0
Breakfast Jack®	126.0	307	18.0	30.0	13	203.0
Cooked Bacon, 2 slices	—	70	3.0	0	6	10.0
Chicken Strips Dinner	180.0	689	40.0	65.0	30	100.0
Shrimp Dinner	165.0	731	22.0	77.0	37	157.0
Sirloin Steak Dinner	—	699	38.0	75.0	27	75.0
Cheese Nachos	—	571	15.0	49.0	35	37.0
Supreme Nachos	—	718	23.0	66.0	40	65.0
Canadian Crescent	134.0	472	18.6	24.6	31	226.0
Pasta Seafood Salad	15.0	394	15.0	32.0	22	47.5
Taco Salad	358.0	377	31.0	10.0	24	102.0
French Fries, reg	68.0	221	2.0	27.0	12	8.0
Onion Rings	108.0	382	5.0	39.0	23	27.0
Hash Brown Potatoes	90.0	68	2.0	15.0	0	0
Vanilla Shake	317.0	320	10.0	57.0	6	25.0
Strawberry Shake	328.0	320	10.0	55.0	7	25.0
Chocolate Shake	322.0	330	11.0	55.0	7	25.0
Apple Turnover	119.0	410	4.0	45.0	24	15.0

Source: Jack in the Box Restaurants, Foodmaker, Inc, San Diego, California. Nutrient analyses by Hazelton Laboratory of America (formerly Raltech Scientific Services Inc), Madison, Wisconsin.

Vitamin A (IU)	Thiamin (mg)	Riboflavin (mg)	Niacin (mg)	Vitamin C (mg)	Calcium (mg)	Iron (mg)	Phosphorus (mg)	Sodium (mg)	Zinc (mg)
50	0.36	0.24	3.20	1.2	70	2.7	—	521	—
300	0.36	0.27	3.30	1.2	160	2.7	—	749	—
348	0.51	0.21	7.03	5.1	97	6.9	—	905	—
750	0.53	0.34	12.0	4.8	250	4.5	—	1665	—
600	0.56	0.51	8.80	3.0	310	4.9	—	1307	—
400	0.45	0.41	6.8	3.0	230	4.7	—	1354	—
430	0.76	0.48	7.6	9.8	268	6.1	—	1330	—
375	0.43	0.28	7.7	2.8	220	5.3	—	906	—
300	0.40	0.25	2.80	×	160	2.2	—	820	—
400	0.07	0.17	1.00	×	100	1.1	—	406	—
600	0.12	0.08	1.40	1.8	150	1.6	—	765	—
250	0.78	0.29	5.89	4.2	80	2.5	—	953	—
450	0.52	0.37	10.6	4.2	240	3.0	—	1582	—
550	0.64	0.54	4.2	×	150	2.7	—	1053	—
550	0.60	0.51	4.6	×	170	2.9	—	1012	—
500	0.60	0.43	5.0	27.0	100	2.7	—	1670	—
750	0.68	0.59	5.0	12.0	250	0.24	—	1110	—
450	0.47	0.41	3.0	×	170	3.1	—	871	—
×	0.03	0.03	0.8	4.0	1	0.38	—	226	—
150	0.45	0.29	18.6	12.0	110	4.0	—	1213	—
150	0.39	0.17	7.0	12.0	370	4.9	—	1510	—
150	0.68	0.51	12.4	7.8	220	9.5	—	969	—
500	0.11	0.19	1.0	3.0	370	1.4	—	1154	—
1000	0.15	0.26	3.2	8.4	410	3.2	—	1782	—
523	0.50	0.40	3.6	3.1	125	3.4	—	851	—
2330	0.38	0.23	1.8	21.0	208	5.9	—	1570	—
1150	0.18	0.53	6.0	6.6	280	4.3	—	1436	—
×	0.07	0.03	1.2	3.0	10	0.5	—	164	—
×	0.21	0.12	1.8	3.0	30	1.4	—	407	—
×	0.03	×	0.8	3.6	×	0.7	—	15	—
×	0.15	0.34	4.0	×	350	—	—	230	—
—	0.15	0.43	4.0	3.3	350	0.4	—	240	—
—	0.15	0.59	4.0	3.2	350	0.7	—	270	—
×	0.23	0.10	2.0	×	×	1.4	—	350	—

Continued.

Fast Foods—Table of Food Composition—cont'd

	Weight (g)	Energy (kcal)	Protein (g)	Carbohydrate (g)	Fat (g)	Cholesterol (mg)
Kentucky Fried Chicken						
Original Recipe®						
Wing*	56.0	181	11.8	5.77	12.3	67.0
Side Breast*	95.0	276	20.0	10.1	17.3	96.0
Center Breast*	107.0	257	25.5	8.0	13.7	93.0
Drumstick*	58.0	147	13.6	3.4	8.82	81.0
Thigh*	96.0	278	18.0	8.4	19.2	122.0
Extra Crispy						
Wing*	57.0	218	11.5	7.81	15.6	63.0
Side Breast*	98.0	354	17.7	17.3	23.7	66.0
Center Breast*	120.0	353	26.9	14.4	20.9	93.0
Drumstick*	60.0	173	12.7	5.9	10.9	65.0
Thigh*	112.0	371	19.6	13.8	26.3	121.0
Kentucky Nuggets (one)	16.0	46	2.82	2.2	2.88	11.9
Kentucky Nugget Sauce (oz)						
Barbeque	1.0**	35	0.3	7.1	0.57	1.0
Sweet and Sour	1.0**	58	0.1	13.0	0.56	1.0
Honey	0.5**	49	0	12.1	0.01	1.0
Mustard	1.0**	36	0.88	6.04	0.91	1.0
Kentucky Fries	119.0	268	4.8	33.3	12.8	1.8
Mashed Potatoes w/Gravy	86.0	62	2.1	10.3	1.4	1.0
Mashed Potatoes	80.0	59	1.9	11.6	0.6	1.0
Chicken Gravy	78.0	59	2.0	4.4	3.7	2.0
Buttermilk Biscuit	75.0	269	5.1	31.6	13.6	1.0
Potato Salad	90.0	141	1.8	12.6	9.27	11.0
Baked Beans	89.0	105	5.1	18.4	1.2	1.0
Corn on the Cob	143.0	176	5.1	31.9	3.1	1.0
Cole Slaw	79.0	103	1.3	11.5	5.7	4.0
Long John Silver's						
3 Pc Fish & Fryes	—	853	43	64	48	106
2 Pc Fish & Fryes	—	651	30	53	36	75
Fish & More	—	978	34	82	58	88
3 Pc Fish Dinner	—	1180	47	93	70	119
3 Pc Chicken Planks Dinner	—	885	32	72	51	25
4 Pc Chicken Planks Dinner	—	1037	41	82	59	25

*Edible portion
**Measured in ounces
Source: Kentucky Fried Chicken Corp. Nutrient Analyses by Hazelton Laboratory of America (formerly Raltech Scientific Services Inc), Madison, Wisconsin.
Source: Long John Silver's Inc, Lexington, Kentucky. Nutrient analyses by Department of Nutrition and Food Science, University of Kentucky.

O

Vitamin A (IU)	Thiamin (mg)	Riboflavin (mg)	Niacin (mg)	Vitamin C (mg)	Calcium (mg)	Iron (mg)	Phosphorus (mg)	Sodium (mg)	Zinc (mg)
56	0.03	0.06	3.2	3.0	37.7	0.45	—	387	—
100	0.07	0.18	6.8	3.0	48.4	0.79	—	654	—
100	0.09	0.14	10.0	3.0	39.3	0.63	—	532	—
100	0.06	0.13	2.9	2.0	12.8	0.597	—	269	—
144	0.08	0.28	4.6	2.0	27.6	1.05	—	517	—
100	0.03	0.07	2.8	2.0	21.4	0.52	—	437	—
100	0.08	0.13	6.5	2.0	31.9	0.86	—	797	—
100	0.10	0.16	10.0	2.2	34.9	0.86	—	842	—
100	0.05	0.14	2.8	2.0	15.2	0.606	—	346	—
102	0.09	0.27	5.2	2.0	46.1	1.21	—	766	—
100	0.02	0.03	1.0	1.5	2.4	0.13	—	140	—
370	0.01	0.014	0.19	0.36	6.05	0.24	—	450	—
60	0.01	0.02	0.04	0.31	4.66	0.16	—	148	—
—	0.01	0.003	0.04	2.5	0.581	0.11	—	15	—
—	0.02	0.008	0.16	1.0	10.2	0.26	—	346	—
—	0.17	0.057	2.7	2.7	24.3	0.94	—	89	—
100	0.01	0.036	1.0	1.0	19.1	0.35	—	297	—
100	0.01	0.038	0.96	1.0	20.6	0.28	—	228	—
—	0.01	0.028	0.47	—	8.58	0.48	—	398	—
100	0.28	0.13	1.8	1.0	77.0	1.22	—	521	—
90	0.07	0.023	0.6	2.7	10.4	0.32	—	396	—
—	0.06	0.039	0.5	2.1	53.6	1.43	—	387	—
272	0.14	0.113	1.8	2.3	7.19	0.39	—	21	—
269	0.03	0.026	0.2	18.7	28.5	0.19	—	171	—
—	—	—	—	—	—	—	—	2025.0	—
—	—	—	—	—	—	—	—	1352.0	—
—	—	—	—	—	—	—	—	2124.0	—
—	—	—	—	—	—	—	—	2797.0	—
—	—	—	—	—	—	—	—	1918.0	—
—	—	—	—	—	—	—	—	2433.0	—

Continued.

O

Fast Foods—Table of Food Composition—cont'd

	Weight (g)	Energy (kcal)	Protein (g)	Carbohydrate (g)	Fat (g)	Cholesterol (mg)
Long John Silver's—cont'd						
6 Pc Chicken Nuggets Dinner	—	699	23	54	45	25
Fish & Chicken	—	935	36	73	55	56
Seafood Platter	—	976	29	85	58	95
Clam Dinner	—	955	22	100	58	27
Batter Fried Shrimp Dinner	—	711	17	60	45	127
Scallop Dinner	—	747	17	66	45	37
Oyster Dinner	—	789	17	78	45	55
3 Pc Kitchen-Breaded Fish Dinner	—	940	35	84	52	101
2 Pc Kitchen-Breaded Fish Dinner	—	818	26	76	46	76
Fish Sandwich Platter	—	835	30	84	42	75
Seafood Salad	—	426	19	22	30	113
Ocean Chef Salad	—	229	27	13	8	64
A La Carte Items						
Batter-Fried Fish	86	202	13	11	12	31
Kitchen-Breaded Fish	58	122	9	8	6	25
Chicken Plank	62	152	9	10	8	×
Batter-Fried Shrimp	17	47	2	3	3	17
Clam Chowder	185	128	7	15	5	17
Cole Slaw	98	182	1	11	15	12
Fryes	85	247	4	31	12	13
Hush Puppies	47	145	3	18	7	1
McDonald's						
Chicken McNuggets®	109	323	19.1	13.7	21.3	72.8
Hamburger	100	263	12.4	28.3	11.3	29.1
Cheeseburger	114	328	15.0	28.5	16.0	40.6
Quarter Pounder®	160	427	24.6	29.3	23.5	81.0
Quarter Pounder® w/Cheese	186	525	29.6	30.5	31.6	107.0
Big Mac®	200	570	24.6	39.2	35.0	83.0
Filet-O-Fish®	143	435	14.7	35.9	25.7	45.2
Mc D.L.T.®	254	680	30.0	40.0	44.0	101.0
French Fries, reg	68	220	3.0	26.1	11.5	8.6
Biscuit w/Sausage, Egg	175	585	19.8	36.4	39.9	285.0
Biscuit w/Bacon, Egg, Cheese	145	483	16.5	33.2	31.6	263.0
Sausage McMuffin®	115	427	17.6	30.0	26.3	59.0

Source: McDonald's Corp, Oak Brook, Illinois. Nutrient analyses by Hazelton Laboratory of America (formerly Raltech Scientific Services Inc), Madison, Wisconsin.

Vitamin A (IU)	Thiamin (mg)	Riboflavin (mg)	Niacin (mg)	Vitamin C (mg)	Calcium (mg)	Iron (mg)	Phosphorus (mg)	Sodium (mg)	Zinc (mg)
—	—	—	—	—	—	—	—	853.0	—
—	—	—	—	—	—	—	—	2076.0	—
—	—	—	—	—	—	—	—	2161.0	—
—	—	—	—	—	—	—	—	1543.0	—
—	—	—	—	—	—	—	—	1297.0	—
—	—	—	—	—	—	—	—	1579.0	—
—	—	—	—	—	—	—	—	763.0	—
—	—	—	—	—	—	—	—	1900.0	—
—	—	—	—	—	—	—	—	1526.0	—
—	—	—	—	—	—	—	—	1402.0	—
—	—	—	—	—	—	—	—	1086.0	—
—	—	—	—	—	—	—	—	986.0	—
—	—	—	—	—	—	—	—	673.0	—
—	—	—	—	—	—	—	—	374.0	—
—	—	—	—	—	—	—	—	515.0	—
—	—	—	—	—	—	—	—	154.0	—
—	—	—	—	—	—	—	—	611.0	—
—	—	—	—	—	—	—	—	367.0	—
—	—	—	—	—	—	—	—	0.6	—
—	—	—	—	—	—	—	—	405.0	—
109	0.16	0.14	7.52	2.1	11	1.25	—	512	—
100	0.31	0.22	4.08	1.8	84	2.85	—	506	—
353	0.30	0.24	4.33	2.1	169	2.84	—	743	—
128	0.35	0.32	7.02	2.6	98	4.30	—	718	—
614	0.37	0.41	7.07	2.8	255	4.84	—	1220	—
380	0.48	0.38	7.20	3.0	203	4.90	—	979	—
186	0.36	0.23	3.0	2.1	133	2.47	—	799	—
508	0.56	0.46	8.0	8.0	230	6.60	—	1030	—
17	0.12	0.02	2.26	12.5	9	0.61	—	109	—
420	0.53	0.49	3.85	1.8	119	3.43	—	1301	—
653	0.30	0.43	2.32	1.6	2	2.57	—	1269	—
380	0.70	0.25	4.14	1.3	168	2.25	—	942	—

Continued.

O

Fast Foods—Table of Food Composition—cont'd

	Weight (g)	Energy (kcal)	Protein (g)	Carbohydrate (g)	Fat (g)	Cholesterol (mg)
McDonald's—cont'd						
Sausage McMuffin® w/Egg	165	517	22.9	32.2	32.9	287.0
Egg McMuffin®	138	340	18.5	31.0	15.8	259.0
Hot Cakes w/Butter, Syrup	214	500	7.9	93.9	10.3	47.1
Scrambled Eggs	98	180	13.2	2.5	13.0	514.0
Sausage	53	210	9.8	0.6	18.6	38.8
English Muffin w/Butter	63	186	5.0	29.5	5.3	15.3
Hash Brown Potatoes	55	125	1.5	14.0	7.0	17.2
Vanilla Shake	291	352	9.3	59.6	8.4	30.6
Chocolate Shake	291	383	9.9	65.5	9.0	29.7
Strawberry Shake	290	362	9.0	62.1	8.7	32.2
Strawberry Sundae	164	320	6.0	54.0	8.7	24.6
Hot Fudge Sundae	164	357	7.0	58.0	10.8	26.6
Caramel Sundae	165	361	7.0	60.8	10.0	31.4
Apple Pie	85	253	1.9	29.3	14.3	12.4
Cherry Pie	88	260	2.0	32.1	13.6	13.4
McDonaldland® Cookies	67	308	4.0	49.0	10.8	10.2
Chocolate Chip Cookies	69	342	4.0	45.0	16.3	17.7
Wendy's						
Single Hamburger, multigrain bun	119	340	25	20	17	67
Single Hamburger, white bun	117	350	21	27	18	65
Double Hamburger, white bun	197	560	41	24	34	125
Bacon Cheeseburger, white bun	147	460	29	23	28	65
Chicken Sandwich, multigrain bun	128	320	25	31	10	59
Kid's Meal Hamburger, 2 oz	75	220	13	11	8	20
Chili, 8 oz	256	260	21	26	8	30
French Fries, reg	98	280	4	35	14	15
Taco Salad	357	390	23	36	18	40
Frosty Dairy Dessert	243	400	8	59	14	50
Hot Stuffed Baked Potatoes						
Plain	250	250	6	52	2	tr
Sour Cream & Chives	310	460	6	53	24	15
Cheese	350	590	17	55	34	22
Chili & Cheese	400	510	22	63	20	22
Bacon & Cheese	350	570	19	57	30	22
Broccoli & Cheese	365	500	13	54	25	22

Source: Wendy's International Inc, Dublin, Ohio. Nutrient analyses: entree items, Hazelton Laboratory of America (formerly Raltech Scientific Services Inc), Madison, Wisconsin; other items, US Department of Agriculture Handbook #8.

Vitamin A (IU)	Thiamin (mg)	Riboflavin (mg)	Niacin (mg)	Vitamin C (mg)	Calcium (mg)	Iron (mg)	Phosphorus (mg)	Sodium (mg)	Zinc (mg)
660	0.84	0.50	4.46	1.6	196	3.47	—	1044	—
591	0.47	0.44	3.77	1.4	226	2.93	—	885	—
257	0.26	0.36	2.27	4.7	103	2.23	—	1070	—
652	0.08	0.47	0.20	1.2	61	2.53	—	205	—
31	0.27	0.11	2.07	0.5	16	0.82	—	423	—
164	0.28	0.49	2.61	0.8	117	1.51	—	310	—
13	0.06	0.01	0.82	4.1	5	0.40	—	325	—
349	0.12	0.70	0.35	3.2	329	0.18	—	201	—
349	0.12	0.44	0.50	2.9	320	0.84	—	300	—
377	0.12	0.44	0.35	4.1	322	0.17	—	207	—
230	0.07	0.30	1.03	2.79	174	0.38	—	90	—
230	0.07	0.31	1.12	2.46	215	0.61	—	170	—
279	0.07	0.31	1.01	3.61	200	0.23	—	145	—
34	0.02	0.02	0.19	0.9	14	0.62	—	398	—
114	0.03	0.02	0.25	0.9	12	0.59	—	427	—
27	0.23	0.23	2.85	0.94	12	1.47	—	358	—
76	0.12	0.21	1.70	1.04	29	1.56	—	313	—
×	0.22	0.17	5	×	16	2.7	—	290	—
—	0.22	0.25	5	—	32	4.5	—	410	—
—	0.22	0.43	9	—	32	6.3	—	575	—
400	0.30	0.26	6	×	120	3.6	—	860	—
×	0.15	0.14	10	×	16	1.4	—	500	—
—	0.09	0.17	3	—	16	1.8	—	265	—
1000	0.15	0.17	3	6	64	4.5	—	1070	—
—	0.15	0.03	3	12	×	1.1	—	95	—
1750	0.15	0.03	3	21	160	4.5	—	1100	—
500	0.12	0.51	—	×	240	1.1	—	220	—
×	0.22	0.10	3	36	16	2.7	—	60	—
500	0.22	0.14	3	36	32	2.7	—	230	—
1000	0.22	0.26	3	36	280	2.7	—	450	—
750	0.30	0.26	4	36	200	3.6	—	610	—
750	0.22	0.17	3	36	160	2.7	—	1180	—
1750	0.30	0.26	4	90	200	2.7	—	430	—

Continued.

Fast Foods—Table of Food Composition—cont'd

	Weight (g)	Energy (kcal)	Protein (g)	Carbohydrate (g)	Fat (g)	Cholesterol (mg)
Wendy's—cont'd						
Ham & Cheese Omelet	114	250	18	6	17	450
Ham, Cheese, & Mushroom Omelet	118	290	18	7	21	355
Ham, Cheese, Onion, & Green Pepper Omelet	128	280	19	7	19	525
Mushroom, Onion, & Green Pepper Omelet	114	210	14	7	15	460
Breakfast Sandwich	129	370	17	33	19	200
French Toast, 2 slices	135	400	11	45	19	115
Home Fries	103	360	4	37	22	20
Whataburger						
Whataburger®	302	580	32	58	24	70
Whataburger® w/Cheese	326	669	36	58	33	96
Whataburger Jr®	153	304	15	31	14	30
Whataburger Jr® w/Cheese	165	351	17	30	18	42
Justaburger®	117	265	12	28	12	25
Justaburger® w/Cheese	129	312	15	28	16	37
Whatacatch®	177	475	14	43	27	34
Whatacatch® w/Cheese	189	522	17	43	31	45
Whataburger® Doublemeat	385	806	51	59	41	154
Whataburger® Doublemeat w/Cheese	409	895	54	59	49	180
Whatachick 'n® Sandwich	288	671	35	61	32	71
French Fries, reg	85	221	4	25	12	1
French Fries, lg	127	332	5	37	18	1
Onion Rings	73	226	4	23	13	1
Apple Pie	39	236	3	30	12	1
Vanilla Shake, sm	254	322	9	50	9	37
Vanilla Shake, med	340	433	12	68	13	49
Vanilla Shake, lg	508	647	18	101	19	74
Vanilla Shake, extra lg	678	861	24	134	25	98
Taquito	125	310	19	17	19	223
Taquito w/Cheese	137	357	22	17	23	235
Egg Omelet Sandwich	120	312	14	29	15	191
Breakfast on a Bun	175	520	23	29	34	234
Pancakes & Sausage, without syrup & butter	153	407	15	38	22	77
Pancakes, without syrup and butter	98	199	6	37	3	34
Sausage	55	208	9	1	19	43
Pecan Danish	63	270	5	28	16	12

Source: Whataburger Inc, Corpus Christi, Texas. Nutrient analyses by Hazelton Laboratory of America Madison, Wisconsin.

Vitamin A (IU)	Thiamin (mg)	Riboflavin (mg)	Niacin (mg)	Vitamin C (mg)	Calcium (mg)	Iron (mg)	Phosphorus (mg)	Sodium (mg)	Zinc (mg)
1000	0.15	0.60	0.8	—	80	2.7	—	405	—
1000	0.23	0.60	1.2	—	80	2.7	—	570	—
1000	0.15	0.60	0.8	6	120	2.7	—	485	—
750	0.09	0.51	×	6	48	2.7	—	200	—
1000	0.45	0.43	3.0	—	120	3.6	—	770	—
500	0.60	0.51	4.0	—	64	1.8	—	850	—
—	0.12	0.03	0.8	5	16	0.7	—	745	—
211	0.79	0.54	9.4	6.3	212	8.7	279	1092	4.6
293	0.77	0.65	9.5	5.9	358	8.0	377	1474	5.0
107	0.37	0.26	3.6	2.9	122	4.1	137	684	2.0
264	0.36	0.28	3.5	3.5	193	4.0	192	921	2.2
35	0.33	0.21	2.8	1.6	106	3.9	113	547	1.6
192	0.33	0.23	2.8	2.2	177	3.9	168	784	1.8
—	0.44	0.23	4.3	2.1	120	3.0	230	722	0.7
—	0.44	0.25	4.3	2.7	191	3.0	285	959	1.0
211	0.81	0.84	13.6	6.3	217	11.2	415	1296	8.1
293	0.79	0.95	13.6	5.9	363	10.5	513	1678	8.4
288	0.78	0.37	17.0	6.3	103	6.4	389	1460	1.5
—	0.15	0.04	2.0	3.2	9	0.6	102	30	0.3
—	0.23	0.07	3.1	4.9	14	0.9	153	45	0.5
—	0.12	0.05	0.7	2.5	21	0.7	67	410	0.3
—	0.16	0.07	1.2	—	9	1.0	55	265	0.1
279	0.10	0.81	0.3	—	261	1.7	233	169	0.8
375	0.14	1.10	0.4	1.0	351	2.3	312	227	1.0
560	0.20	1.63	0.6	—	524	3.4	466	338	1.5
745	0.27	2.17	0.8	—	698	4.5	620	450	2.0
513	0.40	0.36	3.2	—	92	3.1	253	712	1.4
670	0.40	0.38	3.2	—	163	3.1	308	949	1.7
564	0.34	0.55	2.9	—	209	3.4	210	696	1.3
564	0.53	0.71	5.9	—	216	4.1	292	1051	2.3
—	0.45	0.39	5.1	—	60	2.6	401	1029	1.5
—	0.26	0.23	2.1	—	53	1.9	319	674	0.4
—	0.19	0.16	3.0	—	7	0.7	82	355	1.0
223	0.31	0.19	2.5	—	66	1.6	127	419	0.4

O

Continued.

Fast Foods—Table of Food Composition—cont'd

	Weight (g)	Energy (kcal)	Protein (g)	Carbohydrate (g)	Fat (g)	Cholesterol (mg)
Zantigo						
Taco	84.5	198	10.4	12.8	11.7	30.5
Taco Burrito	198.7	415	20.7	41.1	19.0	43.9
Mild Chilito	115.0	330	13.8	36.0	14.7	26.2
Hot Chilito	115.3	329	14.3	35.2	14.5	31.5
Beef Enchilada	184.1	315	18.0	26.0	15.0	49.0
Cheese Enchilada	179.8	390	19.8	26.2	22.8	62.9

	Weight (g)	Energy (kcal)	Protein (g)	Carbohydrate (g)	Fat (g)	Cholesterol (mg)
Coca-Cola						
Coca-Cola Classic®	—	144.0	—	38.0	—	—
Coca-Cola®	—	154.0	—	40.0	—	—
Cherry Coke®	—	154.0	—	40.0	—	—
Diet Coke®**	—	0.9	—	0.3	—	—
Sprite®	—	142.0	—	36.0	—	—
Mr. Pibb®	—	142.0	—	37.0	—	—
Mellow Yello®	—	172.0	—	44.0	—	—
Ramblin' Root Beer®	—	158.0	—	42.0	—	—
Fanta® Orange	—	164.0	—	42.0	—	—
Fanta® Grape	—	168.0	—	42.0	—	—
Fanta® Root Beer	—	158.0	—	42.0	—	—
Fanta® Ginger Ale	—	126.0	—	32.0	—	—
Hi-C® Orange***	—	152.0	—	38.0	—	—
Hi-C® Lemon***	—	142.0	—	36.0	—	—
Hi-C® Punch***	—	154.0	—	40.0	—	—
Hi-C® Grape***	—	164.0	—	40.0	—	—
Tab®**	—	1.0	—	1.0	—	—
Diet Sprite®**	—	3.0	—	0	—	—
Minute Maid® Orange†	—	160.0	—	40.0	—	—

Source: Zantigo Mexican Restaurants, Columbus, Ohio.
Nutritive value of fountain products, 12-oz servings without ice. *Added potassium and sodium; actual content depends on local water supplies. **Sweetened with an aspartame-saccharin blend. Bottled and canned versions of Diet Coke and Diet Sprite are sweetened with 100% NutraSweet, a registered trademark of The NutraSweet Co for aspartame. ***Hi-C soft drinks do not contain fruit juice and are not the same as Hi-C fruit-juice–containing drinks produced by Coca-Cola Foods, a division of The Coca-Cola Co. †Not vitamin enriched. Bottled and canned versions are enriched with vitamins B_6 and C and folic acid. Source: The Coca-Cola Co, Atlanta, Georgia.
Note: There was no data available for calcium and iron.
Source: Young, E.A., Sims, O., Bingham, C., and Brennan, E.H., Fast foods 1986: Nutrient analyses. *Dietetic Currents 13*, No. 6, 1986. Reproduced with the permission of Dr. E.A. Young and Ross Laboratories, Columbus, Ohio, 43216.

O

Vitamin A (IU)	Thiamin (mg)	Riboflavin (mg)	Niacin (mg)	Vitamin C (mg)	Calcium (mg)	Iron (mg)	Phosphorus (mg)	Sodium (mg)	Zinc (mg)
—	—	—	—	—	—	—	—	318	—
—	—	—	—	—	—	—	—	815	—
—	—	—	—	—	—	—	—	505	—
—	—	—	—	—	—	—	—	466	—
—	—	—	—	—	—	—	—	904	—
—	—	—	—	—	—	—	—	759	—

Vitamin A (IU)	Thiamin (mg)	Riboflavin (mg)	Niacin (mg)	Vitamin C (mg)	Phosphorus (mg)	Sodium* (mg)	Zinc (mg)	Caffeine (mg)	Saccharin (mg)	Aspartame (mg)
—	—	—	—	0	60	14	—	46	0	0
—	—	—	—	0	54	6	—	46	0	0
—	—	—	—	0	54	14	—	46	0	0
—	—	—	—	0	28	16	—	46	70	34
—	—	—	—	0	tr	45	—	0	0	0
—	—	—	—	0	42	21	—	40	—	0
—	—	—	—	tr	tr	28	—	51	—	0
—	—	—	—	0	tr	18	—	0	—	0
—	—	—	—	0	tr	12	—	0	—	0
—	—	—	—	0	tr	12	—	0	—	0
—	—	—	—	0	tr	18	—	0	—	0
—	—	—	—	0	tr	26	—	0	—	0
—	—	—	—	120	tr	12	—	0	—	0
—	—	—	—	120	148	100	—	0	—	0
—	—	—	—	120	tr	12	—	0	—	0
—	—	—	—	120	tr	12	—	0	—	0
—	—	—	—	0	45	30	—	46	94	28
—	—	—	—	0	0	9	—	0	70	28
—	—	—	—	0	3	2	—	0	0	0

O

APPENDIX

P

Table of Food Composition

Information from this appendix is useful throughout the book.

Do you want to know your nutrient intake for the past three days? Are apples, popcorn, or yogurt good for you? What percent of the RDA for vitamin A is provided by 1 ounce of cheddar cheese? How many kcalories are in a bagel?

You will find answers to these questions by using a Table of Food Composition. Nutrient intake is obtained by keeping a record of your food intake (Appendix B), and then calculating the nutrient values from this table. To find out if a particular food is "good for you" get the list of nutrients in the food from this table and from those in Appendix J and K. Then express the concentration of the nutrient in the food as a percent of the RDA. This table gives you the food energy (kcalories) in 796 foods and drinks.

A few words on how to get the maximum information from this table:

- Nutritive values are expressed per serving. Notice that the weights of these servings vary. If you want to compare the concentration of nutrients in different foods convert all nutrient values into concentrations per 100 grams (see Appendix B). Now you are comparing equal weights of food.

Item Number	Foods, Approximate Measures, Units, and Weight (edible parts)		Weight (grams)	Water (percent)	Food Energy (calories)	Protein (grams)	Fat (grams)
	Dairy Products (Cheese, Cream, Imitation Cream, Milk, Yogurt)						
	Cheese						
	Natural						
1	Blue	1 oz	28	42	100	6	8
2	Camembert (3 wedges/4-oz container)	1 wedge	38	52	115	8	9
	Cheddar						
3	Cut pieces	1 oz	28	37	115	7	9
4		1 in	17	37	70	4	6
5	Shredded	1 cup	113	37	455	28	37
	Cottage (curd not pressed down)						
	Creamed (cottage cheese, 4% fat)						
6	Large curd	1 cup	225	79	235	28	10
7	Small curd	1 cup	210	79	215	26	9
8	With fruit	1 cup	226	72	280	22	8
9	Lowfat (2%)	1 cup	226	79	205	31	4

- Fatty acids are expressed as saturated, monounsaturated, and polyunsaturated fatty acids. To get the P/S ratio of your diet, or of a particular food, check the calculations in Appendix B. Some people must watch the P/S ratio if they are controlling their intake of saturated fat.
- Carbohydrate values include starches (complex) and sugars (simple).
- Vitamin A values are given as International Units (IU) and as Retinol Equivalents (RE). Nutritionists use RE values. IU values are listed because commercial vitamin supplements use IU values on labels and in advertisements.
- Niacin values are expressed in milligrams. Therefore, these values are for preformed niacin. If values were presented as Niacin Equivalents (NE) it would include the niacin produced from the amino acid tryptophan.
- The sodium, potassium, zinc, selenium, and iodine contents of some foods are presented in Appendix J; the vitamin B_6, vitamin B_{12}, and folacin contents are presented in Appendix K. Refer to these values if you need a more extensive profile of the nutritive value of your diet.
- Tables of food composition do not allow for changes in the bioavailability of nutrients. The positive and negative effects of other dietary components on the digestion, absorption, and utilization of individual nutrients is discussed.
- Footnotes are important—though they may seem bothersome! They refer mainly to major variations in nutritive value due to different methods of food preparation. Another reason for variation is differences within a food type. For example, yellow corn has much more vitamin A than white corn. Other footnotes alert you to which foods have nutrients added.

The nutrient information is from *Composition of Foods,* Agricultural Handbooks Nos. 8-1 through 8-16, U.S. Department of Agriculture, Washington, D.C. Similar information is available in *Nutrient Value of Some Common Foods,* Minister of National Health and Welfare, Health Services and Promotion, Canada 1987.

Fatty Acids							Vitamin A Value					
Satu-rated (grams)	Monoun-saturated (grams)	Polyun-saturated (grams)	Carbo-hydrate (grams)	Calcium (mg)	Phos-phorus (mg)	Iron (mg)	(IU) Inter-national Units	(RE) Retinol Equiv-alents	Thiamin (mg)	Riboflavin (mg)	Niacin (mg)	Vitamin C (mg)
5.3	2.2	0.2	1	150	110	0.1	200	65	0.01	0.11	0.3	0
5.8	2.7	0.3	Tr	147	132	0.1	350	96	0.01	0.19	0.2	0
6.0	2.7	0.3	Tr	204	145	0.2	300	86	0.01	0.11	Tr	0
3.6	1.6	0.2	Tr	123	87	0.1	180	52	Tr	0.06	Tr	0
23.8	10.6	1.1	1	815	579	0.8	1200	342	0.03	0.42	0.1	0
6.4	2.9	0.3	6	135	297	0.3	370	108	0.05	0.37	0.3	Tr
6.0	2.7	0.3	6	126	277	0.3	340	101	0.04	0.34	0.3	Tr
4.9	2.2	0.2	30	108	236	0.2	280	81	0.04	0.29	0.2	Tr
2.8	1.2	0.1	8	155	340	0.4	160	45	0.05	0.42	0.3	Tr

P

Item Number	Foods, Approximate Measures, Units, and Weight (edible parts)		Weight (grams)	Water (percent)	Food Energy (calories)	Protein (grams)	Fat (grams)
	Dairy Products—cont'd						
10	Uncreamed (cottage cheese dry curd, less than ½% fat)	1 cup	145	80	125	25	1
11	Cream	1 oz	28	54	100	2	10
	Mozzarella, made with						
12	Whole milk	1 oz	28	54	80	6	6
13	Part skim milk (low moisture)	1 oz	28	49	80	8	5
14	Muenster	1 oz	28	42	105	7	9
	Parmesan, grated						
15	Cup, not pressed down	1 cup	100	18	455	42	30
16	Tablespoon	1 tbsp	5	18	25	2	2
17	Ounce	1 oz	28	18	130	12	9
18	Provolone	1 oz	28	41	100	7	8
	Ricotta, made with						
19	Whole milk	1 cup	246	72	430	28	32
20	Part skim milk	1 cup	246	74	340	28	19
21	Swiss	1 oz	28	37	105	8	8
	Pasteurized process cheese						
22	American	1 oz	28	39	105	6	9
23	Swiss	1 oz	28	42	95	7	7
24	Pasteurized process cheese food, American	1 oz	28	43	95	6	7
25	Pasteurized process cheese spread, American	1 oz	28	48	80	5	6
	Cream, sweet						
26	Half-and-half (cream and milk)	1 cup	242	81	315	7	28
27		1 tbsp	15	81	20	Tr	2
28	Light, coffee, or table	1 cup	240	74	470	6	46
29		1 tbsp	15	74	30	Tr	3
	Whipping, unwhipped (volume about double when whipped)						
30	Light	1 cup	239	64	700	5	74
31		1 tbsp	15	64	45	Tr	5
32	Heavy	1 cup	238	58	820	5	88
32		1 tbsp	15	58	50	Tr	6
33	Whipped topping, (pressurized)	1 cup	60	61	155	2	13
34		1 tbsp	3	61	10	Tr	1
35	Cream, sour	1 cup	230	71	495	7	48
36		1 tbsp	12	71	25	Tr	3
	Cream products, imitation (made with vegetable fat)						
	Sweet						
	Creamers						
37	Liquid (frozen)	1 tbsp	15	77	20	Tr	1
38	Powdered	1 tsp	2	2	10	Tr	1
	Whipped topping						
39	Frozen	1 cup	75	50	240	1	19
40		1 tbsp	4	50	15	Tr	1
41	Powdered, made with whole milk	1 cup	80	67	150	3	10
42		1 tbsp	4	67	10	Tr	Tr
43	Pressurized	1 cup	70	60	185	1	16
44		1 tbsp	4	60	10	Tr	1

P

Fatty Acids							Vitamin A Value					
Saturated (grams)	Monounsaturated (grams)	Polyunsaturated (grams)	Carbohydrate (grams)	Calcium (mg)	Phosphorus (mg)	Iron (mg)	(IU) International Units	(RE) Retinol Equivalents	Thiamin (mg)	Riboflavin (mg)	Niacin (mg)	Vitamin C (mg)
0.4	0.2	Tr	3	46	151	0.3	40	12	0.04	0.21	0.2	0
6.2	2.8	0.4	1	23	30	0.3	400	124	Tr	0.06	Tr	0
3.7	1.9	0.2	1	147	105	0.1	220	68	Tr	0.07	Tr	0
3.1	1.4	0.1	1	207	149	0.1	180	54	0.01	0.10	Tr	0
5.4	2.5	0.2	Tr	203	133	0.1	320	90	Tr	0.09	Tr	0
19.1	8.7	0.7	4	1376	807	1.0	700	173	0.05	0.39	0.3	0
1.0	0.4	Tr	Tr	69	40	Tr	40	9	Tr	0.02	Tr	0
5.4	2.5	0.2	1	390	229	0.3	200	49	0.01	0.11	0.1	0
4.8	2.1	0.2	1	214	141	0.1	230	75	0.01	0.09	Tr	0
20.4	8.9	0.9	7	509	389	0.9	1210	330	0.03	0.48	0.3	0
12.1	5.7	0.6	13	669	449	1.1	1060	278	0.05	0.46	0.2	0
5.0	2.1	0.3	1	272	171	Tr	240	72	0.01	0.10	Tr	0
5.6	2.5	0.3	Tr	174	211	0.1	340	82	0.01	0.10	Tr	0
4.5	2.0	0.2	1	219	216	0.2	230	65	Tr	0.08	Tr	0
4.4	2.0	0.2	2	163	130	0.2	260	62	0.01	0.13	Tr	0
3.8	1.8	0.2	2	159	202	0.1	220	54	0.01	0.12	Tr	0
17.3	8.0	1.0	10	254	230	0.2	1050	259	0.08	0.36	0.2	2
1.1	0.5	0.1	1	16	14	Tr	70	16	0.01	0.02	Tr	Tr
28.8	13.4	1.7	9	231	192	0.1	1730	437	0.08	0.36	0.1	2
0.8	0.8	0.1	1	14	12	Tr	110	27	Tr	0.02	Tr	Tr
46.2	21.7	2.1	7	166	146	0.1	2690	705	0.06	0.30	0.1	1
2.9	1.4	0.1	Tr	10	9	Tr	170	44	Tr	0.02	Tr	Tr
54.8	25.4	3.3	7	154	149	0.1	3500	1002	0.05	0.26	0.1	1
3.5	1.6	0.2	Tr	10	9	Tr	220	63	Tr	0.02	Tr	Tr
8.3	3.9	0.5	7	61	54	Tr	550	124	0.02	0.04	Tr	0
0.4	0.2	Tr	Tr	3	3	Tr	30	6	Tr	Tr	Tr	0
30.0	13.9	1.8	10	268	195	0.1	1820	448	0.08	0.34	0.2	2
1.6	0.7	0.1	1	14	10	Tr	90	23	Tr	0.02	Tr	Tr
1.4	Tr	Tr	2	1	10	Tr	10^5	1	0.00	0.00	0.0	0
0.7	Tr	Tr	1	Tr	8	Tr	Tr	Tr	0.00	Tr	0.0	0
16.3	1.2	0.4	17	5	6	0.1	650^5	65	0.00	0.00	0.0	0
0.9	0.1	Tr	1	Tr	Tr	Tr	30^5	3	0.00	0.00	0.0	0
8.5	0.7	0.2	13	72	69	Tr	290^5	39	0.02	0.09	Tr	1
0.4	Tr	Tr	1	4	3	Tr	10^5	2	Tr	Tr	Tr	Tr
13.2	1.3	0.2	11	4	13	Tr	330^5	33	0.00	0.00	0.0	0
0.8	0.1	Tr	1	Tr	1	Tr	20^5	2	0.00	0.00	0.0	0

Continued.

Item Number	Foods, Approximate Measures, Units, and Weight (edible parts)		Weight (grams)	Water (percent)	Food Energy (calories)	Protein (grams)	Fat (grams)
	Dairy Products—cont'd						
45	Sour dressing (imitation sour cream type product, nonbutterfat)	1 cup	235	75	415	8	39
46		1 tbsp	12	75	20	Tr	2
	Ice cream. See Milk desserts, frozen (items 74-79).						
	Ice milk. See Milk desserts, frozen (items 80-82).						
	Milk						
	Fluid						
47	Whole (3.3% fat)	1 cup	244	88	150	8	8
	Lowfat (2%)						
48	No milk solids added	1 cup	244	89	120	8	5
49	Milk solids added, label claim less than 10 g of protein per cup	1 cup	245	89	125	9	5
	Lowfat (1%)						
50	No milk solids added	1 cup	244	90	100	8	3
51	Milk solids added, label claim less than 10 g of protein per cup	1 cup	245	90	105	9	2
	Nonfat (skim)						
52	No milk solids added	1 cup	245	91	85	8	Tr
53	Milk solids added, label claim less than 10 g of protein per cup	1 cup	245	90	90	9	1
54	Buttermilk	1 cup	245	90	100	8	2
	Canned						
55	Condensed, sweetened	1 cup	306	27	980	24	27
	Evaporated						
56	Whole milk	1 cup	252	74	340	17	19
57	Skim milk	1 cup	255	79	200	19	1
	Dried						
58	Buttermilk	1 cup	120	3	465	41	7
	Nonfat, instant						
59	Envelope, 3.2 oz, net wt	1 envelope	91	4	325	32	1
60	Cup	1 cup	68	4	245	24	Tr
	Milk beverages						
	Chocolate milk (commercial)						
61	Regular	1 cup	250	82	210	8	8
62	Lowfat (2%)	1 cup	250	84	180	8	5
63	Lowfat (1%)	1 cup	250	85	160	8	3
	Cocoa and chocolate-flavored beverages						
64	Powder containing nonfat dry milk	1 oz	28	1	100	3	1
65	Prepared (6 oz water plus 1 oz powder)	1 serving	206	86	100	3	1
66	Powder without nonfat dry milk	¾ oz	21	1	75	1	1
	Prepared (8 oz whole milk plus ¾ oz powder)	1 serving	265	81	225	9	9
67	Eggnog (commercial)	1 cup	254	74	340	10	19

P

| | Fatty Acids | | | | | | Vitamin A Value | | | | | |
Satu-rated (grams)	Monoun-saturated (grams)	Polyun-saturated (grams)	Carbo-hydrate (grams)	Calcium (mg)	Phos-phorus (mg)	Iron (mg)	(IU) Inter-national Units	(RE) Retinol Equiv-alents	Thiamin (mg)	Riboflavin (mg)	Niacin (mg)	Vitamin C (mg)
31.2	4.6	1.1	11	266	205	0.1	20	5	0.09	0.38	0.2	2
1.6	0.2	0.1	1	14	10	Tr	Tr	Tr	Tr	0.02	Tr	Tr
5.1	2.4	0.3	11	291	228	0.1	310	76	0.09	0.40	0.2	2
2.9	1.4	0.2	12	297	232	0.1	500	139	0.10	0.40	0.2	2
2.9	1.4	0.2	12	313	245	0.1	500	140	0.10	0.42	0.2	2
1.6	0.7	0.1	12	300	235	0.1	500	144	0.10	0.41	0.2	2
1.5	0.7	0.1	12	313	245	0.1	500	145	0.10	0.42	0.2	2
0.3	0.1	Tr	12	302	247	0.1	500	149	0.09	0.34	0.2	2
0.4	0.2	Tr	12	316	255	0.1	500	149	0.10	0.43	0.2	2
1.3	0.6	0.1	12	285	219	0.1	80	20	0.08	0.38	0.1	2
16.8	7.4	1.0	166	868	775	0.6	1000	248	0.28	1.27	0.6	8
11.6	5.9	0.6	25	657	510	0.5	610	136	0.12	0.80	0.5	5
0.3	0.2	Tr	29	738	497	0.7	1000	298	0.11	0.79	0.4	3
4.3	2.0	0.3	59	1421	1119	0.4	260	65	0.47	1.89	1.1	7
0.4	0.2	Tr	47	1120	896	0.3	2160[1]	646[1]	0.38	1.59	0.8	5
0.3	0.1	Tr	35	837	670	0.2	1610[1]	483[1]	0.28	1.19	0.6	4
5.3	2.5	0.3	26	280	251	0.6	300	73	0.09	0.41	0.3	2
3.1	1.5	0.2	26	284	254	0.6	500	143	0.09	0.41	0.3	2
1.5	0.8	0.1	26	287	256	0.6	500	148	0.10	0.42	0.3	2
0.6	0.3	Tr	22	90	88	0.3	Tr	Tr	0.03	0.17	0.2	Tr
0.6	0.3	Tr	22	90	88	0.3	Tr	Tr	0.03	0.17	0.2	Tr
0.3	0.2	Tr	19	7	26	0.7	Tr	Tr	Tr	0.03	0.1	Tr
5.4	2.5	0.3	30	298	254	0.9	310	76	0.10	0.43	0.3	3
11.3	5.7	0.9	34	330	378	0.5	890	203	0.09	0.48	0.3	4

1. Added vitamin A.

Continued.

P

Item Number	Foods, Approximate Measures, Units, and Weight (edible parts)		Weight (grams)	Water (percent)	Food Energy (calories)	Protein (grams)	Fat (grams)
	Dairy Products—cont'd						
	Malted milk						
	Chocolate						
68	Powder	¾ oz	21	2	85	1	1
69	Prepared (8 oz whole milk plus ¾ oz powder)	1 serving	265	81	235	9	9
	Natural						
70	Powder	¾ oz	21	3	85	3	2
71	Prepared (8 oz whole milk plus ¾ oz powder)	1 serving	265	81	235	11	10
	Shakes, thick						
72	Chocolate	10-oz container	283	72	335	9	8
73	Vanilla	10-oz container	283	74	315	11	9
	Milk desserts, frozen						
	Ice cream, vanilla						
	Regular (about 11% fat)						
74	Hardened	½ gal	1064	61	2155	38	115
75		1 cup	133	61	270	5	14
76		3 fl oz	50	61	100	2	5
77	Soft serve (frozen custard)	1 cup	173	60	375	7	23
78	Rich (about 16% fat), hardened	½ gal	1188	59	2805	33	190
79		1 cup	148	59	350	4	24
	Ice milk, vanilla						
80	Hardened (about 4% fat)	½ gal	1048	69	1470	41	45
81		1 cup	131	69	185	5	6
82	Soft serve (about 3% fat)	1 cup	175	70	225	8	5
83	Sherbet (about 2% fat)	½ gal	1542	66	2160	17	31
84		1 cup	193	66	270	2	4
	Yogurt						
	With added milk solids						
	Made with lowfat milk						
85	Fruit-flavored[2]	8-oz container	227	74	230	10	2
86	Plain	8-oz container	227	85	145	12	4
87	Made with nonfat milk	8-oz container	227	85	125	13	Tr
	Without added milk solids						
88	Made with whole milk	8-oz container	227	88	140	8	7

2. Amount of sugar added varies, and therefore, carbohydrate content varies.

P

| Fatty Acids | | | Carbo-hydrate (grams) | Calcium (mg) | Phos-phorus (mg) | Iron (mg) | Vitamin A Value | | Thiamin (mg) | Riboflavin (mg) | Niacin (mg) | Vitamin C (mg) |
Satu-rated (grams)	Monoun-saturated (grams)	Polyun-saturated (grams)					(IU) Inter-national Units	(RE) Retinol Equiv-alents				
0.5	0.3	0.1	18	13	37	0.4	20	5	0.04	0.04	0.4	0
5.5	2.7	0.4	29	304	265	0.5	330	80	0.14	0.43	0.7	2
0.9	0.5	0.3	15	56	79	0.2	70	17	0.11	0.14	1.1	0
6.0	2.9	0.6	27	347	307	0.3	380	93	0.20	0.54	1.3	2
4.8	2.2	0.3	60	374	357	0.9	240	59	0.13	0.63	0.4	0
5.3	2.5	0.3	50	413	326	0.3	320	79	0.08	0.55	0.4	0
71.3	33.1	4.3	254	1406	1075	1.0	4340	1064	0.42	2.63	1.1	6
8.9	4.1	0.5	32	176	134	0.1	540	133	0.05	0.33	0.1	1
3.4	1.6	0.2	12	66	51	Tr	200	50	0.02	0.12	0.1	Tr
13.5	6.7	1.0	38	236	199	0.4	790	199	0.08	0.45	0.2	1
118.3	54.9	7.1	256	1213	927	0.8	7200	1758	0.36	2.27	0.9	5
14.7	6.8	0.9	32	151	115	0.1	900	219	0.04	0.28	0.1	1
28.1	13.0	1.7	232	1409	1035	1.5	1710	419	0.61	2.78	0.9	6
3.5	1.6	0.2	29	176	129	0.2	210	52	0.08	0.35	0.1	1
2.9	1.3	0.2	38	274	202	0.3	175	44	0.12	0.54	0.2	1
19.0	8.8	1.1	469	827	594	2.5	1480	308	0.26	0.71	1.0	31
2.4	1.1	0.1	59	103	74	0.3	190	39	0.03	0.09	0.1	4
1.6	0.7	0.1	43	345	271	0.2	100	25	0.08	0.40	0.2	1
2.3	1.0	0.1	16	415	326	0.2	150	36	0.10	0.49	0.3	2
0.3	0.1	Tr	17	452	355	0.2	20	5	0.11	0.53	0.3	2
4.8	2.0	0.2	11	274	215	0.1	280	68	0.07	0.32	0.2	1

Continued.

P

Item Number	Foods, Approximate Measures, Units, and Weight (edible parts)		Weight (grams)	Water (percent)	Food Energy (calories)	Protein (grams)	Fat (grams)
	Eggs						
	Eggs, large (24 oz/dozen)						
	Raw						
89	Whole, without shell	1 egg	50	75	80	6	6
90	White	1 white	33	88	15	3	Tr
91	Yolk	1 yolk	17	49	65	3	6
	Cooked						
92	Fried in butter	1 egg	46	68	95	6	7
93	Hard-cooked, shell removed	1 egg	50	75	80	6	6
94	Poached	1 egg	50	74	80	6	6
95	Scrambled (milk added) in butter; also, omelet	1 egg	64	73	110	7	8
	Fats and Oils						
	Butter (4 sticks per lb)						
96	Stick	½ cup	113	16	810	1	92
97	Tablespoon (⅛ stick)	1 tbsp	14	16	100	Tr	11
98	Pat (1-in square, ⅓ in high; 90 per lb)	1 pat	5	16	35	Tr	4
99	Fats, cooking (vegetable shortenings)	1 cup	205	0	1810	0	205
100		1 tbsp	13	0	115	0	13
101	Lard	1 cup	205	0	1850	0	205
102		1 tbsp	13	0	115	0	13
	Margarine						
103	Imitation (about 40% fat), soft	8-oz container	227	58	785	1	88
104		1 tbsp	14	58	50	Tr	5
	Regular (about 80% fat)						
	Hard (4 sticks per lb)						
105	Stick	½ cup	113	16	810	1	91
106	Tablespoon (⅛ stick)	1 tbsp	14	16	100	Tr	11
107	Pat (1-in square, ⅓ in high; 90 per lb)	1 pat	5	16	35	Tr	4
108	Soft	8-oz container	227	16	1625	2	183
	Spread (about 60% fat)						
109	Hard (4 sticks per lb)	1 tbsp	14	16	100	Tr	11
110	Stick	½ cup	113	37	610	1	69
111	Tablespoon (⅛ stick)	1 tbsp	14	37	75	Tr	9
112	Pat (1-in square, ⅓ in high; 90 per lb)	1 pat	5	37	25	Tr	3
113	Soft	8-oz container	227	37	1225	1	138
114		1 tbsp	14	37	75	Tr	9

P

	Fatty Acids						Vitamin A Value					
Satu-rated (grams)	Monoun-saturated (grams)	Polyun-saturated (grams)	Carbo-hydrate (grams)	Calcium (mg)	Phos-phorus (mg)	Iron (mg)	(IU) Inter-national Units	(RE) Retinol Equiv-alents	Thiamin (mg)	Riboflavin (mg)	Niacin (mg)	Vitamin C (mg)
1.7	2.2	0.7	1	28	90	1.0	260	78	0.04	0.15	Tr	0
0.0	0.0	0.0	Tr	4	4	Tr	0	0	Tr	0.09	Tr	0
1.7	2.2	0.7	Tr	26	86	0.9	310	94	0.04	0.07	Tr	0
2.7	2.7	0.8	1	29	91	1.1	320	94	0.04	0.14	Tr	0
1.7	2.2	0.7	1	28	90	1.0	260	78	0.04	0.14	Tr	0
1.7	2.2	0.7	1	28	90	1.0	260	78	0.03	0.13	Tr	0
3.2	2.9	0.8	2	54	109	1.0	350	102	0.04	0.18	Tr	Tr
57.1	26.4	3.4	Tr	27	26	0.2	3460	852	0.01	0.04	Tr	0
7.1	3.3	0.4	Tr	3	3	Tr	430	106	Tr	Tr	Tr	0
2.5	1.2	0.2	Tr	1	1	Tr	150	38	Tr	Tr	Tr	0
51.3	91.2	53.5	0	0	0	0.0	0	0	0.00	0.00	0.0	0
3.3	5.8	3.4	0	0	0	0.0	0	0	0.00	0.00	0.0	0
80.4	92.5	23.0	0	0	0	0.0	0	0	0.00	0.00	0.0	0
5.1	5.9	1.5	0	0	0	0.0	0	0	0.00	0.00	0.0	0
17.5	35.6	31.3	1	40	31	0.0	7510[3]	2254[3]	0.01	0.05	Tr	Tr
1.1	2.2	1.9	Tr	2	2	0.0	460[3]	139[3]	Tr	Tr	Tr	Tr
17.9	40.5	28.7	1	34	26	0.1	3740[3]	1122[3]	0.01	0.04	Tr	Tr
2.2	5.0	3.6	Tr	4	3	Tr	460[3]	139[3]	Tr	0.01	Tr	Tr
0.8	1.8	1.3	Tr	1	1	Tr	170[3]	50[3]	Tr	Tr	Tr	Tr
31.3	64.7	78.5	1	60	46	0.0	7510[3]	2254[3]	0.02	0.07	Tr	Tr
1.9	4.0	4.8	Tr	4	3	0.0	460[3]	139[3]	Tr	Tr	Tr	Tr
15.9	29.4	20.5	0	24	18	0.0	3740[3]	1122[3]	0.01	0.03	Tr	Tr
2.0	3.6	2.5	0	3	2	0.0	460[3]	139[3]	Tr	Tr	Tr	Tr
0.7	1.3	0.9	0	1	1	0.0	170[3]	50[3]	Tr	Tr	Tr	Tr
29.1	71.5	31.3	0	47	37	0.0	7510[3]	2254[3]	0.02	0.06	Tr	Tr
1.8	4.4	1.9	0	3	2	0.0	460[3]	139[3]	Tr	Tr	Tr	Tr

3. A minimum amount of vitamin A (15,000 IU/pound) is needed to meet federal specifications. This is achieved by fortifying margarines with vitamin A.

Continued.

P

Item Number	Foods, Approximate Measures, Units, and Weight (edible parts)		Weight (grams)	Water (percent)	Food Energy (calories)	Protein (grams)	Fat (grams)
	Fats and Oils—cont'd						
	Oils, salad or cooking						
115	Corn	1 cup	218	0	1925	0	218
116		1 tbsp	14	0	125	0	14
117	Olive	1 cup	216	0	1910	0	216
118		1 tbsp	14	0	125	0	14
119	Peanut	1 cup	216	0	1910	0	216
120		1 tbsp	14	0	125	0	14
121	Safflower	1 cup	218	0	1925	0	218
122		1 tbsp	14	0	125	0	14
123	Soybean oil, hydrogenated (partially hardened)	1 cup	218	0	1925	0	218
124		1 tbsp	14	0	125	0	14
125	Sunflower	1 cup	218	0	1925	0	218
126		1 tbsp	14	0	125	0	14
	Salad dressings						
	Commercial						
127	Blue cheese	1 tbsp	15	32	75	1	8
	French						
128	Regular	1 tbsp	16	35	85	Tr	9
129	Low calorie	1 tbsp	16	75	25	Tr	2
	Italian						
130	Regular	1 tbsp	15	34	80	Tr	9
131	Low calorie	1 tbsp	15	86	5	Tr	Tr
	Mayonnaise						
132	Regular	1 tbsp	14	15	100	Tr	11
133	Imitation	1 tbsp	15	63	35	Tr	3
134	Mayonnaise type	1 tbsp	15	40	60	Tr	5
135	Tartar sauce	1 tbsp	14	34	75	Tr	8
	Thousand Island						
136	Regular	1 tbsp	16	46	60	Tr	6
137	Low calorie	1 tbsp	15	69	25	Tr	2
	From home recipe						
138	Cooked type	1 tbsp	16	69	25	1	2
139	Vinegar and oil	1 tbsp	16	47	70	0	8
	Fish and Shellfish						
	Clams						
140	Raw, meat only	3 oz	85	82	65	11	1
141	Canned, drained solids	3 oz	85	77	85	13	2
142	Crabmeat, canned (white or king)	1 cup	135	77	135	23	3
143	Fish sticks, frozen, reheated (stick, 4 by 1 by ½ in) (unbreaded)	1 fish stick/1 oz	28	52	70	6	3

| | Fatty Acids | | | | | | Vitamin A Value | | | | | |
Saturated (grams)	Monounsaturated (grams)	Polyunsaturated (grams)	Carbohydrate (grams)	Calcium (mg)	Phosphorus (mg)	Iron (mg)	(IU) International Units	(RE) Retinol Equivalents	Thiamin (mg)	Riboflavin (mg)	Niacin (mg)	Vitamin C (mg)
27.7	52.8	128.0	0	0	0	0.0	0	0	0.00	0.00	0.0	0
1.8	3.4	8.2	0	0	0	0.0	0	0	0.00	0.00	0.0	0
29.2	159.2	18.1	0	0	0	0.0	0	0	0.00	0.00	0.0	0
1.9	10.3	1.2	0	0	0	0.0	0	0	0.00	0.00	0.0	0
36.5	99.8	69.1	0	0	0	0.0	0	0	0.00	0.00	0.0	0
2.4	6.5	4.5	0	0	0	0.0	0	0	0.00	0.00	0.0	0
19.8	26.4	162.4	0	0	0	0.0	0	0	0.00	0.00	0.0	0
1.3	1.7	10.4	0	0	0	0.0	0	0	0.00	0.00	0.0	0
32.5	93.7	82.0	0	0	0	0.0	0	0	0.00	0.00	0.0	0
2.1	6.0	5.3	0	0	0	0.0	0	0	0.00	0.00	0.0	0
22.5	42.5	143.2	0	0	0	0.0	0	0	0.00	0.00	0.0	0
1.4	2.7	9.2	0	0	0	0.0	0	0	0.00	0.00	0.0	0
1.5	1.8	4.2	1	12	11	Tr	30	10	Tr	0.02	Tr	Tr
1.4	4.0	3.5	1	2	1	Tr	Tr	Tr	Tr	Tr	Tr	Tr
0.2	0.3	1.0	2	6	5	Tr	Tr	Tr	Tr	Tr	Tr	Tr
1.3	3.7	3.2	1	1	1	Tr	30	3	Tr	Tr	Tr	Tr
Tr	Tr	Tr	2	1	1	Tr	Tr	Tr	Tr	Tr	Tr	Tr
1.7	3.2	5.8	Tr	3	4	0.1	40	12	0.00	0.00	Tr	0
0.5	0.7	1.6	2	Tr	Tr	0.0	0	0	0.00	0.00	0.0	0
0.7	1.4	2.7	4	2	4	Tr	30	13	Tr	Tr	Tr	0
1.2	2.6	3.9	1	3	4	0.1	30	9	Tr	Tr	0.0	Tr
1.0	1.3	3.2	2	2	3	0.1	50	15	Tr	Tr	Tr	0
0.2	0.4	0.9	2	2	3	0.1	50	14	Tr	Tr	Tr	0
0.5	0.6	0.3	2	13	14	0.1	70	20	0.01	0.02	Tr	Tr
1.5	2.4	3.9	Tr	0	0	0.0	0	0	0.00	0.00	0.0	0
0.3	0.3	0.3	2	59	138	2.6	90	26	0.09	0.15	1.1	9
0.5	0.5	0.4	2	47	116	3.5	90	26	0.01	0.09	0.9	3
0.5	0.8	1.4	1	61	246	1.1	50	14	0.11	0.11	2.6	0
0.8	1.4	0.8	4	11	58	0.3	20	5	0.03	0.05	0.6	0

Continued.

P

Item Number	Foods, Approximate Measures, Units, and Weight (edible parts)		Weight (grams)	Water (percent)	Food Energy (calories)	Protein (grams)	Fat (grams)
	Fish and Shellfish—cont'd						
	Flounder or sole, baked, with lemon juice						
144	With butter	3 oz	85	73	120	16	6
145	With margarine	3 oz	85	73	120	16	6
146	Without added fat	3 oz	85	78	80	17	1
147	Haddock, breaded, fried[4]	3 oz	85	61	175	17	9
148	Herring, pickled	3 oz	85	59	190	17	13
149	Ocean perch, breaded, fried[4]	1 fillet	85	59	185	16	11
	Oysters						
150	Raw, meat only (13-19 medium selects)	1 cup	240	85	160	20	4
151	Breaded, fried[4]	1 oyster	45	65	90	5	5
	Salmon						
152	Canned (pink), solids and liquid	3 oz	85	71	120	17	5
153	Baked (red)	3 oz	85	67	140	21	5
154	Smoked	3 oz	85	59	150	18	8
155	Sardines, Atlantic, canned in oil, drained solids	3 oz	85	62	175	20	9
156	Scallops, breaded, frozen, reheated	6 scallops	90	59	195	15	10
	Shrimp						
157	Canned, drained solids	3 oz	85	70	100	21	1
158	French-fried (7 medium)[6]	3 oz	85	55	200	16	10
159	Trout, broiled, with butter and lemon juice	3 oz	85	63	175	21	9
	Tuna, canned, drained solids						
160	Oil pack, chunk light	3 oz	85	61	165	24	7
161	Tuna salad[7]	1 cup	205	63	375	33	19
	Fruits and Fruit Juices						
	Apples, raw unpeeled, without cores						
162	2¾-in diam (about 3 per lb with cores)	1 apple	138	84	80	Tr	Tr
163	3¼-in diam (about 2 per lb with cores)	1 apple	212	84	125	Tr	1
164	Dried, sulfured	10 rings	64	32	155	1	Tr
165	Apple juice, bottled or canned	1 cup	248	88	115	Tr	Tr
	Applesauce, canned						
166	Sweetened	1 cup	255	80	195	Tr	Tr
167	Unsweetened	1 cup	244	88	105	Tr	Tr

4. Dipped in milk, egg, and bread crumbs; fried in vegetable shortening.
5. Calcium values are much lower if the bones are discarded.
6. Dipped in egg, bread crumbs, and flour, fried in vegetable oil.
7. Ingredients are drained, light tuna, onion, celery, pickle relish, and mayonnaise-type salad dressing.

| | Fatty Acids | | Carbohydrate (grams) | Calcium (mg) | Phosphorus (mg) | Iron (mg) | Vitamin A Value | | Thiamin (mg) | Riboflavin (mg) | Niacin (mg) | Vitamin C (mg) |
Saturated (grams)	Monounsaturated (grams)	Polyunsaturated (grams)					(IU) International Units	(RE) Retinol Equivalents				
3.2	1.5	0.5	Tr	13	187	0.3	210	54	0.05	0.08	1.6	1
1.2	2.3	1.9	Tr	14	187	0.3	230	69	0.05	0.08	1.6	1
0.3	0.2	0.4	Tr	13	197	0.3	30	10	0.05	0.08	1.7	1
2.4	3.9	2.4	7	34	183	1.0	70	20	0.06	0.10	2.9	0
4.3	4.6	3.1	0	29	128	0.9	110	33	0.04	0.18	2.8	0
2.6	4.6	2.8	7	31	191	1.2	70	20	0.10	0.11	2.0	0
1.4	0.5	1.4	8	226	343	15.6	740	223	0.34	0.43	6.0	24
1.4	2.1	1.4	5	49	73	3.0	150	44	0.07	0.10	1.3	4
0.9	1.5	2.1	0	167[5]	243	0.7	60	18	0.03	0.15	6.8	0
1.2	2.4	1.4	0	26	269	0.5	290	87	0.18	0.14	5.5	0
2.6	3.9	0.7	0	12	208	0.8	260	77	0.17	0.17	6.8	0
2.1	3.7	2.9	0	371[5]	424	2.6	190	56	0.03	0.17	4.6	0
2.5	4.1	2.5	10	39	203	2.0	70	21	0.11	0.11	1.6	0
0.2	0.2	0.4	1	98	224	1.4	50	15	0.01	0.03	1.5	0
2.5	4.1	2.6	11	61	154	2.0	90	26	0.06	0.09	2.8	0
4.1	2.9	1.6	Tr	26	259	1.0	230	60	0.07	0.07	2.3	1
1.4	1.9	3.1	0	7	199	1.6	70	20	0.04	0.09	10.1	0
3.3	4.9	9.2	19	31	281	2.5	230	53	0.06	0.14	13.3	6
0.1	Tr	0.1	21	10	10	0.2	70	7	0.02	0.02	0.1	8
0.1	Tr	0.2	32	15	15	0.4	110	11	0.04	0.03	0.2	12
Tr	Tr	0.1	42	9	24	0.9	0	0	0.00	0.10	0.6	2
Tr	Tr	0.1	29	17	17	0.9	Tr	Tr	0.05	0.04	0.2	2[8]
0.1	Tr	0.1	51	10	18	0.9	30	3	0.03	0.07	0.5	4[8]
Tr	Tr	Tr	28	7	17	0.3	70	7	0.03	0.06	0.5	3[8]

Continued.

P

Item Number	Foods, Approximate Measures, Units, and Weight (edible parts)		Weight (grams)	Water (percent)	Food Energy (calories)	Protein (grams)	Fat (grams)
	Fruit and Fruit Juices—cont'd						
	Apricots						
168	Raw, without pits (about 12 per lb with pits)	3 apricots	106	86	50	1	Tr
	Canned (fruit and liquid)						
169	Heavy syrup pack	1 cup	258	78	215	1	Tr
170	Juice pack	1 cup	248	87	120	2	Tr
	Dried						
171	Uncooked (28 large or 37 medium halves per cup)	1 cup	130	31	310	5	1
		Tr					
172	Cooked, unsweetened, fruit and liquid	1 cup	250	76	210	3	Tr
173	Apricot nectar, canned	1 cup	251	85	140	1	Tr
	Avocados, raw, whole, without skin and seed						
174	California (about 2 per lb with skin and seed)	1 avocado	173	73	305	4	30
175	Florida (about 1 per lb with skin and seed)	1 avocado	304	80	340	5	27
	Bananas, raw, without peel						
176	Whole (about 2½ per lb with peel)	1 banana	114	74	105	1	1
177	Blackberries, raw	1 cup	144	86	75	1	1
	Blueberries						
178	Raw	1 cup	145	85	80	1	1
179	Frozen, sweetened	10-oz container	284	77	230	1	Tr
	Cantaloupe. See Melons (item 209).						
	Cherries						
180	Sour, red, pitted, canned, water pack	1 cup	244	90	90	2	Tr
181	Sweet, raw, without pits and stems	10 cherries	68	81	50	1	1
182	Cranberry juice cocktail, bottled, sweetened	1 cup	253	85	145	Tr	Tr
183	Cranberry sauce, sweetened, canned, strained	1 cup	277	61	420	1	Tr
	Dates						
184	Whole, without pits	10 dates	83	23	230	2	Tr
185	Chopped	1 cup	178	23	490	4	1
186	Figs, dried	10 figs	187	28	475	6	2
	Fruit cocktail, canned, fruit and liquid						
187	Heavy syrup pack	1 cup	255	80	185	1	Tr
188	Juice pack	1 cup	248	87	115	1	Tr
	Grapefruit						
189	Raw, without peel, membrane and seeds (3¾-in diam, 1 lb 1 oz, whole, with refuse)	½ grapefruit	120	91	40	1	Tr
190	Canned, sections with syrup	1 cup	254	84	150	1	Tr

P

	Fatty Acids		Carbohydrate (grams)	Calcium (mg)	Phosphorus (mg)	Iron (mg)	Vitamin A Value		Thiamin (mg)	Riboflavin (mg)	Niacin (mg)	Vitamin C (mg)
Saturated (grams)	Monounsaturated (grams)	Polyunsaturated (grams)					(IU) International Units	(RE) Retinol Equivalents				
Tr	0.2	0.1	12	15	20	0.6	2770	277	0.03	0.04	0.6	11
Tr	0.1	Tr	55	23	31	0.8	3170	317	0.05	0.06	1.0	8
Tr	Tr	Tr	31	30	50	0.7	4190	419	0.04	0.05	0.9	12
Tr	0.3	0.1	80	59	152	6.1	9410	941	0.01	0.20	3.9	3
Tr	0.2	0.1	55	40	103	4.2	5910	591	0.02	0.08	2.4	4
Tr	0.1	Tr	36	18	23	1.0	3300	330	0.02	0.04	0.7	2[8]
4.5	19.4	3.5	12	19	73	2.0	1060	106	0.19	0.21	3.3	14
5.3	14.8	4.5	27	33	119	1.6	1860	186	0.33	0.37	5.8	24
0.2	Tr	0.1	27	7	23	0.4	90	9	0.05	0.11	0.6	10
0.2	0.1	0.1	18	46	30	0.8	240	24	0.04	0.06	0.6	30
Tr	0.1	0.3	20	9	15	0.2	150	15	0.07	0.07	0.5	19
Tr	0.1	0.2	62	17	20	1.1	120	12	0.06	0.15	0.7	3
0.1	0.1	0.1	22	27	24	3.3	1840	184	0.04	0.10	0.4	5
0.1	0.2	0.2	11	10	13	0.3	150	15	0.03	0.04	0.3	5
Tr	Tr	0.1	38	8	3	0.4	10	1	0.01	0.04	0.1	108[9]
Tr	0.1	0.2	108	11	17	0.6	60	6	0.04	0.06	0.3	6
0.1	0.1	Tr	61	27	33	1.0	40	4	0.07	0.08	1.8	0
0.3	0.2	Tr	131	57	71	2.0	90	9	0.16	0.18	3.9	0
0.4	0.5	1.0	122	269	127	4.2	250	25	0.13	0.16	1.3	1
Tr	Tr	0.1	48	15	28	0.7	520	52	0.05	0.05	1.0	5
Tr	Tr	Tr	29	20	35	0.5	760	76	0.03	0.04	1.0	7
Tr	Tr	Tr	10	14	10	0.1	10[10]	1[10]	0.04	0.02	0.3	41
Tr	Tr	0.1	39	36	25	1.0	Tr	Tr	0.10	0.05	0.6	54

8. No added vitamin C.
9. With added vitamin C.
10. Values are for white grapefruit; pink grapefruit has about 30 times more vitamin A than white.

Continued.

P

Item Number	Foods, Approximate Measures, Units, and Weight (edible parts)		Weight (grams)	Water (percent)	Food Energy (calories)	Protein (grams)	Fat (grams)
	Fruit and Fruit Juices—cont'd						
	Grapefruit juice						
191	Raw, pink, red, or white	1 cup	247	90	95	1	Tr
	Canned						
192	Unsweetened	1 cup	247	90	95	1	Tr
193	Sweetened	1 cup	250	87	115	1	Tr
	Frozen concentrate, unsweetened						
194	Undiluted	6-fl-oz can	207	62	300	4	1
195	Diluted with 3 parts water by volume	1 cup	247	89	100	1	Tr
	Grapes, European type (adherent skin), raw						
196	Thompson seedless	10 grapes	50	81	35	Tr	Tr
197	Tokay and Emperor, seeded types	10 grapes	57	81	40	Tr	Tr
	Grape juice						
198	Canned or bottled	1 cup	253	84	155	1	Tr
	Frozen concentrate, sweetened						
199	Undiluted	6-fl-oz can	216	54	385	1	1
200	Diluted with 3 parts water by volume	1 cup	250	87	125	Tr	Tr
201	Kiwifruit, raw, without skin, large	1 kiwifruit	76	83	45	1	Tr
202	Lemons, raw, without peel and seeds (about 4 lb with peel and seeds)	1 lemon	58	89	15	1	Tr
	Lemon juice						
203	Raw	1 cup	244	91	60	1	Tr
204	Canned or bottled, unsweetened	1 cup	244	92	50	1	1
205	Frozen, single-strength, unsweetened	6-fl-oz can	244	92	55	1	1
	Lime juice						
206	Raw	1 cup	246	90	65	1	Tr
207	Canned, unsweetened	1 cup	246	93	50	1	1
208	Mangos, raw, without skin and seed (about 1½ per lb with skin and seed)	1 mango	207	82	135	1	1
	Melons, raw, without rind and cavity contents						
209	Cantaloupe, orange-fleshed (5-in diam, 2⅓ lb, whole, with rind and cavity contents)	½ melon	267	90	95	2	1
210	Honeydew (6½-in diam, 5¼ lb, whole, with rind and cavity contents)	⅒ melon	129	90	45	1	Tr
211	Nectarines, raw, without pits (about 3 per lb with pits)	1 nectarine	136	86	65	1	1
	Oranges, raw						
212	Whole, without peel and seeds (2⅝-in diam, about 2½ per lb, with peel and seeds)	1 orange	131	87	60	1	Tr
213	Sections without membranes	1 cup	180	87	85	2	Tr

P

Fatty Acids			Carbo-hydrate (grams)	Calcium (mg)	Phos-phorus (mg)	Iron (mg)	Vitamin A Value		Thiamin (mg)	Riboflavin (mg)	Niacin (mg)	Vitamin C (mg)
Satu-rated (grams)	Monoun-saturated (grams)	Polyun-saturated (grams)					(IU) Inter-national Units	(RE) Retinol Equiv-alents				
Tr	Tr	0.1	23	22	37	0.5	20	2	0.10	0.05	0.5	94
Tr	Tr	0.1	22	17	27	0.5	20	2	0.10	0.05	0.6	72
Tr	Tr	0.1	28	20	28	0.9	20	2	0.10	0.06	0.8	67
0.1	0.1	0.2	72	56	101	1.0	60	6	0.30	0.16	1.6	248
Tr	Tr	0.1	24	20	35	0.3	20	2	0.10	0.05	0.5	83
0.1	Tr	0.1	9	6	7	0.1	40	4	0.05	0.03	0.2	5
0.1	Tr	0.1	10	6	7	0.1	40	4	0.05	0.03	0.2	6
0.1	Tr	0.1	38	23	28	0.6	20	2	0.07	0.09	0.7	Tr[8]
0.2	Tr	0.2	96	28	32	0.8	60	6	0.11	0.20	0.9	179[9]
0.1	Tr	0.1	32	10	10	0.3	20	2	0.04	0.07	0.3	60[9]
Tr	0.1	0.1	11	20	30	0.3	130	13	0.02	0.04	0.4	74
Tr	Tr	0.1	5	15	9	0.3	20	2	0.02	0.01	0.1	31
Tr	Tr	Tr	21	17	15	0.1	50	5	0.07	0.02	0.2	112
0.1	Tr	0.2	16	27	22	0.3	40	4	0.10	0.02	0.5	61
0.1	Tr	0.2	16	20	20	0.3	30	3	0.14	0.03	0.3	77
Tr	Tr	0.1	22	22	17	0.1	20	2	0.05	0.02	0.2	72
0.1	0.1	0.2	16	30	25	0.6	40	4	0.08	0.01	0.4	16
0.1	0.2	0.1	35	21	23	0.3	8060	806	0.12	0.12	1.2	57
0.1	0.1	0.3	22	29	45	0.6	8610	861	0.10	0.06	1.5	113
Tr	Tr	0.1	12	8	13	0.1	50	5	0.10	0.02	0.8	32
0.1	0.2	0.3	16	7	22	0.2	1000	100	0.02	0.06	1.3	7
Tr	Tr	Tr	15	52	18	0.1	270	27	0.11	0.05	0.4	70
Tr	Tr	Tr	21	72	25	0.2	370	37	0.16	0.07	0.5	96

Continued.

P

Item Number	Foods, Approximate Measures, Units, and Weight (edible parts)		Weight (grams)	Water (percent)	Food Energy (calories)	Protein (grams)	Fat (grams)
	Fruit and Fruit Juices—cont'd						
	Orange juice						
214	Raw, all varieties	1 cup	248	88	110	2	Tr
215	Canned, unsweetened	1 cup	249	89	105	1	Tr
	Frozen concentrate						
216	Undiluted	6-fl-oz can	213	58	340	5	Tr
217	Diluted with 3 parts water by volume	1 cup	249	88	110	2	Tr
218	Orange and grapefruit juice, canned	1 cup	247	89	105	1	Tr
219	Papayas, raw, ½-in cubes	1 cup	140	86	65	1	Tr
	Peaches						
	Raw						
220	Whole, 2½-in diam, peeled, pitted (about 4 per lb with peels and pits)	1 peach	87	88	35	1	Tr
221	Sliced	1 cup	170	88	75	1	Tr
	Canned, fruit and liquid						
222	Heavy syrup pack	1 cup	256	79	190	1	Tr
223	Juice pack	1 cup	248	87	110	2	Tr
	Dried						
224	Uncooked	1 cup	160	32	380	6	1
225	Cooked, unsweetened, fruit and liquid	1 cup	258	78	200	3	1
226	Frozen, sliced, sweetened	10-oz container	284	75	265	2	Tr
227		1 cup	250	75	235	2	Tr
	Pears						
	Raw, with skin, cored						
228	Bartlett, 2½-in diam (about 2½ per lb with cores and stems)	1 pear	166	84	100	1	1
229	Bosc, 2½-in diam (about 3 per lb with cores and stems)	1 pear	141	84	85	1	1
230	D'Anjou, 3-in diam (about 2 per lb with cores and stems)	1 pear	200	84	120	1	1
	Canned, fruit and liquid						
231	Heavy syrup pack	1 cup	255	80	190	1	Tr
232	Juice pack	1 cup	248	86	125	1	Tr
	Pineapple						
233	Raw, diced	1 cup	155	87	75	1	1
	Canned, fruit and liquid						
	Heavy syrup pack						
234	Crushed, chunks, tidbits	1 cup	255	79	200	1	Tr
235	Slices	1 slice	58	79	45	Tr	Tr
	Juice pack						
236	Chunks or tidbits	1 cup	250	84	150	1	Tr
237	Slices	1 slice	58	84	35	Tr	Tr
238	Pineapple juice, unsweetened, canned	1 cup	250	86	140	1	Tr

	Fatty Acids						Vitamin A Value					
Satu-rated (grams)	Monoun-saturated (grams)	Polyun-saturated (grams)	Carbo-hydrate (grams)	Calcium (mg)	Phos-phorus (mg)	Iron (mg)	(IU) Inter-national Units	(RE) Retinol Equiv-alents	Thiamin (mg)	Riboflavin (mg)	Niacin (mg)	Vitamin C (mg)
0.1	0.1	0.1	26	27	42	0.5	500	50	0.22	0.07	1.0	124
Tr	0.1	0.1	25	20	35	1.1	440	44	0.15	0.07	0.8	86
0.1	0.1	0.1	81	68	121	0.7	590	59	0.60	0.14	1.5	294
Tr	Tr	Tr	27	22	40	0.2	190	19	0.20	0.04	0.5	97
Tr	Tr	Tr	25	20	35	1.1	290	29	0.14	0.07	0.8	72
0.1	0.1	Tr	17	35	12	0.3	400	40	0.04	0.04	0.5	92
Tr	Tr	Tr	10	4	10	0.1	470	47	0.01	0.04	0.9	6
Tr	0.1	0.1	19	9	20	0.2	910	91	0.03	0.07	1.7	11
Tr	0.1	0.1	51	8	28	0.7	850	85	0.03	0.06	1.6	7
Tr	Tr	Tr	29	15	42	0.7	940	94	0.02	0.04	1.4	9
0.1	0.4	0.6	98	45	190	6.5	3460	346	Tr	0.34	7.0	8
0.1	0.2	0.3	51	23	98	3.4	510	51	0.01	0.05	3.9	10
Tr	0.1	0.2	68	9	31	1.1	810	81	0.04	0.10	1.9	268[9]
Tr	0.1	0.2	60	8	28	0.9	710	71	0.03	0.09	1.6	236[9]
Tr	0.1	0.2	25	18	18	0.4	30	3	0.03	0.07	0.2	7
Tr	0.1	0.1	21	16	16	0.4	30	3	0.03	0.06	0.1	6
Tr	0.2	0.2	30	22	22	0.5	40	4	0.04	0.08	0.2	8
Tr	0.1	0.1	49	13	18	0.6	10	1	0.03	0.06	0.6	3
Tr	Tr	Tr	32	22	30	0.7	10	1	0.03	0.03	0.5	4
Tr	0.1	0.2	19	11	11	0.6	40	4	0.14	0.06	0.7	24
Tr	Tr	0.1	52	36	18	1.0	40	4	0.23	0.06	0.7	19
Tr	Tr	Tr	12	8	4	0.2	10	1	0.05	0.01	0.2	4
Tr	Tr	0.1	39	35	15	0.7	100	10	0.24	0.05	0.7	24
Tr	Tr	Tr	9	8	3	0.2	20	2	0.06	0.01	0.2	6
Tr	Tr	0.1	34	43	20	0.7	10	1	0.14	0.06	0.6	27

Continued.

P

Item Number	Foods, Approximate Measures, Units, and Weight (edible parts)		Weight (grams)	Water (percent)	Food Energy (calories)	Protein (grams)	Fat (grams)
	Fruit and Fruit Juices—cont'd						
	Plantains, without peel						
239	Raw	1 plantain	179	65	220	2	1
240	Cooked, boiled, sliced	1 cup	154	67	180	1	Tr
	Plums, without pits						
	Raw						
241	2⅛-in diam (about 6½ per lb with pits)	1 plum	66	85	35	1	Tr
242	1½-in diam (about 15 per lb with pits)	1 plum	28	85	15	Tr	Tr
	Canned, purple, fruit and liquid						
243	Heavy syrup pack	1 cup	258	76	230	1	Tr
244	Juice pack	1 cup	252	84	145	1	Tr
	Prunes, dried						
245	Uncooked	4 extra large or 5 large prunes	49	32	115	1	Tr
246	Cooked, unsweetened, fruit and liquid	1 cup	212	70	225	2	Tr
247	Prune juice, canned or bottled	1 cup	256	81	180	2	Tr
	Raisins, seedless						
248	Cup, not pressed down	1 cup	145	15	435	5	1
249	Packet, ½ oz (1½ tbsp)	1 packet	14	15	40	Tr	Tr
	Raspberries						
250	Raw	1 cup	123	87	60	1	1
251	Frozen, sweetened	10-oz container	284	73	295	2	Tr
252	Rhubarb, cooked, added sugar	1 cup	240	68	280	1	Tr
	Strawberries						
253	Raw, capped, whole	1 cup	149	92	45	1	1
254	Frozen, sweetened, sliced	10-oz container	284	73	275	2	Tr
	Tangerines						
255	Raw, without peel and seeds (2⅜-in diam, about 4 per lb, with peel and seeds)	1 tangerine	84	88	35	1	Tr
256	Canned, light syrup, fruit and liquid	1 cup	252	83	155	1	Tr
257	Tangerine juice, canned, sweetened	1 cup	249	87	125	1	Tr
	Watermelon, raw, without rind and seeds						
258	Piece (4 by 8 in wedge with rind and seeds; 1/16 of 32⅔-lb melon, 10 by 16 in)	1 piece	482	92	155	3	2

P

	Fatty Acids						Vitamin A Value					
Satu-rated (grams)	Monoun-saturated (grams)	Polyun-saturated (grams)	Carbo-hydrate (grams)	Calcium (mg)	Phos-phorus (mg)	Iron (mg)	(IU) Inter-national Units	(RE) Retinol Equiv-alents	Thiamin (mg)	Riboflavin (mg)	Niacin (mg)	Vitamin C (mg)
0.3	0.1	0.1	57	5	61	1.1	2020	202	0.09	0.10	1.2	33
0.3	Tr	0.1	48	3	43	0.9	1400	140	0.07	0.08	1.2	17
Tr	0.3	0.1	9	3	7	0.1	210	21	0.03	0.06	0.3	6
Tr	0.1	Tr	4	1	3	Tr	90	9	0.01	0.03	0.1	3
Tr	0.2	0.1	60	23	34	2.2	670	67	0.04	0.10	0.8	1
Tr	Tr	Tr	38	25	38	0.9	2540	254	0.06	0.15	1.2	7
Tr	0.2	0.1	31	25	39	1.2	970	97	0.04	0.08	1.0	2
Tr	0.3	0.1	60	49	74	2.4	650	65	0.05	0.21	1.5	6
Tr	0.1	Tr	45	31	64	3.0	10	1	0.04	0.18	2.0	10
0.2	Tr	0.2	115	71	141	3.0	10	1	0.23	0.13	1.2	5
Tr	Tr	Tr	11	7	14	0.3	Tr	Tr	0.02	0.01	0.1	Tr
Tr	0.1	0.4	14	27	15	0.7	160	16	0.04	0.11	1.1	31
Tr	Tr	0.3	74	43	48	1.8	170	17	0.05	0.13	0.7	47
Tr	Tr	0.1	75	348	19	0.5	170	17	0.04	0.06	0.5	8
Tr	0.1	0.3	10	21	28	0.6	40	4	0.03	0.10	0.3	84
Tr	0.1	0.2	74	31	37	1.7	70	7	0.05	0.14	1.1	118
Tr	Tr	Tr	9	12	8	0.1	770	77	0.09	0.02	0.1	26
Tr	Tr	0.1	41	18	25	0.9	2120	212	0.13	0.11	1.1	50
Tr	Tr	0.1	30	45	35	0.5	1050	105	0.15	0.05	0.2	55
0.3	0.2	1.0	35	39	43	0.8	1760	176	0.39	0.10	1.0	46

Continued.

P

Item Number	Foods, Approximate Measures, Units, and Weight (edible parts)		Weight (grams)	Water (percent)	Food Energy (calories)	Protein (grams)	Fat (grams)
	Grain Products						
259	Bagels, plain or water, enriched, 3½-in diam	1 bagel	68	29	200	7	2
260	Barley, pearled, light, uncooked	1 cup	200	11	700	16	2
	Biscuits, baking powder, 2-in diam (enriched flour, vegetable shortening)						
261	From home recipe	1 biscuit	28	28	100	2	5
262	From mix	1 biscuit	28	29	95	2	3
263	From refrigerated dough	1 biscuit	20	30	65	1	2
	Breadcrumbs, enriched						
264	Dry grated	1 cup	100	7	390	13	5
	Soft. See White bread (item 296).						
	Breads						
265	Boston brown bread, canned, slice, 3¼ in by ½ in[11]	1 slice	45	45	95	2	1
	Cracked-wheat bread (¾ enriched wheat flour, ¼ cracked wheat flour)						
266	Loaf, 1 lb	1 loaf	454	35	1190	42	16
267	Slice (18 per loaf)	1 slice	25	35	65	2	1
268	Toasted	1 slice	21	26	65	2	1
	French or vienna bread, enriched						
269	Loaf, 1 lb	1 loaf	454	34	1270	43	18
	Slice						
270	French, 5 by 2½ by 1 in	1 slice	35	34	100	3	1
271	Vienna, 4¾ by ½ in	1 slice	25	34	70	2	1
	Italian bread, enriched						
272	Loaf, 1 lb	1 loaf	454	32	1255	41	4
273	Slice, 4½ by 3¼ by ¾ in	1 slice	30	32	85	3	Tr
	Mixed grain bread, enriched						
274	Loaf, 1 lb	1 loaf	454	37	1165	45	17
275	Slice (18 per loaf)	1 slice	25	37	65	2	1
276	Toasted	1 slice	23	27	65	2	1
277	Pita bread, Arabic or Syrian bread, enriched, white, 6½-in diam	1 pita	60	31	165	6	1
	Pumpernickel (⅔ rye flour, ⅓ enriched wheat flour)[11]						
278	Loaf, 1 lb	1 loaf	454	37	1160	42	16
279	Slice, 5 by 4 by ⅜ in	1 slice	32	37	80	3	1
280	Toasted	1 slice	29	28	80	3	1
	Raisin bread, enriched[11]						
281	Loaf, 1 lb	1 loaf	454	33	1260	37	18
282	Slice (18 per loaf)	1 slice	25	33	65	2	1
283	Toasted	1 slice	21	24	65	2	1

11. Made with vegetable shortening.
12. Made with white cornmeal; the yellow type has 32 IU or 3 RE vitamin A.

| | Fatty Acids | | | | | | Vitamin A Value | | | | | |
Satu-rated (grams)	Monoun-saturated (grams)	Polyun-saturated (grams)	Carbo-hydrate (grams)	Calcium (mg)	Phos-phorus (mg)	Iron (mg)	(IU) Inter-national Units	(RE) Retinol Equiv-alents	Thiamin (mg)	Riboflavin (mg)	Niacin (mg)	Vitamin C (mg)
0.3	0.5	0.7	38	29	46	1.8	0	0	0.26	0.20	2.4	0
0.3	0.2	0.9	158	32	378	4.2	0	0	0.24	0.10	6.2	0
1.2	2.0	1.3	13	47	36	0.7	10	3	0.08	0.08	0.8	Tr
0.8	1.4	0.9	14	58	128	0.7	20	4	0.12	0.11	0.8	Tr
0.6	0.9	0.6	10	4	79	0.5	0	0	0.08	0.05	0.7	0
1.5	1.6	1.0	73	122	141	4.1	0	0	0.35	0.35	4.8	0
0.3	0.1	0.1	21	41	72	0.9	0^{12}	0^{12}	0.06	0.04	0.7	0
3.1	4.3	5.7	227	295	581	12.1	Tr	Tr	1.73	1.73	15.3	Tr
0.2	0.2	0.3	12	16	32	0.7	Tr	Tr	0.10	0.09	0.8	Tr
0.2	0.2	0.3	12	16	32	0.7	Tr	Tr	0.07	0.09	0.8	Tr
3.8	5.7	5.9	230	499	386	14.0	Tr	Tr	2.09	1.59	18.2	Tr
0.3	0.4	0.5	18	39	30	1.1	Tr	Tr	0.16	0.12	1.4	Tr
0.2	0.3	0.3	13	28	21	0.8	Tr	Tr	0.12	0.09	1.0	Tr
0.6	0.3	1.6	256	77	350	12.7	0	0	1.80	1.10	15.0	0
Tr	Tr	0.1	17	5	23	0.8	0	0	0.12	0.07	1.0	0
3.2	4.1	6.5	212	472	962	14.8	Tr	Tr	1.77	1.73	18.9	Tr
0.2	0.2	0.4	12	27	55	0.8	Tr	Tr	0.10	0.10	1.1	Tr
0.2	0.2	0.4	12	27	55	0.8	Tr	Tr	0.08	0.10	1.1	Tr
0.1	0.1	0.4	33	49	60	1.4	0	0	0.27	0.12	2.2	0
2.6	3.6	6.4	218	322	990	12.4	0	0	1.54	2.36	15.0	0
0.2	0.3	0.5	16	23	71	0.9	0	0	0.11	0.17	1.1	0
0.2	0.3	0.5	16	23	71	0.9	0	0	0.09	0.17	1.1	0
4.1	6.5	6.7	239	463	395	14.1	Tr	Tr	1.50	2.81	18.6	Tr
0.2	0.3	0.4	13	25	22	0.8	Tr	Tr	0.08	0.15	1.0	Tr
0.2	0.3	0.4	13	25	22	0.8	Tr	Tr	0.06	0.15	1.0	Tr

Continued.

P

Item Number	Foods, Approximate Measures, Units, and Weight (edible parts)		Weight (grams)	Water (percent)	Food Energy (calories)	Protein (grams)	Fat (grams)
	Grain Products—cont'd						
	Rye bread, light (⅔ enriched wheat flour, ⅓ rye flour)						
284	Loaf, 1 lb	1 loaf	454	37	1190	38	17
285	Slice, 4¾ by 3¾ by ⁷⁄₁₆ in	1 slice	25	37	65	2	1
286	Toasted	1 slice	22	28	65	2	1
	Wheat bread, enriched[11]						
287	Loaf, 1 lb	1 loaf	454	37	1160	43	19
288	Slice (18 per loaf)	1 slice	25	37	65	2	1
289	Toasted	1 slice	23	28	65	3	1
	White bread, enriched[11]						
290	Loaf, 1 lb	1 loaf	454	37	1210	38	18
291	Slice (18 per loaf)	1 slice	25	37	65	2	1
292	Toasted	1 slice	22	28	65	2	1
293	Slice (22 per loaf)	1 slice	20	37	55	2	1
294	Toasted	1 slice	17	28	55	2	1
295	Cubes	1 cup	30	37	80	2	1
296	Crumbs, soft	1 cup	45	37	120	4	2
	Whole-wheat bread[11]						
297	Loaf, 1 lb	1 loaf	454	38	1110	44	20
298	Slice (16 per loaf)	1 slice	28	38	70	3	1
299	Toasted	1 slice	25	29	70	3	1
	Bread stuffing (from enriched bread), prepared from mix						
300	Dry type	1 cup	140	33	500	9	31
301	Moist type	1 cup	203	61	420	9	26
	Breakfast cereals						
	Hot type, cooked						
	Corn (hominy) grits						
302	Regular and quick, enriched	1 cup	242	85	145	3	Tr
303	Instant, plain	1 pkt	137	85	80	2	Tr
	Cream of Wheat®[14]						
304	Regular, quick, instant	1 cup	244	86	140	4	Tr
305	Mix'n Eat, plain	1 pkt	142	82	100	3	Tr
306	Malt-O-Meal®	1 cup	240	88	120	4	Tr
	Oatmeal or rolled oats						
307	Regular, quick, instant, nonfortified	1 cup	234	85	145	6	2
	Instant, fortified						
308	Plain	1 pkt	177	86	105	4	2
309	Flavored	1 pkt	164	76	160	5	2
	Ready to eat						
310	All-Bran® (about ⅓ cup)	1 oz	28	3	70	4	1
311	Cap'n Crunch® (about ¾ cup)	1 oz	28	3	120	1	3
312	Cheerios® (about 1¼ cup)	1 oz	28	5	110	4	2

13. With added amounts of these nutrients.
14. Values computed from label information on this and on all other brands of breakfast cereals.
15. Yellow grits, cooked, contains 145 IU or 14 RE vitamin A.

| | Fatty Acids | | | | | | Vitamin A Value | | | | | |
Saturated (grams)	Monounsaturated (grams)	Polyunsaturated (grams)	Carbohydrate (grams)	Calcium (mg)	Phosphorus (mg)	Iron (mg)	(IU) International Units	(RE) Retinol Equivalents	Thiamin (mg)	Riboflavin (mg)	Niacin (mg)	Vitamin C (mg)
3.3	5.2	5.5	218	363	658	12.3	0	0	1.86	1.45	15.0	0
0.2	0.3	0.3	12	20	36	0.7	0	0	0.10	0.08	0.8	0
0.2	0.3	0.3	12	20	36	0.7	0	0	0.08	0.08	0.8	0
3.9	7.3	4.5	213	572	835	15.8	Tr	Tr	2.09	1.45	20.5	Tr
0.2	0.4	0.3	12	32	47	0.9	Tr	Tr	0.12	0.08	1.2	Tr
0.2	0.4	0.3	12	32	47	0.9	Tr	Tr	0.10	0.08	1.2	Tr
5.6	6.5	4.2	222	572	490	12.9	Tr	Tr	2.13	1.41	17.0	Tr
0.3	0.4	0.2	12	32	27	0.7	Tr	Tr	0.12	0.08	0.9	Tr
0.3	0.4	0.2	12	32	27	0.7	Tr	Tr	0.09	0.08	0.9	Tr
0.2	0.3	0.2	10	25	21	0.6	Tr	Tr	0.09	0.06	0.7	Tr
0.2	0.3	0.2	10	25	21	0.6	Tr	Tr	0.07	0.06	0.7	Tr
0.4	0.4	0.3	15	38	32	0.9	Tr	Tr	0.14	0.09	1.1	Tr
0.6	0.6	0.4	22	57	49	1.3	Tr	Tr	0.21	0.14	1.7	Tr
5.8	6.8	5.2	206	327	1180	15.5	Tr	Tr	1.59	0.95	17.4	Tr
0.4	0.4	0.3	13	20	74	1.0	Tr	Tr	0.10	0.06	1.1	Tr
0.4	0.4	0.3	13	20	74	1.0	Tr	Tr	0.08	0.06	1.1	Tr
6.1	13.3	9.6	50	92	136	2.2	910	273	0.17	0.20	2.5	0
5.3	11.3	8.0	40	81	134	2.0	850	256	0.10	0.18	1.6	0
Tr	0.1	0.2	31	0	29	1.5[13]	0[15]	0[15]	0.24[13]	0.15[13]	2.0[13]	0
Tr	Tr	0.1	18	7	16	1.0[13]	0	0	0.18[13]	0.08[13]	1.3[13]	0
0.1	Tr	0.2	29	54	43	10.9	0	0	0.24	0.07	1.5	0
Tr	Tr	0.1	21	20	20	8.1	1250	376	0.43	0.28	5.0	0
Tr	Tr	0.1	26	5	24	9.6	0	0	0.48	0.24	5.8	0
0.4	0.8	1.0	25	19	178	1.6	40	4	0.26	0.05	0.3	0
0.3	0.6	0.7	18	163[13]	133	6.3[13]	1510[13]	453[13]	0.53[13]	0.28[13]	5.5[13]	0
0.3	0.7	0.8	31	168[13]	148	6.7[13]	1530[13]	460[13]	0.53[13]	0.38[13]	5.9[13]	Tr
0.1	0.1	0.3	21	23	264	4.5	1250	375	0.37	0.43	5.0	15
1.7	0.3	0.4	23	5	36	7.5[13]	40	4	0.50[13]	0.55[13]	6.6[13]	0
0.3	0.6	0.7	20	48	134	4.5	1250	375	0.37	0.43	5.0	15

Continued.

Item Number	Foods, Approximate Measures, Units, and Weight (edible parts)		Weight (grams)	Water (percent)	Food Energy (calories)	Protein (grams)	Fat (grams)
	Grain Products—cont'd						
	Corn Flakes (about 1¼ cup)						
313	Kellogg's®	1 oz	28	3	110	2	Tr
314	Toasties®	1 oz	28	3	110	2	Tr
	40% Bran Flakes						
315	Kellogg's® (about ¾ cup)	1 oz	28	3	90	4	1
316	Post® (about ⅔ cup)	1 oz	28	3	90	3	Tr
	Froot Loops® (about 1 cup)[14]	1 oz	28	3	110	2	1
318	Golden Grahams® (about ¾ cup)[14]	1 oz	28	2	110	2	1
319	Grape-Nuts® (about ¼ cup)[14]	1 oz	28	3	100	3	Tr
320	Honey Nut Cheerios® (about ¾ cup)[14]	1 oz	28	3	105	3	1
321	Lucky Charms® (about 1 cup)[14]	1 oz	28	3	110	3	1
322	Nature Valley® Granola (about ⅓ cup)[14]	1 oz	28	4	125	3	5
323	100% Natural Cereal (about ¼ cup)[14]	1 oz	28	2	135	3	6
324	Product 19® (about ¾ cup)[14]	1 oz	28	3	110	3	Tr
	Raisin Bran:						
325	Kellogg's® (about ¾ cup)[14]	1 oz	28	8	90	3	1
326	Post® (about ½ cup)[14]	1 oz	28	9	85	3	1
327	Rice Krispies® (about 1 cup)[14]	1 oz	28	2	110	2	Tr
328	Shredded Wheat (about ⅔ cup)[14]	1 oz	28	5	100	3	1
329	Special K® (about 1⅓ cup)[14]	1 oz	28	2	110	6	Tr
330	Super Sugar Crisp® (about ⅞ cup)[14]	1 oz	28	2	105	2	Tr
321	Sugar Frosted Flakes, Kellogg's® (about ¾ cup)[14]	1 oz	28	3	110	1	Tr
322	Sugar Smacks® (about ¾ cup)[14]	1 oz	28	3	105	2	1
323	Total® (about 1 cup)[14]	1 oz	28	4	100	3	1
324	Trix® (about 1 cup)[14]	1 oz	28	3	110	2	Tr
325	Wheaties® (about 1 cup)[14]	1 oz	28	5	100	3	Tr
326	Buckwheat flour, light, sifted	1 cup	98	12	340	6	1
327	Bulgur, uncooked	1 cup	170	10	600	19	3
	Cakes prepared from cake mixes with enriched flour[16]						
	Angelfood						
328	Whole cake, 9¾-in diam. tube cake	1 cake	635	38	1510	38	2
329	Piece, ¹⁄₁₂ of cake	1 piece	53	38	125	3	Tr
	Coffeecake, crumb						
330	Whole cake, 7¾ by 5⅝ by 1¼ in	1 cake	430	30	1385	27	41
331	Piece, ⅙ of cake	1 piece	72	30	230	5	7
	Devil's food with chocolate icing						
332	Whole, 2-layer cake, 8- or 9-in diam	1 cake	1107	24	3755	49	136
333	Piece, ¹⁄₁₆ of cake	1 piece	69	24	235	3	8
334	Cupcake, 2½-in diam	1 cupcake	35	24	120	2	4
	Gingerbread						
335	Whole cake, 8 in square	1 cake	570	37	1575	18	39
336	Piece, ⅑ of cake	1 piece	63	37	175	2	4

P

	Fatty Acids						Vitamin A Value					
Satu- rated (grams)	Monoun- saturated (grams)	Polyun- saturated (grams)	Carbo- hydrate (grams)	Calcium (mg)	Phos- phorus (mg)	Iron (mg)	(IU) Inter- national Units	(RE) Retinol Equiv- alents	Thiamin (mg)	Riboflavin (mg)	Niacin (mg)	Vitamin C (mg)
Tr	Tr	Tr	24	1	18	1.8	1250	375	0.37	0.43	5.0	15
Tr	Tr	Tr	24	1	12	0.7	1250	375	0.37	0.43	5.0	0
0.1	0.1	0.3	22	14	139	8.1	1250	375	0.37	0.43	5.0	0
0.1	0.1	0.2	22	12	179	4.5	1250	375	0.37	0.43	5.0	0
0.2	0.1	0.1	25	3	24	4.5	1250	375	0.37	0.43	5.0	15
0.7	0.1	0.2	24	17	41	4.5	1250	375	0.37	0.43	5.0	15
Tr	Tr	0.1	23	11	71	1.2	1250	375	0.37	0.43	5.0	0
0.1	0.3	0.3	23	20	105	4.5	1250	375	0.37	0.43	5.0	15
0.2	0.4	0.4	23	32	79	4.5	1250	375	0.37	0.43	5.0	15
3.3	0.7	0.7	19	18	89	0.9	20	2	0.10	0.05	0.2	0
4.1	1.2	0.5	18	49	104	0.8	20	2	0.09	0.15	0.6	0
Tr	Tr	0.1	24	3	40	18.0	5000	1501	1.50	1.70	20.0	60
0.1	0.1	0.3	21	10	105	3.5	960	288	0.28	0.34	3.9	0
0.1	0.1	0.3	21	13	119	4.5	1250	375	0.37	0.43	5.0	0
Tr	Tr	0.1	25	4	34	1.8	1250	375	0.37	0.43	5.0	15
0.1	0.1	0.3	23	11	100	1.2	0	0	0.07	0.08	1.5	0
Tr	Tr	Tr	21	8	55	4.5	1250	375	0.37	0.43	5.0	15
Tr	Tr	0.1	26	6	52	1.8	1250	375	0.37	0.43	5.0	0
Tr	Tr	Tr	26	1	21	1.8	1250	375	0.37	0.43	5.0	15
0.1	0.1	0.2	25	3	31	1.8	1250	375	0.37	0.43	5.0	15
0.1	0.1	0.3	22	48	118	18.0	5000	1501	1.50	1.70	20.0	60
0.2	0.1	0.1	25	6	19	4.5	1250	375	0.37	0.43	5.0	15
0.1	Tr	0.2	23	43	98	4.5	1250	375	0.37	0.43	5.0	15
0.2	0.4	0.4	78	11	86	1.0	0	0	0.08	0.04	0.4	0
1.2	0.3	1.2	129	49	575	9.5	0	0	0.48	0.24	7.7	0
0.4	0.2	1.0	342	527	1086	2.7	0	0	0.32	1.27	1.6	0
Tr	Tr	0.1	29	44	91	0.2	0	0	0.03	0.11	0.1	0
11.8	16.7	9.6	225	262	748	7.3	690	194	0.82	0.90	7.7	1
0.2	2.8	1.6	38	44	125	1.2	120	32	0.14	0.15	1.3	Tr
55.6	51.4	19.7	645	653	1162	22.1	1660	498	1.11	1.66	10.0	1
3.5	3.2	1.2	40	41	72	1.4	100	31	0.07	0.10	0.6	Tr
1.8	1.6	0.6	20	21	37	0.7	50	16	0.04	0.05	0.3	Tr
9.6	16.4	10.5	291	513	570	10.8	0	0	0.86	1.03	7.4	1
1.1	1.8	1.2	32	57	63	1.2	0	0	0.09	0.11	0.8	Tr

P

Continued.

Item Number	Foods, Approximate Measures, Units, and Weight (edible parts)		Weight (grams)	Water (percent)	Food Energy (calories)	Protein (grams)	Fat (grams)
	Grain Products—cont'd						
	Yellow with chocolate icing						
337	Whole, 2-layer cake, 8- or 9-in diam	1 cake	1108	26	3735	45	125
338	Piece, 1/16 of cake	1 piece	69	26	235	3	8
	Cakes prepared from home recipes using enriched flour[16]						
	Carrot, with cream cheese icing[17]						
339	Whole cake, 10-in diam tube cake	1 cake	1536	23	6175	63	328
340	Piece, 1/16 of cake	1 piece	96	23	385	4	21
	Fruitcake, dark[17]						
341	Whole cake, 7½-in diam, 2¼-in high tube cake	1 cake	1361	18	5185	74	228
342	Piece, 1/32 of cake, ⅔-in arc	1 piece	43	18	165	2	7
	Plain sheet cake						
	Without icing						
343	Whole cake, 9-in square	1 cake	777	25	2830	35	108
344	Piece, ⅑ of cake	1 piece	86	25	315	4	12
	With uncooked white icing						
345	Whole cake, 9-in square	1 cake	1096	21	4020	37	129
346	Piece, ⅑ of cake	1 piece	121	21	445	4	14
	Pound						
347	Loaf, 8½ by 3¼ in	1 loaf	514	22	2025	33	94
348	Slice, 1/17 of loaf	1 slice	30	22	120	2	5
	Cheesecake						
349	Whole cake, 9-in diam	1 cake	1110	46	3350	60	213
350	Piece, 1/12 of cake	1 piece	92	46	280	5	18
	Cookies made with enriched flour						
	Brownies with nuts						
351	Commercial, with icing, 1½ by 1¾ by ⅞ in	1 brownie	25	13	100	1	4
352	From home recipe, 1¾ by 1¾ by ⅞ in[17]	1 brownie	20	10	95	1	6
	Chocolate chip						
353	Commercial, 2¼-in diam, ⅜ in thick	4 cookies	42	4	180	2	9
354	From home recipe, 2⅓-in diam[11]	4 cookies	40	3	185	2	11
355	Fig bars, square, 1⅝ by 1⅝ by ⅜ in or rectangular, 1½ by 1¾ by ½ in	4 cookies	56	12	210	2	4
356	Oatmeal with raisins, 2⅝-in diam, ¼ in thick	4 cookies	52	4	245	3	10
357	Peanut butter cookie, from home recipe, 2⅝-in diam[11]	4 cookies	48	3	245	4	14
358	Sandwich type (chocolate or vanilla), 1¾-in diam, ⅜ in thick	4 cookies	40	2	195	2	8
	Shortbread						
359	Commercial	4 small cookies	32	6	155	2	8
360	From home recipe[18]	2 large cookies	28	3	145	2	8

16. All cakes, except angel food, made from mixes containing vegetable shortening. The icings were made with margarine.

17. Make with vegetable oil.

18. Made with margarine.

Fatty Acids			Carbohydrate (grams)	Calcium (mg)	Phosphorus (mg)	Iron (mg)	Vitamin A Value		Thiamin (mg)	Riboflavin (mg)	Niacin (mg)	Vitamin C (mg)
Saturated (grams)	Monounsaturated (grams)	Polyunsaturated (grams)					(IU) International Units	(RE) Retinol Equivalents				
47.8	48.8	21.8	638	1008	2017	15.5	1550	465	1.22	1.66	11.1	1
3.0	3.0	1.4	40	63	126	1.0	100	29	0.08	0.10	0.7	Tr
66.0	135.2	107.5	775	707	998	21.0	2240	246	1.83	1.97	14.7	23
4.1	8.4	6.7	48	44	62	1.3	140	15	0.11	0.12	0.9	1
47.6	113.0	51.7	783	1293	1592	37.6	1720	422	2.41	2.55	17.0	504
1.5	3.6	1.6	25	41	50	1.2	50	13	0.08	0.08	0.5	16
29.5	45.1	25.6	434	497	793	11.7	1320	373	1.24	1.40	10.1	2
3.3	5.0	2.8	48	55	88	1.3	150	41	0.14	0.15	1.1	Tr
41.6	50.4	26.3	694	548	822	11.0	2190	647	1.21	1.42	9.9	2
4.6	5.6	2.9	77	61	91	1.2	240	71	0.13	0.16	1.1	Tr
21.1	40.9	26.7	265	339	473	9.3	3470	1033	0.93	1.08	7.8	1
1.2	2.4	1.6	15	20	28	0.5	200	60	0.05	0.06	0.5	Tr
119.9	65.5	14.4	317	622	977	5.3	2820	833	0.33	1.44	5.1	56
9.9	5.4	1.2	26	52	81	0.4	230	69	0.03	0.12	0.4	5
1.6	2.0	0.6	16	13	26	0.6	70	18	0.08	0.07	0.3	Tr
1.4	2.8	1.2	11	9	26	0.4	20	6	0.05	0.05	0.3	Tr
2.9	3.1	2.6	28	13	41	0.8	50	15	0.10	0.23	1.0	Tr
3.9	4.3	2.0	26	13	34	1.0	20	5	0.06	0.06	0.6	0
1.0	1.5	1.0	42	40	34	1.4	60	6	0.08	0.07	0.7	Tr
2.5	4.5	2.8	36	18	58	1.1	40	12	0.09	0.08	1.0	0
4.0	5.8	2.8	28	21	60	1.1	20	5	0.07	0.07	1.9	0
2.0	3.6	2.2	29	12	40	1.4	0	0	0.09	0.07	0.8	0
2.9	3.0	1.1	20	13	39	0.8	30	8	0.10	0.09	0.9	0
1.3	2.7	3.4	17	6	31	0.6	300	89	0.08	0.06	0.7	Tr

P

Continued.

Item Number	Foods, Approximate Measures, Units, and Weight (edible parts)		Weight (grams)	Water (percent)	Food Energy (calories)	Protein (grams)	Fat (grams)
	Grain Products—cont'd						
361	Sugar cookie, from refrigerated dough, 2½-in diam, ¼ in thick	4 cookies	48	4	235	2	12
362	Vanilla wafers, 1¾-in diam, ¼ in thick	10 cookies	40	4	185	2	7
363	Corn chips	1-oz package	28	1	155	2	9
	Cornmeal						
364	Whole-ground, unbolted, dry form	1 cup	122	12	435	11	5
365	Bolted (nearly whole-grain), dry form	1 cup	122	12	440	11	4
	Degermed, enriched						
366	Dry form	1 cup	138	12	500	11	2
367	Cooked	1 cup	240	88	120	3	Tr
	Crackers[19]						
	Cheese						
368	Plain, 1 in square	10 crackers	10	4	50	1	3
369	Sandwich type (peanut butter)	1 sandwich	8	3	40	1	2
370	Graham, plain, 2½ in square	2 crackers	14	5	60	1	1
371	Rye wafers, whole-grain, 1⅞ by 3½ in	2 wafers	14	5	55	1	1
372	Saltines[20]	4 crackers	12	4	50	1	1
	Snack-type, standard	1 round cracker	3	3	15	Tr	1
374	Wheat, thin	4 crackers	8	3	35	1	1
375	Whole wheat wafers	2 crackers	8	4	35	1	2
376	Croissants, made with enriched flour, 4½ by 4 by 1¾ in	1 croissant	57	22	235	5	12
	Danish pastry, made with enriched flour						
	Plain without fruit or nuts						
377	Packaged ring, 12 oz	1 ring	340	27	1305	21	71
378	Round piece, about 4¼-in diam, 1 in high	1 pastry	57	27	220	4	12
379	Fruit, round piece	1 pastry	65	30	235	4	13
	Doughnuts, made with enriched flour						
380	Cake type, plain, 3¼-in diam, 1 in high	1 doughnut	50	21	210	3	12
381	Yeast-leavened, glazed, 3¾-in diam, 1¼ in high	1 doughnut	60	27	235	4	13
382	English muffins, plain, enriched	1 muffin	57	42	140	5	1
383	Toasted	1 muffin	50	29	140	5	1
384	French toast, from home recipe	1 slice	65	53	155	6	7

19. Made with enriched flour—exceptions are rye wafers and whole-wheat wafers.
20. Made with lard.

P

Fatty Acids			Carbo-hydrate (grams)	Calcium (mg)	Phos-phorus (mg)	Iron (mg)	Vitamin A Value		Thiamin (mg)	Riboflavin (mg)	Niacin (mg)	Vitamin C (mg)
Satu-rated (grams)	Monoun-saturated (grams)	Polyun-saturated (grams)					(IU) Inter-national Units	(RE) Retinol Equiv-alents				
2.3	5.0	3.6	31	50	91	0.9	40	11	0.09	0.06	1.1	0
1.8	3.0	1.8	29	16	36	0.8	50	14	0.07	0.10	1.0	0
1.4	2.4	3.7	16	35	52	0.5	110	11	0.04	0.05	0.4	1
0.5	1.1	2.5	90	24	312	2.2	620	62	0.46	0.13	2.4	0
0.5	0.9	2.2	91	21	272	2.2	590	59	0.37	0.10	2.3	0
0.2	0.4	0.9	108	8	137	5.9	610	61	0.61	0.36	4.8	0
Tr	0.1	0.2	26	2	34	1.4	140	14	0.14	0.10	1.2	0
0.9	1.2	0.3	6	11	17	0.3	20	5	0.05	0.04	0.4	0
0.4	0.8	0.3	5	7	25	0.3	Tr	Tr	0.04	0.03	0.6	0
0.4	0.6	0.4	11	6	20	0.4	0	0	0.02	0.03	0.6	0
0.3	0.4	0.3	10	7	44	0.5	0	0	0.06	0.03	0.5	0
0.5	0.4	0.2	9	3	12	0.5	0	0	0.06	0.05	0.6	0
0.2	0.4	0.1	2	3	6	0.1	Tr	Tr	0.01	0.01	0.1	0
0.5	0.5	0.4	5	3	15	0.3	Tr	Tr	0.04	0.03	0.4	0
0.5	0.6	0.4	5	3	22	0.2	0	0	0.02	0.03	0.4	0
3.5	6.7	1.4	27	20	64	2.1	50	13	0.17	0.13	1.3	0
21.8	28.6	15.6	152	360	347	6.5	360	99	0.95	1.02	8.5	Tr
3.6	4.8	2.6	26	60	58	1.1	60	17	0.16	0.17	1.4	Tr
3.9	5.2	2.9	28	17	80	1.3	40	11	0.16	0.14	1.4	Tr
2.8	5.0	3.0	24	22	111	1.0	20	5	0.12	0.12	1.1	Tr
5.2	5.5	0.9	26	17	55	1.4	Tr	Tr	0.28	0.12	1.8	0
0.3	0.2	0.3	27	96	67	1.7	0	0	0.26	0.19	2.2	0
0.3	0.2	0.3	27	96	67	1.7	0	0	0.23	0.19	2.2	0
1.6	2.0	1.6	17	72	85	1.3	110	32	0.12	0.16	1.0	Tr

Continued.

P

Item Number	Foods, Approximate Measures, Units, and Weight (edible parts)		Weight (grams)	Water (percent)	Food Energy (calories)	Protein (grams)	Fat (grams)
	Grain Products—cont'd						
	Macaroni, enriched, cooked (cut lengths, elbows, shells)						
385	Firm stage (hot)	1 cup	130	64	190	7	1
	Tender stage						
386	Cold	1 cup	105	72	115	4	Tr
387	Hot	1 cup	140	72	155	5	1
	Muffins made with enriched flour, 2½-in diam, 1½ in high						
	From home recipe						
388	Blueberry[11]	1 muffin	45	37	135	3	5
389	Bran[17]	1 muffin	45	35	125	3	6
390	Corn (enriched, degermed cornmeal and flour)[11]	1 muffin	45	33	145	3	5
	From commercial mix (egg and water added)						
391	Blueberry	1 muffin	45	33	140	3	5
392	Bran	1 muffin	45	28	140	3	4
393	Corn	1 muffin	45	30	145	3	6
394	Noodles (egg noodles), enriched, cooked	1 cup	160	70	200	7	2
395	Noodles, chow mein, canned	1 cup	45	11	220	6	11
	Pancakes, 4-in diam.						
396	Buckwheat, from mix (with buckwheat and en-riched flours), egg and milk added	1 pancake	27	58	55	2	2
	Plain						
397	From home recipe using enriched flour	1 pancake	27	50	60	2	2
398	From mix (with enriched flour), egg, milk, and oil added	1 pancake	27	54	60	2	2
	Piecrust, made with enriched flour and vegetable shortening, baked						
399	From home recipe, 9-in diam	1 pie shell	180	15	900	11	60
400	From mix, 9-in diam	Piecrust for 2-crust pie	320	19	1485	20	93
	Pies, piecrust made with enriched flour, vegetable shortening, 9-in diam.						
	Apple						
401	Whole	1 pie	945	48	2420	21	105
402	Piece, ⅙ of pie	1 piece	158	48	405	3	18
	Blueberry						
403	Whole	1 pie	945	51	2285	23	102
404	Piece, ⅙ of pie	1 piece	158	51	380	4	17
	Cherry						
405	Whole	1 pie	945	47	2465	25	107
406	Piece, ⅙ of pie	1 piece	158	47	410	4	18

P

Saturated (grams)	Monounsaturated (grams)	Polyunsaturated (grams)	Carbohydrate (grams)	Calcium (mg)	Phosphorus (mg)	Iron (mg)	(IU) International Units	(RE) Retinol Equivalents	Thiamin (mg)	Riboflavin (mg)	Niacin (mg)	Vitamin C (mg)
0.1	0.1	0.3	39	14	85	2.1	0	0	0.23	0.13	1.8	0
0.1	0.1	0.2	24	8	53	1.3	0	0	0.15	0.08	1.2	0
0.1	0.1	0.2	32	11	70	1.7	0	0	0.20	0.11	1.5	0
1.5	2.1	1.2	20	54	46	0.9	40	9	0.10	0.11	0.9	1
1.4	1.6	2.3	19	60	125	1.4	230	30	0.11	0.13	1.3	3
1.5	2.2	1.4	21	66	59	0.9	80	15	0.11	0.11	0.9	Tr
1.4	2.0	1.2	22	15	90	0.9	50	11	0.10	0.17	1.1	Tr
1.3	1.6	1.0	24	27	182	1.7	100	14	0.08	0.12	1.9	0
1.7	2.3	1.4	22	30	128	1.3	90	16	0.09	0.09	0.8	Tr
0.5	0.6	0.6	37	16	94	2.6	110	34	0.22	0.13	1.9	0
2.1	7.3	0.4	26	14	41	0.4	0	0	0.05	0.03	0.6	0
0.9	0.9	0.5	6	59	91	0.4	60	17	0.04	0.05	0.2	Tr
0.5	0.8	0.5	9	27	38	0.5	30	10	0.06	0.07	0.5	Tr
0.5	0.9	0.5	8	36	71	0.7	30	7	0.09	0.12	0.8	Tr
14.8	25.9	15.7	79	25	90	4.5	0	0	0.54	0.40	5.0	0
22.7	41.0	25.0	141	131	272	9.3	0	0	1.06	0.80	9.9	0
27.4	44.4	26.5	360	76	208	9.5	280	28	1.04	0.76	9.5	9
4.6	7.4	4.4	60	13	35	1.6	50	5	0.17	0.13	1.6	2
25.5	44.4	27.4	330	104	217	12.3	850	85	1.04	0.85	10.4	38
4.3	7.4	4.6	55	17	36	2.1	140	14	0.17	0.14	1.7	6
28.4	46.3	27.4	363	132	236	9.5	4160	416	1.13	0.85	9.5	0
4.7	7.7	4.6	61	22	40	1.6	700	70	0.19	0.14	1.6	0

Continued.

Item Number	Foods, Approximate Measures, Units, and Weight (edible parts)		Weight (grams)	Water (percent)	Food Energy (calories)	Protein (grams)	Fat (grams)
	Grain Products—cont'd						
	Cream						
407	Whole	1 pie	910	43	2710	20	139
408	Piece, ⅙ of pie	1 piece	152	43	455	3	23
	Custard						
409	Whole	1 pie	910	58	1985	56	101
410	Piece, ⅙ of pie	1 piece	152	58	330	9	17
	Lemon meringue						
411	Whole	1 pie	840	47	2140	31	86
412	Piece, ⅙ of pie	1 piece	140	47	355	5	14
	Peach						
413	Whole	1 pie	945	48	2410	24	101
414	Piece, ⅙ of pie	1 piece	158	48	405	4	17
	Pecan						
415	Whole	1 pie	825	20	3450	42	189
416	Piece, ⅙ of pie	1 piece	138	20	575	7	32
	Pumpkin						
417	Whole	1 pie	910	59	1920	36	102
418	Piece, ⅙ of pie	1 piece	152	59	320	6	17
	Pies, fried						
419	Apple	1 pie	85	43	255	2	14
420	Cherry	1 pie	85	42	250	2	14
	Popcorn, popped						
421	Air-popped, unsalted	1 cup	8	4	30	1	Tr
422	Popped in vegetable oil, salted	1 cup	11	3	55	1	3
423	Coated with sugar syrup	1 cup	35	4	135	2	1
	Pretzels, made with enriched flour						
424	Stick, 2¼ in long	10 pretzels	3	3	10	Tr	Tr
425	Twisted, Dutch, 2¾ by 2⅝ in	1 pretzel	16	3	65	2	1
	Rice						
426	Brown, cooked, served hot	1 cup	195	70	230	5	1
	White, enriched						
	Commercial varieties, all types						
427	Cooked, served hot	1 cup	205	73	225	4	Tr
428	Instant, ready-to-serve, hot	1 cup	165	73	180	4	0
	Parboiled						
429	Cooked, served hot	1 cup	175	73	185	4	Tr
	Rolls, enriched						
	Commercial						
430	Dinner, 2½-in diam, 2 in high	1 roll	28	32	85	2	2
431	Frankfurter and hamburger (8 per 11½-oz pkg)	1 roll	40	34	115	3	2
432	Hard, 3¾-in diam, 2 in high	1 roll	50	25	155	5	2
433	Hoagie or submarine, 11½ by 3 by 2½ in	1 roll	135	31	400	11	8
	From home recipe						
434	Dinner, 2½-in diam, 2 in high	1 roll	35	26	120	3	3

| Fatty Acids | | | | | | | Vitamin A Value | | | | | |
Saturated (grams)	Monounsaturated (grams)	Polyunsaturated (grams)	Carbohydrate (grams)	Calcium (mg)	Phosphorus (mg)	Iron (mg)	(IU) International Units	(RE) Retinol Equivalents	Thiamin (mg)	Riboflavin (mg)	Niacin (mg)	Vitamin C (mg)
90.1	23.7	6.4	351	273	919	6.8	1250	391	0.36	0.89	6.4	0
15.0	4.0	1.1	59	46	154	1.1	210	65	0.06	0.15	1.1	0
33.7	40.0	19.1	213	874	1028	9.1	2090	573	0.82	1.91	5.5	0
5.6	6.7	3.2	36	146	172	1.5	350	96	0.14	0.32	0.9	0
26.0	34.4	17.6	317	118	412	8.4	1430	395	0.59	0.84	5.0	25
4.3	5.7	2.9	53	20	69	1.4	240	66	0.10	0.14	0.8	4
24.6	43.5	26.5	361	95	274	11.3	6900	690	1.04	0.95	14.2	28
4.1	7.3	4.4	60	16	46	1.9	1150	115	0.17	0.16	2.4	5
28.1	101.5	47.0	423	388	850	27.2	1320	322	1.82	0.99	6.6	0
4.7	17.0	7.9	71	65	142	4.6	220	54	0.30	0.17	1.1	0
38.2	40.0	18.2	223	464	628	8.2	22,480	2493	0.82	1.27	7.3	0
6.4	6.7	3.0	37	78	105	1.4	3750	416	0.14	0.21	1.2	0
5.8	6.6	0.6	31	12	34	0.9	30	3	0.09	0.06	1.0	1
5.8	6.7	0.6	32	11	41	0.7	190	19	0.06	0.06	0.6	1
Tr	0.1	0.2	6	1	22	0.2	10	1	0.03	0.01	0.2	0
5.0	1.4	1.2	6	3	31	0.3	20	2	0.01	0.02	0.1	0
0.1	0.3	0.6	30	2	47	0.5	30	3	0.13	0.02	0.4	0
Tr	Tr	Tr	2	1	3	0.1	0	0	0.01	0.01	0.1	0
0.1	0.2	0.2	13	4	15	0.3	0	0	0.05	0.04	0.7	0
0.3	0.3	0.4	50	23	142	1.0	0	0	0.18	0.04	2.7	0
1.1	0.1	0.1	50	21	57	1.8	0	0	0.23	0.02	2.1	0
0.1	0.1	0.1	40	5	31	1.3	0	0	0.21	0.02	1.7	0
Tr	Tr	0.1	41	33	100	1.4	0	0	0.19	0.02	2.1	0
0.5	0.8	0.6	14	33	44	0.8	Tr	Tr	0.14	0.09	1.1	Tr
0.5	0.8	0.6	20	54	44	1.2	Tr	Tr	0.20	0.13	1.6	Tr
0.4	0.5	0.6	30	24	46	1.4	0	0	0.20	0.12	1.7	0
1.8	3.0	2.2	72	100	115	3.8	0	0	0.54	0.33	4.5	0
0.8	1.2	0.9	20	16	36	1.1	30	8	0.12	0.12	1.2	0

P

Continued.

Item Number	Foods, Approximate Measures, Units, and Weight (edible parts)		Weight (grams)	Water (percent)	Food Energy (calories)	Protein (grams)	Fat (grams)
	Grain Products—cont'd						
	Spaghetti, enriched, cooked						
435	Firm stage, "al dente," served hot	1 cup	130	64	190	7	1
436	Tender stage, served hot	1 cup	140	73	155	5	1
437	Toaster pastries	1 pastry	54	13	210	2	6
438	Tortillas, corn	1 tortilla	30	45	65	2	1
	Waffles, made with enriched flour, 7-in diam						
439	From home recipe	1 waffle	75	37	245	7	13
440	From mix, egg and milk added	1 waffle	75	42	205	7	8
	Wheat flours						
	All-purpose or family flour, enriched						
441	Sifted, spooned	1 cup	115	12	420	12	1
442	Unsifted, spooned	1 cup	125	12	455	13	1
443	Cake or pastry flour, enriched, sifted, spooned	1 cup	96	12	350	7	1
444	Self-rising enriched, unsifted, spooned	1 cup	125	12	440	12	1
445	Whole-wheat, from hard wheats, stirred	1 cup	120	12	400	16	2
	Legumes, Nuts and Seeds						
	Almonds, shelled						
446	Slivered, packed	1 cup	135	4	795	27	70
447	Whole	1 oz	28	4	165	6	15
	Beans, dry						
	Cooked, drained						
448	Black (turtle beans)	1 cup	171	66	225	15	1
449	Great Northern	1 cup	180	69	210	14	1
450	Lima	1 cup	190	64	260	16	1
451	Pea (navy)	1 cup	190	69	225	15	1
452	Pinto	1 cup	180	65	265	15	1
	Canned, solids and liquid						
	White with						
453	Frankfurters (sliced)	1 cup	255	71	365	19	18
454	Pork and tomato sauce	1 cup	255	71	310	16	7
455	Pork and sweet sauce	1 cup	255	66	385	16	12
456	Red kidney	1 cup	255	76	230	15	1
457	Black-eyed peas, dry, cooked (with residual cooking liquid)	1 cup	250	80	190	13	1
458	Brazil nuts, shelled	1 oz	28	3	185	4	19
459	Carob flour	1 cup	140	3	255	6	Tr
	Cashew nuts, salted						
460	Dry roasted	1 cup	137	2	785	21	63
461	Roasted in oil	1 cup	130	4	750	21	63
462	Chestnuts, European (Italian), roasted, shelled	1 cup	143	40	350	5	3

P

	Fatty Acids		Carbo-hydrate (grams)	Calcium (mg)	Phos-phorus (mg)	Iron (mg)	Vitamin A Value		Thiamin (mg)	Riboflavin (mg)	Niacin (mg)	Vitamin C (mg)
Satu-rated (grams)	Monoun-saturated (grams)	Polyun-saturated (grams)					(IU) Inter-national Units	(RE) Retinol Equiv-alents				
0.1	0.1	0.3	39	14	85	2.0	0	0	0.23	0.13	1.8	0
0.1	0.1	0.2	32	11	70	1.7	0	0	0.20	0.11	1.5	0
1.7	3.6	0.4	38	104	104	2.2	520	52	0.17	0.18	2.3	4
0.1	0.3	0.6	13	42	55	0.6	80	8	0.05	0.03	0.4	0
4.0	4.9	2.6	26	154	135	1.5	140	39	0.18	0.24	1.5	Tr
2.7	2.9	1.5	27	179	257	1.2	170	49	0.14	0.23	0.9	Tr
0.2	0.1	0.5	88	18	100	5.1	0	0	0.73	0.46	6.1	0
0.2	0.1	0.5	95	20	109	5.5	0	0	0.80	0.50	6.6	0
0.1	0.1	0.3	76	16	70	4.2	0	0	0.58	0.38	5.1	0
0.2	0.1	0.5	93	331	583	5.5	0	0	0.80	0.50	6.6	0
0.3	0.3	1.1	85	49	446	5.2	0	0	0.66	0.14	5.2	0
6.7	45.8	14.8	28	359	702	4.9	0	0	0.28	1.05	4.5	1
1.4	9.6	3.1	6	75	147	1.0	0	0	0.06	0.22	1.0	Tr
0.1	0.1	0.5	41	47	239	2.9	Tr	Tr	0.43	0.05	0.9	0
0.1	0.1	0.6	38	90	266	4.9	0	0	0.25	0.13	1.3	0
0.2	0.1	0.5	49	55	293	5.9	0	0	0.25	0.11	1.3	0
0.1	0.1	0.7	40	95	281	5.1	0	0	0.27	0.13	1.3	0
0.1	0.1	0.5	49	86	296	5.4	Tr	Tr	0.33	0.16	0.7	0
7.4	8.8	0.7	32	94	303	4.8	330	33	0.18	0.15	3.3	Tr
2.4	2.7	0.7	48	138	235	4.6	330	33	0.20	0.08	1.5	5
4.3	4.9	1.2	54	161	291	5.9	330	33	0.15	0.10	1.3	5
0.1	0.1	0.6	42	74	278	4.6	10	1	0.13	0.10	1.5	0
0.2	Tr	0.3	35	43	238	3.3	30	3	0.40	0.10	1.0	0
4.6	6.5	6.8	4	50	170	1.0	Tr	Tr	0.28	0.03	0.5	Tr
Tr	0.1	0.1	126	390	102	5.7	Tr	Tr	0.07	0.07	2.2	Tr
12.5	37.4	10.7	45	62	671	8.2	0	0	0.27	0.27	1.9	0
12.4	36.9	10.6	37	53	554	5.3	0	0	0.55	0.23	2.3	0
0.6	1.1	1.2	76	41	153	1.3	30	3	0.35	0.25	1.9	37

P

Continued.

Item Number	Foods, Approximate Measures, Units, and Weight (edible parts)		Weight (grams)	Water (percent)	Food Energy (calories)	Protein (grams)	Fat (grams)
	Legumes, Nuts, and Seeds—cont'd						
463	Chickpeas, cooked, drained	1 cup	163	60	270	15	4
	Coconut						
	Raw						
464	Piece, about 2 by 2 by ½ in	1 piece	45	47	160	1	15
465	Shredded or grated	1 cup	80	47	285	3	27
466	Dried, sweetened, shredded	1 cup	93	13	470	3	33
467	Filberts (hazelnuts), chopped	1 cup	115	5	725	15	72
468	Lentils, dry, cooked	1 cup	200	72	215	16	1
469	Macadamia nuts, roasted in oil, salted	1 cup	134	2	960	10	103
	Mixed nuts, with peanuts, salted						
470	Dry roasted	1 oz	28	2	170	5	15
471	Roasted in oil	1 oz	28	2	175	5	16
472	Peanuts, roasted in oil, salted	1 cup	145	2	840	39	71
473	Peanut butter	1 tbsp	16	1	95	5	8
474	Peas, split, dry, cooked	1 cup	200	70	230	16	1
475	Pecans, halves	1 cup	108	5	720	8	73
476	Pine nuts (pinyons), shelled	1 oz	28	6	160	3	17
477	Pistachio nuts, dried, shelled	1 oz	28	4	165	6	14
478	Pumpkin and squash kernels, dry, hulled	1 oz	28	7	155	7	13
479	Refried beans, canned	1 cup	290	72	295	18	3
480	Sesame seeds, dry, hulled	1 tbsp	8	5	45	2	4
481	Soybeans, dry, cooked, drained	1 cup	180	71	235	20	10
	Soy products						
482	Miso	1 cup	276	53	470	29	13
483	Tofu, piece 2½ by 2¾ by 1 in	1 piece	120	85	85	9	5
484	Sunflower seeds, dry, hulled	1 oz	28	5	160	6	14
485	Tahini (tahini butter)	1 tbsp	15	3	90	3	8
	Walnuts						
486	Black, chopped	1 cup	125	4	760	30	71
573	English or Persian, pieces or chips	1 cup	120	4	770	17	74

	Fatty Acids		Carbo-hydrate (grams)	Calcium (mg)	Phos-phorus (mg)	Iron (mg)	Vitamin A Value		Thiamin (mg)	Riboflavin (mg)	Niacin (mg)	Vitamin C (mg)
Satu-rated (grams)	Monoun-saturated (grams)	Polyun-saturated (grams)					(IU) Inter-national Units	(RE) Retinol Equiv-alents				
0.4	0.9	1.9	45	80	273	4.9	Tr	Tr	0.18	0.09	0.9	0
13.4	0.6	0.2	7	6	51	1.1	0	0	0.03	0.01	0.2	1
23.8	1.1	0.3	12	11	90	1.9	0	0	0.05	0.02	0.4	3
29.3	1.4	0.4	44	14	99	1.8	0	0	0.03	0.02	0.4	1
5.3	56.5	6.9	18	216	359	3.8	80	8	0.58	0.13	1.3	1
0.1	0.2	0.5	38	50	238	4.2	40	4	0.14	0.12	1.2	0
15.4	80.9	1.8	17	60	268	2.4	10	1	0.29	0.15	2.7	0
2.0	8.9	3.1	7	20	123	1.0	Tr	Tr	0.06	0.06	1.3	0
2.5	9.0	3.8	6	31	131	0.9	10	1	0.14	0.06	1.4	Tr
9.9	35.5	22.6	27	125	734	2.8	0	0	0.42	0.15	21.5	0
1.4	4.0	2.5	3	5	60	0.3	0	0	0.02	0.02	2.2	0
0.1	0.1	0.3	42	22	178	3.4	80	8	0.30	0.18	1.8	0
5.9	45.5	18.1	20	39	314	2.3	140	14	0.92	0.14	1.0	2
2.7	6.5	7.3	5	2	10	0.9	10	1	0.35	0.06	1.2	1
1.7	9.3	2.1	7	38	143	1.9	70	7	0.23	0.05	0.3	Tr
2.5	4.0	5.9	5	12	333	4.2	110	11	0.06	0.09	0.5	Tr
0.4	0.6	1.4	51	141	245	5.1	0	0	0.14	0.16	1.4	17
0.6	1.7	1.9	1	11	62	0.6	10	1	0.06	0.01	0.4	0
1.3	1.9	5.3	19	131	322	4.9	50	5	0.38	0.16	1.1	0
1.8	2.6	7.3	65	188	853	4.7	110	11	0.17	0.28	0.8	0
0.7	1.0	2.9	3	108	151	2.3	0	0	0.07	0.04	0.1	0
1.5	2.7	9.3	5	33	200	1.9	10	1	0.65	0.07	1.3	Tr
1.1	3.0	3.5	3	21	119	0.7	10	1	0.24	0.02	0.8	1
4.5	15.9	46.9	15	73	580	3.8	370	37	0.27	0.14	0.9	Tr
6.7	17.0	47.0	22	133	380	2.9	150	15	0.46	0.18	1.3	4

Continued.

P

Item Number	Foods, Approximate Measures, Units, and Weight (edible parts)		Weight (grams)	Water (percent)	Food Energy (calories)	Protein (grams)	Fat (grams)
	Meat and Meat Products						
	Beef, cooked[21]						
	Cuts braised, simmered, or pot roasted						
	Relatively fat, such as chuck blade						
487	Lean and fat, piece, 2½ by 2½ by ¾ in	3 oz	85	43	325	22	26
488	Lean only (from item 487)	2.2 oz	62	53	170	19	9
	Ground beef, broiled, patty, 3 by ⅝ in						
489	Lean	3 oz	85	56	230	21	16
490	Regular	3 oz	85	54	245	20	18
491	Liver, fried, one slice, 6½ by 2⅜ by ⅜ in[22]	3 oz	85	56	185	23	7
	Roast, oven cooked, no liquid added						
	Relatively fat, such as rib						
492	Lean and fat, 2 pieces, 4⅛ by 2¼ by ¼ in	3 oz	85	46	315	19	26
493	Lean only (from item 492)	2.2 oz	61	57	150	17	9
	Relatively lean, such as eye of round						
494	Lean and fat, 2 pieces, 2½ by 2½ by ⅜ in	3 oz	85	57	205	23	12
495	Lean only (from item 494)	2.6 oz	75	63	135	22	5
	Steak						
	Sirloin, broiled						
496	Lean and fat, piece, 2½ by 2½ by ¾ in	3 oz	85	53	240	23	15
497	Lean only (from item 496)	2.5 oz	72	59	150	22	6
498	Beef, canned, corned	3 oz	85	59	185	22	10
499	Beef, dried, chipped	2.5 oz	72	48	145	24	4
	Lamb, cooked						
	Chops, (3 per lb with bone)						
	Arm, braised						
500	Lean and fat	2.2 oz	63	44	220	20	15
501	Lean only (from item 500)	1.7 oz	48	49	135	17	7
	Loin, broiled						
502	Lean and fat	2.8 oz	80	54	235	22	16
503	Lean only (from item 502)	2.3 oz	64	61	140	19	6
	Leg, roasted						
504	Lean and fat, 2 pieces, 4⅛ by 2¼ by ¼ in	3 oz	85	59	205	22	13
505	Lean only (from item 504)	2.6 oz	73	64	140	20	6
	Rib, roasted						
506	Lean and fat, 3 pieces, 2½ by 2½ by ¼ in	3 oz	85	47	315	18	26
507	Lean only (from item 506)	2 oz	57	60	130	15	7
	Pork, cured, cooked						
	Bacon						
508	Regular	3 medium slices	19	13	110	6	9
509	Canadian-style	2 slices	46	62	85	11	4

21. About ½ inch of fat.
22. Fried in vegetable shortening.
23. Values vary widely.

	Fatty Acids						Vitamin A Value					
Satu-rated (grams)	Monoun-saturated (grams)	Polyun-saturated (grams)	Carbo-hydrate (grams)	Calcium (mg)	Phos-phorus (mg)	Iron (mg)	(IU) Inter-national Units	(RE) Retinol Equiv-alents	Thiamin (mg)	Riboflavin (mg)	Niacin (mg)	Vitamin C (mg)
10.8	11.7	0.9	0	11	163	2.5	Tr	Tr	0.06	0.19	2.0	0
3.9	4.2	0.3	0	8	146	2.3	Tr	Tr	0.05	0.17	1.7	0
6.2	6.9	0.6	0	9	134	1.8	Tr	Tr	0.04	0.18	4.4	0
6.9	7.7	0.7	0	9	144	2.1	Tr	Tr	0.03	0.16	4.9	0
2.5	3.6	1.3	7	9	392	5.3	30,690[23]	9120[23]	0.18	3.52	12.3	23
10.8	11.4	0.9	0	8	145	2.0	Tr	Tr	0.06	0.16	3.1	0
3.6	3.7	0.3	0	5	127	1.7	Tr	Tr	0.05	0.13	2.7	0
4.9	5.4	0.5	0	5	177	1.6	Tr	Tr	0.07	0.14	3.0	0
1.9	2.1	0.2	0	3	170	1.5	Tr	Tr	0.07	0.13	2.8	0
6.4	6.9	0.6	0	9	186	2.6	Tr	Tr	0.10	0.23	3.3	0
2.6	2.8	0.3	0	8	176	2.4	Tr	Tr	0.09	0.22	3.1	0
4.2	4.9	0.4	0	17	90	3.7	Tr	Tr	0.02	0.20	2.9	0
1.8	2.0	0.2	0	14	287	2.3	Tr	Tr	0.05	0.23	2.7	0
6.9	6.0	0.9	0	16	132	1.5	Tr	Tr	0.04	0.16	4.4	0
2.9	2.6	0.4	0	12	111	1.3	Tr	Tr	0.03	0.13	3.0	0
7.3	6.4	1.0	0	16	162	1.4	Tr	Tr	0.09	0.21	5.5	0
2.6	2.4	0.4	0	12	145	1.3	Tr	Tr	0.08	0.18	4.4	0
5.6	4.9	0.8	0	8	162	1.7	Tr	Tr	0.09	0.24	5.5	0
2.4	2.2	0.4	0	6	150	1.5	Tr	Tr	0.08	0.20	4.6	0
12.1	10.6	1.5	0	19	139	1.4	Tr	Tr	0.08	0.18	5.5	0
3.2	3.0	0.5	0	12	111	1.0	Tr	Tr	0.05	0.13	3.5	0
3.3	4.5	1.1	Tr	2	64	0.3	0	0	0.13	0.05	1.4	6
1.3	1.9	0.4	1	5	136	0.4	0	0	0.38	0.09	3.2	10

Continued.

P

Item Number	Foods, Approximate Measures, Units, and Weight (edible parts)		Weight (grams)	Water (percent)	Food Energy (calories)	Protein (grams)	Fat (grams)
	Meat and Meat Products—cont'd						
	Ham, light cure, roasted						
510	Lean and fat, 2 pieces, 4⅛ by 2¼ by ¼ in	3 oz	85	58	205	18	14
511	Lean only (from item 510)	2.4 oz	68	66	105	17	4
512	Ham, canned, roasted, 2 pieces, 4⅛ by 2¼ by ¼ in	3 oz	85	67	140	18	7
	Luncheon meat						
513	Canned, spiced or unspiced, slice, 3 by 2 by ½ in	2 slices	42	52	140	5	13
514	Chopped ham (8 slices per 6-oz pkg)	2 slices	42	64	95	7	7
	Cooked ham (8 slices per 8-oz pkg)						
515	Regular	2 slices	57	65	105	10	6
516	Extra lean	2 slices	57	71	75	11	3
	Ham (leg), roasted						
517	Lean and fat, piece, 2½ by 2½ by ¾ in	3 oz	85	53	250	21	18
518	Lean only (from item 517)	2.5 oz	72	60	160	20	8
	Shoulder cut, braised						
519	Lean and fat, 3 pieces, 2½ by 2½ by ¼ in	3 oz	85	47	295	23	22
520	Lean only (from item 519)	2.4 oz	67	54	165	22	8
	Sausages (See also Luncheon meats, items 513-516)						
521	Bologna, slice (8 per 8-oz pkg)	2 slices	57	54	180	7	16
522	Braunschweiger, slice (6 per 6-oz pkg)	2 slices	57	48	205	8	18
523	Brown and serve (10-11 per 8-oz pkg), browned	1 link	13	45	50	2	5
524	Frankfurter (10 per 1-lb pkg), cooked (re-heated)	1 frank-furter	45	54	145	5	13
525	Pork link (16 per 1-lb pkg), cooked	1 link	13	45	50	3	4
	Salami						
526	Cooked type, slice (8 per 8-oz pkg)	2 slices	57	60	145	8	11
527	Dry type, slice (12 per 4-oz pkg)	2 slices	20	35	85	5	7
528	Sandwich spread (pork, beef)	1 tbsp	15	60	35	1	3
529	Vienna sausage (per 4-oz can)	1 sausage	16	60	45	2	4
	Veal, medium fat, cooked, bone removed						
530	Cutlet, 4⅛ by 2¼ by ½ in, braised or broiled	3 oz	85	60	185	23	9
531	Rib, 2 pieces, 4⅛ by 2¼ by ¼ in, roasted	3 oz	85	55	230	23	14
	Mixed dishes						
532	Beef and vegetable stew, from home recipe	1 cup	245	82	220	16	11
533	Beef pot pie, from home recipe, baked, piece, ⅓ of 9-in diam pie[24]	1 piece	210	55	515	21	30
534	Chicken a la king, cooked, from home recipe	1 cup	245	68	470	27	34
535	Chicken and noodles, cooked, from home recipe	1 cup	240	71	365	22	18

24. Vegetable shortening and enriched flour used in making the crust.

	Fatty Acids						Vitamin A Value					
Satu-rated (grams)	Monoun-saturated (grams)	Polyun-saturated (grams)	Carbo-hydrate (grams)	Calcium (mg)	Phos-phorus (mg)	Iron (mg)	(IU) Inter-national Units	(RE) Retinol Equiv-alents	Thiamin (mg)	Riboflavin (mg)	Niacin (mg)	Vitamin C (mg)
5.1	6.7	1.5	0	6	182	0.7	0	0	0.51	0.19	3.8	0
1.3	1.7	0.4	0	5	154	0.6	0	0	0.46	0.17	3.4	0
2.4	3.5	0.8	Tr	6	188	0.9	0	0	0.82	0.21	4.3	19
4.5	6.0	1.5	1	3	34	0.3	0	0	0.15	0.08	1.3	Tr
2.4	3.4	0.9	0	3	65	0.3	0	0	0.27	0.09	1.6	8
1.9	2.8	0.7	2	4	141	0.6	0	0	0.49	0.14	3.0	16
0.9	1.3	0.3	1	4	124	0.4	0	0	0.53	0.13	2.8	15
6.4	8.1	2.0	0	5	210	0.9	10	2	0.54	0.27	3.9	Tr
2.7	3.6	1.0	0	5	202	0.8	10	1	0.50	0.25	3.6	Tr
7.9	10.0	2.4	0	6	162	1.4	10	3	0.46	0.26	4.4	Tr
2.8	3.7	1.0	0	5	151	1.3	10	1	0.40	0.24	4.0	Tr
6.1	7.6	1.4	2	7	52	0.9	0	0	0.10	0.08	1.5	12
6.2	8.5	2.1	2	5	96	5.3	8010	2405	0.14	0.87	4.8	6
1.7	2.2	0.5	Tr	1	14	0.1	0	0	0.05	0.02	0.4	0
4.8	6.2	1.2	1	5	39	0.5	0	0	0.09	0.05	1.2	12
1.4	1.8	0.5	Tr	4	24	0.2	0	0	0.10	0.03	0.6	Tr
4.6	5.2	1.2	1	7	66	1.5	0	0	0.14	0.21	2.0	7
2.4	3.4	0.6	1	2	28	0.3	0	0	0.12	0.06	1.0	5
0.9	1.1	0.4	2	2	9	0.1	10	1	0.03	0.02	0.3	0
1.5	2.0	0.3	Tr	2	8	0.1	0	0	0.01	0.02	0.3	0
4.1	4.1	0.6	0	9	196	0.8	Tr	Tr	0.06	0.21	4.6	0
6.0	6.0	1.0	0	10	211	0.7	Tr	Tr	0.11	0.26	6.6	0
4.4	4.5	0.5	15	29	184	2.9	5690	568	0.15	0.17	4.7	17
7.9	12.9	7.4	39	29	149	3.8	4220	517	0.29	0.29	4.8	6
12.9	13.4	6.2	12	127	358	2.5	1130	272	0.10	0.42	5.4	12
5.1	7.1	3.9	26	26	247	2.2	430	130	0.50	0.17	4.3	Tr

Continued.

P

Item Number	Foods, Approximate Measures, Units, and Weight (edible parts)		Weight (grams)	Water (percent)	Food Energy (calories)	Protein (grams)	Fat (grams)
	Meat and Meat Products—cont'd						
	Chicken chow mein:						
536	Canned	1 cup	250	89	95	7	Tr
537	From home recipe	1 cup	250	78	255	31	10
538	Chicken pot pie, from home recipe, baked, piece, 1/3 of 9-in diam pie	1 piece	232	57	545	23	31
539	Chili con carne with beans, canned	1 cup	255	72	340	19	16
540	Chop suey with beef and pork, from home recipe	1 cup	250	75	300	26	17
	Macaroni (enriched) and cheese						
541	Canned	1 cup	240	80	230	9	10
542	From home recipe[18]	1 cup	200	58	430	17	22
543	Quiche Lorraine, 1/8 of 8-in diam quiche[24]	1 slice	176	47	600	13	48
	Spaghetti (enriched) in tomato sauce with cheese						
544	Canned	1 cup	250	80	190	6	2
545	From home recipe	1 cup	250	77	260	9	9
	Spaghetti (enriched) with meatballs and tomato sauce						
546	Canned	1 cup	250	78	260	12	10
547	From home recipe	1 cup	248	70	330	19	12
	Poultry and Poultry Products						
	Chicken						
	Fried, flesh, with skin[22]						
	Batter dipped						
548	Breast, 1/2 breast (5.6 oz with bones)	4.9 oz	140	52	365	35	18
549	Drumstick (3.4 oz with bones)	2.5 oz	72	53	195	16	11
	Roasted, flesh only						
550	Breast, 1/2 breast (4.2 oz with bones and skin)	3.0 oz	86	65	140	27	3
551	Drumstick, (2.9 oz with bones and skin)	1.6 oz	44	67	75	12	2
552	Stewed, flesh only, light and dark meat, chopped or diced	1 cup	140	67	250	38	9
553	Chicken liver, cooked	1 liver	20	68	30	5	1
554	Duck, roasted, flesh only	1/2 duck	221	64	445	52	25
	Turkey, roasted, flesh only						
555	Dark meat, piece, 2 1/2 by 1 5/8 by 1/4 in	4 pieces	85	63	160	24	6
556	Light meat, piece, 4 by 2 by 1/4 in	2 pieces	85	66	135	25	3
	Poultry food products						
	Chicken						
557	Canned, boneless	5 oz	142	69	235	31	11
558	Frankfurter (10 per 1-lb pkg)	1 frankfurter	45	58	115	6	9
559	Roll, light (6 slices per 6-oz pkg)	2 slices	57	69	90	11	4

P

| Fatty Acids | | | | | | | Vitamin A Value | | | | | |
Saturated (grams)	Monounsaturated (grams)	Polyunsaturated (grams)	Carbohydrate (grams)	Calcium (mg)	Phosphorus (mg)	Iron (mg)	(IU) International Units	(RE) Retinol Equivalents	Thiamin (mg)	Riboflavin (mg)	Niacin (mg)	Vitamin C (mg)
0.1	0.1	0.8	18	45	85	1.3	150	28	0.05	0.10	1.0	13
4.1	4.9	3.5	10	58	293	2.5	280	50	0.08	0.23	4.3	10
10.3	15.5	6.6	42	70	232	3.0	7220	735	0.32	0.32	4.9	5
5.8	7.2	1.0	31	82	321	4.3	150	15	0.08	0.18	3.3	8
4.3	7.4	4.2	13	60	248	4.8	600	60	0.28	0.38	5.0	33
4.7	2.9	1.3	26	199	182	1.0	260	72	0.12	0.24	1.0	Tr
9.8	7.4	3.6	40	362	322	1.8	860	232	0.20	0.40	1.8	1
23.2	17.8	4.1	29	211	276	1.0	1640	454	0.11	0.32	Tr	Tr
0.4	0.4	0.5	39	40	88	2.8	930	120	0.35	0.28	4.5	10
3.0	3.6	1.2	37	80	135	2.3	1080	140	0.25	0.18	2.3	13
2.4	3.9	3.1	29	53	113	3.3	1000	100	0.15	0.18	2.3	5
3.9	4.4	2.2	39	124	236	3.7	1590	159	0.25	0.30	4.0	22
4.9	7.6	4.3	13	28	259	1.8	90	28	0.16	0.20	14.7	0
3.0	4.6	2.7	6	12	106	1.0	60	19	0.08	0.15	3.7	0
0.9	1.1	0.7	0	13	196	0.9	20	5	0.06	0.10	11.8	0
0.7	0.8	0.6	0	5	81	0.6	30	8	0.03	0.10	2.7	0
2.6	3.3	2.2	0	20	210	1.6	70	21	0.07	0.23	8.6	0
0.4	0.3	0.2	Tr	3	62	1.7	3270	983	0.03	0.35	0.9	3
9.2	8.2	3.2	0	27	449	6.0	170	51	0.57	1.04	11.3	0
2.1	1.4	1.8	0	27	173	2.0	0	0	0.05	0.21	3.1	0
0.9	0.5	0.7	0	16	186	1.1	0	0	0.05	0.11	5.8	0
3.1	4.5	2.6	0	20	158	2.2	170	48	0.02	0.18	9.0	3
2.5	3.8	1.8	3	43	48	0.9	60	17	0.03	0.05	1.4	0
1.1	1.7	0.9	1	24	89	0.6	50	14	0.04	0.07	3.0	0

Continued.

P

Item Number	Foods, Approximate Measures, Units, and Weight (edible parts)		Weight (grams)	Water (percent)	Food Energy (calories)	Protein (grams)	Fat (grams)
	Poultry and Poultry Products—cont'd						
	Turkey						
560	Gravy and turkey, frozen	5-oz package	142	85	95	8	4
561	Ham, cured turkey thigh meat (8 slices per 8-oz pkg)	2 slices	57	71	75	11	3
562	Loaf, breast meat (8 slices per 6-oz pkg)	2 slices	42	72	45	10	1
563	Roast, boneless, frozen, seasoned, light and dark meat, cooked	3 oz	85	68	130	18	5
	Soups, Sauces, and Gravies						
	Soups						
	Canned, condensed						
	Prepared with equal volume of milk						
564	Clam chowder, New England	1 cup	248	85	165	9	7
565	Cream of chicken	1 cup	248	85	190	7	11
566	Cream of mushroom	1 cup	248	85	205	6	14
567	Tomato	1 cup	248	85	160	6	6
	Prepared with equal volume of water						
568	Bean with bacon	1 cup	253	84	170	8	6
569	Beef broth, bouillon, consomme	1 cup	240	98	15	3	1
570	Beef noodle	1 cup	244	92	85	5	3
571	Chicken noodle	1 cup	241	92	75	4	2
572	Chicken rice	1 cup	241	94	60	4	2
573	Cream of chicken	1 cup	244	91	115	3	7
574	Cream of mushroom	1 cup	244	90	130	2	9
575	Minestrone	1 cup	241	91	80	4	3
576	Tomato	1 cup	244	90	85	2	2
577	Vegetable beef	1 cup	244	92	80	6	2
578	Vegetarian	1 cup	241	92	70	2	2
	Sauces						
	From dry mix						
579	Cheese, prepared with milk	1 cup	279	77	305	16	17
580	Hollandaise, prepared with water	1 cup	259	84	240	5	20
581	White sauce, prepared with milk	1 cup	264	81	240	10	13
	From home recipe						
582	White sauce, medium	1 cup	250	73	395	10	30
	Ready-to-serve						
583	Barbecue	1 tbsp	16	81	10	Tr	Tr
584	Soy	1 tbsp	18	68	10	2	0
	Gravies						
	Canned						
585	Beef	1 cup	233	87	125	9	5
586	Chicken	1 cup	238	85	190	5	14
587	Mushroom	1 cup	238	89	120	3	6
	From dry mix						
588	Brown	1 cup	261	91	80	3	2
589	Chicken	1 cup	260	91	85	3	2

P

| | Fatty Acids | | | | | | Vitamin A Value | | | | | |
Satu-rated (grams)	Monoun-saturated (grams)	Polyun-saturated (grams)	Carbo-hydrate (grams)	Calcium (mg)	Phos-phorus (mg)	Iron (mg)	(IU) Inter-national Units	(RE) Retinol Equiv-alents	Thiamin (mg)	Riboflavin (mg)	Niacin (mg)	Vitamin C (mg)
1.2	1.4	0.7	7	20	115	1.3	60	18	0.03	0.18	2.6	0
1.0	0.7	0.9	Tr	6	108	1.6	0	0	0.03	0.14	2.0	0
0.2	0.2	0.1	0	3	97	0.2	0	0	0.02	0.05	3.5	0
1.6	1.0	1.4	3	4	207	1.4	0	0	0.04	0.14	5.3	0
3.0	2.3	1.1	17	186	156	1.5	160	40	0.07	0.24	1.0	3
4.6	4.5	1.6	15	181	151	0.7	710	94	0.07	0.26	0.9	1
5.1	3.0	4.6	15	179	156	0.6	150	37	0.08	0.28	0.9	2
2.9	1.6	1.1	22	159	149	1.8	850	109	0.13	0.25	1.5	68
1.5	2.2	1.8	23	81	132	2.0	890	89	0.09	0.03	0.6	2
0.3	0.2	Tr	Tr	14	31	0.4	0	0	Tr	0.05	1.9	0
1.1	1.2	0.5	9	15	46	1.1	630	63	0.07	0.06	1.1	Tr
0.7	1.1	0.6	9	17	36	0.8	710	71	0.05	0.06	1.4	Tr
0.5	0.9	0.4	7	17	22	0.7	660	66	0.02	0.02	1.1	Tr
2.1	3.3	1.5	9	34	37	0.6	560	56	0.03	0.06	0.8	Tr
2.4	1.7	4.2	9	46	49	0.5	0	0	0.05	0.09	0.7	1
0.6	0.7	1.1	11	34	55	0.9	2340	234	0.05	0.04	0.9	1
0.4	0.4	1.0	17	12	34	1.8	690	69	0.09	0.05	1.4	66
0.9	0.8	0.1	10	17	41	1.1	1890	189	0.04	0.05	1.0	2
0.3	0.8	0.7	12	22	34	1.1	3010	301	0.05	0.05	0.9	1
9.3	5.3	1.6	23	569	438	0.3	390	117	0.15	0.56	0.3	2
11.6	5.9	0.9	14	124	127	0.9	730	220	0.05	0.18	0.1	Tr
6.4	4.7	1.7	21	425	256	0.3	310	92	0.08	0.45	0.5	3
9.1	11.9	7.2	24	292	238	0.9	1190	340	0.15	0.43	0.8	2
Tr	0.1	0.1	2	3	3	0.1	140	14	Tr	Tr	0.1	1
0.0	0.0	0.0	2	3	38	0.5	0	0	0.01	0.02	0.6	0
2.7	2.3	0.2	11	14	70	1.6	0	0	0.07	0.08	1.5	0
3.4	6.1	3.6	13	48	69	1.1	880	264	0.04	0.10	1.1	0
1.0	2.8	2.4	13	17	36	1.6	0	0	0.08	0.15	1.6	0
0.9	0.8	0.1	14	66	47	0.2	0	0	0.04	0.09	0.9	0
0.5	0.9	0.4	14	39	47	0.3	0	0	0.05	0.15	0.8	3

Continued.

P

Item Number	Foods, Approximate Measures, Units, and Weight (edible parts)		Weight (grams)	Water (percent)	Food Energy (calories)	Protein (grams)	Fat (grams)
	Sugars and Sweets						
	Candy						
590	Caramels, plain or chocolate	1 oz	28	8	115	1	3
	Chocolate						
591	Milk, plain	1 oz	28	1	145	2	9
592	Milk, with almonds	1 oz	28	2	150	3	10
593	Milk, with peanuts	1 oz	28	1	155	4	11
594	Semisweet, small pieces (60 per oz)	1 cup or 6 oz	170	1	860	7	61
595	Sweet (dark)	1 oz	28	1	150	1	10
596	Fondant, uncoated (mints, candy corn, other)	1 oz	28	3	105	Tr	0
597	Fudge, chocolate, plain	1 oz	28	8	115	1	3
598	Gum drops	1 oz	28	12	100	Tr	Tr
599	Hard candy	1 oz	28	1	110	0	0
600	Jelly beans	1 oz	28	6	105	Tr	Tr
601	Marshmallows	1 oz	28	17	90	1	0
602	Custard, baked	1 cup	265	77	305	14	15
603	Gelatin dessert prepared with gelatin dessert powder and water	½ cup	120	84	70	2	0
604	Honey, strained or extracted	1 cup	339	17	1030	1	0
605	Jams and preserves	1 tbsp	20	29	55	Tr	Tr
606	Jellies	1 tbsp	18	28	50	Tr	Tr
607	Popsicle, 3-fl-oz size	1 popsicle	95	80	70	0	0
	Puddings						
	Canned						
608	Chocolate	5-oz can	142	68	205	3	11
609	Tapioca	5-oz can	142	74	160	3	5
610	Vanilla	5-oz can	142	69	220	2	10
	Dry mix, prepared with whole milk						
	Chocolate						
611	Instant	½ cup	130	71	155	4	4
612	Regular (cooked)	½ cup	130	73	150	4	4
613	Rice	½ cup	132	73	155	4	4
614	Tapioca	½ cup	130	75	145	4	4
	Vanilla						
615	Instant	½ cup	130	73	150	4	4
616	Regular (cooked)	½ cup	130	74	145	4	4
	Sugars						
617	Brown, pressed down	1 cup	220	2	820	0	0
	White						
618	Granulated	1 cup	200	1	770	0	0
619		1 pkt	6	1	25	0	0

| Fatty Acids | | | Carbo-hydrate (grams) | Calcium (mg) | Phos-phorus (mg) | Iron (mg) | Vitamin A Value | | Thiamin (mg) | Riboflavin (mg) | Niacin (mg) | Vitamin C (mg) |
Satu-rated (grams)	Monoun-saturated (grams)	Polyun-saturated (grams)					(IU) Inter-national Units	(RE) Retinol Equiv-alents				
2.2	0.3	0.1	22	42	35	0.4	Tr	Tr	0.01	0.05	0.1	Tr
5.4	3.0	0.3	16	50	61	0.4	30	10	0.02	0.10	0.1	Tr
4.8	4.1	0.7	15	65	77	0.5	30	8	0.02	0.12	0.2	Tr
4.2	3.5	1.5	13	49	83	0.4	30	8	0.07	0.07	1.4	Tr
36.2	19.9	1.9	97	51	178	5.8	30	3	0.10	0.14	0.9	Tr
5.9	3.3	0.3	16	7	41	0.6	10	1	0.01	0.04	0.1	Tr
0.0	0.0	0.0	27	2	Tr	0.1	0	0	Tr	Tr	Tr	0
2.1	1.0	0.1	21	22	24	0.3	Tr	Tr	0.01	0.03	0.1	Tr
Tr	Tr	0.1	25	2	Tr	0.1	0	0	0.00	Tr	Tr	0
0.0	0.0	0.0	28	Tr	2	0.1	0	0	0.10	0.00	0.0	0
Tr	Tr	0.1	26	1	1	0.3	0	0	0.00	Tr	Tr	0
0.0	0.0	0.0	23	1	2	0.5	0	0	0.00	Tr	Tr	0
6.8	5.4	0.7	29	297	310	1.1	530	146	0.11	0.50	0.3	1
0.0	0.0	0.0	17	2	23	Tr	0	0	0.00	0.00	0.0	0
0.0	0.0	0.0	279	17	20	1.7	0	0	0.02	0.14	1.0	3
0.0	Tr	Tr	14	4	2	0.2	Tr	Tr	Tr	0.01	Tr	Tr
Tr	Tr	Tr	13	2	Tr	0.1	Tr	Tr	Tr	0.01	Tr	1
0.0	0.0	0.0	18	0	0	Tr	0	0	0.00	0.00	0.0	0
9.5	0.5	0.1	30	74	117	1.2	100	31	0.04	0.17	0.6	Tr
4.8	Tr	Tr	28	119	113	0.3	Tr	Tr	0.03	0.14	0.4	Tr
9.5	0.2	0.1	33	79	94	0.2	Tr	Tr	0.03	0.12	0.6	Tr
2.3	1.1	0.2	27	130	329	0.3	130	33	0.04	0.18	0.1	1
2.4	1.1	0.1	25	146	120	0.2	140	34	0.05	0.20	0.1	1
2.3	1.1	0.1	27	133	110	0.5	140	33	0.10	0.18	0.6	1
2.3	1.1	0.1	25	131	103	0.1	140	34	0.04	0.18	0.1	1
2.2	1.1	0.2	27	129	273	0.1	140	33	0.04	0.17	0.1	1
2.3	1.0	0.1	25	132	102	0.1	140	34	0.04	0.18	0.1	1
0.0	0.0	0.0	22	3	Tr	0.1	0	0	0.00	0.00	0.0	0
0.0	0.0	0.0	199	Tr	Tr	Tr	0	0	0.00	0.00	0.0	0
0.0	0.0	0.0	6	1	Tr	Tr	0	0	0.00	0.00	0.0	0

Continued.

P

Item Number	Foods, Approximate Measures, Units, and Weight (edible parts)		Weight (grams)	Water (percent)	Food Energy (calories)	Protein (grams)	Fat (grams)
	Sugars and Sweets—cont'd						
	Syrups						
	Chocolate-flavored syrup or topping						
620	Thin type	2 tbsp	38	37	85	1	Tr
621	Fudge type	2 tbsp	38	25	125	2	5
622	Molasses, cane, blackstrap	2 tbsp	40	24	85	0	0
623	Table syrup (corn and maple)	2 tbsp	42	25	122	0	0
	Vegetables and Vegetable Products						
	Asparagus, green						
	Cooked, drained						
	From raw						
624	Cuts and tips	1 cup	180	92	45	5	1
625	Spears, ½-in diam at base	4 spears	60	92	15	2	Tr
	From frozen						
626	Cuts and tips	1 cup	180	91	50	5	1
627	Spears, ½-in diam at base	4 spears	60	91	15	2	Tr
628	Canned, spears, ½-in diam at base	4 spears	80	95	10	1	Tr
629	Bamboo shoots, canned, drained	1 cup	131	94	25	2	1
	Beans						
	Lima, immature seeds, frozen, cooked, drained						
630	Thick-seeded types (Ford hooks)	1 cup	170	74	170	10	1
631	Thin-seeded types (baby limas)	1 cup	180	72	190	12	1
	Snap						
	Cooked, drained						
632	From raw (cut and French style)	1 cup	125	89	45	2	Tr
633	From frozen (cut)	1 cup	135	92	35	2	Tr
634	Canned, drained solids (cut)	1 cup	135	93	25	2	Tr
	Beans, mature (See Beans, dry, items 448-456; and Black-eyed peas, dry, item 457).						
	Bean sprouts (mung)						
635	Raw	1 cup	104	90	30	3	Tr
636	Cooked, drained	1 cup	124	93	25	3	Tr
	Beets						
	Cooked, drained						
637	Diced or sliced	1 cup	170	91	55	2	Tr
638	Whole beets, 2-in diam	2 beets	100	91	30	1	Tr
639	Canned, drained solids, diced or sliced	1 cup	170	91	55	2	Tr
640	Beet greens, leaves and stems, cooked, drained	1 cup	144	89	40	4	Tr
	Black-eyed peas, immature seeds, cooked and drained						
641	From raw	1 cup	165	72	180	13	1
642	From frozen	1 cup	170	66	225	14	1

| | Fatty Acids | | Carbo-hydrate (grams) | Calcium (mg) | Phos-phorus (mg) | Iron (mg) | Vitamin A Value | | Thiamin (mg) | Riboflavin (mg) | Niacin (mg) | Vitamin C (mg) |
Satu-rated (grams)	Monoun-saturated (grams)	Polyun-saturated (grams)					(IU) Inter-national Units	(RE) Retinol Equiv-alents				
0.2	0.1	0.1	21	38	60	0.5	40	13	0.02	0.08	0.10	0
3.1	1.7	0.2	22	274	34	10.1	0	0	0.04	0.08	0.8	0
0.0	0.0	0.0	32	1	4	Tr	0	0	0.00	0.00	0.0	0
0.0	0.0	0.0	212	187	56	4.8	0	0	0.02	0.07	0.2	0
0.1	Tr	0.2	8	43	110	1.2	1490	149	0.18	0.22	1.9	49
Tr	Tr	0.1	3	14	37	0.4	500	50	0.06	0.07	0.6	16
0.2	Tr	0.3	9	41	99	1.2	1470	147	0.12	0.19	1.9	44
0.1	Tr	0.1	3	14	33	0.4	490	49	0.04	0.06	0.6	15
Tr	Tr	0.1	2	11	30	0.5	380	38	0.04	0.07	0.7	13
0.1	Tr	0.2	4	10	33	0.4	10	1	0.03	0.03	0.2	1
0.1	Tr	0.3	32	37	107	2.3	320	32	0.13	0.10	1.8	22
0.1	Tr	0.3	35	50	202	3.5	300	30	0.13	0.10	1.4	10
0.1	Tr	0.2	10	58	49	1.6	830	83	0.09	0.12	0.8	12
Tr	Tr	0.1	8	61	32	1.1	710	71	0.06	0.10	0.6	11
Tr	Tr	0.1	6	35	26	1.2	470	47	0.02	0.08	0.3	6
Tr	Tr	0.1	6	14	56	0.9	20	2	0.09	0.13	0.8	14
Tr	Tr	Tr	5	15	35	0.8	20	2	0.06	0.13	1.0	14
Tr	Tr	Tr	11	19	53	1.1	20	2	0.05	0.02	0.5	9
Tr	Tr	Tr	7	11	31	0.6	10	1	0.03	0.01	0.3	6
Tr	Tr	0.1	12	26	29	3.1	20	2	0.02	0.07	0.3	7
Tr	0.1	0.1	8	164	59	2.7	7340	734	0.17	0.42	0.7	36
0.3	0.1	0.6	30	46	196	2.4	1050	105	0.11	0.18	1.8	3
0.3	0.1	0.5	40	39	207	3.6	130	13	0.44	0.11	1.2	4

Continued.

Item Number	Foods, Approximate Measures, Units, and Weight (edible parts)		Weight (grams)	Water (percent)	Food Energy (calories)	Protein (grams)	Fat (grams)
	Broccoli						
643	Raw	1 spear	151	91	40	4	1
	Cooked, drained						
	From raw						
644	Spear, medium	1 spear	180	90	50	5	1
645	Spears, cut into ½-in pieces	1 cup	155	90	45	5	Tr
	From frozen						
646	Piece, 4½ to 5 in long	1 piece	30	91	10	1	Tr
647	Chopped	1 cup	185	91	50	6	Tr
	Brussels sprouts, cooked, drained						
648	From raw, 7 to 8 sprouts, 1¼ to 1½-in diam	1 cup	155	87	60	4	1
649	From frozen	1 cup	155	87	65	6	1
	Cabbage, common varieties						
650	Raw, coarsely shredded or sliced	1 cup	70	93	15	1	Tr
651	Cooked, drained	1 cup	150	94	30	1	Tr
	Carrots						
	Raw, without crowns and tips, scraped						
652	Whole, 7½ by 1⅛ in, or strips, 2½ to 3 in long	1 carrot, or 18 strips	72	88	30	1	Tr
653	Grated	1 cup	110	88	45	1	Tr
	Cooked, sliced, drained						
654	From raw	1 cup	156	87	70	2	Tr
655	From frozen	1 cup	146	90	55	2	Tr
656	Canned, sliced, drained solids	1 cup	146	93	35	1	Tr
	Cauliflower						
657	Raw, (flowerets)	1 cup	100	92	25	2	Tr
	Cooked, drained						
658	From raw (flowerets)	1 cup	125	93	30	2	Tr
659	From frozen (flowerets)	1 cup	180	94	35	3	Tr
	Celery, pascal type, raw						
660	Stalk, large outer, 8 by 1½ in (at root end)	1 stalk	40	95	5	Tr	Tr
661	Pieces, diced	1 cup	120	95	20	1	Tr
	Collards, cooked, drained						
662	From raw (leaves without stems)	1 cup	190	96	25	2	Tr
663	From frozen (chopped)	1 cup	170	88	60	5	1
	Corn, sweet						
	Cooked, drained						
664	From raw, ear, 5 by 1¾ in	1 ear	77	70	85	3	1
	From frozen						
665	Ear, trimmed to about 3½ in long	1 ear	63	73	60	2	Tr
666	Kernels	1 cup	165	76	135	5	Tr
	Canned						
667	Cream style	1 cup	256	79	185	4	1
668	Whole kernel, vacuum pack	1 cup	210	77	165	5	1

25. Values are for green varieties, yellow varieties contain about one third of this amount.
26. White varieties contain only a trace of vitamin A.

P

Fatty Acids							Vitamin A Value					
Satu-rated (grams)	Monoun-saturated (grams)	Polyun-saturated (grams)	Carbo-hydrate (grams)	Calcium (mg)	Phos-phorus (mg)	Iron (mg)	(IU) Inter-national Units	(RE) Retinol Equiv-alents	Thiamin (mg)	Riboflavin (mg)	Niacin (mg)	Vitamin C (mg)
0.1	Tr	0.3	8	72	100	1.3	2330	233	0.10	0.18	1.0	141
0.1	Tr	0.2	10	205	86	2.1	2540	254	0.15	0.37	1.4	113
0.1	Tr	0.2	9	177	74	1.8	2180	218	0.13	0.32	1.2	97
Tr	Tr	Tr	2	15	17	0.2	570	57	0.02	0.02	0.1	12
Tr	Tr	0.1	10	94	102	1.1	3500	350	0.10	0.15	0.8	74
0.2	0.1	0.4	13	56	87	1.9	1110	111	0.17	0.12	0.9	96
0.1	Tr	0.3	13	37	84	1.1	910	91	0.16	0.18	0.8	71
Tr	Tr	0.1	4	33	16	0.4	90	9	0.04	0.02	0.2	33
Tr	Tr	0.2	7	50	38	0.6	130	13	0.09	0.08	0.3	36
Tr	Tr	0.1	7	19	32	0.4	20,250	2025	0.07	0.04	0.7	7
Tr	Tr	0.1	11	30	48	0.6	30,940	3094	0.11	0.06	1.0	10
0.1	Tr	0.1	16	48	47	1.0	38,300	3830	0.05	0.09	0.8	4
Tr	Tr	0.1	12	41	38	0.7	25,850	2585	0.04	0.05	0.6	4
0.1	Tr	0.1	8	37	35	0.9	20,110	2011	0.03	0.04	0.8	4
Tr	Tr	0.1	5	29	46	0.6	20	2	0.08	0.06	0.6	72
Tr	Tr	0.1	6	34	44	0.5	20	2	0.08	0.07	0.7	69
0.1	Tr	0.2	7	31	43	0.7	40	4	0.07	0.10	0.6	56
Tr	Tr	Tr	1	14	10	0.2	50	5	0.01	0.01	0.1	3
Tr	Tr	0.1	4	43	31	0.6	150	15	0.04	0.04	0.4	8
0.1	Tr	0.2	5	148	19	0.8	4220	422	0.03	0.08	0.4	19
0.1	0.1	0.4	12	357	46	1.9	10,170	1017	0.08	0.20	1.1	45
0.2	0.3	0.5	19	2	79	0.5	170[26]	17[26]	0.17	0.06	1.2	5
0.1	0.1	0.2	14	2	47	0.4	130[26]	13[26]	0.11	0.04	1.0	3
Tr	Tr	0.1	34	3	78	0.5	410[26]	41[26]	0.11	0.12	2.1	4
0.2	0.3	0.5	46	8	131	1.0	250[26]	25[26]	0.06	0.14	2.5	12
0.2	0.3	0.5	41	11	134	0.9	510[26]	51[26]	0.09	0.15	2.5	17

P

Continued.

Item Number	Foods, Approximate Measures, Units, and Weight (edible parts)	Weight (grams)	Water (percent)	Food Energy (calories)	Protein (grams)	Fat (grams)
	Vegetables and Vegetable Products—cont'd					
	Cowpeas (See Black-eyed peas, immature, items 641, 642; and mature, item 457)					
669	Cucumber, with peel, slices, ⅛ in thick (large, 2⅛-in diam; small, 1¾-in diam)	6 large or 8 small slices	28	96	5	Tr	Tr
670	Dandelion greens, cooked, drained	1 cup	105	90	35	2	1
671	Eggplant, cooked, steamed	1 cup	96	92	25	1	Tr
672	Endive, curly (including escarole), raw, small pieces	1 cup	50	94	10	1	Tr
	Lettuce, raw					
	Butterhead, as Boston types					
673	Head, 5-in diam	1 head	163	96	20	2	Tr
674	Leaves	1 outer or 2 inner leaves	15	96	Tr	Tr	Tr
	Crisphead, as iceberg					
675	Head, 6-in diam	1 head	539	96	70	5	1
676	Wedge, ¼ of head	1 wedge	135	96	20	1	Tr
677	Pieces, chopped or shredded	1 cup	55	96	5	1	Tr
678	Looseleaf (bunching varieties including romaine or cos), chopped or shredded pieces	1 cup	56	94	10	1	Tr
	Mushrooms					
679	Raw, sliced or chopped	1 cup	70	92	20	1	Tr
680	Cooked, drained	1 cup	156	91	40	3	1
681	Canned, drained solids	1 cup	156	91	35	3	Tr
682	Mustard greens, without stems and mid-ribs, cooked, drained	1 cup	140	94	20	3	Tr
683	Okra pods, 3 by ⅝ in, cooked	8 pods	85	90	25	2	Tr
	Onions					
	Raw					
684	Chopped	1 cup	160	91	55	2	Tr
685	Sliced	1 cup	115	91	40	1	Tr
686	Cooked (whole or sliced), drained	1 cup	210	92	60	2	Tr
687	Onions, spring, raw, bulb (⅜-in diam) and white portion of top	6 onions	30	92	10	1	Tr
688	Onion rings, breaded, parfried, frozen, prepared	2 rings	20	29	80	1	5
	Parsley					
689	Raw	10 sprigs	10	88	5	Tr	Tr
690	Freeze-dried	1 tbsp	0.4	2	Tr	Tr	Tr

P

| | Fatty Acids | | Carbo-hydrate (grams) | Calcium (mg) | Phos-phorus (mg) | Iron (mg) | Vitamin A Value | | Thiamin (mg) | Riboflavin (mg) | Niacin (mg) | Vitamin C (mg) |
Satu-rated (grams)	Monoun-saturated (grams)	Polyun-saturated (grams)					(IU) Inter-national Units	(RE) Retinol Equiv-alents				
Tr	Tr	Tr	1	4	5	0.1	10	1	0.01	0.01	0.1	1
0.1	Tr	0.3	7	147	44	1.9	12,290	1229	0.14	0.18	0.5	19
Tr	Tr	0.1	6	6	21	0.3	60	6	0.07	0.02	0.6	1
Tr	Tr	Tr	2	26	14	0.4	1030	103	0.04	0.04	0.2	3
Tr	Tr	0.2	4	52	38	0.5	1580	158	0.10	0.10	0.5	13
Tr	Tr	Tr	Tr	5	3	Tr	150	15	0.01	0.01	Tr	1
0.1	Tr	0.5	11	102	108	2.7	1780	178	0.25	0.16	1.0	21
Tr	Tr	0.1	3	26	27	0.7	450	45	0.06	0.04	0.3	5
Tr	Tr	0.1	1	10	11	0.3	180	18	0.03	0.02	0.1	2
Tr	Tr	0.1	2	38	14	0.8	1060	106	0.03	0.04	0.2	10
Tr	Tr	0.1	3	4	73	0.9	0	0	0.07	0.31	2.9	2
0.1	Tr	0.3	8	9	136	2.7	0	0	0.11	0.47	7.0	6
0.1	Tr	0.2	8	17	103	1.2	0	0	0.13	0.03	2.5	0
Tr	0.2	0.1	3	104	57	1.0	4240	424	0.06	0.09	0.6	35
Tr	Tr	Tr	6	54	48	0.4	490	49	0.11	0.05	0.7	14
0.1	0.1	0.2	12	40	46	0.6	0	0	0.10	0.02	0.2	13
0.1	Tr	0.1	8	29	33	0.4	0	0	0.07	0.01	0.1	10
0.1	Tr	0.1	13	57	48	0.4	0	0	0.09	0.02	0.2	12
Tr	Tr	Tr	2	18	10	0.6	1500	150	0.02	0.04	0.1	14
1.7	2.2	1.0	8	6	16	0.3	50	5	0.06	0.03	0.7	Tr
Tr	Tr	Tr	1	13	4	0.6	520	52	0.01	0.01	0.1	9
Tr	Tr	Tr	Tr	1	2	0.2	250	25	Tr	0.01	Tr	1

Continued.

P

Item Number	Foods, Approximate Measures, Units, and Weight (edible parts)		Weight (grams)	Water (percent)	Food Energy (calories)	Protein (grams)	Fat (grams)
	Vegetables and Vegetable Products—cont'd						
691	Parsnips, cooked (diced or 2 in lengths), drained	1 cup	156	78	125	2	Tr
692	Peas, edible pod, cooked, drained	1 cup	160	89	65	5	Tr
	Peas, green						
693	Canned, drained solids	1 cup	170	82	115	8	1
694	Frozen, cooked, drained	1 cup	160	80	125	8	Tr
	Peppers (red)						
695	Hot chili, raw	1 pepper	45	88	20	1	Tr
	Sweet (about 5 per lb, whole), stem and seeds removed						
696	Raw	1 pepper	74	93	20	1	Tr
697	Cooked, drained	1 pepper	73	95	15	Tr	Tr
	Potatoes, cooked						
	Baked (about 2 per lb, raw)						
698	With skin	1 potato	202	71	220	5	Tr
699	Flesh only	1 potato	156	75	145	3	Tr
	Boiled (about 3 per lb, raw)						
700	Peeled after boiling	1 potato	136	77	120	3	Tr
701	Peeled before boiling	1 potato	135	77	115	2	Tr
	French fried, strip, 2 to 3½ in long, frozen						
702	Oven heated	10 strips	50	53	110	2	4
703	Fried in vegetable oil	10 strips	50	38	160	2	8
	Potato products, prepared						
	Au gratin						
704	From dry mix	1 cup	245	79	230	6	10
705	Hash brown, from frozen	1 cup	156	56	340	5	18
	Mashed						
	From home recipe						
706	Milk added	1 cup	210	78	160	4	1
707	Milk and margarine added	1 cup	210	76	225	4	9
708	From dehydrated flakes (without milk), water, milk, butter, and salt added	1 cup	210	76	235	4	12
709	Potato salad, made with mayonnaise	1 cup	250	76	360	7	21
	Scalloped						
710	From dry mix	1 cup	245	79	230	5	11
711	Potato chips	10 chips	20	3	105	1	7
	Pumpkin						
712	Cooked from raw, mashed	1 cup	245	94	50	2	Tr
713	Canned	1 cup	245	90	85	3	1
714	Radishes, raw, stem ends, rootlets cut off	4 radishes	18	95	5	Tr	Tr
715	Sauerkraut, canned, solids and liquid	1 cup	236	93	45	2	Tr

27. Green peppers contain about 14 times less vitamin A.

	Fatty Acids		Carbo-hydrate (grams)	Calcium (mg)	Phos-phorus (mg)	Iron (mg)	Vitamin A Value		Thiamin (mg)	Riboflavin (mg)	Niacin (mg)	Vitamin C (mg)
Satu-rated (grams)	Monoun-saturated (grams)	Polyun-saturated (grams)					(IU) Inter-national Units	(RE) Retinol Equiv-alents				
0.1	0.2	0.1	30	58	108	0.9	0	0	0.13	0.08	1.1	20
0.1	Tr	0.2	11	67	88	3.2	210	21	0.20	0.12	0.9	77
0.1	0.1	0.3	21	34	114	1.6	1310	131	0.21	0.13	1.2	16
0.1	Tr	0.2	23	38	144	2.5	1070	107	0.45	0.16	2.4	16
Tr	Tr	Tr	4	8	21	0.5	4840[27]	484[27]	0.04	0.04	0.4	109
Tr	Tr	0.2	4	4	16	0.9	390[27]	39[27]	0.06	0.04	0.4	95
Tr	Tr	0.1	3	3	11	0.6	280[27]	28[27]	0.04	0.03	0.3	81
0.1	Tr	0.1	51	20	115	2.7	0	0	0.22	0.07	3.3	26
Tr	Tr	0.1	34	8	78	0.5	0	0	0.16	0.03	2.2	20
Tr	Tr	0.1	27	7	60	0.4	0	0	0.14	0.03	2.0	18
Tr	Tr	0.1	27	11	54	0.4	0	0	0.13	0.03	1.8	10
2.1	1.8	0.3	17	5	43	0.7	0	0	0.06	0.02	1.2	5
2.5	1.6	3.8	20	10	47	0.4	0	0	0.09	0.01	1.6	5
6.3	2.9	0.3	31	203	233	0.8	520	76	0.05	0.20	2.3	8
7.0	8.0	2.1	44	23	112	2.4	0	0	0.17	0.03	3.8	10
0.7	0.3	0.1	37	55	101	0.6	40	12	0.18	0.08	2.3	14
2.2	3.7	2.5	35	55	97	0.5	360	42	0.18	0.08	2.3	13
7.2	3.3	0.5	32	103	118	0.5	380	44	0.23	0.11	1.4	20
3.6	6.2	9.3	28	48	130	1.6	520	83	0.19	0.15	2.2	25
6.5	3.0	0.5	31	88	137	0.9	360	51	0.05	0.14	2.5	8
1.8	1.2	3.6	10	5	31	0.2	0	0	0.03	Tr	0.8	8
0.1	Tr	Tr	12	37	74	1.4	2650	265	0.08	0.19	1.0	12
0.4	0.1	Tr	20	64	86	3.4	54,040	5404	0.06	0.13	0.9	10
Tr	Tr	Tr	1	4	3	0.1	Tr	Tr	Tr	0.01	0.1	4
0.1	Tr	0.1	10	71	47	3.5	40	4	0.05	0.05	0.3	35

Continued.

P

Item Number	Foods, Approximate Measures, Units, and Weight (edible parts)		Weight (grams)	Water (percent)	Food Energy (calories)	Protein (grams)	Fat (grams)
	Vegetables and Vegetable Products—cont'd						
	Seaweed						
716	Kelp, raw	1 oz	28	82	10	Tr	Tr
717	Spirulina, dried	1 oz	28	5	80	16	2
	Southern peas. See Black-eyed peas, immature (items 641, 642), mature (item 457).						
	Spinach						
718	Raw, chopped	1 cup	55	92	10	2	Tr
	Cooked, drained						
719	From raw	1 cup	180	91	40	5	Tr
720	From frozen (leaf)	1 cup	190	90	55	6	Tr
721	Canned, drained solids	1 cup	214	92	50	6	1
722	Spinach souffle	1 cup	136	74	220	11	18
	Squash, cooked						
723	Summer (all varieties), sliced, drained	1 cup	180	94	35	2	1
724	Winter (all varieties), baked, cubed	1 cup	205	89	80	2	1
	Sweet potatoes						
	Cooked (raw, 5 by 2 in; about 2½ per lb):						
725	Baked in skin, peeled	1 potato	114	73	115	2	Tr
726	Boiled, without skin	1 potato	151	73	160	2	Tr
727	Candied, 2½ by 2 in, one piece	1 piece	105	67	145	1	3
	Canned						
728	Solid pack (mashed)	1 cup	255	74	260	5	1
729	Vacuum pack, piece 2¾ by 1 in	1 piece	40	76	35	1	Tr
	Tomatoes						
730	Raw, 2⅗-in diam (3 per 12-oz pkg)	1 tomato	123	94	25	1	Tr
731	Canned, solids and liquid	1 cup	240	94	50	2	1
732	Tomato juice, canned	1 cup	244	94	40	2	Tr
	Tomato products, canned						
733	Paste	1 cup	262	74	220	10	2
734	Puree	1 cup	250	87	105	4	Tr
735	Sauce	1 cup	245	89	75	3	Tr
736	Turnips, cooked, diced	1 cup	156	94	30	1	Tr
737	Vegetable juice cocktail, canned	1 cup	242	94	45	2	Tr
	Vegetables, mixed						
738	Canned, drained solids	1 cup	163	87	75	4	Tr
739	Frozen, cooked, drained	1 cup	182	83	105	5	Tr
740	Water chestnuts, canned, raw	1 cup	140	86	70	1	Tr

P

	Fatty Acids						Vitamin A Value					
Satu-rated (grams)	Monoun-saturated (grams)	Polyun-saturated (grams)	Carbo-hydrate (grams)	Calcium (mg)	Phos-phorus (mg)	Iron (mg)	(IU) Inter-national Units	(RE) Retinol Equiv-alents	Thiamin (mg)	Riboflavin (mg)	Niacin (mg)	Vitamin C (mg)
0.1	Tr	Tr	3	48	12	0.8	30	3	0.01	0.04	0.1	(¹)
0.8	0.2	0.6	7	34	33	8.1	160	16	0.67	1.04	3.6	3
Tr	Tr	0.1	2	54	27	1.5	3690	369	0.04	0.10	0.4	15
0.1	Tr	0.2	7	245	101	6.4	14,740	1474	0.17	0.42	0.9	18
0.1	Tr	0.2	10	277	91	2.9	14,790	1479	0.11	0.32	0.8	23
0.2	Tr	0.4	7	272	94	4.9	18,780	1878	0.03	0.30	0.8	31
7.1	6.8	3.1	3	230	231	1.3	3460	675	0.09	0.30	0.5	3
0.1	Tr	0.2	8	49	70	0.6	520	52	0.08	0.07	0.9	10
0.3	0.1	0.5	18	29	41	0.7	7290	729	0.17	0.05	1.4	20
Tr	Tr	0.1	28	32	63	0.5	24,880	2488	0.08	0.14	0.7	28
0.1	Tr	0.2	37	32	41	0.8	25,750	2575	0.08	0.21	1.0	26
1.4	0.7	0.2	29	27	27	1.2	4400	440	0.02	0.04	0.4	7
0.1	Tr	0.2	59	77	133	3.4	38,570	3857	0.07	0.23	2.4	13
Tr	Tr	Tr	8	9	20	0.4	3190	319	0.01	0.02	0.3	11
Tr	Tr	0.1	5	9	28	0.6	1390	139	0.07	0.06	0.7	22
0.1	0.1	0.2	10	62	46	1.5	1450	145	0.11	0.07	1.8	36
Tr	Tr	0.1	10	22	46	1.4	1360	136	0.11	0.08	1.6	45
0.3	0.4	0.9	49	92	207	7.8	6470	647	0.41	0.50	8.4	111
Tr	Tr	0.1	25	38	100	2.3	3400	340	0.18	0.14	4.3	88
0.1	0.1	0.2	18	34	78	1.9	2400	240	0.16	0.14	2.8	32
Tr	Tr	0.1	8	34	30	0.3	0	0	0.04	0.04	0.5	18
Tr	Tr	0.1	11	27	41	1.0	2830	283	0.10	0.07	1.8	67
0.1	Tr	0.2	15	44	68	1.7	18,990	1899	0.08	0.08	0.9	8
0.1	Tr	0.1	24	46	93	1.5	7780	778	0.13	0.22	1.5	6
Tr	Tr	Tr	17	6	27	1.2	10	1	0.02	0.03	0.5	2

Continued.

P

Item Number	Foods, Approximate Measures, Units, and Weight (edible parts)		Weight (grams)	Water (percent)	Food Energy (calories)	Protein (grams)	Fat (grams)
	Miscellaneous Items						
	Baking powders for home use						
	Sodium aluminum sulfate						
741	With monocalcium phosphate monohydrate	1 tsp	3	2	5	Tr	0
742	With monocalcium phosphate monohydrate, calcium sulfate	1 tsp	2.9	1	5	Tr	0
743	Straight phosphate	1 tsp	3.8	2	5	Tr	0
744	Low sodium	1 tsp	4.3	1	5	Tr	0
745	Catsup	1 cup	273	69	290	5	1
746	Chili powder	1 tsp	2.6	8	10	Tr	Tr
	Chocolate						
747	Bitter or baking	1 oz	28	2	145	3	15
	Semisweet; see Candy (item 594).						
748	Cinnamon	1 tsp	2.3	10	5	Tr	Tr
749	Curry powder	1 tsp	2	10	5	Tr	Tr
750	Garlic powder	1 tsp	2.8	6	10	Tr	Tr
760	Gelatin, dry	1 envelope	7	13	25	6	Tr
761	Mustard, prepared, yellow	1 tsp or individual pkt	5	80	5	Tr	Tr
	Olives, canned						
762	Green	4 medium or 3 extra large	13	78	15	Tr	2
763	Ripe, Mission, pitted	3 small or 2 large	9	73	15	Tr	2
764	Paprika	1 tsp	2.1	10	5	Tr	Tr
765	Pepper, black	1 tsp	2.1	11	5	Tr	Tr
	Pickles, cucumber						
766	Dill, medium, whole, 3¾ in long, 1¼-in diam	1 pickle	65	93	5	Tr	Tr
767	Fresh-pack, slices 1½-in diam, ¼ in thick	2 slices	15	79	10	Tr	Tr
768	Sweet, gherkin, small, whole, about 2½ in long, ¾-in diam	1 pickle	15	61	20	Tr	Tr
	Popcorn (See Grain products, items 421-423)						
769	Relish, finely chopped, sweet	1 tbsp	15	63	20	Tr	Tr
770	Salt	1 tsp	5.5	0	0	0	0
771	Vinegar, cider	1 tbsp	15	94	Tr	Tr	0
	Yeast						
772	Baker's, dry, active	1 pkg	7	5	20	3	Tr
773	Brewer's, dry	1 tbsp	8	5	25	3	Tr

| | Fatty Acids | | | | | | Vitamin A Value | | | | | |
Satu-rated (grams)	Monoun-saturated (grams)	Polyun-saturated (grams)	Carbo-hydrate (grams)	Calcium (mg)	Phos-phorus (mg)	Iron (mg)	(IU) Inter-national Units	(RE) Retinol Equiv-alents	Thiamin (mg)	Riboflavin (mg)	Niacin (mg)	Vitamin C (mg)
0.0	0.0	0.0	1	58	87	0.0	0	0	0.00	0.00	0.0	0
0.0	0.0	0.0	1	183	45	0.0	0	0	0.00	0.00	0.0	0
0.0	0.0	0.0	1	239	359	0.0	0	0	0.00	0.00	0.0	0
0.0	0.0	0.0	1	207	314	0.0	0	0	0.00	0.00	0.0	0
0.2	0.2	0.4	69	60	137	2.2	3820	382	0.	0.19	4.4	41
0.1	0.1	0.2	1	7	8	0.4	910	91	0.01	0.02	0.2	2
9.0	4.9	0.5	8	22	109	1.9	10	1	0.01	0.07	0.4	0
Tr	Tr	Tr	2	28	1	0.9	10	1	Tr	Tr	Tr	1
—	—	—	1	10	7	0.6	20	2	0.01	0.01	0.1	Tr
Tr	Tr	Tr	2	2	12	0.1	0	0	0.01	Tr	Tr	Tr
Tr	Tr	Tr	0	1	0	0.0	0	0	0.00	0.00	0.0	0
Tr	0.2	Tr	Tr	4	4	0.1	0	0	Tr	0.01	Tr	Tr
0.2	1.2	0.1	Tr	8	2	0.2	40	4	Tr	Tr	Tr	0
0.3	1.3	0.2	Tr	10	2	0.2	10	1	Tr	Tr	Tr	0
Tr	Tr	0.2	1	4	7	0.5	1270	127	0.01	0.04	0.3	1
Tr	Tr	Tr	1	9	4	0.6	Tr	Tr	Tr	0.01	Tr	0
Tr	Tr	0.1	1	17	14	0.7	70	7	Tr	0.01	Tr	4
Tr	Tr	Tr	3	5	4	0.3	20	2	Tr	Tr	Tr	1
Tr	Tr	Tr	5	2	2	0.2	10	1	Tr	Tr	Tr	1
Tr	Tr	Tr	5	3	2	0.1	20	2	Tr	Tr	0.0	1
0.0	0.0	0.0	0	14	3	Tr	0	0	0.00	0.00	0.0	0
0.0	0.0	0.0	1	1	1	0.1	0	0	0.00	0.00	0.0	0
Tr	0.1	Tr	3	3	90	1.1	Tr	Tr	0.16	0.38	2.6	Tr
Tr	Tr	0.0	3	17	140	1.4	Tr	Tr	1.25	0.34	3.0	Tr

Continued.

Item Number	Foods, Approximate Measures, Units, and Weight (edible parts)		Weight (grams)	Water (percent)	Food Energy (calories)	Protein (grams)	Fat (grams)
	Beverages						
	Alcoholic						
	Beer						
774	Regular	12 fl oz	360	92	150	1	0
775	Light	12 fl oz	355	95	95	1	0
	Gin, rum, vodka, whiskey						
776	80-proof	1½ fl oz	42	67	95	0	0
777	86-proof	1½ fl oz	42	64	105	0	0
778	90-proof	1½ fl oz	42	62	110	0	0
	Wines						
779	Dessert	3½ fl oz	103	77	140	Tr	0
	Table						
780	Red	3½ fl oz	102	88	75	Tr	0
781	White	3½ fl oz	102	87	80	Tr	0
	Carbonated[28]						
782	Club soda	12 fl oz	370	89	151	0	0
	Cola type						
783	Regular	12 fl oz	355	100	0	0	0
784	Diet, artificially sweetened	12 fl oz	355	100	Tr	0	0
785	Ginger ale	12 fl oz	366	91	125	0	0
786	Grape	12 fl oz	372	88	160	0	0
787	Lemon-lime	12 fl oz	372	89	150	0	0
787	Orange	12 fl oz	372	88	180	0	0
789	Pepper type	12 fl oz	369	89	150	0	0
790	Root beer	12 fl oz	370	89	150	0	0
	Cocoa and chocolate-flavored beverages. See Dairy Products (items 64-66).						
	Coffee						
791	Brewed	6 fl oz	180	100	Tr	Tr	Tr
792	Instant, prepared (2 tsp powder plus 6 fl oz water)	6 fl oz	182	99	Tr	Tr	Tr
	Fruit drinks, noncarbonated						
	Canned						
792	Fruit punch drink	6 fl oz	190	88	85	Tr	0
793	Grape drink	6 fl oz	187	86	100	Tr	0
794	Pineapple-grapefruit juice drink	6 fl oz	187	87	90	Tr	Tr
	Frozen						
	Lemonade concentrate						
795	Undiluted	6-fl-oz can	219	49	425	Tr	Tr
796	Diluted with 4⅓ parts water by volume	6 fl oz	185	89	80	Tr	Tr
	Fruit juices. See type under Fruits and Fruit Juices.						
	Milk beverages. See Dairy Products (items 61-73).						
	Tea						
797	Brewed	8 fl oz	240	100	Tr	Tr	Tr
	Instant, powder, prepared						
	Unsweetened (1 tsp powder plus 8 fl oz water)	8 fl oz	241	100	Tr	Tr	Tr
799	Sweetened (3 tsp powder plus 8 fl oz water)	8 fl oz	262	91	85	Tr	Tr

28. Water source influences the mineral content.

P

| Fatty Acids | | | Carbo-hydrate (grams) | Calcium (mg) | Phos-phorus (mg) | Iron (mg) | Vitamin A Value | | Thiamin (mg) | Riboflavin (mg) | Niacin (mg) | Vitamin C (mg) |
Satu-rated (grams)	Monoun-saturated (grams)	Polyun-saturated (grams)					(IU) Inter-national Units	(RE) Retinol Equiv-alents				
0.0	0.0	0.0	13	14	50	0.1	0	0	0.02	0.09	1.8	0
0.0	0.0	0.0	5	14	43	0.1	0	0	0.03	0.11	1.4	0
0.0	0.0	0.0	Tr	Tr	Tr	Tr	0	0	Tr	Tr	Tr	0
0.0	0.0	0.0	Tr	Tr	Tr	Tr	0	0	Tr	Tr	Tr	0
0.0	0.0	0.0	Tr	Tr	Tr	Tr	0	0	Tr	Tr	Tr	0
0.0	0.0	0.0	8	8	9	0.2	—	—	0.01	0.02	0.2	0
0.0	0.0	0.0	3	8	18	0.4	—	—	0.00	0.03	0.1	0
0.0	0.0	0.0	3	9	14	0.3	—	—	0.00	0.01	0.1	0
0.0	0.0	0.0	0	18	0	Tr	0	0	0.00	0.00	0.0	0
0.0	0.0	0.0	41	11	52	0.2	0	0	0.00	0.00	0.0	0
0.0	0.0	0.0	Tr	14	39	0.2	0	0	0.00	0.00	0.0	0
0.0	0.0	0.0	32	11	0	0.1	0	0	0.00	0.00	0.0	0
0.0	0.0	0.0	46	15	0	0.4	0	0	0.00	0.00	0.0	0
0.0	0.0	0.0	39	7	0	0.4	0	0	0.00	0.00	0.0	0
0.0	0.0	0.0	46	15	4	0.3	0	0	0.00	0.00	0.0	0
0.0	0.0	0.0	41	11	41	0.1	0	0	0.00	0.00	0.0	0
0.0	0.0	0.0	42	15	0	0.2	0	0	0.00	0.00	0.0	0
Tr	Tr	Tr	Tr	4	2	Tr	0	0	0.00	0.02	0.4	0
Tr	Tr	Tr	1	2	6	0.1	0	0	0.00	0.00	0.6	0
0.0	0.0	0.0	22	15	2	0.4	20	2	0.03	0.04	Tr	61[9]
0.0	0.0	0.0	26	2	2	0.3	Tr	Tr	0.01	0.01	Tr	64[9]
Tr	Tr	Tr	23	13	7	0.9	60	6	0.06	0.04	0.5	110[9]
Tr	Tr	Tr	112	9	13	0.4	40	4	0.04	0.07	0.7	66
Tr	Tr	Tr	21	2	2	0.1	10	1	0.01	0.02	0.2	13
Tr	Tr	Tr	Tr	0	2	Tr	0	0	0.00	0.03	Tr	0
Tr	Tr	Tr	1	1	4	Tr	0	0	0.00	0.02	0.1	0
Tr	Tr	Tr	22	1	3	Tr	0	0	0.00	0.04	0.1	0

Glossary

Absorption Transfer of nutrients and other substances into the body or into cells. (18)

Acne Inflammation of the skin causing pimples, cysts, and scars. (417)

Additives Chemicals added to food, either intentionally (sweeteners, nutrients) or unintentionally during growing or processing of foods. (345)

Adenosine Triphosphate (ATP) A storage form of energy; used as an immediate source of energy. (276)

Amenorrhea Absence or suppression of menstruation. (316)

Amino Acids Naturally occurring chemicals that act as the building blocks of protein in the human body and in foods; there are about 20. (34)

Amniotic Fluid Fluid that protects the fetus from injury and helps maintain an even temperature in the womb. (245)

Anemia Low oxygen-carrying capacity of blood; often caused by low hemoglobin because of insufficient dietary iron. (10)

Anorexia Eating disorder involving loss of appetite or self-starvation due to distorted body image. (294)

Anthropometric Measurements May include body weight, height, arm and head circumference, and skinfold thickness. (38)

Antibodies Blood proteins that inactivate proteins foreign to the body. (11)

Antioxidant Protects other compounds from the harmful effects of oxygen. (15)

Atherosclerosis Deposit of plaques in the inner walls of arteries. (124)

Autism A self-centered mental state from which reality tends to be excluded. (412)

Basal Energy Energy needed to maintain life. (270)

BHT, BHA Butylated hydroxytoluene, butylated hydroxyanisole; food additives that are antioxidants. (107)

Bile A liquid made in the liver and stored in the gallbladder that is secreted into small intestine. Bile aids in fat digestion. (91)

Bioavailability The amount of a nutrient that can be used by the body. (205)

Body Mass Index A meaningful measure of ideal body weight that includes body weight (in kilograms) divided by height (in meters squared). (297)

Bonding The formation of a close relationship between infant and parents. (382)

Brown Adipose Tissue (BAT) Helps maintain body temperature so that less energy is lost in heat loss from the body. (274)

Bulimia Eating large quantities of food at one time (binging), followed by artificial elimination of the food (purging) by vomiting, laxatives, etc. (294)

Calipers An instrument with spring-loaded arms that measures folds of body fat. (298)

Calories See kilocalorie. (37)

Carbohydrates Contain carbon, hydrogen, and oxygen arranged as monosaccharides, disaccharides, and polysaccharides. (69)

Carotenoids A group of yellow and red pigments structurally related to carotene; some are converted into retinol in the body. (177)

Carrier A chemical that provides transportation for another chemical across a membrane. (144)

Catabolism The breakdown of complex molecules. (29)

Cell Membrane The cell wall around the outside of cells. (104)

Cellulose Polysaccharide containing glucose; found in plants; indigestible by humans. (69)

Chlorophyll Green pigment in plants; uses sunlight to make carbohydrates from carbon dioxide and water. (75)

Cholesterol Substance found in the body; related to lipids; made in the body and consumed in some foods of animal origin. A human adult body has about 140 g. Most kinds of cholesterol are found in all membranes. Cholesterol is the raw material in the synthesis of sex hormones, vitamin D, and bile salts. (54)

Crohn's Disease Chronic inflammation of the intestine. (444)

Cirrhosis Degenerative disease of the liver seen often in alcoholics. (256)

Coenzymes Substances needed by some enzymes before enzyme activity occurs; several are B-complex vitamins. (34)

Collagen A protein; acts as the "scaffolding" around cells; a major part of tendons. (33)

Colostrum Breast milk secreted during the first 2 or 3 days after delivery of the infant. (384)

Complementary or Supplementary Proteins When two or more food proteins *together* have the proportion of essential amino acids needed by the body. (153)

Cretinism Mental and physical retardation in children caused by iodine deficiency during pregnancy. (42)

Crude Fiber A number expressing the fiber content of a food; obtained from older methods. This value should not be used now, although it is still found on labels. (80)

Cystic Fibrosis Hereditary disease that affects most glands, causing abnormal secretions. (444)

Degree of Saturation Saturated means all carbons have their maximum amount of hydrogens; unsaturated fat has some carbons without the maximum amount of hydrogen. (105)

Denatures Changes in the shape of a protein molecule. Usually produced by heat, acid, alkali, alcohol. (144)

Dental Caries Cavities in teeth; one of the most common health problems in the world. Oral bacteria produce acid by fermenting dietary carbohydrates; the acid destroys tooth enamel. (71)

Diabetes Type I (insulin-dependent or juvenile) diabetes is a genetic condition, usually first seen in childhood; the pancreas fails to produce enough insulin to control blood sugar levels. Type II (non-insulin-dependent or maturity-onset) diabetes is seen especially in obesity; the pancreas produces sufficient insulin, but there is interference in glucose uptake by cells with the help of insulin; it can often be corrected by weight loss. (38)

Diastolic Pressure Blood pressure measured when the heart is relaxed. (441)

Dietary Fiber Realistic measure of what happens to fiber in the digestive tract. (80)

Dietary Thermogenesis Body heat produced by metabolizing food. (270)

Digestion The breakdown of nutrients in ingested foods into a form suitable for absorption from the gastrointestinal tract into the blood. (18)

Dipeptides, Tripeptides Two and three amino acids, respectively, joined by peptide bonds. (144)

Disaccharide Simple sugars with two monosaccharides linked together—sucrose, lactose, maltose (di = two). (69)

Diuretics Agents that increase the volume of urine. (247)

DNA Deoxyribonucleic acid; found in the nucleus of cells and determines the hereditary makeup of an individual. (34)

Down's Syndrome Preferred name for mongolism; a form of mental retardation. (444)

Dysgeusia Impairment or perversion of the normal sense of taste. (444)

Edema Accumulation of an excessive amount of watery fluid in cells. (163)

Emulsifier Allows water and fatty substances to mix; breaks large fat globules into many smaller ones. (104)

Endocrine Another name for hormonal. (319)

Enzymes Proteins that speed up biochemical reactions. (33)

Epinephrine A hormone secreted by the adrenal gland in emergencies to speed the release of glucose; better known as *adrenaline*. (83)

Epithelial Cells The cells that form the outermost part of the body (skin) and line body cavities (gastrointestinal, respiratory, genitourinary tracts). (178)

Essential Amino Acid An amino acid that cannot be synthesized by the body at a rate required for adequate growth and maintenance. (137)

Essential Fatty Acid Linoleic acid; cannot be made by the body in an amount sufficient for normal needs of the body. (33)

Estrogens Female sex hormones. (191)

Fatty Acid An organic acid containing carbon and hydrogen; forms a lipid when combined with glycerol. (104)

Fetal Alcohol Syndrome (FAS) Abnormalities in newborns born to alcoholic mothers. (379)

Fetus A child in utero from the third month to birth. Until the third month it is called an embryo. (365)

Fiber Part of plants indigestible to humans, but digestible by bacteria, cattle, and some other animals; example, cellulose. (72)

Fructose A monosaccharide found mainly in fruits and honey. (69)

Galactose A monosaccharide found mainly as part of the disaccharide lactose. (69)

Geophagy or pica Eating clay, starch, ashes, or plaster. (202)

Glucagon Hormone secreted by the pancreas; it has the opposite function to insulin—helping the breakdown of glycogen and fat. (83)

Glucose A monosaccharide; the essential carbohydrate. (69)

Glycemic Index (GI) Measures changes in blood glucose caused by different foods eaten by diabetics; high GI values mean higher blood glucose levels. (85)

Glycerol All fats and oils have glycerol as part of their structure; has three carbon chains that can attach to three fatty acids. (104)

Glycogen A polysaccharide consisting of many glucose units joined together; storage form of carbohydrate in muscles and liver. (69)

Goiter Enlargement of the thyroid gland from iodine deficiency. (42)

Gout A type of painful arthritis affecting especially the toes and fingers. May be genetic, but associated usually with the "good life"—high intakes of protein and alcohol. Treated by diet change or with drugs. (54)

Health Food Term used on labels; these foods have no special health-giving properties. (11)

Hemoglobin Iron-containing protein in red blood cells; carries oxygen to the cells and carbon dioxide back to the lungs. (34)

Hemolytic Anemia An anemia caused by the breaking down of red blood cells. (182)

Hormones Chemical messengers secreted by certain glands; may affect metabolism at other sites in the body. (33)

Hydrogenation Addition of hydrogen to unsaturated fat; used to harden oils in some manufactured foods, such as margarines. (107)

Hydrolyze To use water in the chemical breakdown of a substance; for example, digestion is the hydrolysis of carbohydrate, fat, and protein. (88)

Hydroxyapatite The hard substance between cells in bones and teeth; contains calcium, phosphorus, hydrogen, and oxygen. (209)

Hypercarotenemia High levels of carotene (vitamin A percursor) in the blood. (319)

Hypertension High blood pressure. (7)

IgA Antibody A major antibody in the blood. (140)

Insulin Hormone produced by the pancreas. It removes excess glucose from blood, helps glucose enter cells, and helps in storing excess as glycogen or fat. (83)

Jejunoileal The jejunum is the second portion, and the ileum is the lower three fifths of the small intestine. (311)

Keratinization A hardening of the skin caused by a lack of mucus. (178)

Ketones When carbohydrates are not available, fat is broken down incompletely to ketones. The presence of high levels of ketones in urine and blood is known as ketosis. (84)

Ketosis High levels of ketones in the blood. (84)

Kilocalorie (kcal) A unit of heat used to measure energy in food and in the body. (37)

Kwashiorkor A deficiency disease mainly in children caused by a diet deficient in protein but adequate in energy. (322)

Lean Body Mass The soft tissue—for example, heart, muscles, liver; excludes adipose tissue and bone. (147)

Lecithin A phospholipid made in the liver; an important part of cell membranes; an emulsifier in the body and in foods; high amounts are present in soy and egg yolks. (104)

Legumes Plants of the bean and pea families. (43)

Linoleic Acid Essential fatty acid, polyunsaturated, in highest amounts in foods from plants. (108)

Lipids Fats, oils, and related substances, including cholesterol and phospholipids. (104)

Lipoprotein Combination of lipids with protein; water-insoluble lipids are transported in the blood in water-soluble form as lipoproteins. (108)

Lymphatic System Transports some lipids and some other nutrients after ab-

sorption from the gastrointestinal tract; it drains eventually into the blood. (114)

Macromineral Essential mineral whose RDA is over 100 mg per day. (203)

Marasmus Deficiency of protein and energy (starvation). (322)

Megaloblastic Anemia An anemia, or lack of oxygen-carrying capacity of the blood, caused by large, irregularly shaped red blood cells. (191)

Metabolism Chemical changes occurring in tissues; consists of anabolism (buildup) and catabolism (breakdown) of molecules. (29)

Micelles Combination of lipids and bile salts that bring lipids from the gastrointestinal tract into contact with the intestinal cell wall; from there, the lipids are absorbed into the circulation. (114)

Micromineral or Trace Element Essential mineral whose RDA is less than 20 mg per day (223)

Milk bank Expressed human milk saved for future use. (384)

Monosaccharide Simple sugar with five or six carbon atoms—glucose, fructose, galactose (mono = one). (69)

Multiple Sclerosis A chronic, slowly progressive disease of the central nervous system. (443)

Myoglobin Transports oxygen and carbon dioxide in muscles; it gives muscle its red color. (203)

Natural Food Unprocessed food. (11)

Neurological Pertaining to the nervous system. (208)

Neurotransmitters Chemicals produced by the body to transmit nerve impulses between nerve cells. (141)

Nutrients Chemicals in food needed to maintain life. (3)

Obesity More than 20% over ideal body weight. (32)

Omega-3 Fatty Acids A group of polyunsaturated fatty acids; in highest amounts in fish oils. (123)

Organic Food Food produced without artificial fertilizers, pesticides, or additives. (11)

Osmosis Passage of certain fluids through a membrane. (163)

Osteomalacia Softening of bones, caus-

ing deformities; occurs in adults because of deficiencies of calcium and vitamin D. (181)

Osteoporosis Loss of bone in adults, especially postmenopausal women. (10)

Overweight Between 10% and 20% over ideal body weight. (48)

Pellagra Deficiency of miacin; most common when corn (maize) is a major part of the diet. (169)

Peptide Bond The link between amino acids that allows formation of a protein molecule. (138)

Periodontal Disease Disease of the bone and gums supporting teeth. (442)

pH Measure of the degree of acidity or alkalinity. (245)

Phospholipids One of three fatty acids in a triglyceride is replaced by a phosphorus-containing unit. (104)

Pica See Geophagy. (202)

Placenta The part of the uterus through which the fetus receives its nutrients. (378)

Plaque Deposits of cholesterol and calcium in the smooth muscle lining arteries. (123)

Polysaccharides Complex carbohydrates formed from many monosaccharides linked together—starch, dextrin, glycogen, cellulose (poly = many). (69)

Precursors Substances available in food that can be converted into the active form of the vitamin in the body; also called provitamins. (177)

Premenstrual Syndrome (PMS) Several unpleasant symptoms occurring before and thought to be related to menstruation. (431)

Protein Complex combinations of amino acids that are essential parts of all living cells. (135)

Protein-Energy Malnutrition Deficiency of protein and energy; severe effects in children; one of the most common nutrition disorders. Also called protein-calorie malnutrition (PCN). (136)

Recommended Dietary Allowance (RDA) Recommended nutrient intake to maintain health of people in the United States. (44)

Retinol An active form of vitamin A found in foods of animal origin. (177)

Ribosome Subcellular part of the cell involved in protein synthesis. (30)

Rickets Defective formation of bone caused by vitamin D deficiency. (180)

RNA Ribonucleic acid; found mainly outside the nucleus of the cell; controls manufacture of body proteins, including enzymes. (34)

Rods Light-sensitive cells in the retina of the eye. (178)

Salicylates Organic compounds occurring naturally in many foods of plant origin. (412)

Saliva The fluid in the mouth. (90)

Scurvy Vitamin C deficiency. (169)

Starch Polysaccharides containing glucose; found in plants; digestible by humans. (69)

Sterols Fat-related substances, including cholesterol, sex hormones, vitamin D; soluble in fat solvents. (104)

Subcutaneous Fat Fat that is nearest to the skin. (115)

Sucrose Disaccharide composed of glucose and fructose; table sugar. (69)

Suction Lipectomy Removal of fat from under the skin (subcutaneous). (311)

Sugar Alcohols Structures similar to simple sugars that are used as sweeteners. (71)

Systolic Pressure Blood pressure measured when the heart is contracting. (441)

Tannin Naturally occurring chemical found in tea and unripe fruits; decreases iron absorption. (254)

Thyroid Hormones Produced by thyroid gland in neck; require iodine for activity; control energy metabolism. (34)

Total Parenteral Nutrition Infusion of all nutrients through a vein. (417)

Toxemia The condition caused by the presence of toxic substances in the blood; symptoms include edema and hypertension during pregnancy. (373)

Toxicants Chemicals that harm the human body. (13)

Trace Element See Microminerals. (223)

Trans Fatty Acids Some polyunsaturated fatty acids twisted into unusual shapes during hydrogenation; enzymes involved in fat metabolism cannot react on these unusual shapes. (119)

Triglycerides Three fatty acids attached to one molecule of glycerol; most of the fat and oil in our food and body are triglycerides. (105)

Underweight Less than ideal body weight. (314)

Vegan A person who does not eat foods of animal origin (meat, fish, poultry, milk, eggs). (405)

Vegetarian A person who does not eat meat, fish, or poultry. (415)

Vitamin An organic substance that cannot be synthesized by the body; required in small amounts and essential for body functions. (166)

Women's, Infants', and Children's Program (WIC) Nutritional and medical support from federal funds for low-income women with high-risk pregnancies. (405)

Xerophthalmia Hardening of the epithelium of the eye, leading to blindness; usually caused by vitamin A deficiency. (178)

Zygote A fertilized ovum (egg). (377)

Index

Page numbers in *italics* indicate illustrations. Page numbers
followed by *t* indicate tables.

Credits

Front matter *p. i*, Michael Furman Ltd.; *p. ii*, Michael Furman Ltd.; *p. v (top)*, Nancy Brown/Image Bank; *(bottom)*, Doug Menuez/Picture Group; *p. vi*, Tom Tracy/Stock Shop; *p. vii*, Jon Riley/Stock Shop; *p. viii*, © Yanotti/Stock Shop; *p. ix*, Adina Tovy/Stock Shop; *p. x*, Jaques M. Chenet/Woodfin Camp & Assoc.; *p. xi*, FourByFive; *p. xii*, Michael Hamashita/Stock Shop; *p. xiii*, Dick Luria/Stock Shop; *p. xiv*, Ken Lax/Stock Shop; *p. xv*, Charles William Bush/Stock Shop; *p. xvi*, W. Bokelburg/Image Bank; *p. xvii*, Tom Tracy/Stock Shop; *p. xviii*, Murray Alcosser/Image Bank; *p. xix*, FourByFive; *p. xx*, Frank Siteman/Picture Cube; *p. xxi*, Murray Alcosser/Image Bank; *p. xxii*, FourByFive; *p. xxiii*, June Harrison/Stock Shop; *p. xxiv*, David Vance/Image Bank; *p. xxv*, FourByFive; *p. xxvi*, Jeffrey Reed/Stock Shop; *p. xxvii*, Jeffrey Reed/Stock Shop; *p. xxviii*, Lester Sloan/Woodfin Camp & Assoc.; *p. xxix*, NASA Lyndon B. Johnson Center.

Chapter 1 Fig. 1-2, adapted from Harlan, J.R., Scientific American, September 1976; *Fig. 1-3*, from National Restaurant Association 1983 telephone survey results, Food Engineering, April, 1984; *p. 8 (bottom)*, H. Armstrong Roberts; *p. 9 (top)*, H. Armstrong Roberts; *(bottom)*, American Source Photography; *p. 12 (top)*, Ken Regan/Camera 5; *(bottom)*, Doug Menuez/Picture Group; *Table 1-2*, from ACSH News & Views, 3(1): 1,1982, reprinted from Vickery, C.E., Philips, J.A., and Crenshaw, M.A., Health Values 9:13, 1985; *Fig. 1-8*, adapted from Hegsted, D.M., and Ausman, L.J., Sole foods and some not so scientific experiments, Nutrition Today, 8:22, 1973; *Fig. 1-10*, adapted from Finean, J.B., and others: Membranes and their cellular functions, John Wiley & Sons, Inc., New York, 1978.

Chapter 2 Table 2-2, human data from Grande, F., and Keys, A.: Body weight, body composition and calorie status. In Modern Nutrition in Health and Disease, 6th ed., editors, Goodhart, R.S., and Shils, M.E., Lea & Febiger, Philadelphia, 1980. Food composition data from Composition of Foods, Agricultural Handbook No. 8, U.S. Department of Agriculture, 1963; *Fig. 2-2*, adapted from America's changing diet, FDA Consumer, p. 4, Oct. 1985; *Fig. 2-3*, 1985 Agriculture Chartbook, Agricultural Handbook No. 652, and 1984 Handbook of Agricultural Charts, Agricultural Handbook No. 637, from U.S. Department of Agriculture; *Fig. 2-4*, Smil, V., China's food, Scientific American, December 1985; *Table 2-3*, adapted from Latham, M.C., International nutrition problems and policies. In World Food Issues, ed. 2, editor, Drosdoff, M., Center for the Analysis of World Food Issues, Cornell University, 1984. *Table 2-4*, from Franz, M.J., and others: Exchange lists (revised 1986), Journal of the American Dietetic Association, **87**:28, 1987; *Table 2-6*, adapted from Guthrie, H.: Introductory nutrition, ed. 6, Times Mirror/Mosby College Publishing, St. Louis, 1986; *p. 52 (top)*, Image Bank; *(bottom)*, FourbyFive; *Table 2-7*, adapted from McNutt, K.W., and others: Consumer perceptions on consumer protection, Food, Drug, Cosmetic Law Journal, **39**:86, 1984; *Fig. 2-8*, Peterkin, B.B.: Making food dollars count, Family Economics Review, **4**:23, 1983; *p. 59*, FourbyFive.

Chapter 3 *p. 68 (quote)*, Yudkin, J., Sweet—and sour, *Nature*, **316**:770, 1985; *Table 3-2*, adapted from Ensminger, A.H., and others: Food for health—a nutrition encyclopedia, Pegus Press, Clovis, CA, 1986; *Table 3-3*, adapted from Dahlquist, A.: Carbohydrates. In Present knowledge in nutrition, ed. 5, The Nutrition Foundation, Inc., Washington, D.C., 1984. *Table 3-4*, values obtained from Tufts University Diet and Nutrition Letter, 3(3), May, 1985; *Fig. 3-5*, adapted from Lanza, E., and Butrum, R.R.: A critical review of food fiber analysis and data, Journal of the American Dietetic Association, **86**:732, 1986; *Fig. 3-6*, adapted from Welsh, S.O., and Marston, R.M.: Review of trends in food use in the United States—1909-13 to 1980, Journal of the American Dietetic Association, **81**:120, 1982; *Fig. 3-8*, from Linder, M.C., editor: Nutritional biochemistry and metabolism, Elsevier, NY, 1985; *Table 3-6*, adapted from Jenkins, D.J.A., and others: The glycemic response to carbohydrate foods, *Lancet ii*:388,

1984; *p. 92 (left)*, Kathryn Dudek/Photo News; *(right)*, © David Madison 1987.

Chapter 4 *p. 102 (quote)*, Klein, F.C., Embargo aftermath, The Wall Street Journal, Sept. 7, 1978; *Fig. 4-1*, adapted from Bunch, K.L.: Consumption trends favor fresh, lowfat, and sweet, National Food Review, Winter 1986; *Fig. 4-2*, adapted from Welsh, S.O., and Marston, R.M.: Review of trends in food use in the United States, 1909 to 1980, Journal of the American Dietetic Association, **81**:120, 1982; *Table 4-1*, Economic Research Service, U.S. Department of Agriculture; *Table 4-3*, adapted from Hepburn, F.N., and others: Provisional tables on the content of omega-3 fatty acids and other fat components of selected foods, Journal of the American Dietetic Association, **86**:788, 1986; *Table 4-4*, adapted from Hoeg, J.M., and others: An approach to the management of hyperlipoproteinemia, Journal of the American Medical Association, **255**:512, 1986; *p. 115*, Randee Ladden, Chicago, IL; *Fig. 4-5 (top)*, adapted from Lohman, T.G.: Body composition, The Physician and Sportsmedicine, **14**:144, March 1986; *(bottom)*, Cohn, S.H., and others: Improved models for determination of body fat by in vivo neutron activation, American Journal of Clinical Nutrition, **40**: 255, 1984; *p. 119*, Bill Gallery/Stock, Boston; *Fig. 4-7*, National Cancer Institute; *Fig. 4-9*, adapted from Ahrens, E.H., and Boucher, C.A.: The composition of a simulated American diet, Journal of the American Dietetic Association, **73**:613, 1978; *p. 124*, from Gernsheim Collection, Harry Ranson Humanities Research Center, University of Texas at Austin; *Fig. 4-10*, Stallones, R.: Ischemic heart disease and lipids in blood and diet, *Annual Review of Public Health*, 1983.

Chapter 5 *p. 136 (quote)*, Ballentine, C., The essential guide to amino acids, FDA Consumer, p. 23, Sept. 1985; *Fig. 5-5*, adapted from Pellett, P.L., and Young, V.R., editors: Nutritional evaluation of protein foods, Food and Nutrition Bulletin, (suppl.) **4**:30, 1980; *Fig. 5-6*, National Food Review, Winter, 1986.

Chapter 6 *p. 165* (quote), Fried, J., Vitamin Politics, New York, Prometheus Books, 1984; *Table 6-4*, adapted from Hathcock, J.N.: Quantitative evaluation of vitamin safety, Pharmacy Times, May 1985; *Fig. 6-2*, adapted from Hathcock, J.: Vitamin safety: a current appraisal, Vitamin Issues, **5**(1):4; *Table 6-6*, adapted from Alhadeff, L., and others: Toxic effects of water-soluble vitamins, Nutrition Reviews, **42**:33, 1984; *Table 6-8*, adapted from Roe, D.A.: Nutrient and drug interactions, Nutrition Reviews, **42**:141, 1984; *Fig. 6-4*, data from Harris, R.S., and Von Loesecke, H.: Nutritional evaluation of food processing, John Wiley and Sons, Inc., New York, 1960; *p. 176 (top)*, Tom Tracy/Medichrome; *(bottom)*, FourbyFive; *Fig. 6-10*, Schilling, R.F.: Is nitrous oxide a dangerous anesthetic for vitamin B$_{12}$ deficient subjects? Journal of the American Medical Association, **255**:1605, 1986; *Fig. 6-11*, from U.S. Department of Agriculture; *Fig. 6-13*, adapted from Linder, M.C., Nutritional Biochemistry and Metabolism, Elsevier, New York, 1985; *Fig. 6-14*, data from Peterkin, B.B., and others: Changes in dietary patterns, Journal of the American Dietetics Association, **78**:453, 1981.

Chapter 7 *p. 202* (quote), Frate, P.A., Last of the earth eaters, The Sciences, p. 34, Nov./Dec., 1984; Table 7-1, adapted from Linder, M.C.: Nutritional biochemistry and metabolism, Elsevier, New York, 1985; *Fig. 7-2*, adapted from Pennington, J.A.T., and others: Selected mineral in food surveys, 1974 to 1981/1982, Journal of the American Dietetic Association, **84**:771, 1984; *Table 7-2*, adapted from Pennington, J.A.T, and others: Selected mineral in food surveys, 1974 to 1981/1982, Journal of the American Dietetic Association, **84**:771, 1984; *p. 209*, from Thibodeau, G.A.: Anatomy and physiology, Times Mirror/Mosby College Publishing, St. Louis, 1987; *Fig. 7-4*, data from U.S. Department of Agriculture, 1985 Agricultural Chartbook, Agricultural Handbook No. 652, p. 44, 1985; *p. 211*, Bernard Gotfryd/Woodfin Camp & Assoc.; *Figs. 7-5 and 7-7*, from Calcuin, A., Summary of current research for the health professional, National Dairy Council, Rosemont, IL, 1984; *Table 7-5*, U.S. Department of Agriculture, Home and Garden Bulletin No. 232-6, April, 1986; *Table 7-10*, adapted from Hathcock, J.N.: Quantitative evaluation of vitamin safety, Pharmacy Times, May 1985; *p. 227*, courtesy Dr. Eduardo Gaitan, University of Mississippi Medical Center. In Hickman, C.P., Roberts, L.S., and Hickman, F.: Integrated principles of zoology, ed. 8, Times Mirror/Mosby College

Publishing, St. Louis, 1988; *p. 232*, Bernard Gotfryd/Woodfin Camp & Assoc.; *Fig. 7-11*, from Guthrie, H.: Introductory nutrition, ed. 6, Times Mirror/Mosby College Publishing, St. Louis, 1986.

Chapter 8 *p. 237* (quote), Anonymous, Getting the most from the most essential nutrient, Tufts University Diet and Nutrient Newsletter, 4, No. 8, Oct. 1986; p. 238 (quote), Crick, F., Life Itself: Its origin and nature, Simon & Schuster, New York, 124, 1982; *Table 8-1*, adapted from Banks, P., and others: The biochemistry of the tissues, ed. 2, John Wiley & Sons, Inc., London, 1976; *Table 8-2*, the author gratefully acknowledges the following people who provided data in 1985 from which this information was obtained: Quana E. Caldwell, City of Atlanta Department of Water and Pollution Control; Seattle Water Department; Al Bishop, Bureau of Water Management, Florida; Charles F. Kennedy, Division of Water Resources, Massachusetts; Dorothy L. Bennett, Division of Public Water Supplies, Illinois Environmental Protection Agency; *Fig. 8-1*, based on data from Getting the most from the most essential nutrient, Tufts University Diet & Nutrition Letter, **4**(8) October, 1968; *Table 8-4*, from Nutritive value of American foods, Agriculture Handbook No. 456, Agricultural Research Service, U.S. Department of Agriculture, Washington, D.C., 1975; *Table 8-5*, adapted from Nutrition for sport success, AAHPERD (The American Alliance for Health, Physical Education, Recreation and Dance), Reston, VA, 1984; *Fig. 8-4, A* adapted from Anderson, B., and others: Regulation of water intake, Annual Review of Nutrition 2:73, 1982; *Fig. 8-4, B*, Sheetz, M., and others: Journal of Cellular Biology 70:193, 1976. Also from Greenleaf, J.E., and Harrison, H.H.: Water and electrolytes. In Nutrition and aerobic exercise, editor, Layman, D.K., American Chemical Society, Washington, D.C., 1986; *Table 8-6*, adapted from Fallert, R.F., and Boyton, R.D.: Milk: fitness that could change, National Food Review, Fall, 1985; *p. 248*, H. Armstrong Roberts; *p. 253*, Stock Shop; *Table 8-7*, adapted from Smith, J.C., Jr.: Marginal nutritional states and conditioned deficiencies. In Research monograph No. 2; Alcohol and Nutrition, U.S. Department of Health, Education, and Welfare, Rockville, MD, 1979; *Table 8-8*, United States Department of Agriculture, Human Nutrition Information Service, Home and Garden Bulletin No. 232-7, April 1986; *Figs. 8-8 and 8-9*, Lieber, C.S.: Alcohol and malnutrition in the pathogenesis of liver disease, Journal of the American Medical Association **233**:1077, 1975.

Chapter 9, *p. 266* (quote), Aykroyd, W.R., The conquest of famine, Reader's Digest Press, New York, 1975; Stunkard, A.J., The pain of obesity, Bull Publishing Co., Palo Alto, CA, 1976; Kris-Etherton, P.M., Nutrition and the exercising female, Nutrition Today, p. 6, March/April, 1986; *Fig. 9-1*, adapted from Bray, G.A.: The obese patient, W.B. Saunders Co., Philadelphia, 1976; *Table 9-2*, data on ancient diet from Eaton, S.B., and Konner, M.: Paleolithic nutrition, New England Journal of Medicine **312**:283, 1985; *Table 9-3*, from Welsh, S.O., and Marston, R.M.: Review of trends in food use in the United States, 1909 to 1980, Journal of the American Dietetic Association **81**:120, 1982; *Table 9-4*, data on reference man adapted from McArdle, W.D., and others: Exercise physiology, ed. 2, Lea & Febiger, Philadelphia, 1986; *p. 272 (top)*, David Madison, 1987; *(middle)*, Picture Cube; *(bottom)*, Stock, Boston; *Table 9-6*, adapted from Kris-Etherton, P.M.: Nutrition and the exercising female, Nutrition Today, p. 6, March/April, 1986; *p. 274*, from Guthrie, H.: Introductory nutrition, ed. 6, Times Mirror/Mosby College Publishing, St. Louis, 1986; *Figs. 9-3, 9-4*, and 9-5, data from Davidson, S., and others: Human nutrition and dietetics, ed. 7, Churchill Livingstone, New York, 1979; *Table 9-7*, from Miller, R.W.: The fight against heart disease, FDA Consumer, p. 8, February 1986; *Table 9-8*, from Kris-Etherton, P.M.: Nutrition and the exercising female, Nutrition Today, p. 6, March/April 1986; *Fig. 9-6*, adapted from Short, S.H., and Short, W.R.: Four-year study of university athletes' dietary intake, Journal of the American Dietetic Association, **82**:632, 1983; *Figs. 9-7 and 9-8*, adapted from Koivisto, V.A.: The physiology of marathon running, Science Progress, **70**:109, 1986; *Table 9-9*, from Clark, N.: The athlete's kitchen, CBI Publishing Co., Inc. Reprinted by permission, Van Nostrand Reinhold Co., Inc., New York, 1981.

Chapter 10 *p. 292* (quotes), Stunkard, A.J., The pain of obesity, Bull Publishing Co., Palo Alto, CA, p. 74, 1976; Aykroyd, W.R., The conquest of famine, Reader's Digest Press, New York, p. 12, 1975; p. 293 (quote), Crisp, A.H., In: Eating and its disorders, Stunkard, A.J., and Stellar, E., Raven Press, New York, p. 226, 1984; *Table 10-1*, adapted from 1983 Metropolitan height and weight tables, reprinted with permission of the Metropolitan Life Insurance Company; *p. 304 (top)*; from Williams, S.R.: Nutrition and diet therapy, ed. 5, 1985, Times Mirror/Mosby College Publishing; *(bottom)*, Picture Cube; *p. 309*, from Prentice, W.E., and Bucher, C.A.: Fitness for college and life, ed. 2, Times Mirror/ Mosby College Publishing, St. Louis, 1988; *Table 10-5*, Classification taken from Vasseli, J.R., and others: Obesity. In Present knowledge in nutrition, ed. 5, p. 35, The Nutrition Foundation, Inc., 1984, Washington, D.C.; *Table 10-7*, adapted from Mitchell, J.E., and others: Characteristics of 275 patients with bulimia, American Journal of Psychiatry, **142**:482, 1985; *Table 19-8*, from Helmi, K.A.: adapted from Classification of the eating disorders, Journal of Psychiatric Research, **19**:113, 1985; *Fig. 10-6*, from Dane, C.: Family therapy for families containing an anorectic youngster. In Understanding anorexia nervosa and bulimia, p. 28, Ross Laboratories, Columbus, OH, 1981; *Table 10-7*, adapted from Mitchell, J.E., and others: Characteristics of 275 patients with bulimia, American Journal of Psychiatry, **142**:482, 1985; *Table 10-8*, adapted from Halmi, K.A.: Classification of the eating disorders, Journal of Psychiatric Research, **19**:113, 1985; *Fig. 10-6*, from Dane, C.: Family therapy for families containing an anorectic youngster. In Understanding anorexia nervosa and bulimia, Ross Laboratories, Columbus, OH, 1981; *Table 10-9*, adapted from Herzog, D.B., and Copeland, P.M.: Eating disorders, New England Journal of Medicine, **313**:295, 1985; *Table 10-10*, from Rosen, L.W., and others: Pathologic weight-control behavior in female athletes, Physician and Sportsmedicine, **14**:79, 1986; *Table 10-11*, from Rosen, L.W., and others: Pathologic weight-control behavior in female athletes, Physician and Sportsmedicine, **14**:79, 1986; *Fig. 10-8*, Bronwell, K.D., and others: Weight loss competitions at the work site: impact on weight, morale and cost-effectiveness, American Journal of Public Health, **74**:1283, 1984.

Chapter 11 *p. 332* (quotes), Jarvis, W.T., The myth of the healthy savage, Nutrition Today, p. 14, March/April, 1981; Scrimshaw, N.S., Food nutrition and nuclear war, New England Journal of Medicine, **311**:272, 1984; *Table 11-1*, from Borgstrom, G.: The hungry planet: the modern world at the edge of famine, Collier Books, New York, 1972; *p. 333 (top)*, H. Armstrong Roberts; *(bottom)*, Image Bank; *p. 334*, Doug Menuez/Picture Group; *p. 337*, FourbyFive; *Fig. 11-1*, 1984 Handbook of Agriculture, Agriculture Handbook No. 637, U.S. Department of Agriculture, Washington, D.C., 1984; *Fig. 11-2*, based on June 1985 U.S. average retail prices from the Bureau of Labor Statistics, U.S. Department of Labor, and the National Marine Fisheries Service, U.S. Department of Commerce; *p. 343*, Peter Menzel/Stock, Boston; *Table 11-5*,

adapted from Noah, N.D.: Food poisoning, British Medical Journal **291**:879, 1985: *Table 11-4*, *from Bender, A.E. Health or hoax? The truth about health food and diets, Elvendon Press, Goring-on-Thames, England, 1985. ** from Hambraeus, L.: Naturally occurring toxicants in food. In Adverse effects of food, editors, Jelliffe, E.P.F., and Jelliffe, D.B., Plenum Press, New York, 1982; *Table 11-4*, adapted from Noah, N.D., Food poisoning, British Medical Journal, **291**:879, 1985; *p. 357*, Woodfin Camp & Assoc.; *p. 358*, Tom Tracy/Stock Shop.

Chapter 12 *p. 364* (quotes), Widdowson, E.M., Food and health from conception to extreme old age. In: Food and Health: Science and Technology, editors Birch, G.G., and Parker, K.J., Applied Sciences Publishers, Ltd., London, p. 1, 1980; Beal, V.A., Nutrition in the life span, John Wiley and Sons, New York, p. 265, 1980; *Fig. 12-1*, from National Research Council, Recommended Dietary Allowances, ed. 9, National Academy of Sciences, Washington, D.C., 1980; *p. 366*, from Denney, N., and Quadagno, D.: Human sexuality, Times Mirror/Mosby College Publishing, St. Louis, 1988; *Table 12-1*, adapted from Wegman, M.E.: Annual summary of vital statistics, 1985, Pediatrics **78**:983, 1986; *p. 369* FourbyFive, *p. 370* H. Armstrong Roberts; *Table 12-2*, data for 1983 provided by Dr. James Haughton, Director of Public Health, Houston, TX; *p. 373*, H. Armstrong Roberts; *Table 12-3*, from Williams, S.R.: Nutrition and diet therapy, ed. 5, Times Mirror/Mosby College Publishing, St. Louis, 1985; *Table 12-4*, modified from Nutrition during pregnancy and lactation, Sacramento, CA, 1975, California Department of Health, from Worthington, B.S., Vermeersch, J. and Williams, S.R.: Nutrition in pregnancy and lactation, ed. 3, Times Mirror/Mosby College Publishing, St. Louis, 1985; *p. 379*, from Streissguth, A., and others: Tertogenic effects of alcohol in human and laboratory animals, Science **109**:353, 1980, © 1980 American Association for the Advancement of Science; *Table 12-5*, adapted from Widdowson, E.M.: Food and health from conception to extreme old age. In Food and health: science and technology, editors, Birch, G.G., and Parker, K.J., Applied Science Publishers, Ltd., London, 1980; p. 384, Jeffrey Reed/Medichrome *Table 12-6*, from Widdowson, E.M.: Development of the digestive system comparative animal studies, American Journal of Clinical Nutrition **11**:384, 1985; p. 387, H. Armstrong Roberts; *Table 12-9*, adapted from Pipes, P.L.: Nutrition in infancy and childhood, ed. 3, Times Mirror/Mosby College Publishing, St. Louis, 1985.

Chapter 13 p. 399 (quote), Durnin, J.V., Energy balance in childhood and adolescence, *Proceedings of the nutrition society*, 43:271, 1984; *Fig. 13-1*, from Caliendo, M.A., and Sanjur, D.: Journal of Nutrition Education, **19**:69, 1978; *Fig. 13-2*, from Beal, V.A.: Nutrition in the life span, John Wiley and Sons, Inc., New York, 1980; *Table 13-2*, from Lowengerg, M.E.: The development of food patterns in young children. In Nutrition in infancy and childhood, editor, Pipes, P.E., Times Mirror/Mosby College Publishing, St. Louis, 1985; *Table 13-3*, from Food and Nutrition Service, Department of Agriculture: National school lunch program regulations, Nov. 16, 1982, Federal Register; *p. 409*, Ellis Herwig/Stock, Boston; *p. 414*, H. Armstrong Roberts.

Chapter 14 *p. 425* (quotes), Harper, A.E., Nutrition, aging and longevity, *American Journal of Clinical Nutrition*, 36:737, 1982; Widdowson, E.M., Food and health from conception to extreme old age. In: Food and Health: Science and Technology, editors Birch, G.G., and Parker, K.J., Applied Sciences Publishers, Ltd., London, p. 1, 1980; *Fig. 14-1*, from U.S. Bureau of the Census (1984). From Leveille, G.A., and Cloutier, P.F.: Role of the food industry in meeting the nutritional needs of the elderly, Food Technology, **40**:82, February, 1986; *Fig. 14-2*, Leveille, G.A., and Cloutier, P.F.: Role of the food industry in meeting the nutritional needs of the elderly, Food Technology, **40**:82, February 1986; Jeff Reinking, 1986 *Fig. 14-3*, data based on the U.S. Department of Agriculture Nationwide Food Consumption Survey, 1977-1978, adapted from Peterkin, B.B., in Nutrition in the 1980's: constraints on our knowledge, editors, Selvey, N.L., and White, P.L., Alan R. Liss, Inc., New York, 1981; *Fig. 14-4*, from Week, E.: The dangerous burden of obesity, FDA Consumer, November, 1986; *Fig. 14-5*, from Millar, W.J., and Stephens, T.: The prevalence of overweight and obesity in Britain, Canada, and United States, American Journal of Public Health, **77**:38, 1987; *Fig. 14-7*, from Hegsted, D.M.: Calcium and osteoporosis, Journal of Nutrition, **116**:2316, 1986; *Fig. 14-8*, from Castelli, W.P., and Anderson, K.: A population at risk: prevalence of high cholesterol levels in hypertensive patients in the Framingham Study, American Journal of Medicine, **80**(suppl. 2A):23, 1986; *Fig. 14-9*, The Economist, Sept. 6, 1985; *p. 440*, Jeff Reinking, 1986; *Figs. 14-10 and 14-11*, Leveille, G.A., and Cloutier, P.F.: Role of the food industry in meeting the nutritional needs of the elderly, Food Technology, **40**:82, February 1986; *p. 448*, *The Picture Cube p. 451*, FourbyFive; *p. 452*, Image Bank.

Chapter 15 *p. 461,* D'Lites; *p. 462,* FourbyFive; *Fig. 15-1,* adapted from Krames Communications, Daly City, CA; *Table 15-1,* adapted from Liebman, B.: Stress pills: burning the consumer at both ends, Nutrition Action *12*:1, April 1985; *Table 15-2,* adapted from Berdanier, C.D.: The many faces of stress, Nutrition Today, p. 12, March-April 1987; *Table 15-3,* Chernoff, R.: Aging and nutrition, Nutrition Today *22*:4, March-April, 1987; *Fig. 15-2,* from Shoaf, L.R., and others: Nutrition knowledge, interests and information sources of male athletes, Journal of Nutrition Education, *18*:243, 1986; *Table 15-4,* Cinque, C.: Are Americans fit?: survey date conflict, Physician and Sportsmedicine *14*:26, November 1986; *Fig. 15-3,* from Sallis, J.F., and others: Moderate-intensity physical activity and cardiovascular risk factors, Preventive Medicine, *15*:561, 1986; *Table 15-5,* adapted from McSherry, J.A.: The diagnostic challenge of anorexia nervosa, American Family Physician *29*:141, 1984; *p. 472,* Stock Shop; *p. 473,* (top), Arthur Sirdofsky/Stock Shop, (bottom), Mike Ellis/Stock Shop; *Table 15-6,* from Hecht, A.: Healthy lunches for the brown bag set, FDA Consumer, September 1986; *Fig. 15-6,* adapted from USA Today, Jan. 6, 1986, USA Today; *Fig. 15-4,* Bureau of Economic Analysis, U.S. Department of Commerce; *Fig. 15-5,* adapted from Krames Communications, Daly City, CA; *Table 15-7,* from Morris, C.E., and others: Mergers fuel a healthy industry, Food Engineering, p. 65, June, 1987.

Chapter 16 *p. 487* (quotes), Tannahill, R., Food in history, Stein and Day, New York, 1973; Orlans, H., On knowledge, policy, practice and fate, Federation proceedings, *38*:2553, 1979; Whelan, E., Wall Street Journal, April 9, 1985; *Table 16-1,* adapted from Darby, W.J.: Some personal reflections of a half century of nutrition science—1930s to 1980s, Annual Review of Nutrition *5*:1, 1985; *Fig. 16-1,* adapted from Lenaire, W.H., Food in the Year 2000, Food Engineering, p. 90, May, 1985; *p. 498,* from NASA Lyndon B. Johnson Center; *p. 499,* Fred Ward/Black Star; *Table 16-2,* adapted from Pennington, J.: Revision of the total diet study food list and diets, Journal of the American Dietetic Association *82*:166, 1983; *pp. 500-501,* Peter DeSeve, New York; *Fig. 16-3,* Tompkins, A.M., Protein-energy malnutrition and risk of infection, Proceedings of the nutrition society, *45*:289, 1986; *Table 16-3,* adapted from Mellor, J.S.: Prediction and prevention of famine, Federation Proceedings *45*:2427, 1986; *Table 16-4,* adapted from Sorenson, A.W., and others: Health objectives for the nation: moving toward the 1990s, Journal of the American Dietetic Association *87*:920, 1987.